Eye Diseases: Clinical Perspectives

Eye Diseases: Clinical Perspectives

Editor: Aubrey Hopper

MURPHY & MOORE
www.murphy-moorepublishing.com

www.murphy-moorepublishing.com

MURPHY & MOORE

Cataloging-in-Publication Data

Eye diseases : clinical perspectives / edited by Aubrey Hopper.
p. cm.
Includes bibliographical references and index.
ISBN 978-1-63987-793-5
1. Eye--Diseases--Diagnosis. 2. Eye--Diseases--Treatment. 3. Eye--Abnormalities.
4. Eye--Care and hygiene. I. Hopper, Aubrey.
RE46 .D53 2023
617.7--dc23

Murphy & Moore Publishing
1 Rockefeller Plaza,
New York City,
NY 10020, USA

ISBN 978-1-63987-793-5

Contents

Preface

An eye disease can refer to any of the diseases or disorders that affect the human eye. Eye problems are treated within the field of ophthalmology. Age-related eye diseases are the leading cause of blindness and low vision. A few major eye diseases are macular degeneration, cataract, diabetic retinopathy and glaucoma. Macular degeneration is an eye disease which involves damage to the center area of the retina, which enables a person to see fine details. Cataracts are caused due to the development of a cloud film in one or both eyes. Most eye diseases have no early symptoms. The patient might not notice any pain or changes in the vision until the disease has become quite advanced. The book aims to shed light on some of the unexplored aspects of eye diseases. It includes contributions of experts and researchers which will provide clinical perspectives on these diseases. In this book, using case studies and examples, constant effort has been made to make the understanding of the clinical perspectives on eye diseases as easy and informative as possible, for the readers.

This book unites the global concepts and researches in an organized manner for a comprehensive understanding of the subject. It is a ripe text for all researchers, students, scientists or anyone else who is interested in acquiring a better knowledge of this dynamic field.

I extend my sincere thanks to the contributors for such eloquent research chapters. Finally, I thank my family for being a source of support and help.

Editor

1

Is Peripheral Motion Detection Affected by Myopia?

Junhan Wei[1†], Deying Kong[1†], Xi Yu[1], Lili Wei[1], Yue Xiong[1], Adeline Yang[2,3], Björn Drobe[2,3], Jinhua Bao[1,2], Jiawei Zhou[1], Yi Gao[2,3*] and Zhifen He[1*]*

[1] State Key Laboratory of Ophthalmology, Optometry and Vision Science, School of Ophthalmology and Optometry, Affiliated Eye Hospital, Wenzhou Medical University, Wenzhou, China, [2] WEIRC, WMU-Essilor International Research Centre, Wenzhou, China, [3] R&D AMERA, Essilor International, Singapore, Singapore

***Correspondence:**
Jiawei Zhou
zhcujw@mail.eye.ac.cn
Yi Gao
yi.gao@essilor.com
Zhifen He
zhifen0821@163.com

† These authors share first authorship

Purpose: The current study was to investigate whether myopia affected peripheral motion detection and whether the potential effect interacted with spatial frequency, motion speed, or eccentricity.

Methods: Seventeen young adults aged 22–26 years participated in the study. They were six low to medium myopes [spherical equivalent refractions −1.0 to −5.0 D (diopter)], five high myopes (<-5.5 D) and six emmetropes (+0.5 to −0.5 D). All myopes were corrected by self-prepared, habitual soft contact lenses. A four-alternative forced-choice task in which the subject was to determine the location of the phase-shifting Gabor from the four quadrants (superior, inferior, nasal, and temporal) of the visual field, was employed. The experiment was blocked by eccentricity (20° and 27°), spatial frequency (0.6, 1.2, 2.4, and 4.0 cycles per degree (c/d) for 20° eccentricity, and 0.6, 1.2, 2.0, and 3.2 c/d for 27° eccentricity), as well as the motion speed [2 and 6 degree per second (d/s)].

Results: Mixed-model analysis of variances showed no significant difference in the thresholds of peripheral motion detection between three refractive groups at either 20° ($F[2,14] = 0.145$, $p = 0.866$) or 27° ($F[2,14] = 0.475$, $p = 0.632$). At 20°, lower motion detection thresholds were associated with higher myopia ($p < 0.05$) mostly for low spatial frequency and high-speed targets in the nasal and superior quadrants, and for high spatial frequency and high-speed targets in the temporal quadrant in myopic viewers. Whereas at 27°, no significant correlation was found between the spherical equivalent and the peripheral motion detection threshold under all conditions (all $p > 0.1$). Spatial frequency, speed, and quadrant of the visual field all showed significant effect on the peripheral motion detection threshold.

Conclusion: There was no significant difference between the three refractive groups in peripheral motion detection. However, lower motion detection thresholds were associated with higher myopia, mostly for low spatial frequency targets, at 20° in myopic viewers.

Keywords: myopia, peripheral vision, motion perception, motion speed, eccentricity

INTRODUCTION

The human visual system is not fully functional at birth. During early postnatal development, the eye grows toward emmetropia (Banks, 1980; Mohindra and Held, 1980). Abnormal development of the visual system can lead to different types of eye disorders, the most widespread of which is myopia (Wiesel and Raviola, 1977; Wallman et al., 1978; Siegwart and Norton, 2011). Myopia is a benign disorder in which visual images come to a focus in front of the retina mostly due to the elongation of the eye horizontally. The condition is mainly manifested as a reduction of distance visual acuity (Morgan et al., 2012). The global prevalence of myopia has reached very high as reported in multiple epidemiological studies (Grosvenor and Scott, 1993, 1994; Dirani et al., 2009; Lim et al., 2012), particularly in Asian populations (Wang et al., 2020; Xie et al., 2020). It was predicted that almost half of the world population would have myopia by 2050 (Holden et al., 2016).

Besides poor visual acuity, myopes also show abnormalities in spatial visual processing including contrast sensitivity (Stoimenova, 2007; Ehsaei et al., 2013), blur perception (Gwiazda et al., 1993; Rosenfield and Abraham-Cohen, 1999; Vasudevan et al., 2006; Maiello et al., 2017; Ang et al., 2020), color vision (Garcia-Domene et al., 2018), binocular vision (Vera-Diaz et al., 2018), and attention (Kerber et al., 2016). Myopes may also have abnormal temporal visual processing abilities. For example, Vera-Diaz et al. (2018) found that myopes had poorer performance than emmetropes in perceiving flickered binocular stimuli at lower temporal frequencies. Another study found that critical flicker frequency was lower in high myopes compared to emmetropes; and in a large range (5–60 Hz) of temporal frequency, the contrast modulation threshold of flickering stimuli was higher in high myopes (Chen et al., 2000). A recent study using a psychophysical multichannel functional test (Antón et al., 2012) to study the sensitivity of visual pathways in high myopes (Garcia-Domene et al., 2018) found that the sensitivity of the magnocellular pathway, which is mainly responsible for the motion perception (Merigan and Maunsell, 1990), decreased. Therefore, it suggested myopia may have impaired motion perception.

Most of the aforementioned studies focused on the central vision. Recent studies have shown that myopia also causes abnormal changes in the morphology of the peripheral retina (Ohno-Matsui et al., 2016; Nagra et al., 2018), and peripheral defocus is closely related to the development of myopia (Smith et al., 2005, 2010). In general, peripheral vision refers to the area outside 2° eccentricity of the fovea and parafovea (Strasburger et al., 2011). Many myopia progression control lenses have been designed based on the finding of myopic peripheral defocus slowing down the elongation of the eyeball (Sankaridurg et al., 2019; Tarutta et al., 2019; Kaphle et al., 2020; Lam et al., 2020). Studying the characteristics of visual information processing in the periphery of myopic vision is thus of great significance to our understanding of myopia.

To understand temporal information processing in the peripheral visual field of myopes, peripheral motion detection is a good starting point. Peripheral motion perception, as a fundamental visual function of humans, affects a range of higher-level cognitive functions, including orienting, balance, visually guided action, and mobility (Marron and Bailey, 1982; Nakayama, 1985; Geruschat et al., 1998; Marigold, 2008), and closely relates to daily activities (Henderson et al., 2013). Previous studies on the effect of myopia on peripheral motion perception did not reach consistent conclusions. To illustrate, Leibowitz et al. (1972) and Johnson and Leibowitz (1974) found no significant difference between myopes and emmetropes in motion discrimination task at 10°–80° eccentricities in the temporal visual field. McKee and Nakayama (1984) found that correcting peripheral refractive errors in myopes did not improve the performance of differential motion perception tasks in the lower peripheral visual field. A recent study (Kuo et al., 2018) assessed central and peripheral motion perception (at 3.65° and 12° eccentricities) using the random-dot paradigm also did not find significant differences in peripheral motion perception tasks including minimum displacement (Dmin), maximum displacement (Dmax), and motion coherence tasks between young myopic and emmetropic adults. However, they have found a small but significant correlation between the peripheral Dmin threshold in the superior-temporal visual field and the axial length, as well as the macular thickness of the corresponding inferior-nasal retina. The latter finding suggested that peripheral motion perception might be affected by myopia.

These studies have enriched our knowledge of the link between myopia and peripheral motion perception. However, considering that motion perception is influenced by a variety of factors, such as eccentricity (Leibowitz et al., 1972; Rogers, 1972; Johnson and Leibowitz, 1974; Koenderink et al., 1978a,b; McKee and Nakayama, 1984; van de Grind et al., 1987; Wesemann and Norcia, 1992), spatial frequency (Koenderink et al., 1978a,b; van de Grind et al., 1987; Boulton and Baker, 1991; Beard et al., 1997; Bex and Dakin, 2003; Lappin et al., 2009), speed (Lagae et al., 1993; Lappin et al., 2009; Ananyev et al., 2019), and the area in the different visual fields (Kuo et al., 2018), it remains unclear that whether myopia affects peripheral motion processing and if so, whether the potential effect varied with these factors. In this study, we directly addressed this issue by measuring the motion detection thresholds of gratings in a four-alternative forced-choice task in blocks of eccentricity, spatial frequency, and speed in young adults with low to high myopia and emmetropes.

MATERIALS AND METHODS

Participants

Six adults [mean age: 25.17 ± 0.37 years old; mean ± standard deviation (SD)] with low to medium myopia [LM group; spherical equivalent refraction (SER) between −1.0 and −5.0 D (diopter)], five adults (mean age: 25.4 ± 0.8 years old) with high myopia (HM group; SER less than −5.5 D) and six controls (EM group; mean age: 23.83 ± 1.07 years old) with SER between +0.5 and −0.5 D, participated in the current study. Refraction was done for each subject at the beginning of the study. Subjects were then grouped according to the refraction (Flitcroft et al., 2019). All myopes wore self-prepared, habitual soft contact lenses

TABLE 1 | Clinical details of the participants.

	Emmetropes (EM)	Low to medium myopes (LM)	High myopes (HM)
n	6	6	5
Age (y)	23.83 ± 1.07	25.17 ± 0.37	25.4 ± 0.8
Gender (female/male) (*n*)	4/2	4/2	5/0
Best-corrected visual acuity (logMAR)	−0.11 ± 0.11	−0.08 ± 0.09	−0.06 ± 0.06
Refraction (D)	−0.04 ± 0.31	−3.13 ± 1.19	−6.03 ± 0.75
Refraction of contact lenses (DE)	–	−2.96 ± 1.14	−5.65 ± 0.8

Data are mean ± SD.
DE, dominant eye: the logMAR VA of LM and HM were measured with the soft contact lens correction.

during the experimental session. Subjects' best-corrected visual acuity was equal to or better than log MAR 0.0. All subjects had no history of ocular surgery, or other eye diseases. Observer's dominant eye, which was determined using the card-in-the-hole test (Dane and Dane, 2004), was tested in this study. Details of the dominant eyes of participants are provided in **Table 1**.

This study adhered to the Declaration of Helsinki. Informed consent was obtained from all subjects after explaining the nature and possible consequences of the study. The study was approved by the Ethics Committee of the affiliated eye hospital of Wenzhou Medical University.

Apparatus

Stimuli were generated and controlled by a PC running Matlab R2016b (MathWorks, Inc., Natick, MA, United States) with Psychtoolbox 3.0.14 (Brainard, 1997; Pelli, 1997; Kleiner et al., 2007). The stimuli were presented on a gamma-corrected ASUS PG278QR LED screen (ASUS Corp., China) with a 2,560 × 1,440 resolution and a 60-Hz refresh rate. The average background luminance was 37.5 cd/on the screen. During the measurement, observers viewed the screen monocularly with their dominant eye at a viewing distance of 27 cm. The untested eye was covered with an opaque patch. The whole experiment was carried out in a dark room to ensure the only light source was the display.

Stimuli

As shown in **Figure 1**, the target stimulus was a Gabor, which was a phase-shifting grating within a two-dimensional Gaussian window (sigma: 1.2° of visual angle; diameter: 4° of visual angle). The grating moved from the far periphery inward in the Gaussian window. The stimulus was presented randomly in one of the four quadrants of the visual field (**Figure 1B**), namely nasal, temporal, superior and inferior, at one of the two eccentricities (20° and 27°) on a uniform gray background. To be consistent with the major motion direction of environmental objects during locomotion, the motion direction of the target in each quadrant was aligned with its meridian. To avoid location or eccentricity change of the target, phase-shifting Gabors whose orientations were perpendicular to their motion directions were employed. Therefore, the orientation of the grating was vertical if the nasal and temporal visual fields were tested, or horizontal if the superior and inferior visual fields were tested. The spatial frequencies (SF) of the stimuli were 0.6, 1.2, 2.4, and 4.0 cycle per degree (c/d) at 20° eccentricity, and 0.6, 1.2, 2.0, and 3.2 c/d at 27° eccentricity (**Figure 1C**). Two speeds, 2 and 6 degrees per second (d/s) (**Figure 1D**), were tested.

Procedure

All subjects underwent dark adaptation for 5 min in the darkroom before the measurements. Subjects were asked to look straight ahead, with their dominant eye, at a fixation cross in the center of the screen while performing the task. The non-dominant eye was covered with an opaque patch. A chin rest was used to minimize head movements to ensure the viewing distance and the eccentricities of the stimuli were corrected. The experiment was done in blocks of two eccentricities, four SFs, and two speeds with two repetitions in each combined condition, i.e., in total 32 runs. In each run, a four-alternative forced-choice task was employed.

Figure 1A shows the procedure of two trials. In each trial, a stimulus was presented randomly in one of the four quadrants of the visual field for 600 ms. We asked subjects to determine in which quadrant the target was presented, and to respond by pressing the "2," "4," "6," and "8" keys on the keyboard, respectively. There was a constant 400 ms interval between the button press and the onset of the next stimulus. Two 2-down 1-up staircases were interleaved for each run to determine the contrast level of the gratings (Cornsweet, 1962). The step size of the staircase was 1 dB [Decibel, dB = $20*\log_{10}$ (C), C represents contrast (%)]. The contrast was started from the highest (100%), decreased with two consecutive, correct responses, and increased by one level with a single incorrect response. A reversal was defined as a change of direction of the staircases between increasing and decreasing. Each block was terminated after 50 trials or 10 reversals. The detection threshold was calculated as the mean level of the last five reversals of all four staircases under each condition. From the pilot testing, we found that the levels of contrast that were requested during the staircases at any spatial frequency, speed, and eccentricity in the current study did not exceed the resolution of the eight-bit graphic card's capacity. Therefore, no special procedure to achieve extra bits was carried out.

One 5-min practice run was applied before the start of the test. Each run lasted about 5 mins. Subjects normally finished the test (which took 3.5–4 h in total) on two or three separate days within 1 week. Measures were taken during each session to prevent visual fatigue, including 2-min mandatory breaks after every one or two runs, and applying hydrating eye drops (Bausch

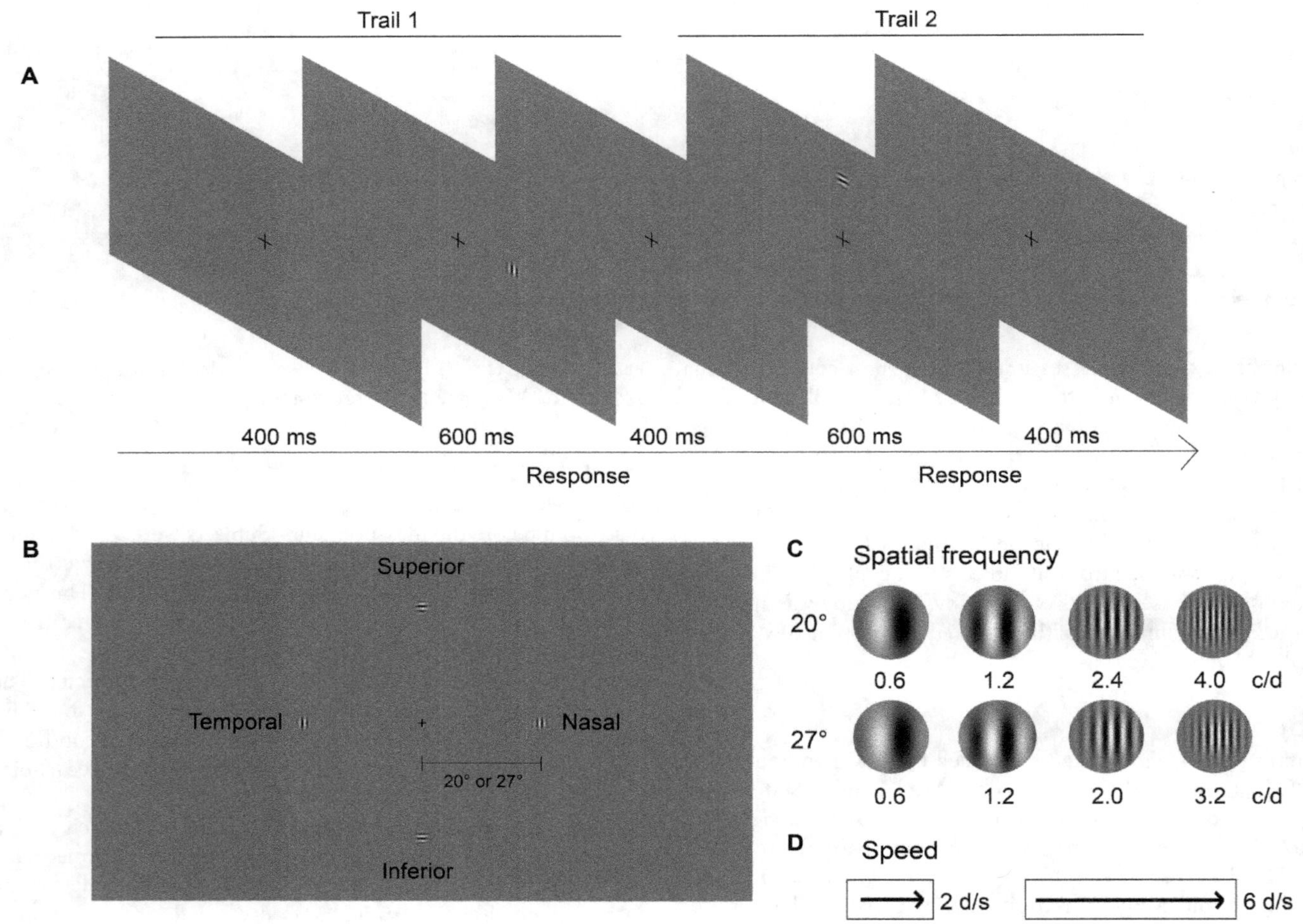

FIGURE 1 | Illustration of the experiment design. **(A)** The peripheral motion detection procedure. In each trail, the stimulus was randomly presented in one of the four quadrants of the visual field for 600 ms. Then subjects were asked to determine in which quadrant the grating was presented, followed by a 400 ms interval before the onset of the next stimulus. **(B)** Examples of four quadrants (superior, inferior, nasal, and temporal) of the visual field. The cross in the center of the screen was for fixation. **(C)** Examples of SFs for two eccentricities, SF were 0.6, 1.2, 2.4, and 4.0 cycle/degree (c/d) at 20° eccentricity, and 0.6, 1.2, 2.0, and 3.2 c/d at 27° eccentricity. **(D)** Two speeds of grating moving were tested, 2 and 6 degree/second (d/s).

& Lomb Incorporated) prepared by the authors for each subject who wore contact lenses.

Statistical Analysis

Contrast thresholds of motion detection were used for statistical analysis. Two mixed-model analysis of variances (ANOVAs) were used to test the effects of one between-subjects factor-refractive group, and three within-subject factors-spatial frequency, speed, and quadrant of the visual field for each eccentricity. By Pearson correlation coefficient (ranging between −1 and 1; two-tailed) and empirical p values from permutation tests (based on 10,000 permutations of the data), which have been used to calculate the p values for multiple comparison correction, the correlation between the average motion detection threshold and the spherical equivalent were calculated. Statistical analysis was performed using Matlab and IBM-SPSS 23.0 (IBM Inc., Armonk, NY, United States).

RESULTS

The Effect of Myopia on the Peripheral Motion Detection Threshold at 20° Eccentricity

In **Figure 2**, we plotted the average motion detection thresholds at 20° across visual fields, speeds, SFs for EM (green), LM (blue), and HM (red). LM group had larger peripheral motion detection thresholds than other groups at 0.6 c/d. At 1.2 c/d, the threshold of the nasal quadrant was higher in the EM group, and the threshold of temporal and superior quadrants at low speed were higher in the LM group. While at high SFs (i.e., 2.4 and 4.0 c/d), there was no obvious difference in the thresholds among the three groups. We conducted a four-factor, mixed model ANOVA with one between-subject factor (refractive group) and three within-subject factors (quadrant, SF, and speed), on peripheral motion detection thresholds. However,

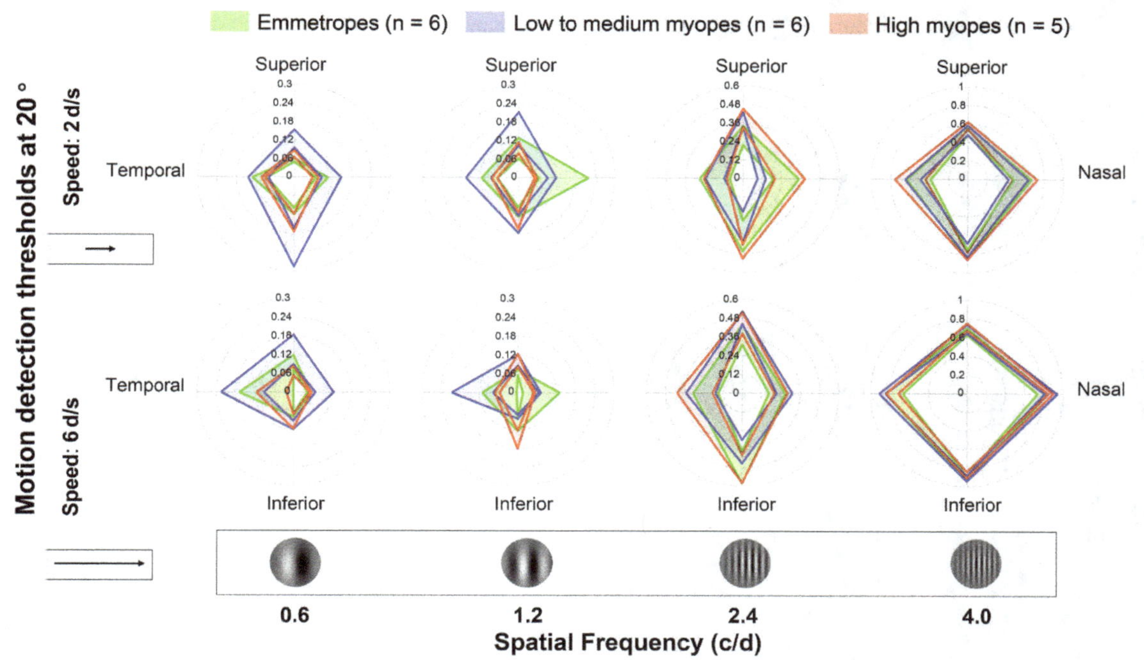

FIGURE 2 | Average motion detection thresholds at 20° for emmetropes, low to medium myopes and high myopes. Data were plotted for different visual fields (in different quadrants), spatial frequencies (in different columns), and speeds (in different rows). The green, blue, and red lines and shadows represent three refractive groups (EM, LM, and HM). The width of the band represents the range between "mean ± standard error [SE]".

the ANOVA revealed no significant main effect for the refractive group ($F[2,14] = 0.145, p = 0.866$), nor interaction between group and other within-subject factors (for all, $F < 1.391$; $p > 0.25$). There were significant main effects for all within-subject factors: quadrant ($F[3,42] = 6.009$, $p = 0.002$), SF ($F[3,12] = 328.848$, $p < 0.001$), and speed ($F[1,14] = 62.216$, $p < 0.001$). We also found significant interactions between quadrant and SF ($F[9,6] = 39.263, p < 0.001$), quadrant and speed ($F[3,12] = 3.961$, $p = 0.036$), SF and speed ($F[3,12] = 15.571$, $p < 0.001$), and significant three-way interaction between quadrant, SF and speed ($F[9,6] = 8.383, p = 0.009$).

The Effect of Myopia on the Peripheral Motion Detection Threshold at 27° Eccentricity

Figure 3 illustrates the average motion detection thresholds at 27° for the three groups. Overall, no differences were observed among the three groups under any of the conditions in **Figure 3**. A four-factor mixed ANOVA, with quadrant, SF and speed as within-subject factors and refractive group as between-subject factor, also revealed no significant difference between group ($F[2,14] = 0.475$, $p = 0.632$), nor interaction between group and factors (for all, $F < 0.403$; $p > 0.097$). There were significant main effects for quadrant ($F[3,42] = 19.139, p < 0.001$) and SF ($F[3,12] = 233.346$, $p < 0.001$), and significant interactions between quadrant and SF ($F[9,6] = 26.15, p < 0.001$), quadrant and speed ($F[3,12] = 7.388$, $p < 0.001$), SF and speed ($F[3,12] = 19.394$, $p < 0.001$) and three-way interaction between quadrant, SF and speed ($F[9,6] = 2.023$, $p = 0.042$). While no significant main effect for speed ($F[1,14] = 1.26, p = 0.281$) was found.

Correlation Analysis of the Motion Detection Threshold and the Spherical Equivalent of Myopes

We further performed Pearson correlation analysis and used empirical p values from permutation tests to determine the significance of the correlation between the motion detection threshold and the spherical equivalent of myopic subjects in LM and HM. Results at 20° are shown in **Figure 4**. At 20°, significantly positive correlations between motion detection thresholds and refractive error were found at low SF (i.e., 0.6 and 1.2 c/d) and mainly high speed (6 d/s) in the nasal visual field (for all, $p < 0.05$). This means that patients with higher myopia had lower motion detection thresholds. Such pattern was also found at low SF (0.6 c/d) and high speed (6 d/s) in the superior visual field ($r = 0.575, p = 0.034$). While at high SF (4.0 c/d), significant correlation only occurred at high speed (6 d/s) in the temporal visual field ($r = 0.556, p = 0.032$). At 27°, no significant correlation was found in any condition (for all, $p > 0.1$). Results for 27° are attached in **Supplementary Material**.

DISCUSSION

In this study, we investigated the effect of myopia on peripheral motion detection in young adults, and to see if it varied with

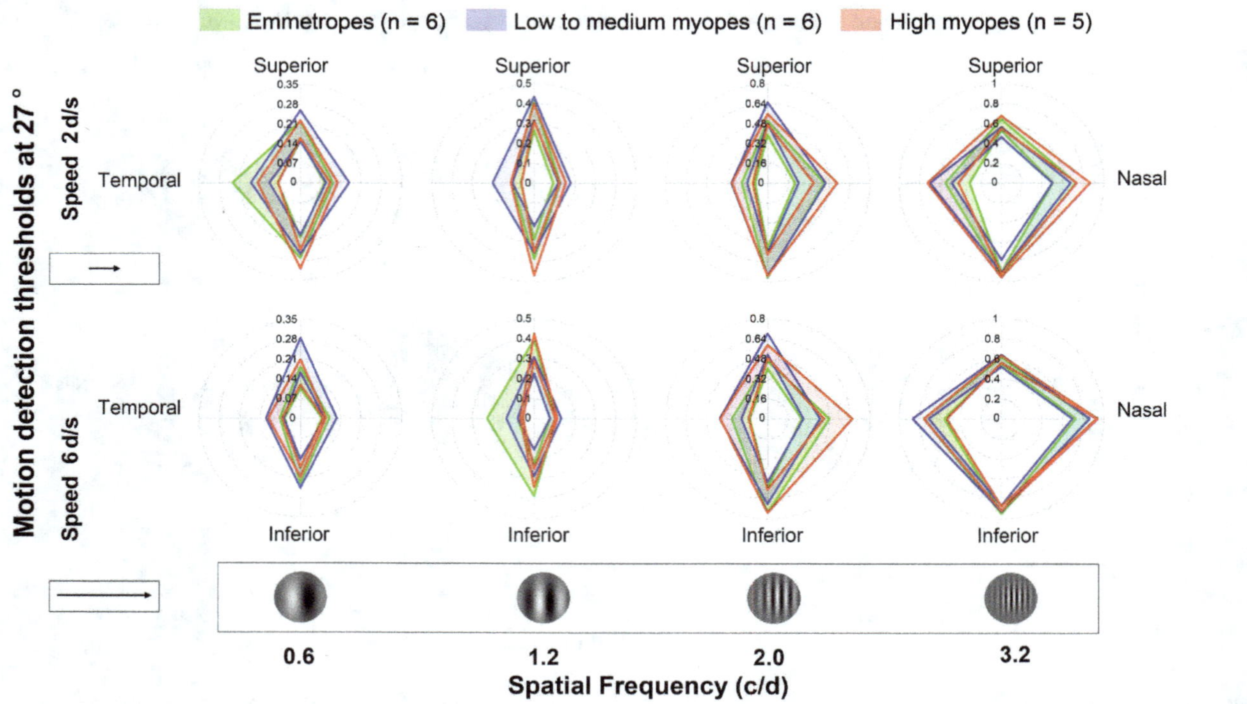

FIGURE 3 | Average motion detection thresholds at 27° for emmetropes, low to medium myopes and high myopes. Data were plotted for different visual fields (in different quadrants), spatial frequencies (in different columns), and speeds (in different rows). The green, blue, and red lines and shadows represent three refractive groups (EM, LM, and HM). The width of the band represents the range between "mean ± SE".

eccentricity, spatial frequency, speed, as well as location in the visual field. We found no statistically significant difference in the peripheral motion detection threshold between emmetropes, low to medium myopes, and high myopes. Further analysis revealed that lower motion detection thresholds were associated with higher myopia, mostly for low spatial frequency target, at 20° in myopic viewers.

Although there was evidence that peripheral visual deficit existed in myopes compared to emmetropes, it was contrast-dependent. For example, Ehsaei et al. (2013) found reduced peripheral acuity at a high contrast level (100%) but not at a low contrast of 14%. Contrast detection thresholds in the periphery were found not to differ between myopes and emmetropes in Kerber et al. (2016) study where they measured peripheral contrast detection thresholds binocularly by using vertical Gabor stimuli presented at three eccentricities, 8°, 17°, and 30°. These findings, together with ours, suggest that the difference of peripheral perception between myopes and emmetropes is minimal at low contrast.

The fact that no statistical difference in the behavioral task performance between myopes and emmetropes cannot rule out the potential effect of myopia on peripheral motion perception. In fact, we still found significant correlations between the spherical equivalent of myopia and the peripheral motion detection threshold, mostly in the nasal and superior visual fields at low SF. The correlations suggest the myopic impact on peripheral motion perception. This finding is consistent with a previous study in which Kuo et al. (2018) used random-dot patterns to assess dot motion perception using Dmin, Dmax, and motion coherence tasks in both central and peripheral visual fields in young myopic and emmetropic adults. They also found that the Dmin threshold in the superior-temporal visual field was correlated positively with the axial length and negatively with the macular thickness of the corresponding retina, despite the fact that no difference was found between myopes and emmetropes, regardless of the tasks used, in the periphery. This correlation suggested that the severer myopia, the worse the performance of the Dmin task at the near periphery. Although the direction of correlations between the severity of myopia and the peripheral motion detection task performance was opposite to that in our study, it could be due to, first, the difference in eccentricity which was 3.65° in their study, 20° and 27° in our study; second, the nature of the task which was global motion processing in their study and local motion processing in ours; and third, the SF of the stimuli that covered the full range by the dots in their study and more narrowly filtered in our Gabor stimuli for the current study, whereas the myopic impact on contrast sensitivity has been demonstrated to be uneven across the spatial frequency range (Risse et al., 1996; Jaworski et al., 2006).

The negative correlations we found between the myopia severity and the peripheral motion detection threshold mostly at the low spatial frequency in the nasal and superior visual field have some interesting implications about myopic vision and the myopization process. First, findings from visual search tasks suggested that myopes tend to adopt the local processing strategy over the global processing strategy (Mascetti et al., 2001), or focus their attention more locally (McKone et al., 2008; Kerber et al., 2016) compared to their emmetropic counterparts. Therefore, patients with severer myopia may perform better in the current peripheral motion detection task which required local instead of global processing. Second, myopic vision may try to compensate for its loss in the central vision, especially at high SF (Risse et al., 1996; Jaworski et al., 2006), by improving peripheral vision at low SF. Compensation of central vision loss by peripheral vision has been discovered in several brain plasticity studies (Cummings et al., 1985; Timberlake et al., 1986; Maniglia et al., 2020). Third, there is consensus that visual performance varies in different parts of the visual field (Wertheim, 1980; Fahle and Schmid, 1988). For example, it was found that peripheral visual acuity was better in the nasal and superior retinal regions than the temporal and inferior regions for both myopic and emmetropic groups (Ehsaei et al., 2013). The finding of the current study that correlations between myopia severity and the peripheral motion detection were mostly found in the nasal and superior

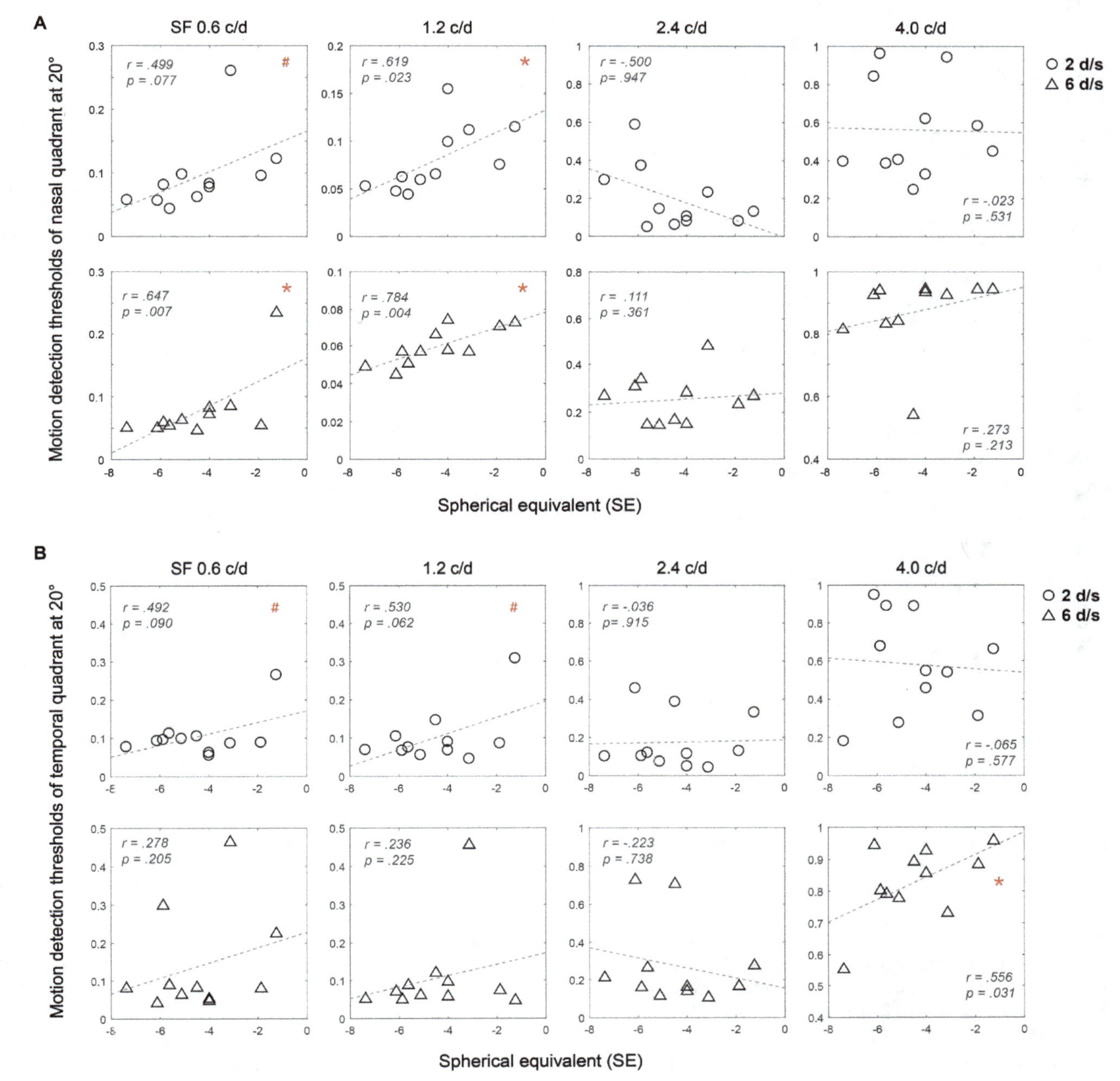

FIGURE 4 | Continued

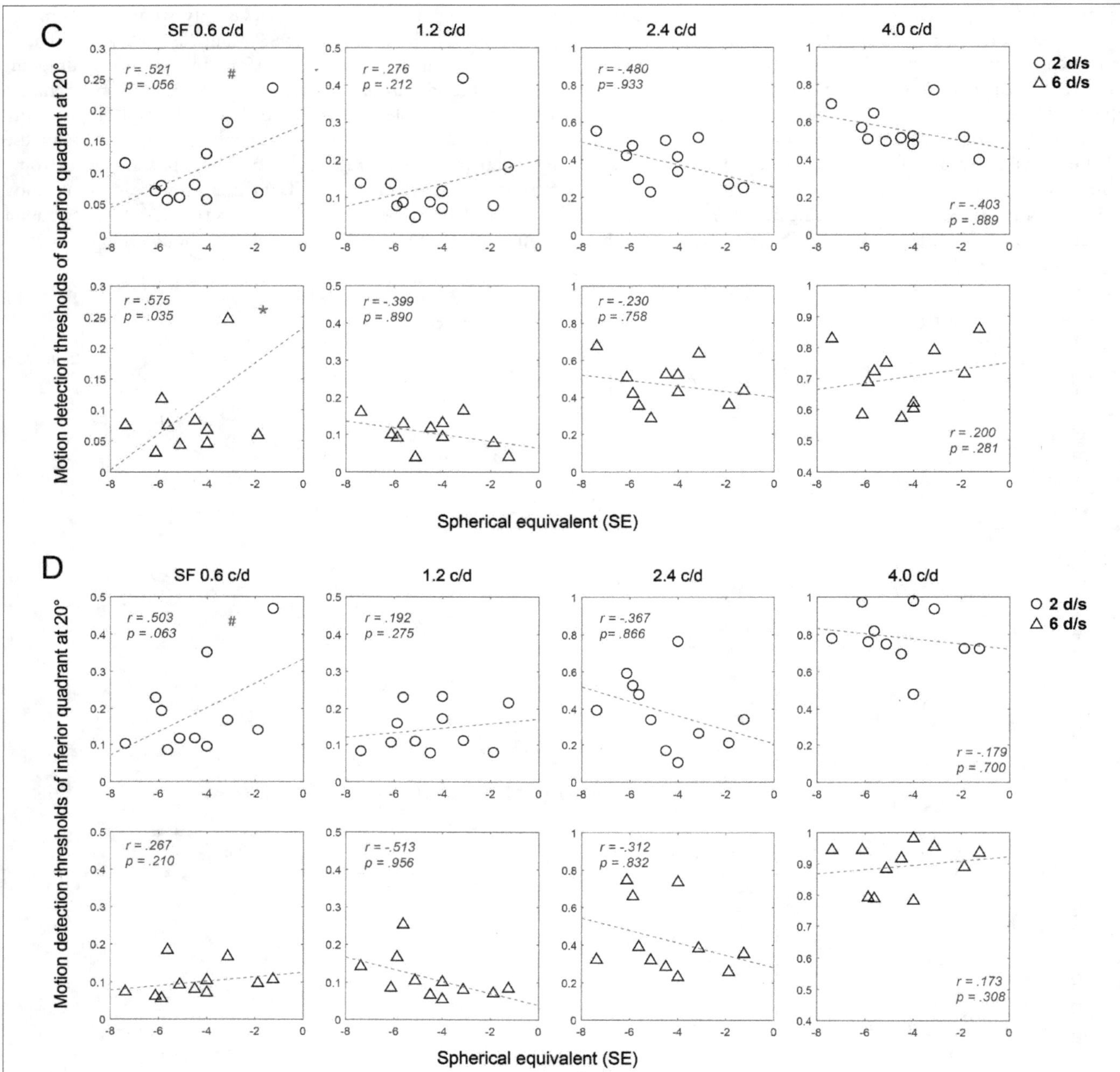

FIGURE 4 | Relationship between the motion detection thresholds and the spherical equivalent (SE) of myopes in the nasal **(A)**, temporal **(B)**, superior **(C)** and inferior **(D)** visual field at 20°. Each point represents one participant, the circles represent 2 d/s, and the triangles represent 6 d/s. Pearson correlation coefficients and empirical p values from permutation tests (based on 10,000-time simulation) are shown. $\#p < 0.1$; $^*p < 0.05$.

visual field and only at 20°, not 27°, further suggested that the myopic influence on visual performance also varies across the whole visual field. This uneven distribution of the myopic impact in the visual field is also consistent with the finding in Kuo et al. (2018) study that only in the superior-temporal visual field the correlations between Dmin task performance and myopia severity were significant. Besides, the correlation we found was mainly at low SF. This indicated that the effect of myopia varies across the SF range, which is consistent with Diez et al. (2020) research. They found that the changes of accommodation response were SF-dependent, too. In particular, the changes of accommodation response of emmetropes and myopes were similar after the induction of stimulation of high SF, while there was an opposite direction of accommodation response changes between the two groups after low SF stimulation.

In this study, we did not measure or correct the subjects' peripheral refractive status like some previous studies, which used an adaptive optics vision system (Ghosh et al., 2016; Zheleznyak et al., 2016). Peripheral vision was affected by multiple ocular and physical factors, including refractive error, diffraction, scattering, aberration, and the form of the palpebral fissure (Rosenholtz, 2016). Many studies have shown that refractive errors distribute unevenly across the whole retina, and conventional correction methods including single vision spectacle lenses and soft contact lenses do not correct the refractive errors in the whole visual field evenly either (Shen et al., 2010). It is possible that uncorrected peripheral refraction might have influenced the threshold of the peripheral motion detection. However, previous studies have found that the relative peripheral refraction is larger when the central corrective power used is higher with both contact lenses (Shen et al., 2010; Moore et al., 2017) and spectacles (Lin et al., 2010). This means that more severe myopic eyes corrected with soft contact lenses suffer from more peripheral refractive errors, thus more blur in the peripheral vision. This is opposite to the negative correlation between myopia severity and peripheral motion detection threshold. Thus, the correlation we found could not be completely explained by refractive status in the peripheral retina.

Compared with previous studies, we did not take additional measures [e.g., blind spot (Leibowitz et al., 1972; Johnson and Leibowitz, 1974; Kuo et al., 2018), bright-colored afterimage (McKee and Nakayama, 1984), and pupil tracking camera (Venkataraman et al., 2015), etc.] to monitor subjects' eye movements. In our experiment, stimulus was randomly presented in one of four visual quadrants to minimize the effect of expected eye movements. Previous studies have shown that the response time of the human eye to the moving target is 150–250 ms on the horizontal meridian, which increased with the decrease of motion speed (Westheimer, 1954), and the latency of a voluntary saccade in a visual search was found to be 200–250 ms (Araujo et al., 2001). This means that the duration of the stimulus-600 ms, was not long enough for the subjects to scan all four possible locations in the four visual quadrants to look for the target with central vision. It was possible that the gaze moved toward the target location unintentionally upon the detection of the target. It was the consequent reaction following the detection of the target with peripheral vision, instead of planned voluntary eye movements to see the target with central vision. In addition, the statistical difference of motion detection thresholds between the two eccentricities, and among the four visual quadrants also indicated that the detection was not performed by central vision.

The viewing distance was 27 cm in our study. We have adjusted eccentricity with viewing distance due to the size of the screen and proximal accommodation (PA). The distance of PA in emmetropes is generally 25 cm, and shorter in myopic patients (Maiello et al., 2014). In order to measure the largest eccentricity and to avoid the occurrence of PA with our experimental setup, 27° were selected as the largest eccentricity to test, and 27 cm as the viewing distance.

The orientations and motion directions of the Gabor targets in the current study were designed intentionally. Previous studies (Berkley et al., 1975; Venkataraman et al., 2016; Zheleznyak et al., 2016) have shown that peripheral vision measured with gratings oriented parallel to the meridian performs better than those using perpendicular gratings. While in the current study, by using Gabors oriented perpendicular to the meridians, we kept the motion direction at each location consistent with the major relative motion direction of environmental objects during locomotion. To keep the location of the target constant, phase-shifting Gabors were used. If the orientation was parallel to the motion direction, one would not tell that the target was moving. Thus, the orientation of the Gabor at each location had to be perpendicular to its motion direction. What's more, aligning the motion direction with the meridian also avoids bias toward one of the quadrants at the other meridian. For example, a Gabor moving horizontally at the superior location presents a bias toward the temporal or nasal field depending on the viewing eye. To achieve these aforementioned goals, also considering that the orientation sensitivity of different meridian is different (Berkley et al., 1975; Venkataraman et al., 2016; Zheleznyak et al., 2016), we intentionally used Gabors oriented perpendicular to its motion direction.

Note that all our myopic subjects were young adults with stable refraction status. The peripheral motion perception in myopic children whose refractive status is still developing is an interesting topic for further research for two main reasons. First, peripheral defocus plays an important role in myopia progression (Smith et al., 2005, Smith et al., 2010; Mutti et al., 2007). Second, previous studies showed different development rates of peripheral vision from central vision (Bjerre et al., 2014), and more constricted visual field in children compared to adults (Aspinall, 1976). Whether the maturation of peripheral visual functions is affected by myopia and how it is different from the central vision will provide insight into the myopization process.

CONCLUSION

In summary, no significant difference was found in the peripheral motion detection threshold between myopic and emmetropic observers, however, we showed significant correlations between the spherical equivalent of myopia and the peripheral motion detection threshold, mostly in the nasal and superior visual fields at low SF, and in the temporal quadrant at high spatial frequency and high speed in myopic viewers at 20°. The higher the myopia, the lower the motion detection thresholds. We speculate it might be related to adaptation and compensation in the process of myopia development. Future research on the effect of myopia on peripheral motion perception in children will contribute to further understanding of the myopization process.

AUTHOR CONTRIBUTIONS

JW, DK, AY, BD, JB, JZ, YG, and ZH conceived the experiments. JW, DK, XY, LW, and YX performed the experiments. JW, DK,

ZH, YG, and JZ analyzed and interpreted the data and wrote the manuscript. All authors contributed to manuscript revision, read, and approved the submitted version.

SUPPLEMENTARY MATERIAL

Correlation Analysis of the Motion Detection Threshold and the Spherical Equivalent (SE) of Myopes at 27

We also performed Pearson correlation analysis and used empirical p values from permutation tests to determine the significance of the correlation between the motion detection threshold and the SE of myopic subjects in LM and HM at 27°. As shown in **Supplementary Figure**, no significant correlation was found under all conditions (for all, $p > 0.1$).

Supplementary Figure | Relationship between the motion detection thresholds and the spherical equivalent (SE) of myopes in the nasal **(A)**, temporal **(B)**, superior **(C)** and inferior **(D)** visual field at 27°. Each point represents one participant, the circles represent 2 d/s, and the triangles represent 6 d/s. Pearson correlation coefficients and empirical p values from permutation tests (based on 10,000-time simulation) are shown.

REFERENCES

Ananyev, E., Yong, Z., and Hsieh, P.-J. (2019). Center-surround velocity-based segmentation: speed, eccentricity, and timing of visual stimuli interact to determine interocular dominance. *J. Vis.* 19:3. doi: 10.1167/19.13.3

Ang, B. C. H., Cheong, K. X., Tan, M. M. H., Lim, E. W. L., Tey, F. L. K., Tan, C. S. H., et al. (2020). Correlation of myopia severity with visual performance. *Int. Ophthalmol.* 40, 2201–2211. doi: 10.1007/s10792-020-01403-7

Antón, A., Capilla, P., Morilla-Grasa, A., Luque, M. J., Artigas, J. M., and Felipe, A. (2012). Multichannel functional testing in normal subjects, glaucoma suspects, and glaucoma patients. *Invest. Ophthalmol. Vis. Sci.* 53, 8386–8395. doi: 10.1167/iovs.12-9944

Araujo, C., Kowler, E., and Pavel, M. (2001). Eye movements during visual search: the costs of choosing the optimal path. *Vis. Res.* 41, 3613–3625. doi: 10.1016/s0042-6989(01)00196-1

Aspinall, P. A. (1976). Peripheral vision in children. *Ophthalmologica* 173, 364–374.

Banks, M. S. (1980). Infant refraction and accommodation. *Int. Ophthalmol. Clin.* 20, 205–232. doi: 10.1097/00004397-198002010-00010

Beard, B. L., Klein, S. A., and Carney, T. (1997). Motion thresholds can be predicted from contrast discrimination. *J. Opt. Soc. Am. A Opt. Image Sci. Vis.* 14, 2449–2470. doi: 10.1364/josaa.14.002449

Berkley, M. A., Kitterle, F., and Watkins, D. W. (1975). Grating visibility as a function of orientation and retinal eccentricity. *Vis. Res.* 15, 239–244. doi: 10.1016/0042-6989(75)90213-8

Bex, P. J., and Dakin, S. C. (2003). Motion detection and the coincidence of structure at high and low spatial frequencies. *Vis. Res.* 43, 371–383. doi: 10.1016/s0042-6989(02)00497-2

Bjerre, A., Codina, C., and Griffiths, H. (2014). Peripheral visual fields in children and young adults using semi-automated kinetic perimetry: feasibility of testing, normative data, and repeatability. *Neuro Ophthalmol. (Aeolus Press)* 38, 189–198. doi: 10.3109/01658107.2014.902971

Boulton, J. C., and Baker, C. L. (1991). Motion detection is dependent on spatial frequency not size. *Vis. Res.* 31, 77–87. doi: 10.1016/0042-6989(91)90075-g

Brainard, D. H. (1997). The psychophysics toolbox. *Spatial Vis.* 10, 433–436. doi: 10.1163/156856897x00357

Chen, P. C., Woung, L. C., and Yang, C. F. (2000). Modulation transfer function and critical flicker frequency in high myopia patients. *J. Formos. Med. Assoc.* 99, 45–48.

Cornsweet, T. N. (1962). The staircase-method in psychophysics. *Am. J. Psychol.* 75, 485–491. doi: 10.2307/1419876

Cummings, R. W., Whittaker, S. G., Watson, G. R., and Budd, J. M. (1985). Scanning characters and reading with a central scotoma. *Am. J. Optom. Physiol. Opt.* 62, 833–843. doi: 10.1097/00006324-198512000-00004

Dane, A., and Dane, S. (2004). Correlations among handedness, eyedness, monocular shifts from binocular focal point, and nonverbal intelligence in university mathematics students. *Percept. Mot. Skills* 99, 519–524. doi: 10.2466/pms.99.2.519-524

Diez, P. S., Schaeffel, F., Wahl, S., and Ohlendorf, A. (2020). Accommodation responses following contrast adaptation. *Vis. Res.* 170, 12–17. doi: 10.1016/j.visres.2020.03.003

Dirani, M., Tong, L., Gazzard, G., Zhang, X., Chia, A., Young, T. L., et al. (2009). Outdoor activity and myopia in Singapore teenage children. *Br. J. Ophthalmol.* 93, 997–1000. doi: 10.1136/bjo.2008.150979

Ehsaei, A., Chisholm, C. M., Pacey, I. E., and Mallen, E. A. H. (2013). Visual performance fall-off with eccentricity in myopes versus emmetropes. *J. Optom.* 6, 36–44. doi: 10.1016/j.optom.2012.07.001

Fahle, M., and Schmid, M. (1988). Naso-temporal asymmetry of visual perception and of the visual cortex. *Vis. Res.* 28, 293–300. doi: 10.1016/0042-6989(88)90157-5

Flitcroft, D. I., He, M., Jonas, J. B., Jong, M., Naidoo, K., Ohno-Matsui, K., et al. (2019). IMI – defining and classifying myopia: a proposed set of standards for clinical and epidemiologic studies. *Invest. Ophthalmol. Vis. Sci.* 60, M20–M30. doi: 10.1167/iovs.18-25957

Garcia-Domene, M. C., Luque, M. J., Diez-Ajenjo, M. A., Desco-Esteban, M. C., and Artigas, J. M. (2018). Chromatic and achromatic visual fields in relation to choroidal thickness in patients with high myopia: a pilot study. *J. Fr. Dophtalmol.* 41, 109–115. doi: 10.1016/j.jfo.2017.07.006

Geruschat, D. R., Turano, K. A., and Stahl, J. W. (1998). Traditional measures of mobility performance and retinitis pigmentosa. *Optom. Vis. Sci. Off. Publ. Am. Acad. Optom.* 75, 525–537. doi: 10.1097/00006324-199807000-00022

Ghosh, A., Zheleznyak, L., Barbot, A., Jung, H. W., and Yoon, G. (2016). Neural adaptation to peripheral blur in myopes and emmetropes. *Vis. Res.* 132:69. doi: 10.1016/j.visres.2016.07.011

Grosvenor, T., and Scott, R. (1993). Three-year changes in refraction and its components in youth-onset and early adult-onset myopia. *Optom. Vis. Sci. Off. Publ. Am. Acad. Optom.* 70, 677–683. doi: 10.1097/00006324-199308000-00017

Grosvenor, T., and Scott, R. (1994). Role of the axial length/corneal radius ratio in determining the refractive state of the eye. *Optom. Vis. Sci. Off. Publ. Am. Acad. Optom.* 71, 573–579. doi: 10.1097/00006324-199409000-00005

Gwiazda, J., Thorn, F., Bauer, J., and Held, R. (1993). Myopic children show insufficient accommodative response to blur. *Invest. Ophthalmol. Vis. Sci.* 34, 690–694. doi: 10.1097/00004397-199303320-00025

Henderson, S., Gagnon, S., Collin, C., Tabone, R., and Stinchcombe, A. (2013). Near peripheral motion contrast threshold predicts older drivers' simulator performance. *Accid. Anal. Prev.* 50, 103–109. doi: 10.1016/j.aap.2012.03.035

Holden, B. A., Fricke, T. R., Wilson, D. A., Jong, M., Naidoo, K. S., Sankaridurg, P., et al. (2016). Global prevalence of myopia and high myopia and temporal trends from 2000 through 2050. *Ophthalmology* 123, 1036–1042. doi: 10.1016/j.ophtha.2016.01.006

Jaworski, A., Gentle, A., Zele, A. J., Vingrys, A. J., and Mcbrien, N. A. (2006). Altered visual sensitivity in axial high myopia: a local postreceptoral phenomenon? *Invest. Ophthalmol. Vis. Sci.* 47, 3695–3702. doi: 10.1167/iovs.05-1569

Johnson, C. A., and Leibowitz, H. W. (1974). Practice, refractive error, and feedback as factors influencing peripheral motion thresholds. *Percept. Psychophys.* 15, 276–280. doi: 10.3758/BF03213944

Kaphle, D., Atchison, D. A., and Schmid, K. L. (2020). Multifocal spectacles in childhood myopia: are treatment effects maintained? A systematic review and meta-analysis. *Surv. Ophthalmol.* 65, 239–249. doi: 10.1016/j.survophthal.2019.10.001

Kerber, K. L., Thorn, F., Bex, P. J., and Vera-Diaz, F. A. (2016). Peripheral contrast sensitivity and attention in myopia. *Vis. Res.* 125, 49–54. doi: 10.1016/j.visres.2016.05.004

Kleiner, M. B., Brainard, D. H., Pelli, D. G., Ingling, A., and Broussard, C. (2007). What's new in Psychtoolbox-3? *Perception* 36, 301–307. doi: 10.1068/v070821

Koenderink, J. J., Bouman, M. A., Bueno De Mesquita, A. E., and Slappendel, S. (1978a). Perimetry of contrast detection thresholds of moving spatial sine patterns. II. The far peripheral visual field (eccentricity 0 degrees-50 degrees). *J. Opt. Soc. Am.* 68, 850–854. doi: 10.1364/josa.68.000850

Koenderink, J. J., Bouman, M. A., Bueno De Mesquita, A. E., and Slappendel, S. (1978b). Perimetry of contrast detection thresholds of moving spatial sine wave patterns. I. The near peripheral visual field (eccentricity 0 degrees-8 degrees). *J. Opt. Soc. Am.* 68, 845–849. doi: 10.1364/josa.68.000845

Kuo, H. Y., Atchison, D. A., and Schmid, K. L. (2018). Dot motion perception in young adult emmetropes and myopes. *Optom. Vis. Sci. Off. Publ. Am. Acad. Optometry* 95, 498–504. doi: 10.1097/OPX.0000000000001223

Lagae, L., Raiguel, S., and Orban, G. A. (1993). Speed and direction selectivity of macaque middle temporal neurons. *J. Neurophysiol.* 69, 19–39. doi: 10.1152/jn.1993.69.1.19

Lam, C. S. Y., Tang, W. C., Tse, D. Y.-Y., Lee, R. P. K., Chun, R. K. M., Hasegawa, K., et al. (2020). Defocus Incorporated Multiple Segments (DIMS) spectacle lenses slow myopia progression: a 2-year randomised clinical trial. *Br. J. Ophthalmol.* 104, 363–368. doi: 10.1136/bjophthalmol-2018-313739

Lappin, J. S., Tadin, D., Nyquist, J. B., and Corn, A. L. (2009). Spatial and temporal limits of motion perception across variations in speed, eccentricity, and low vision. *J. Vis.* 9, 3001–3014. doi: 10.1167/9.1.30

Leibowitz, H. W., Johnson, C. A., and Isabelle, E. (1972). Peripheral motion detection and refractive error. *Science* 177, 1207–1208. doi: 10.1126/science.177.4055.1207

Lim, H. T., Yoon, J. S., Hwang, S. S., and Lee, S. Y. (2012). Prevalence and associated sociodemographic factors of myopia in Korean children: the 2005 third Korea National Health and Nutrition Examination Survey (KNHANES III). *Jpn. J. Ophthalmol.* 56, 76–81. doi: 10.1007/s10384-011-0090-7

Lin, Z., Martinez, A., Chen, X., Li, L., Sankaridurg, P., Holden, B. A., et al. (2010). Peripheral defocus with single-vision spectacle lenses in myopic children. *Optom. Vis. Sci.* 87, 4–9. doi: 10.1097/OPX.0b013e3181c078f1

Maiello, G., Chessa, M., Solari, F., and Bex, P. J. (2014). Simulated disparity and peripheral blur interact during binocular fusion. *J. Vis.* 14:13. doi: 10.1167/14.8.13

Maiello, G., Walker, L., Bex, P. J., and Vera-Diaz, F. A. (2017). Blur perception throughout the visual field in myopia and emmetropia. *J. Vis.* 17, 1–13. doi: 10.1167/17.5.3

Maniglia, M., Jogin, R., Visscher, K. M., and Seitz, A. R. (2020). We don't all look the same; detailed examination of peripheral looking strategies after simulated central vision loss. *J. Vis.* 20:5. doi: 10.1167/jov.20.13.5

Marigold, D. S. (2008). Role of peripheral visual cues in online visual guidance of locomotion. *Exerc. Sport Sci. Rev.* 36, 145–151. doi: 10.1097/JES.0b013e31817bff72

Marron, J. A., and Bailey, I. L. (1982). Visual factors and orientation-mobility performance. *Am. J. Optom. Physiol. Opt.* 59, 413–426. doi: 10.1097/00006324-198205000-00009

Mascetti, G. G., Turatto, M., and Facoetti, A. (2001). Four paradigms to study visual-spatial attention of myopic subjects. *Brain Res. Protoc.* 7, 241–247. doi: 10.1016/s1385-299x(01)00070-8

McKee, S. P., and Nakayama, K. (1984). The detection of motion in the peripheral visual field. *Vis. Res.* 24, 25–32. doi: 10.1016/0042-6989(84)90140-8

McKone, E., Davies, A. A., and Fernando, D. (2008). Blurry means good focus: myopia and visual attention. *Perception* 37, 1765–1768. doi: 10.1068/p6156

Merigan, W. H., and Maunsell, J. H. (1990). Macaque vision after magnocellular lateral geniculate lesions. *Vis. Neurosci.* 5, 347–352. doi: 10.1017/s0952523800000432

Mohindra, I., and Held, R. (1980). "Refraction in humans from birth to five years," in *Proceedings of the 3rd International Conference on Myopia Copenhagen*, Vol. 28, eds H. C. Fledelius, P. H. Alsbirk, and E. Goldschmidt (Dordrecht: Springer), 19–27. doi: 10.1007/978-94-009-8662-6_4

Moore, K. E., Benoit, J. S., and Berntsen, D. A. (2017). Spherical soft contact lens designs and peripheral defocus in myopic eyes. *Optom. Vis. Sci.* 94, 370–379. doi: 10.1097/OPX.0000000000001053

Morgan, I. G., Ohno-Matsui, K., and Saw, S. M. (2012). Ophthalmology 2 myopia. *Lancet* 379, 1739–1748. doi: 10.1016/s0140-6736(12)60272-4

Mutti, D. O., Hayes, J. R., Mitchell, G. L., Jones, L. A., Moeschberger, M. L., Cotter, S. A., et al. (2007). Refractive error, axial length, and relative peripheral refractive error before and after the onset of myopia. *Invest. Ophthalmol. Vis. Sci.* 48, 2510–2519. doi: 10.1167/iovs.06-0562

Nagra, M., Gilmartin, B., Logan, N. S., and Anderson, S. J. (2018). The effects of severe myopia on the properties of sampling units in peripheral retina. *Optom. Vis. Sci.* 95, 399–404. doi: 10.1097/OPX.0000000000001199

Nakayama, K. (1985). Biological image motion processing: a review. *Vis. Res.* 25, 625–660. doi: 10.1016/0042-6989(85)90171-3

Ohno-Matsui, K., Lai, T. Y. Y., Lai, C.-C., and Cheung, C. M. G. (2016). Updates of pathologic myopia. *Prog. Retinal Eye Res.* 52, 156–187. doi: 10.1016/j.preteyeres.2015.12.001

Pelli, D. G. (1997). The VideoToolbox software for visual psychophysics: transforming numbers into movies. *Spat. Vis.* 10, 437–442. doi: 10.1163/156856897X00366

Risse, J. F., Saint-Blancat, P., Boissonnot, M., and Grillot, L. (1996). Spatial contrast sensitivity in patients with severe myopia. *J. Fr. d'Ophtalmol.* 19, 271–277.

Rogers, J. G. (1972). Peripheral contrast thresholds for moving images. *Hum. Fact.* 14, 199–205.

Rosenfield, M., and Abraham-Cohen, J. A. (1999). Blur sensitivity in myopes. *Optom. Vis. Sci.* 76, 303–307. doi: 10.1097/00006324-199905000-00018

Rosenholtz, R. (2016). Capabilities and limitations of peripheral vision. *Annu. Rev. Vis. Sci.* 2, 437–457. doi: 10.1146/annurev-vision-082114-035733

Sankaridurg, P., Bakaraju, R. C., Naduvilath, T., Chen, X., Weng, R., Tilia, D., et al. (2019). Myopia control with novel central and peripheral plus contact lenses and extended depth of focus contact lenses: 2 year results from a randomised clinical trial. *Ophthalmic Physiol. Opt.* 39, 294–307. doi: 10.1111/opo.12621

Shen, J., Clark, C. A., Soni, P. S., and Thibos, L. N. (2010). Peripheral refraction with and without contact lens correction. *Optom. Vis. Sci.* 87, 642–655. doi: 10.1097/OPX.0b013e3181ea16ea

Siegwart, J. T., and Norton, T. T. (2011). Perspective : how might emmetropization and genetic factors produce myopia in normal eyes? *Optom. Vis. Sci.* 88, 365–372. doi: 10.1097/OPX.0b013e31820b053d

Smith, E. L. III, Hung, L.-F., Huang, J., Blasdel, T. L., Humbird, T. L., and Bockhorst, K. H. (2010). Effects of optical defocus on refractive development in monkeys: evidence for local, regionally selective mechanisms. *Invest. Ophthalmol. Vis. Sci.* 51, 3864–3873. doi: 10.1167/iovs.09-4969

Smith, E. L., Kee, C. S., Ramamirtham, R., Qiao-Grider, Y., and Hung, L. F. (2005). Peripheral vision can influence eye growth and refractive development in infant monkeys. *Invest. Ophthalmol. Vis. Sci.* 46, 3965–3972. doi: 10.1167/iovs.05-0445

Stoimenova, B. D. (2007). The effect of myopia on contrast thresholds. *Invest. Ophthalmol. Vis. Sci.* 48, 2371–2374. doi: 10.1167/iovs.05-1377

Strasburger, H., Rentschler, I., and Jüttner, M. (2011). Peripheral vision and pattern recognition: a review. *J. Vis.* 11:13. doi: 10.1167/11.5.13

Tarutta, E. P., Proskurina, O. V., Tarasova, N. A., Milash, S. V., and Markosyan, G. A. (2019). Long-term results of perifocal defocus spectacle lens correction in children with progressive myopia. *Vestn. Oftalmol.* 135, 46–53. doi: 10.17116/oftalma201913505146

Timberlake, G. T., Mainster, M. A., Peli, E., Augliere, R. A., Essock, E. A., and Arend, L. E. (1986). Reading with a macular scotoma. I. Retinal location of scotoma and fixation area. *Invest. Ophthalmol. Vis. Sci.* 27, 1137–1147.

van de Grind, W. A., Koenderink, J. J., and Van Doorn, A. J. (1987). Influence of contrast on foveal and peripheral detection of coherent motion in moving random-dot patterns. *J. Opt. Soc. Am. A Opt. Image Sci.* 4, 1643–1652. doi: 10.1364/josaa.4.001643

Vasudevan, B., Ciuffreda, K. J., and Wang, B. (2006). Objective blur thresholds in free space for different refractive groups. *Curr. Eye Res.* 31, 111–118. doi: 10.1080/02713680500514669

Venkataraman, A. P., Winter, S., Rosén, R., and Lundström, L. (2016). Choice of grating orientation for evaluation of peripheral vision. *Optom. Vis. Sci.* 93, 567–574. doi: 10.1097/OPX.0000000000000832

Venkataraman, A. P., Winter, S., Unsbo, P., and Lundström, L. (2015). Blur adaptation: contrast sensitivity changes and stimulus extent. *Vis. Res.* 110, 100–106. doi: 10.1016/j.visres.2015.03.009

Vera-Diaz, F. A., Bex, P. J., Ferreira, N., and Kosovicheva, A. (2018). Binocular temporal visual processing in myopia. *J. Vis.* 18, 1–12. doi: 10.1167/18.11.17

Wallman, J., Turkel, J., and Trachtman, J. (1978). Extreme myopia produced by modest change in early visual experience. *Science (New York, N.Y.)* 201, 1249–1251.

Wang, X., He, H., Wang, X., Shan, G., Tao, Z., Pan, L., et al. (2020). Prevalence and risk factors of myopia in Han and Yugur older adults in Gansu,

China: a cross-sectional study. *Sci. Rep.* 10:8249. doi: 10.1038/s41598-020-65078-x

Wertheim, T. (1980). Peripheral visual acuity: Th. Wertheim. *Am. J. Optom. Physiol. Opt.* 57, 915–924.

Wesemann, W., and Norcia, A. M. (1992). Contrast dependence of the oscillatory motion threshold across the visual field. *J. Opt. Soc. Am. A Opt. Image Sci.* 9, 1663–1671. doi: 10.1364/josaa.9.001663

Westheimer, G. (1954). Eye movement responses to a horizontally moving visual stimulus. *AMA Arch. Ophthalmol.* 52, 932–941. doi: 10.1001/archopht.1954.00920050938013

Wiesel, T. N., and Raviola, E. (1977). Myopia and eye enlargement after neonatal lid fusion in monkeys. *Nature* 266, 66–68. doi: 10.1038/266066a0

Xie, Z. H., Long, Y., Wang, J. X., Li, Q. Q., and Zhang, Q. (2020). Prevalence of myopia and associated risk factors among primary students in Chongqing: multilevel modeling. *BMC Ophthalmol.* 20:8. doi: 10.1186/s12886-020-01410-3

Zheleznyak, L., Barbot, A., Ghosh, A., and Yoon, G. (2016). Optical and neural anisotropy in peripheral vision. *J. Vis.* 16:1. doi: 10.1167/16.5.1

2

Meridian-Specific and Post-Optical Deficits of Spatial Vision in Human Astigmatism: Evidences from Psycho-Physical and EEG Scalings

Li Gu[1†], Yiyao Wang[1†], Lei Feng[1], Saiqun Li[1], Mengwei Zhang[1], Qingqing Ye[1], Yijing Zhuang[1], Zhong-Lin Lu[2,3,4], Jinrong Li[1] and Jin Yuan[1*]*

[1] State Key Laboratory of Ophthalmology, Zhongshan Ophthalmic Center, Sun Yat-sen University, Guangzhou, China, [2] Division of Arts and Sciences, NYU Shanghai, Shanghai, China, [3] Center for Neural Science, Department of Psychology, New York University, New York, NY, United States, [4] NYU-ECNU Institute of Cognitive Neuroscience, NYU Shanghai, Shanghai, China

***Correspondence:**
Jin Yuan
yuanjincornea@126.com
Jinrong Li
lijingr3@mail.sysu.edu.cn

† These authors have contributed equally to this work

Previous studies have demonstrated that orientation-specific deprivation in early life can lead to neural deficits of spatial vision in certain space, and can even result in meridional amblyopia (MA). Individuals with astigmatism are the optimal and natural models for exploring this asymmetric development of spatial vision in the human visual system. This study aims to assess the contrast sensitivity function (CSF) and EEG signals along two principal meridians in participants with regular astigmatism when being optimal optical corrected. Twelve participants with astigmatism (AST group, 20 eyes) and thirteen participants with (MA group, 19 eyes) were recruited in the current study. CSFs and spatial sweep visual evoked potentials (sVEP) were measured with vertical and horizontal sinewave gratings along two principal meridians monocularly. Area under log CSF (AULCSF), spatial frequency threshold corresponding to 80% contrast gratings (SF threshold at 80% ctr), and CSF acuity were calculated from CSF test. In addition, sVEP amplitudes and thresholds were calculated with the recursive least square method. Participants with astigmatism exhibited marked vertical-horizontal resolution disparities even after they were corrected with optimal optical corrections. CSF tests showed that AULCSF along weak meridian (measured with horizontal gratings) was lower than that along strong meridian (measured with vertical gratings) in both groups. Significant meridional disparity of CSF acuity was also found in both groups. In addition, the MA group showed larger meridional disparity compared to the AST group. Spatial sVEP thresholds also supported the existence of marked meridional disparity. Our results suggest that meridian-specific partial deprivation in early life might lead to monocularly asymmetric development of spatial vision in the human visual system. In terms of application, we tested the feasibility and reliability of adopting psychophysical and EEG scalings to investigate the asymmetric development of spatial vision related to astigmatism. These paradigms are potentially applicable to reduce and even eliminate the meridional disparity in the primary visual cortex by adopting perceptual learning or other vision-related interventions.

Keywords: contrast sensitivity, sVEP, astigmatism, meridional amblyopia, spatial vision

INTRODUCTION

The development of visual system is extraordinary sensitive to early visual experience (Berardi et al., 2000; Knudsen, 2004; Kiorpes, 2016). Abnormal visual experience will result in functional and structural deficits in the visual pathway and cerebral cortex, such as deprivation amblyopia (Kiorpes and McKee, 1999; Kiorpes, 2006). In the past decades, psychophysical, electrophysiological, and neuro-imaging techniques make the exploration of neural mechanism underlying human amblyopia feasible and fruitful. However, less attention has been given to meridional amblyopia (MA) resulting from astigmatism. Animal studies have consistently demonstrated that visual deprivation along one orientation would lead to orientation-specific deficits in the visual pathway and cerebral cortex (Blakemore and Cooper, 1970; Hirsch and Spinelli, 1970). However, systematic and comprehensive investigation of meridian-specific deficits in the human visual system is still lacking.

Individuals with astigmatism are the optimal model for investigating the asymmetric meridional development of spatial vision in the human neural system. Astigmatism is a common condition of refractive error in which the eye's refractive power differs in various meridians, with maximum and minimum powers mutually perpendicular (Read et al., 2014). There are two categories of astigmatism, regular, and irregular astigmatism. The former is normally from abnormal development of corneal curvature, and the latter is from the influence of ocular disease on the components of optical media. Astigmatism has a high prevalence (over 25%) in eastern Asia population most probably due to the different anatomical structure between eyelid, orbit, and eyeball (He et al., 2004, 2007; Rim et al., 2016; Nakamura et al., 2018; Wang et al., 2019).

For regular astigmatism, the parallel rays of light entering the eye are brought to a focus at two distinct focal lines perpendicular to each other rather than to a single focal point (Read et al., 2014). The asymmetrical input of visual signal in perpendicular meridians will affect visual functions, and may even result in MA (Mitchell et al., 1973; Gwiazda et al., 1985). Patients with MA have substandard corrected visual acuity behaviorally, and more notably, astigmatic individuals and amblyopes showed the abnormal development of spatial vision in the visual system (Fiorentini and Maffei, 1973; Freeman and Thibos, 1973; Mitchell et al., 1973; Freeman, 1975). Freeman and his collaborators (Freeman et al., 1972) first demonstrated that astigmatism may contribute to meridian-specific neural deficits in spatial vision, since certain astigmatic participants showed substantial vertical-horizontal resolution differences, even when being fully corrected optically. Since then, researchers further reported on an extensive investigation of the meridional differences in resolution with contrast sensitivity and electrophysiological evidence (Fiorentini and Maffei, 1973; Mitchell et al., 1973; Freeman, 1975). These results indicated that meridian-specific partial deprivation may lead to an analogous modification in the organization of neurons in the human visual system (Freeman et al., 1972). Following previous studies, we used the meridional disparity to represent the resolution differences between vertical and horizontal meridians. However, psychophysical and electrophysiological evidence from a recent study (Yap et al., 2019) demonstrated that non-amblyopic children with and without astigmatism also showed meridional disparity.

Contrast sensitivity and visual evoked potentials (VEPs) have been widely used to investigate the influence of stimulus orientation on the spatial tuning function in healthy subjects and patients (Freeman and Thibos, 1973; Tobimatsu et al., 1993; Arakawa et al., 2000; Tobimatsu and Celesia, 2006; Yap et al., 2019, 2020a). The computerized contrast sensitivity function (CSF) paradigm assesses spatial vision over a wide range of spatial frequencies and contrast levels, and has been demonstrated to be a suitable and applicable paradigm for detecting and diagnosing deficits in spatial vision by a handful of studies (Zhou et al., 2006; Yenice et al., 2007; Huang et al., 2008). Spatial sweep visual evoked potentials (sVEP) has been adopted to measure spatial acuity (Regan, 1977; Tyler, 1979; Norcia and Tyler, 1985; Good and Hou, 2006; Hou et al., 2011; Norcia et al., 2015). The combination of both two scalings would furnish subjective and objective paradigm to future studies related to the improvement of spatial vision, such as diminishing the meridional disparity via perceptual learning in the future study.

Therefore, the goal of the present study was to verify the feasibility and reliability of combining psycho-physical and EEG scalings to build human model of asymmetrical spatial vision development in individuals with astigmatism. To this end, the computerized CSF and sVEP tests were employed. CSF paradigm was adopted to assess spatial vision over a wide range of spatial frequencies and contrast levels (Zhou et al., 2006; Yenice et al., 2007; Huang et al., 2008) and spatial sVEP was adopted to measure spatial acuity (Regan, 1977; Tyler, 1979; Norcia and Tyler, 1985; Good and Hou, 2006; Hou et al., 2011; Norcia et al., 2015). Here, the Area under log CSF (AULCSF), spatial frequency threshold corresponding to 80% contrast gratings (SF threshold at 80% ctr), and CSF acuity were calculated from CSF tests, and the sVEP thresholds were calculated to evaluate meridional disparity in spatial acuity. In these two different paradigms, grating stimuli were presented either along the vertical or the horizontal meridian. Notably, the meridional disparity was quantified under full optical correction with spectacles or contact lenses to eliminate the influence from optical errors. From this, we expect to explore the asymmetrical visual development in human astigmatism in a comprehensive and systematic way.

MATERIALS AND METHODS

Participants

Twelve participants with astigmatism (AST group, 20 eyes, 6 males, mean age = 9.10 ± 1.37 years, age range:) and thirteen astigmatic participants with substandard corrected visual acuity (VA; defined as meridional amblyopia, MA group, 19 eyes, 7 males, mean age = 13.08 ± 6.75 years) were also recruited in the current study. Their refractive profiles were summarized in **Table 1**, and clinical demographics details were provided in **Supplementary Table 1**. Five amblyopes entered this study within a few years (3.89 ± 1.79) of completing conventional amblyopia therapy (i.e., patching therapy). Individuals with

TABLE 1 | Summary of the refractive profile of MA and AST groups in this study showing the mean refractive error (in DS and DC), power range (in DS and DC), spherical equivalent (in D), the refractive and occlusion history of the participants.

	AST	MA
N	10 (20 eyes);3/10 astigmatism with anisometropia	13 (19 eyes);6/13 meridional amblyopia with anisometropia
Age	Mean 9.10 ± 1.37	Mean 13.08 ± 6.75
	median 9	median 11
	age range 8–12	age range 7–26
BCVA	OD −0.00 ± 0.04	OD 0.22 ± 0.10
	OS 0.01 ± 0.04	OS 0.16 ± 0.06
VA	OD 0.31 ± 0.19	OD 0.50 ± 0.21
	OS 0.34 ± 0.23	OS 0.41 ± 0.14
Mean refractive error (DS/DC)	OD + 1.15 DS/−3.08 DC	OD + 1.78 DS/−3.56 DC
	OS + 1.03 DS/−3.13 DC	OS + 1.66 DS/−3.30 DC
Power range (DS/DC)	OD −2.50 to + 2.50 DS/−6.00 to −1.75 DC	OD −3.75 to + 6.50 DS/−5.50 to −1.50 DC
	OS −2.75 to + 2.75 DS/−6.00 to −1.50 DC	OS −4.00 to + 5.75 DS/−6.00 to −2.00 DC
Spherical equivalent (mean ± SD)	OD 0 ± 3.51 D	OD −0.39 ± 1.41 D
	OS 0.01 ± 3.29 D	OS −0.54 ± 1.69 D
Refractive history	Current spectacle wearers	Current spectacle wearers
Occlusion history	N.A.	5/13 were treated with patching therapy (3.89 ± 1.79 years)

N, number of participants; OD, right eye; OS, left eye; and N.A., not applicable.

regular astigmatism were recruited under the inclusion criteria (Chuck et al., 2018) for eyes in the AST and MA groups. Participants in the study went through careful ocular health examination, VA, autorefraction, manifest subjective refraction, motility examination (including cover-uncover and alternate-cover testing), near stereopsis (marked as Vision Assessment Cooperation™ V01, United States), distance stereopsis (Stereo Optical Distance Randot® Stereotest, United States), and corneal topography assessments. Cases of strabismus or micro-strabismus, ocular diseases, and/or abnormalities were excluded.

All participants completed the CSF tests, and nine participants in the AST group (13 eyes) and twelve participants in the MA group (16 eyes) completed the EEG scalings. Other participants did not complete the EEG scalings for personal reasons (e.g., limited time, low willing for receiving EEG scalings). This study followed the tenets of the Declaration of Helsinki and was approved by the Zhongshan Ophthalmic Center Ethics Committee. Informed consent was obtained from all participants (or their guardian) prior to data collection. All the participants were wearing 1 month new spectacles or contact lenses under optimal optical corrections prescribed by the same experienced optometrist (author FL) at Zhongshan Ophthalmic Center, in order to avoid the influence of new optical adaptation and previous incorrect optical fitting.

Procedure

Stimuli were displayed on a gamma-corrected AOC G2460PQU/BR LCD computer monitor (120 Hz refresh rate, 1920 × 1080 resolution, and 53.1 cm × 29.8 cm). All experiments were controlled by a PC running MATLAB (Mathworks Inc. Natick, MA, United States) and Psychophysics Toolbox (Brainard, 1997; Pelli, 1997). A special circuit was used to produce 14-bit gray-level resolution (Li et al., 2003; Li and Lu, 2012). The mean background luminance was 27 cd/m^2. During the whole experiment, the participant put the head on a chin rest and viewed the stimuli monocularly in a dimly lit room, with the tested eye watching while another eye occluded.

Participants went through a battery of measurements, including EDTRS VA, CSF tests along two perpendicular meridians (i.e., horizontal and vertical meridian, to match the distribution of regular astigmatism), and sVEP tests along the same two perpendicular meridians. Both the CSFs and sVEPs were measured monocularly.

The Tasks

CSF Test

The CSF paradigm was applied to assess the CSF along two meridians. While measuring CSF, the display subtended 4° × 4° at a viewing distance of 1.50 m for participants. To minimize edge effects, a half-Gaussian ramp (σ = 0.5°) was used to blend the gratings into the background. We measured contrast thresholds in a two-interval forced choice grating detection task at seven spatial frequencies (0.5, 1, 2, 4, 8, 12, and 16 c/d) using a three-down one-up staircase procedure that decreased signal contrast by 10% (multiplied the previous value by 0.9) after every three consecutive correct responses and increased signal contrast by 10% after every incorrect response, converging to a performance level of 79.3% correct (Huang et al., 2008; Lu and Dosher, 2014). Following previous studies, each trial started with a 200-ms fixation cross in the center of the display. This was followed by two 200-ms intervals, signaled by a brief tone in the beginning of each and separated by 500 ms. A grating was randomly presented in one of the two intervals. The other interval was blank. Participants indicated the signal interval by pressing one of the keys (F/J keypress) with index finger. The response also initiated the next trial. A reversal results when the staircase changes from increasing to decreasing contrast or vice versa. Usually, one block of three-down one-up staircase with a

10% step size produces about a dozen reversals in 80 trials (Zhang et al., 2019). To make sure getting enough reversals, we set 100 trials to measure the contrast threshold at each spatial frequency. Following the standard practice, we averaged the contrasts of an even number of reversals to estimate the contrast threshold after excluding the first three or four reversals.

Vertical and horizontal sinusoidal gratings were adopted to measure CSF along two meridians, respectively. The seven spatial frequency conditions were randomly mixed, with two meridian blocks completed in random order under each spatial frequency condition. Thus, there were fourteen blocks with 100 trials per block. A 10 min demo program was applied to run before formal data collection to avoid learning effect. A formal testing session of about 1.5 h was required to complete the CSF test in each eye. The sequence of the CSF tests in the two eyes was randomized and counterbalanced across participants.

EEG Data Acquisition and sVEP Test

Participants were seated in a shielded room. The EEG signals were amplified and digitized using an Active Two 64-channel Amplifier with the 64-channel Cap in accordance to the international 10–20 system (Biosemi, Netherland), which provided fast and simple electrode placement. Signals from 64 electrodes were recorded and the impedance of each electrode was kept below 10 kV. Horizontal and vertical electrooculograms (HEOG and VEOG) were also recorded to monitor eye movements. Two reference electrodes were used. The data were sampled at 2048 Hz and filtered with a 0.16–100 Hz band-pass filter.

For spatial sVEP, sweeps of spatial frequency at high contrast were adopted (see **Figure 1**), and the parameters of stimulus refer to previous research (Hou et al., 2011). An 80% contrast, 6-Hz, phase-reversing cosine grating (shown as a square-wave grating) was swept from 2 to 16 cyc/deg in 10 linear steps. The sweep duration was 10 s. The display subtended 10° × 10° at a viewing distance of 0.90 m for participants. Spatial sVEP test was also monocularly conducted, and the non-viewing eye was occluded with a black eye patch.

Data Analysis

CSF Data

The AULCSF and CSF acuity were calculated (Dorr et al., 2018). Both the spatial frequency and the contrast sensitivity in the logarithmic value were generated. We computed the area under the log CSF (AULCSF) for spatial frequencies ranging from 1.5 to 18 cpd using the trapezoid method. We also computed CSF Acuity, i.e., the intersection of the CSF with the x axis (where contrast threshold is 100%). Additionally, the SF threshold at 80% ctr was calculated and extracted in order to investigate the relationship between CSF and sVEP tests.

sVEP Data

The EEG was analyzed using a customized toolbox (mfeeg. http://sourceforge.net/p/mfeeg) programmed with MATLAB (The Mathworks, Natick, MA, United States). Continuous EEG recordings were band-pass filtered from 1 to 30 Hz.

The stimulus is presented at a given temporal frequency (6 Hz in this study) that drives visual cortical neurons at that frequency and at exact integer multiples of that frequency, as well as the stimulus is in the visible range. The visual response synchronized to the display is sampled with appropriately positioned leads, and the VEP amplitude versus stimulus intensity function is measured as the stimulus-driven response drops into the background EEG noise. In this study, swept parameter presentations were repeated ten times.

To measure the response functions, sVEP recordings for each 10-s trial were divided into 10 sequential epochs that corresponded to the swept stimulus values. For each epoch, a recursive least square (RLS) adaptive filter was used to generate a series of complex valued spectral coefficients representing the amplitude and phase of response components tuned to its multiples of the stimulus frequency (Tang and Norcia, 1995). The signals from three electrodes (Oz, O1, and O2) were averaged for further analysis and we focused on the second harmonics (12 Hz in the current study) of the temporal frequency (Almoqbel et al., 2008, 2011; Hou et al., 2018). These spectral coefficients for each epoch were coherently averaged across trials for each subject and stimulus conditions (Hou et al., 2018). These functions were also used to estimate thresholds for each subject's individual conditions.

sVEP Threshold Estimation

Response thresholds were estimated by regression of amplitudes from the trial-average epochs for each swept stimulus condition of each subject (Hou et al., 2018). We applied the regression procedure to the sweep response function of each individual subject. For those individuals whose response functions along two meridians both passed the regression criteria, we calculated the resultant thresholds. The regression criteria was adopted from previous research (Norcia and Tyler, 1985), which chose an SNR (signal to noise ratio) of $>3:1$ (i.e., the amplitude of the peak response signal has to be at least three times larger than the adjacent noise frequency) as a criterion (Norcia and Tyler, 1985).

We also calculated the amplitudes by averaging the sweep response functions of individual participants for a given stimulus condition. In this analysis, each participant contributed equally to all conditions. Error bars in the figures depicting sweep responses are vector standard errors of the vector mean (Hou et al., 2007).

Statistical Analysis

The statistical software package SPSS (version 19; IBM Corp, Armonk, NY, United States) was used for analysis. In order to account for right and left eye-related data (Glynn and Rosner, 2012), linear mixed models (LMMs) analysis was used to investigate the effect of stimulus meridian (strong or weak meridian) and group on the outcome measures. Bonferroni correction was applied to multiple paired comparisons to correct for family-wise error. According to previous research (Huang et al., 2018), monocular data from two eyes was in the same comparison group in the current study design, making F-test of LMMs no better than two sample t-test. Moreover, t-test using the average of two eyes would not perform best considering the

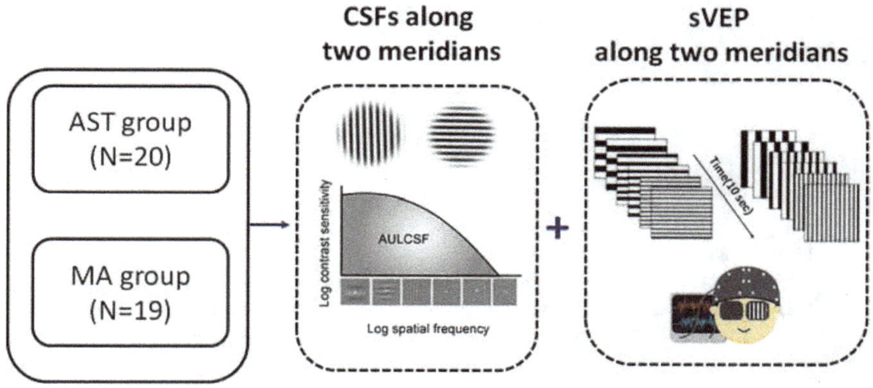

FIGURE 1 | Experimental flowchart. We measured the CSF and sVEP signals along two principal meridians (i.e., horizontal meridian and vertical meridian, to match the distribution of with-the-rule astigmatic subjects in the study) monocularly in all participants. *N* indicates the number of eyes. See also **Supplementary Table 1** for clinical details.

small sample size. Thus, comparisons between two meridians were reported with two sample *t*-test.

RESULTS

CSF Results

Contrast sensitivity function results along two meridians were shown in **Table 2**, and meridional disparity was present in the AST group (**Figure 2A**) and MA group (**Figure 2B**). Individual CSF result for each participant was provided in **Supplementary Figure 1**. LMMs analysis was used to investigate the effect of stimulus meridian (strong or weak meridian) and group on the AULCSF and Cutoff acuity.

We first evaluated the meridional disparity of AULCSF. LMMs analysis showed a significant effect of meridian ($F_{1,52.44}$ = 46.812, p < 0.001), a marginal significant main effect of group ($F_{1,20.22}$ = 3.176, p = 0.090), and a marginal significant interaction between the two factors ($F_{1,52.44}$ = 3.461, p = 0.070). *F*-test of LMMs based on estimated marginal means indicated a significant meridional disparity of AULCSF (M_{diff} = 0.223 ± 0.033, $F_{1,52.44}$ = 46.812, and p < 0.001). Significant meridional disparity of AULCSF was found in the AST (M_{diff} = 0.163 ± 0.032, t_{19} = 5.030, and p < 0.001; **Figure 3A**) and MA (M_{diff} = 0.284 ± 0.028, t_{18} = 10.209, and p < 0.001; **Figure 3B**) groups. In addition, the MA group showed larger meridional disparity of AULCSF compared to the AST group (t_{37} = 2.834, p = 0.007).

We then evaluated the meridional disparity of CSF acuity. LMMs analysis showed a significant effect of meridian ($F_{1,51.33}$ = 18.142, p < 0.001), and group ($F_{1,18.58}$ = 10.793, p = 0.004). The interaction between the two factors was not significant ($F_{1,51.33}$ = 1.425, p = 0.238). *F*-test of LMMs based on estimated marginal means indicated a significant meridional disparity of CSF acuity (M_{diff} = 0.107 ± 0.025, $F_{1,51.33}$ = 18.142, and p < 0.001). Significant meridional disparity of CSF acuity was found in the AST (M_{diff} = 0.077 ± 0.033, t_{19} = 2.362, and p = 0.029; **Figure 4A**) and MA group (M_{diff} = 0.138 ± 0.029, t_{18} = 4.707, and p < 0.001; **Figure 4B**). Meanwhile, there was no significant difference between meridional disparity of CSF acuity in two groups (t_{37} = 1.367, p = 0.180).

Furthermore, we evaluated the meridional disparity of contrast sensitivity corresponding to individual SF. LMMs analysis showed a significant main effect of meridian ($F_{1,496.69}$ = 90.249, p < 0.001), a significant main effect of SF ($F_{6,496.69}$ = 174.645, p < 0.001), a marginal significant main effect of group ($F_{1,20.57}$ = 3.053, p = 0.096), a significant interaction effect between meridian and group ($F_{1,496.69}$ = 6.292, p = 0.012), a significant interaction effect between SF and group ($F_{6,496.69}$ = 8.155, p < 0.001), a significant interaction effect between meridian and SF ($F_{6,496.69}$ = 3.060, p = 0.006), and but a non-significant interaction between the three factors ($F_{6,496.69}$ = 0.563, p = 0.759). *F*-test of LMMs further showed the existence of meridional disparity of contrast sensitivity corresponding to several spatial frequencies (2, 4, 8, 12, and 16 c/d), $F_{1,496.69}$ = 11.069, p = 0.001; $F_{1,496.69}$ = 24.160, p < 0.001; $F_{1,496.69}$ = 22.923, p < 0.001; $F_{1,496.69}$ = 22.604, p < 0.001; and $F_{1,496.69}$ = 25.119, p < 0.001, respectively. *Post hoc* comparisons between two meridians are listed in **Table 2**.

sVEP Results

For sVEP data, we first evaluated the meridional disparity of sVEP thresholds (**Table 2**). LMMs analysis showed a significant effect of meridian ($F_{1,54}$ = 16.234, p < 0.001), and group ($F_{1,54}$ = 10.354, p = 0.002). The interaction between the two factors was not significant ($F_{1,54}$ = 0.050, p = 0.825). *F*-test of LMMs based on estimated marginal means indicated a significant meridional disparity of sVEP thresholds (M_{diff} = 2.445 ± 0.607, $F_{1,54}$ = 16.234, and p < 0.001). Significant meridional disparity of sVEP threshold was found in the AST (M_{diff} = 2.580 ± 0.881, t_{12} = 2.928, and p = 0.013) and MA (M_{diff} = 2.310 ± 0.610, t_{15} = 3.789, and p = 0.002) groups. Meanwhile, the meridional disparity of sVEP threshold in the MA group was no larger than that in the AST group (t_{27} = 0.259, p = 0.798).

We then examined the meridional disparity of amplitudes for spatial frequencies presented (**Figure 5**; also see **Table 2**).

TABLE 2 | Mean values of sVEP threshold, amplitudes at target frequency (12 Hz), and CSF tests along two meridians.

	Strong meridian (Mean ± SE)	Weak meridian (Mean ± SE)	Difference (Mean ± SE)	*t*-value	*p*-value
sVEP results at 12 Hz					
AST group					
Threshold (*N* = 13)	19.201 ± 0.675	16.621 ± 0.569	2.580 ± 0.881	2.928	0.013*
sf1(2 cpd)	4.235 ± 0.362	3.580 ± 0.500	0.292 ± 0.814	0.359	0.729
sf2(3.6 cpd)	3.539 ± 0.288	3.274 ± 0.254	0.362 ± 0.190	1.907	0.073
sf3(5.1 cpd)	4.211 ± 0.379	2.997 ± 0.273	1.214 ± 0.258	4.713	<0.001**
sf4(6.7 cpd)	4.096 ± 0.391	2.909 ± 0.244	1.265 ± 0.298	4.240	<0.001**
sf5(8.2 cpd)	3.857 ± 0.394	2.898 ± 0.192	0.921 ± 0.372	2.475	0.024*
sf6(9.8 cpd)	3.276 ± 0.307	2.303 ± 0.192	1.051 ± 0.298	3.529	0.002*
sf7(11.3 cpd)	2.909 ± 0.258	2.385 ± 0.164	0.586 ± 0.309	1.896	0.076
sf8(12.9 cpd)	2.304 ± 0.183	2.269 ± 0.172	0.092 ± 0.231	0.396	0.697
sf9(14.4 cpd)	2.214 ± 0.201	2.230 ± 0.124	0.096 ± 0.181	0.529	0.605
sf10(16 cpd)	2.080 ± 0.111	2.262 ± 0.197	−0.272 ± 0.224	−1.216	0.243
MA group					
Threshold (*N* = 16)	17.113 ± 0.634	14.803 ± 0.529	2.310 ± 0.610	3.789	0.002*
sf1(2 cpd)	3.997 ± 0.432	4.558 ± 0.356	−1.453 ± 0.512	−2.835	0.025*
sf2(3.6 cpd)	3.524 ± 0.293	3.018 ± 0.149	0.506 ± 0.292	1.735	0.100
sf3(5.1 cpd)	3.834 ± 0.379	2.911 ± 0.193	0.923 ± 0.362	2.552	0.020*
sf4(6.7 cpd)	3.859 ± 0.338	2.655 ± 0.193	1.204 ± 0.293	4.111	0.001*
sf5(8.2 cpd)	3.480 ± 0.352	2.376 ± 0.204	1.104 ± 0.289	3.826	0.001*
sf6(9.8 cpd)	3.123 ± 0.383	2.149 ± 0.198	1.050 ± 0.376	2.791	0.013*
sf7(11.3 cpd)	2.823 ± 0.388	2.082 ± 0.163	0.741 ± 0.378	1.959	0.066
sf8(12.9 cpd)	2.439 ± 0.253	1.968 ± 0.173	0.450 ± 0.231	1.951	0.068
sf9(14.4 cpd)	2.024 ± 0.207	1.937 ± 0.176	0.103 ± 0.243	0.422	0.679
sf10(16 cpd)	2.360 ± 0.207	1.977 ± 0.173	0.256 ± 0.218	1.176	0.261
CSF measures					
AST group					
SF threshold	41.919 ± 2.786	34.681 ± 2.114	7.238 ± 2.829	2.558	0.019*
AULCSF	1.574 ± 0.050	1.411 ± 0.054	0.163 ± 0.032	5.030	<0.001**
CSF acuity	1.642 ± 0.028	1.565 ± 0.026	0.077 ± 0.033	2.362	0.029*
0.5 cpd	1.212 ± 0.029	1.153 ± 0.048	0.059 ± 0.038	1.563	0.135
1 cpd	1.473 ± 0.033	1.443 ± 0.035	0.031 ± 0.025	1.212	0.240
2 cpd	1.626 ± 0.043	1.558 ± 0.038	0.068 ± 0.040	1.718	0.102
4 cpd	1.648 ± 0.057	1.454 ± 0.070	0.194 ± 0.056	3.464	0.003*
8 cpd	1.446 ± 0.056	1.227 ± 0.071	0.219 ± 0.049	4.444	<0.001**
12 cpd	1.245 ± 0.070	1.097 ± 0.079	0.149 ± 0.065	2.287	0.034*
16 cpd	0.859 ± 0.065	0.686 ± 0.050	0.173 ± 0.065	2.667	0.015*
MA group					
SF threshold	32.107 ± 3.014	21.949 ± 1.478	10.158 ± 2.143	4.740	<0.001**
AULCSF	1.397 ± 0.066	1.113 ± 0.077	0.284 ± 0.028	10.209	<0.001**
CSF acuity	1.508 ± 0.042	1.370 ± 0.026	0.138 ± 0.029	4.707	<0.001**
0.5 cpd	1.238 ± 0.053	1.185 ± 0.036	0.052 ± 0.037	1.400	0.178
1 cpd	1.426 ± 0.047	1.343 ± 0.041	0.083 ± 0.033	2.554	0.020
2 cpd	1.604 ± 0.042	1.351 ± 0.078	0.253 ± 0.050	5.060	<0.001**
4 cpd	1.512 ± 0.063	1.232 ± 0.085	0.280 ± 0.043	6.505	<0.001**
8 cpd	1.212 ± 0.093	0.968 ± 0.087	0.243 ± 0.052	4.717	<0.001**
12 cpd	0.960 ± 0.083	0.650 ± 0.087	0.310 ± 0.058	5.337	<0.001**
16 cpd	0.624 ± 0.090	0.313 ± 0.057	0.311 ± 0.045	6.946	<0.001**

*Post hoc comparisons between strong meridian and weak meridian are also presented. A single asterisk * indicates a significance level of $p < 0.05$. Two asterisks ** indicate a significance level of $p < 0.001$.*

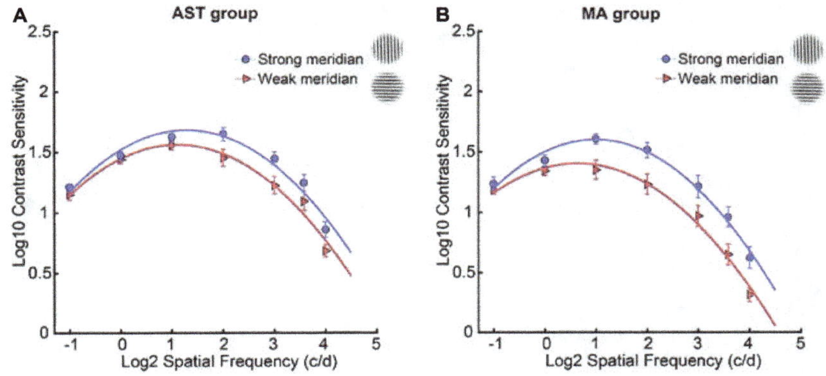

FIGURE 2 | CSF results along two meridians. Participants showed meridional disparity in the AST group **(A)** and MA group **(B)**. Error bars stand for ± S.E.M.

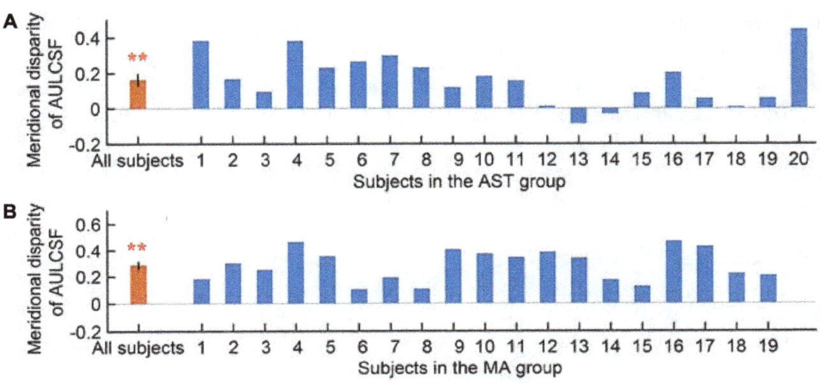

FIGURE 3 | Meridional disparity of AULCSF in the AST group **(A)** and the MA group **(B)**. Error bars represent ± S.E.M. Two asterisks ** indicate a significance level of $p < 0.001$.

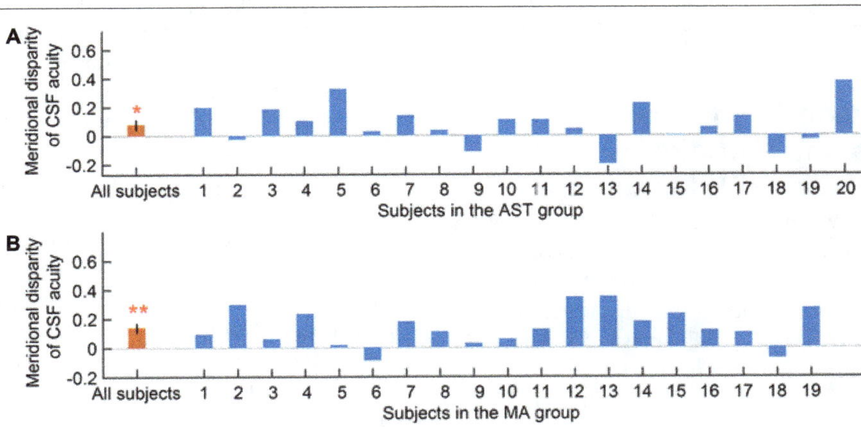

FIGURE 4 | Meridional disparity of CSF acuity in the AST group **(A)** and the MA group **(B)**. Error bars represent ± S.E.M. An asterisk * indicates a significance level of $p < 0.05$. Two asterisks ** indicate a significance level of $p < 0.001$.

LMMs analysis showed a significant main effect of meridian ($F_{1,665.08} = 64.807$, $p < 0.001$), a significant main effect of SF ($F_{9,665.05} = 34.494$, $p < 0.001$), a significant interaction effect between meridian and SF ($F_{9,665.12} = 4.959$, $p < 0.001$, but a non-significant main effect of group ($F_{1,20.75} = 0.241$, $p = 0.628$). No significant interaction between meridian and group ($F_{1,665.08} = 0.043$, $p = 0.835$), between SF and group ($F_{9,665.05} = 1.025$, $p = 0.418$), or between the three factors

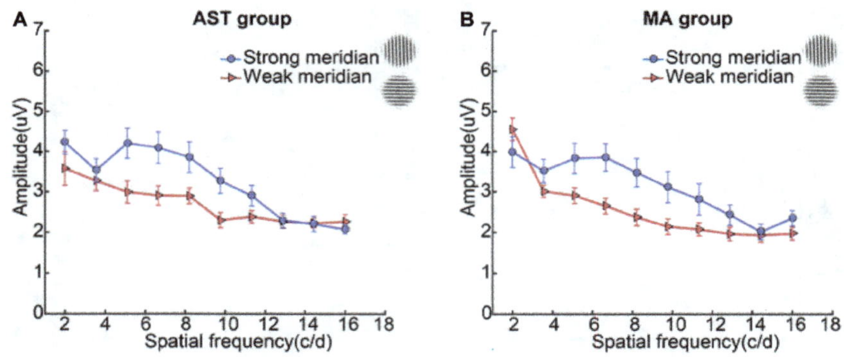

FIGURE 5 | Spatial sVEP voltage response at the second harmonic of the test stimulus reversal rate is plotted as a function of spatial frequency of the test stimulus in the AST group **(A)** and the MA group **(B)**. Error bars represent ± S.E.M.

($F_{9,665.12} = 0.950$, $p = 0.481$) was found. Multiple comparison analysis further showed the existence of meridional disparity of amplitudes corresponding to medium SF (5.1, 6.7, 8.2, 9.8, and 11.3 c/d), $F_{1,664.87} = 25.053$, $p < 0.001$; $F_{1,664.89} = 32.381$, $p < 0.001$; $F_{1,664.89} = 23.397$, $p < 0.001$; $F_{1,665.01} = 22.570$, $p < 0.001$; and $F_{1,664.95} = 10.252$, $p = 0.001$, respectively. *Post hoc* comparisons between two meridians are listed in **Table 2**.

Correlation Between CSF and sVEP Tests

Most interestingly, we found measurable correlations between CSF (SF threshold at 80% ctr) and sVEP (sVEP threshold) tests. Results showed that there was a significant correlation between SF threshold at 80% ctr and the sVEP threshold in the AST ($r = 0.578$, $p = 0.002$; **Figure 6A**) and MA ($r = 0.671$, $p < 0.001$; **Figure 6C**) groups. Moreover, the meridional disparity of SF threshold at 80% ctr and meridional disparity of the sVEP threshold was also significantly correlated in the AST ($r = 0.569$, $p = 0.043$; **Figure 6B**) and MA ($r = 0.532$, $p = 0.034$; **Figure 6D**) groups.

Correlation Between Cylindrical Refractive Errors and Meridional Disparities of CSF or sVEP Measures

In a final analysis, we examined the relationship between cylindrical refractive errors and meridional disparities of CSF or sVEP measures. There was no significant correlation between cylindrical refractive errors and meridional disparities of any CSF or sVEP measure (AULCSF, CSF acuity, SF threshold at 80% ctr, and sVEP threshold; all $p > 0.050$). Consistent with previous study (Yap et al., 2020a), this indicated that cylindrical refractive error alone does not constitute the decisive factor for the level of meridional disparity, and other factors may also be related to the asymmetric development in the visual system.

DISCUSSION

The current study investigated the asymmetric development of spatial vision related to astigmatism in the human visual system via combining psycho-physical and EEG scalings. We assessed the CSF and sVEP along two principal meridians in participants with astigmatism when being optimally corrected with spectacles, and confirmed the horizontal and vertical asymmetry of spatial vision in human astigmatism. This finding was in line with animal studies (Blakemore and Cooper, 1970; Hirsch and Spinelli, 1970) and other human studies (Freeman et al., 1972; Fiorentini and Maffei, 1973; Mitchell et al., 1973; Freeman, 1975), suggesting that the meridian-specific partial deprivation in early life can lead to monocularly asymmetric development of spatial vision in the visual system.

Neurons in the primary visual cortex, responsive to the retina mapping projection from optical input, is highly sensitive to visual experience during the critical period (Wiesel, 1963; Morishita and Hensch, 2008). Astigmatism without appropriate optical corrections before the critical period would permanently modify the visual system and result in monocularly and binocularly abnormal visual perception (Freeman et al., 1972). It has been reported that abnormal visual input in early life would affect the establishment of visual perception, and may even lead to MA (Hubel and Wiesel, 1962; Shapley et al., 2003). In this study, converging evidence from CSF and sVEP results suggested that meridional disparity on participants with astigmatism are of neural, rather than optical, origin. In addition, we found that the meridional disparity of AULCSF was more remarkable in MA group. As the AULCSF is a summary measure of spatial vision (Applegate et al., 1998; Oshika et al., 2006; Lesmes et al., 2010), we speculated that this finding indicated a higher level of abnormal spatial vision in meridional amblyopes than astigmats, and that the phenomenon that astigmats had normal corrected VA but showed meridional disparity of spatial vision might be due to the compensation of neural system. It should be noted that higher level of meridional disparity was only found in the AULCSF measurement but not in other measures (CSF acuity, SF threshold at 80% ctr, sVEP threshold, and sVEP amplitudes). Meridional amblyopes would generally be expected to have much greater magnitude of meridional disparities. We speculated that it may be due to low severity of amblyopia or the treatment history of amblyopes. All the amblyopes were

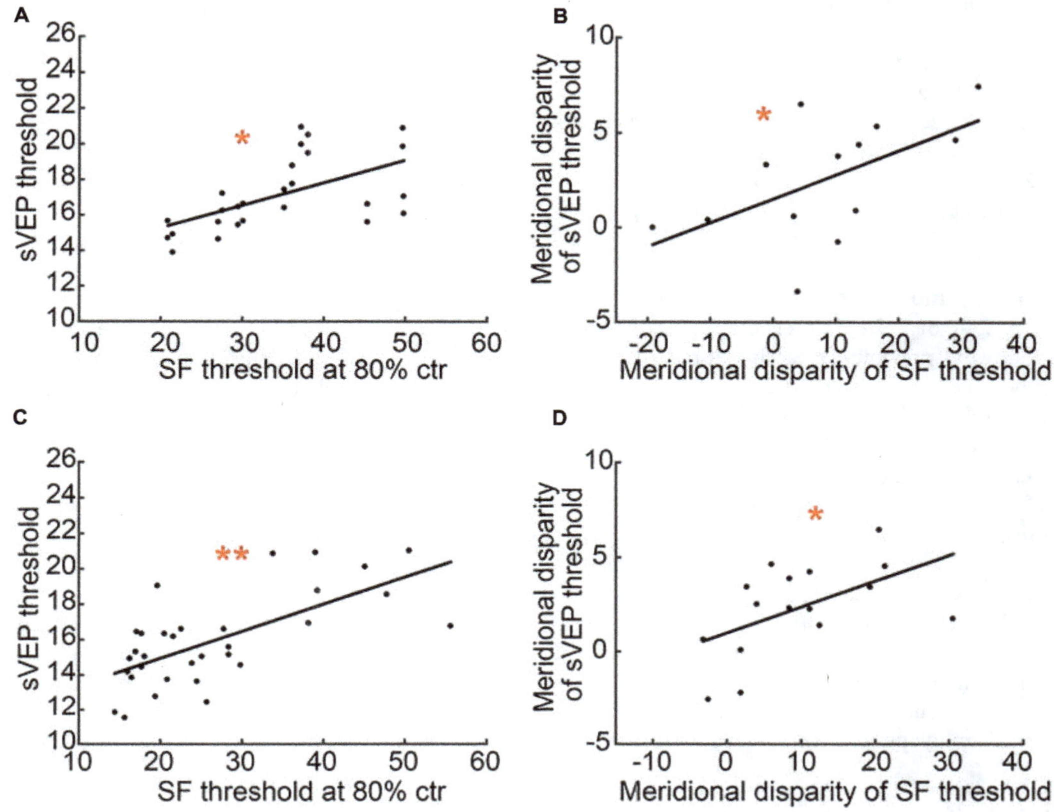

FIGURE 6 | A scatter plot of CSF and sVEP measures. **(A)** SF threshold at 80% ctr and the sVEP threshold in the AST group; **(B)** meridional disparity of SF threshold at 80% ctr and meridional disparity of the sVEP threshold in the AST group; **(C)** SF threshold at 80% ctr and the sVEP threshold in the MA group; and **(D)** meridional disparity of SF threshold at 80% ctr and meridional disparity of the sVEP threshold in the MA group. An asterisk * indicates a significance level of $p < 0.05$. Two asterisks ** indicate a significance level of $p < 0.001$.

already treated via wearing spectacles prior to the measuring of the VEPs, which helped to improve the visual performance (Gao et al., 2018).

The finding that the horizontal meridian was weaker than vertical meridian in the current study, may be attributed to a horizontal effect. Horizontal effect indicated that the horizontal meridian is less sensitive than the rest of meridians. This finding was consistent with previous study showing that horizontal effect existed in both astigmats and non-astigmats (Yap et al., 2019). Therefore, it should be noted that the horizontal effect might be confounding. All the participants included in the current study were with-the-rule astigmatic, which might limit the explanation. Future research could include individuals with other types of regular astigmatism and further clarify the relationship between astigmatism type and meridional disparity.

Consistent with previous study (Yap et al., 2020a), our results demonstrated that astigmatism alone is not the decisive factor on the magnitude of their meridional disparity. We speculated that meridional disparity of spatial vision might result not only from meridional optical blur alone, but also from many alternative mechanisms, such as neural suppression of amblyopia if existed (Hess et al., 2014). Meanwhile, there exists differences between the current study and Yap's study. They recruited newly diagnosed amblyopic children who have never worn spectacles, and this current study investigated subjects who have worn spectacles for at least a few months prior to testing. Considering that the duration of astigmatic blur (Keech and Kutschke, 1995) and treatment history (Gao et al., 2018) also influenced the magnitude of meridional disparity, the finding that meridional amblyopes demonstrated the horizontal effect in the current study might suggest a consequence of treatment or recovery. Besides, the horizontal effect was only observed in children (3–7 years old) in Yap's study, and the meridional disparity was observed in subjects of older age range (7–26 years old) in our study. According to recent studies (Yap et al., 2019, 2020b; Yap and Boon, 2020), the horizontal effect is an indicator of normality. It is important to separate the meridian-specific deficit from the normal physiological phenomenon (i.e., horizontal effect), thus future study could include newly diagnosed amblyopes and meridional amblyopes with other types of regular astigmatism to further clarify it.

For the combination of psycho-physical methods and EEG scalings, the spatial sVEP was adopted, instead of contrast sVEP

For the combination of psycho-physical methods and EEG scalings, the spatial sVEP was adopted, instead of contrast sVEP which measured contrast sensitivity, causing the mismatch of two paradigms. We adopted seven spatial frequencies in the CSF test and ten spatial frequencies in the sVEP test, which also caused the mismatching of grating stimuli in two paradigms. Even though the SF thresholds at 80% ctr and the sVEP thresholds were significantly correlated, it is not applicable to explore the relationship between contrast sensitivity and sVEP amplitude of gratings on each spatial frequency. CSF and sVEP tests with the same set of grating stimuli are expected in future research. Though we set an SNR of >3:1 as a criterion to control the overestimation following previous research (Norcia and Tyler, 1985), it is acknowledged that sweep VEPs might overestimate spatial resolution thresholds (Hamilton et al., 2020).

In the current study design, monocular data from two eyes was included in the same group. A larger sample size and data from randomly selected eye may help to clarify these observations. Other limitations of the study include: (1) the age range (7–26 years old) was relatively wide; (2) some amblyopes had VA reduction in both eyes without an interocular acuity difference significantly; (3) several amblyopes with anisometropia were not specifically excluded from this present study, which may contribute to an alternative neural mechanism of amblyopia, such as neural suppression (Hess et al., 2014); and (4) several amblyopes received occlusion treatment for years, which may already compensate for the magnitude of their meridional disparity.

Individuals with astigmatism are the optimal and natural models for exploring the asymmetric development of spatial vision, and further investigations are expected based on our current findings. Firstly, we could carry out more explorations to investigate the occurrence and development of astigmatism and MA. For instance, we could measure CSF in the real-world scenarios, or apply other neuroimaging tools, such as functional magnetic resonance imaging (fMRI) and functional near infrared spectroscopy (fNIRS). Secondly, we could reduce and even eliminate the visual deficit in the primary visual cortex by adopting perceptual learning or other vision-related interventions. Furthermore, we expect individuals with astigmatism to fully restore visual functions even without optical corrections by taking advantage of visual neural plasticity.

AUTHOR CONTRIBUTIONS

JY, JL, and LG designed the research. LG, YW, and LF performed the research. LG analyzed the data and drafted the manuscript. JY, JL, and Z-LL revised the manuscript. All authors commented on and edited the manuscript, and approved the final version of the manuscript.

REFERENCES

Almoqbel, F. M., Leat, S. J., and Irving, E. (2008). The technique, validity and clinical use of the sweep VEP. *Ophthalmic Physiol. Opt.* 28, 393–403. doi: 10.1111/j.1475-1313.2008.00591.x

Almoqbel, F. M., Yadav, N. K., Leat, S. J., Head, L. M., and Irving, E. L. (2011). Effects of sweep VEP parameters on visual acuity and contrast thresholds in children and adults. *Graefes Arch. Clin. Exp. Ophthalmol.* 249, 613–623. doi: 10.1007/s00417-010-1469-8

Applegate, R. A., Howland, H. C., Sharp, R. P., Cottingham, A. J., and Yee, R. W. (1998). Corneal aberrations and visual performance after radial keratotomy. *J. Refract. Surg.* 14, 397–407. doi: 10.3928/1081-597X-19980701-05

Arakawa, K., Tobimatsu, S., Kurita-Tashima, S., Nakayama, M., Kira, J.-I., and Kato, M. (2000). Effects of stimulus orientation on spatial frequency function of the visual evoked potential. *Exp. Brain Res.* 131, 121–125. doi: 10.1007/s002219900274

Berardi, N., Pizzorusso, T., and Maffei, L. (2000). Critical periods during sensory development. *Curr. Opin. Neurobiol.* 10, 138–145.

Blakemore, C., and Cooper, G. F. (1970). Development of the brain depends on the visual environment. *Nature* 228, 477–478.

Brainard, D. H. (1997). The psychophysics toolbox. *Spat. Vis.* 10, 433–436.

Chuck, R. S., Jacobs, D. S., Lee, J. K., Afshari, N. A., Vitale, S., Shen, T. T., et al. (2018). Refractive errors & refractive surgery preferred practice pattern® . *Ophthalmology* 125, P1–P104. doi: 10.1016/j.ophtha.2017.10.003

Dorr, M., Elze, T., Wang, H., Lu, Z.-L., Bex, P. J., and Lesmes, L. A. (2018). New precision metrics for contrast sensitivity testing. *IEEE J. Biomed. Health Inform.* 22, 919–925. doi: 10.1109/JBHI.2017.2708745

Fiorentini, A., and Maffei, L. (1973). Evoked potentials in astigmatic subjects. *Vis. Res.* 13, 1781–1783. doi: 10.1016/0042-6989(73)90095-3

Freeman, R. D. (1975). Contrast sensitivity in meridional amblyopia. *Invest. Ophthalmol. Vis. Sci.* 14, 78–81.

Freeman, R. D., Mitchell, D. E., and Millodot, M. A. (1972). A neural effect of partial visual deprivation in humans. *Science* 175, 1384–1386.

Freeman, R. D., and Thibos, L. N. (1973). Electrophysiological evidence that abnormal early visual experience can modify the human brain. *Science* 180, 876–878. doi: 10.1126/science.180.4088.876

Gao, T. Y., Anstice, N., Babu, R. J., Black, J. M., Bobier, W. R., Dai, S., et al. (2018). Optical treatment of amblyopia in older children and adults is essential prior to enrolment in a clinical trial. *Ophthalmic Physiol. Opt.* 38, 129–143. doi: 10.1111/opo.12437

Glynn, R. J., and Rosner, B. (2012). Regression methods when the eye is the unit of analysis. *Ophthalmic Epidemiol.* 19, 159–165. doi: 10.3109/09286586.2012.674614

Good, W. V., and Hou, C. (2006). Sweep visual evoked potential grating acuity thresholds paradoxically improve in low-luminance conditions in children with cortical visual impairment. *Invest. Opthalmol. Vis. Sci.* 47:3220. doi: 10.1167/iovs.05-1252

Gwiazda, J., Mohindra, I., Brill, S., and Held, R. (1985). Infant astigmatism and meridional amblyopia. *Vis. Res.* 25, 1269–1276. doi: 10.1016/0042-6989(85)90042-2

Hamilton, R., Bach, M., Heinrich, S. P., Hoffmann, M. B., Odom, J. V., McCulloch, D. L., et al. (2020). VEP estimation of visual acuity: a systematic review. *Doc. Ophthalmol.* 142, 25–74. doi: 10.1007/s10633-020-09770-3

He, M., Huang, W., Zheng, Y., Huang, L., and Ellwein, L. B. (2007). Refractive error and visual impairment in school children in rural Southern China. *Ophthalmology* 114, 374–382. doi: 10.1016/j.ophtha.2006.08.020

He, M., Zeng, J., Liu, Y., Xu, J., Pokharel, G. P., and Ellwein, L. B. (2004). Refractive error and visual impairment in urban children in Southern China. *Invest. Opthalmol. Vis. Sci.* 45:793. doi: 10.1167/iovs.03-1051

Hess, R. F., Thompson, B., and Baker, D. H. (2014). Binocular vision in amblyopia: structure, suppression and plasticity. *Ophthalmic Physiol. Opt.* 34, 146–162. doi: 10.1111/opo.12123

Hirsch, H. V. B., and Spinelli, D. N. (1970). visual experience modifies distribution of horizontally and vertically oriented receptive fields in cats. *Science* 168, 869–871. doi: 10.1126/science.168.3933.869

Hou, C., Good, W. V., and Norcia, A. M. (2007). Validation study of VEP vernier acuity in normal-vision and amblyopic adults. *Invest. Opthalmol. Vis. Sci.* 48:4070. doi: 10.1167/iovs.06-1368

Hou, C., Good, W. V., and Norcia, A. M. (2018). Detection of amblyopia using sweep VEP vernier and grating acuity. *Invest. Ophthalmol. Vis. Sci.* 59, 1435–1442.

Hou, C., Norcia, A. M., Madan, A., Tith, S., Agarwal, R., and Good, W. V. (2011). Visual cortical function in very low birth weight infants without retinal or cerebral pathology. *Invest. Opthalmol. Vis. Sci.* 52:9091. doi: 10.1167/iovs.11-7458

Huang, C.-B., Zhou, Y., and Lu, Z.-L. (2008). Broad bandwidth of perceptual learning in the visual system of adults with anisometropic amblyopia. *Proc. Natl. Acad. Sci.* 105, 4068–4073.

Huang, J., Huang, J., Chen, Y., and Ying, G. (2018). Evaluation of approaches to analyzing continuous correlated eye data when sample size is small. *Ophthalmic Epidemiol.* 25, 45–54. doi: 10.1080/09286586.2017.1339809

Hubel, D. H., and Wiesel, T. N. (1962). Receptive fields, binocular interaction and functional architecture in the cat's visual cortex. *J. Physiol.* 160, 106–154.

Keech, R. V., and Kutschke, P. J. (1995). Upper age limit for the development of amblyopia. *J. Pediatr. Ophthalmol. Strabismus* 32, 89–93. doi: 10.3928/0191-3913-19950301-07

Kiorpes, L. (2006). Visual processing in amblyopia: animal studies. *Strabismus* 14, 3–10. doi: 10.1080/09273970500536193

Kiorpes, L. (2016). The puzzle of visual development: behavior and neural limits. *J. Neurosci.* 36, 11384–11393. doi: 10.1523/JNEUROSCI.2937-16.2016

Kiorpes, L., and McKee, S. P. (1999). Neural mechanisms underlying amblyopia. *Curr. Opin. Neurobiol.* 9, 480–486.

Knudsen, E. I. (2004). Sensitive periods in the development of the brain and behavior. *J. Cogn. Neurosci.* 16, 1412–1425. doi: 10.1162/0898929042304796

Lesmes, L. A., Lu, Z.-L., Baek, J., and Albright, T. D. (2010). Bayesian adaptive estimation of the contrast sensitivity function: the quick CSF method. *J. Vis.* 10, 1–21. doi: 10.1167/10.3.17

Li, X., and Lu, Z. L. (2012). Enabling high grayscale resolution displays and accurate response time measurements on conventional computers. *J. Vis. Exp.* 60:e3312.

Li, X., Lu, Z. L., Xu, P., Jin, J., and Zhou, Y. (2003). Generating high gray-level resolution monochrome displays with conventional computer graphics cards and color monitors. *J. Neurosci. Methods* 130, 9–18.

Lu, Z.-L., and Dosher, B. (2014). *Visual Psychophysics: From Laboratory to Theory.* Cambridge, MA: The MIT Press.

Mitchell, D. E., Freeman, R. D., Millodot, M., and Haegerstrom, G. (1973). Meridional amblyopia: evidence for modification of the human visual system by early visual experience. *Vis. Res.* 13, 535–558. doi: 10.1016/0042-6989(73)90023-0

Morishita, H., and Hensch, T. (2008). Critical period revisited: impact on vision. *Curr. Opin. Neurobiol.* 18, 101–107.

Nakamura, Y., Nakamura, Y., Higa, A., Sawaguchi, S., Tomidokoro, A., Iwase, A., et al. (2018). Refractive errors in an elderly rural Japanese population: the Kumejima study. *PLoS One* 13:e0207180. doi: 10.1371/journal.pone.0207180

Norcia, A. M., Appelbaum, L. G., Ales, J. M., Cottereau, B. R., and Rossion, B. (2015). The steady-state visual evoked potential in vision research: a review. *J. Vis.* 15:4.

Norcia, A. M., and Tyler, C. W. (1985). Spatial frequency sweep VEP: visual acuity during the first year of life. *Vis. Res.* 25, 1399–1408.

Oshika, T., Okamoto, C., Samejima, T., Tokunaga, T., and Miyata, K. (2006). Contrast sensitivity function and ocular higher-order wavefront aberrations in normal human eyes. *Ophthalmology* 113, 1807–1812. doi: 10.1016/j.ophtha.2006.03.061

Pelli, D. G. (1997). The VideoToolbox software for visual psychophysics: transforming numbers into movies. *Spat. Vis.* 10, 437–442.

Read, S. A., Vincent, S. J., and Collins, M. J. (2014). The visual and functional impacts of astigmatism and its clinical management. *Ophthalmic Physiol. Opt.* 34, 267–294. doi: 10.1111/opo.12128

Regan, D. (1977). Speedy assessment of visual acuity in amblyopia by the evoked potential method. *Ophthalmologica* 175, 159–164.

Rim, T. H., Kim, S.-H., Lim, K. H., Choi, M., Kim, H. Y., Baek, S.-H., et al. (2016). Refractive errors in koreans: the korea national health and nutrition examination survey 2008-2012. *Korean J. Ophthalmol.* 30:214. doi: 10.3341/kjo.2016.30.3.214

Shapley, R., Hawken, M., and Ringach, D. L. (2003). Dynamics of orientation selectivity in the primary visual cortex and the importance of cortical inhibition. *Neuron* 38, 689–699. doi: 10.1016/S0896-6273(03)00332-5

Tang, Y., and Norcia, A. M. (1995). An adaptive filter for steady-state evoked responses. *Electroencephalogr. Clin. Neurophysiol.* 96, 268–277. doi: 10.1016/0168-5597(94)00309-3

Tobimatsu, S., and Celesia, G. G. (2006). Studies of human visual pathophysiology with visual evoked potentials. *Clin. Neurophysiol.* 117, 1414–1433. doi: 10.1016/j.clinph.2006.01.004

Tobimatsu, S., Kurita-Tashima, S., Nakayama, M., and Kato, M. (1993). Effects of spatial frequency on transient and steady state VEPs: stimulation with checkerboard, square-wave grating and sinusoidal grating patterns. *J. Neurol. Sci.* 118, 17–24. doi: 10.1016/0022-510X(93)90239-U

Tyler, C. W. (1979). Rapid assessment of visual function: an electronic sweep technique for the pattern visual evoked potential. *Invest. Ophthalmol. Vis. Sci.* 18, 703–713.

Wang, M., Ma, J., Pan, L., Chen, T., Wang, H. L., Wang, Y. H., et al. (2019). Prevalence of and risk factors for refractive error: a cross-sectional study in Han and Mongolian adults aged 40–80 years in Inner Mongolia, China. *Eye* 33, 1722–1732. doi: 10.1038/s41433-019-0469-0

Wiesel, T. N. (1963). Single-cell responses in striate cortex of kittens deprived of vision in one eye. *J. Neurophysiol.* 26, 1002–1017.

Yap, T. P., and Boon, M. Y. (2020). Electrodiagnosis and treatment monitoring of children with refractive amblyopia. *Adv. Ophthalmol. Optom.* 5, 1–24. doi: 10.1016/j.yaoo.2020.04.001

Yap, T. P., Luu, C. D., Suttle, C., Chia, A., and Boon, M. Y. (2020a). Effect of stimulus orientation on visual function in children with refractive amblyopia. *Invest. Opthalmol. Vis. Sci.* 61:5. doi: 10.1167/iovs.61.5.5

Yap, T. P., Luu, C. D., Suttle, C. M., Chia, A., and Boon, M. Y. (2019). Electrophysiological and psychophysical studies of meridional anisotropies in children with and without astigmatism. *Invest. Opthalmol. Vis. Sci.* 60:1906. doi: 10.1167/iovs.18-25924

Yap, T. P., Luu, C. D., Suttle, C. M., Chia, A., and Boon, M. Y. (2020b). Characterising the orientation-specific pattern-onset visual evoked potentials in children with bilateral refractive amblyopia and non-amblyopic controls. *Doc. Ophthalmol.* 1–15. doi: 10.1007/s10633-020-09794-9

Yenice, O., Onal, S., Incili, B., Temel, A., Afsar, N., and Tanrida Gcaron, T. (2007). Assessment of spatial-contrast function and short-wavelength sensitivity deficits in patients with migraine. *Eye* 21, 218–223. doi: 10.1038/sj.eye.6702251

Zhang, P., Zhao, Y., Dosher, B. A., and Lu, Z.-L. (2019). Evaluating the performance of the staircase and quick change detection methods in measuring perceptual learning. *J. Vis.* 19:14. doi: 10.1167/19.7.14

Zhou, Y., Huang, C.-B., Xu, P., Tao, L., Qiu, Z., Li, X., et al. (2006). Perceptual learning improves contrast sensitivity and visual acuity in adults with anisometropic amblyopia. *Vis. Res.* 46, 739–750. doi: 10.1016/j.visres.2005.07.031

3

Altered Effective Connectivity of Children and Young Adults with Unilateral Amblyopia: A Resting-State Functional Magnetic Resonance Imaging Study

Peishan Dai[1,2], Xiaoyan Zhou[1,2], Yilin Ou[1,2], Tong Xiong[1,2], Jinlong Zhang[1,2], Zailiang Chen[1,2], Beiji Zou[1,2], Xin Wei[3,4], Ying Wu[3,4] and Manyi Xiao[3,4]**

[1] School of Computer Science and Engineering, Central South University, Changsha, China, [2] Hunan Engineering Research Center of Machine Vision and Intelligent Medicine, Central South University, Changsha, China, [3] Department of Ophthalmology, The Second Xiangya Hospital, Central South University, Changsha, China, [4] Hunan Clinical Research Center of Ophthalmic Disease, Changsha, China

***Correspondence:**
Ying Wu
wuying216@csu.edu.cn
Manyi Xiao
13973119862@163.com

The altered functional connectivity (FC) in amblyopia has been investigated by many studies, but the specific causality of brain connectivity needs to be explored further to understand the brain activity of amblyopia. We investigated whether the effective connectivity (EC) of children and young adults with amblyopia was altered. The subjects included 16 children and young adults with left eye amblyopia and 17 healthy controls (HCs). The abnormalities between the left/right primary visual cortex (PVC) and the other brain regions were investigated in a voxel-wise manner using the Granger causality analysis (GCA). According to the EC results in the HCs and the distribution of visual pathways, 12 regions of interest (ROIs) were selected to construct an EC network. The alteration of the EC network of the children and young adults with amblyopia was analyzed. In the voxel-wise manner analysis, amblyopia showed significantly decreased EC between the left/right of the PVC and the left middle frontal gyrus/left inferior frontal gyrus compared with the HCs. In the EC network analysis, compared with the HCs, amblyopia showed significantly decreased EC from the left calcarine fissure, posterior cingulate gyrus, left lingual gyrus, right lingual gyrus, and right fusiform gyrus to the right calcarine fissure. Amblyopia also showed significantly decreased EC from the right inferior frontal gyrus and right lingual gyrus to the left superior temporal gyrus compared with the HCs in the EC network analysis. The results may indicate that amblyopia altered the visual feedforward and feedback pathway, and amblyopia may have a greater relevance with the feedback pathway than the feedforward pathway. Amblyopia may also correlate with the feedforward of the third visual pathway.

Keywords: resting-state, fMRI, unilateral amblyopia, effective connectivity, granger causality analysis

INTRODUCTION

Amblyopia (also called lazy eye) can be defined as a disorder that is associated with dysfunction of the processing of visual information, and the dysfunction can be detected and evident as reduced recognition visual acuity (Holmes and Clarke, 2006). It usually occurs in just one eye, when there is a breakdown in the working mode of the brain and eyes, and the brain cannot recognize the sight of the lazy eye, resulting in the brain relying more on the other eye[1]. Amblyopia is associated with abnormal visual function in the brain, especially the function of the visual cortex (Huang et al., 2017). It is a developmental visual disease whose visual defects cannot be improved by refractive correction, and the structural abnormalities accompanied by visual impairment are insignificant (Roper-Hall, 2007). It starts in early childhood, which is the critical period of treatment (Tailor et al., 2016), and affects approximately 2%–5% of the general population (Guo et al., 2016).

In general, amblyopia is a neurodevelopmental problem, not an eye organic problem (Li et al., 2012). As functional magnetic resonance imaging (fMRI) can be used to investigate brain activity non-invasively, it has been extensively used to assess visual deficits including amblyopia (Brown et al., 2016). There are two main ways to analyze the brain activity of amblyopia using fMRI data: the regional brain activity analysis [including the amplitude of low-frequency fluctuation (ALFF) (Liang et al., 2016; Min et al., 2018) and the regional homogeneity (ReHo) (Lin et al., 2012; Yang et al., 2019)] and interregional connectivity analysis [including functional connectivity (FC) and effective connectivity (EC)].

Functional connectivity describes the statistical dependence of spatially isolated neuronal events, thereby reflecting the altered interactions among the brain regions in amblyopia. Ding et al. (2013) used resting-state fMRI to study the FC differences between patients with amblyopia and normal controls and found that the cerebellum and the inferior parietal lobule showed altered FC with the primary visual area in individuals with amblyopia. Wang et al. (2014) analyzed the abnormalities of amblyopia patients by both the seed-based FC with the left/right primary visual cortex (PVC) and the network constructed throughout the whole brain and found decreased FC to superior occipital gyrus, lingual gyrus, and several areas in the temporal cortex. Zhou et al. (2015) analyzed the resting-state fMRI of children with strabismus amblyopia and found that the brain FC of patients is lower than the healthy controls (HCs) in the occipital lobe, temporal lobe, posterior cerebellar lobe, parietal lobe, frontal lobe, and cingulate gyrus. Mendola et al. (2018) used resting-state fMRI to study the FC of adult amblyopia in V1, V2, and V3 in a subcortical area manner and found decreased FC within V1, V2, and V3. Lu et al. (2019) used resting-state fMRI to study the FC networks between patients with amblyopia and normal controls and found a decrease of both network functional correlations and local efficiencies in the extra-striate visual networks. Dai et al. (2019) used resting-state fMRI to study the FC networks between patients with amblyopia and normal controls. They found reduced FC in the dorsal and ventral visual pathways. These studies found many altered FCs in or out of the visual pathway, but as different data sets and different data analysis strategies were used, these results are with no high comparability.

Functional connectivity does not reflect the specific causality of brain regions, whereas EC makes up this deficiency. EC depends on the mechanism of the causal effects that generated from the data, which can reflect the specific strength and direction of interaction information in the brain region (Stephan and Friston, 2010). Some researchers began to apply EC to fMRI analysis (Sharaev et al., 2016; Wang et al., 2016; Park et al., 2017; Chen et al., 2018; Ma et al., 2018). EC can be analyzed by various methods. Ohta et al. (2018) explored the causal relationship between the psychosocial aspects of subjective quality of life, symptoms, cognitive functions, and salience network dysfunction in schizophrenia by establishing a structural equation model. Hofmann and Straube (2019) used a dynamic causal model to estimate the EC between BNST and amygdala nuclei and found that there were positive EC between all amygdala nuclei. These studies are model-driven methods that require considerable prior knowledge. In this study, we used Granger causality analysis (GCA), which is a data-driven EC calculation method and can be directly applied to the resting-state data (Liu et al., 2018; Ning et al., 2018; Shi et al., 2019). It has been widely used for time-directed prediction between BOLD fMRI time series to measure the causal effects among brain regions (Jiao et al., 2011).

Few researchers have analyzed altered EC in amblyopia. To the best of our knowledge, only Li et al. (2011) investigated the altered EC of task fMRI of amblyopia and found reduced EC in both feedforward and feedback pathway in the lateral geniculate nucleus and visual cortex when driven by the amblyopic eye. However, this research studied the EC within the lateral geniculate nucleus and visual cortex, which are just part of the visual pathway, with only six amblyopia and there were no HCs. The subjects were a mixture of three types of amblyopia, and they have been receiving different treatments. The cortical impairment in amblyopia is not only limited to the visual cortex but also related to the visual pathway and other complex networks (Wu and Liu, 2017).

In this study, we investigated the altered EC of children and young adults with unilateral amblyopia compared to the HCs using resting-state fMRI. In current researches in amblyopia, the amblyopia group (AMs) usually includes left eye, right eye, and bilateral amblyopia. To reduce the sample interference by the mixture of the left, right, and bilateral eye amblyopia, we chose children and young adults with unilateral amblyopia as the research object. We hypothesized that unilateral amblyopia may affect causal connectivity, which can be measured by the alteration of brain EC, and the brain regions with altered EC may not just be limited to the dorsal and ventral pathways, as there may exist a third visual pathway on the lateral brain surface that is anatomically segregated from the two pathways (Pitcher and Ungerleider, 2020). Our study may reveal some alterations of visual feedforward and feedback pathway of amblyopia.

[1] https://www.nei.nih.gov/learn-about-eye-health/eye-conditions-and-diseases/amblyopia-lazy-eye

MATERIALS AND METHODS

Participants

The experiment in this paper was approved by the ethics committee of the Second Xiangya Hospital, Central South University. The HCs had no amblyopia-related diseases, with a corrected visual acuity of $\leq$0.1 logMAR. All the subjects understood the purpose of this study and signed the written informed consent, and all participants received the same detailed eye examinations. A total of 16 children and young adults with amblyopia and 17 HCs were recruited. We used the thresholds 2 mm translation/2 deg rotation to exclude the subjects with big head movements. As a result, 13 individuals were retained in the amblyopia group (AMs), and 13 individuals were retained in the HCs. All of the subjects had no history of other ocular diseases, surgery, or other treatments. The demographic information of the participants is summarized in **Table 1**.

Data Acquisition

The data acquisition was performed with a Philips 3.0-T nuclear magnetic resonance scanner. The subjects were scanned by the MRI scanner in the resting state. All participants were asked to close their eyes, relax their bodies, and have no thinking tasks or external stimuli during the whole scanning process. The lights were dimmed and the participants were asked to wear earmuffs to reduce noise during scanning. The participants' heads were fixed with foam blocks to reduce head movements during testing. The T1-weighted anatomical data were obtained with the parameters as follows: TE = 2.7 ms, TR = 5.8 ms, FA = 8°, voxel size = 1 mm^3. The fMRI data were obtained by echo-planar imaging, and the parameters are as follows: TR = 2,000 ms, TE = 30 ms, FA = 90°, number of slices = 36, slice thickness = 4 mm, FOV = 240 mm × 240 mm × 144 mm, and time points = 189, acquisition time = 6 min 18 s.

Data Processing

The data in this paper were preprocessed based on the DPARSF tool in the SPM8 toolkit[2] (Yan et al., 2016). The specific preprocessing steps included data format conversion, removal of the first 10 time points, slice timing, head motion correction (Friston 24-parameter model), and spatial normalization to the Montreal Neurological Institute (MNI) Template. The structural

[2]http://rfmri.org/DPARSF

TABLE 1 | Demographic information of subjects.

Subject	Gender	Age	Amblyopic type	Amblyopic eye	CVA (LogMAR)		History of treatment
					OD	OS	
Amb 01	F	12	ANA	OS	−0.1	0.7	None
Amb 02	M	5	ANA	OS	0.1	0.4	None
Amb 03	F	14	ANA	OS	0.0	1.0	None
Amb 04	M	8	AMA	OS	−0.1	0.5	None
Amb 05	M	6	ANA; AMA	OS	0.0	1.0	None
Amb 06	M	13	ANA	OS	0.0	0.4	None
Amb 07	M	8	ANA; AMA	OS	0.1	0.7	None
Amb 08	M	10	ANA; AMA	OS	0.0	0.7	None
Amb 09	F	14	ANA; AMA	OS	0.0	0.5	None
Amb 10	M	12	ANA	OS	0.0	1.2	None
Amb 11	F	8	ANA	OS	0.0	0.7	None
Amb 12	M	24	AMA	OS	0.0	0.2	None
Amb 13	M	15	AMA	OS	0.0	0.5	None
Control 01	F	6	None	None	0.2	0.1	None
Control 02	F	14	None	None	0.0	0.0	None
Control 03	F	12	None	None	0.0	0.0	None
Control 04	F	12	None	None	0.0	0.0	None
Control 05	M	9	None	None	0.0	0.0	None
Control 06	F	8	None	None	0.0	0.0	None
Control 07	M	13	None	None	0.0	0.0	None
Control 08	M	14	None	None	0.0	0.0	None
Control 09	F	14	None	None	−0.2	−0.1	None
Control 10	F	11	None	None	0.0	0.0	None
Control 11	M	10	None	None	−0.1	−0.2	None
Control 12	M	7	None	None	0.0	−0.1	None
Control 13	M	10	None	None	−0.2	−0.1	None

Amb, amblyopia group; F, female; M, male; CVA, corrected visual acuity; OD, oculus dexter; OS, oculus sinister; ANA, anisometropic amblyopia; AMA, ametropic amblyopia.

image was coregistered to the mean functional image and then the structural image was segmented into gray matter, white matter, and cerebrospinal fluid by using a unified segmentation algorithm (New segment). The EPI images were spatially normalized to the MNI space using the normalization parameters estimated in DARTEL. Nuisance covariates (head motion, white matter signal, and cerebrospinal fluid signal) were regressed out, and then we performed smoothing (4 mm full width at half maximum of Gaussian kernel to decrease the spatial noise), linear trends, and band-pass filtering (0.01 Hz $< f <$ 0.08 Hz).

EC Calculation Using Granger Causality Model

We used REST-GCA version 1.8 (a MatLab toolkit for GCA) (Song et al., 2011; Zang et al., 2012) for EC analysis, using a signed-path coefficient algorithm. REST-GCA using the Granger causality model was used to calculate EC. Granger causality model (Granger, 1969, 2001) can be used to analyze the causality among multiple time series. If we define two time series $X(t)$ and $Y(t)$ their autoregressive models are as follows:

$$X(t) = \alpha_{11}X(t-1) + \alpha_{12}X(t-2) + \cdots + \alpha_{1p}X(t-p) + \varepsilon_1(t). \tag{1}$$

$$Y(t) = \beta_{11}Y(t-1) + \beta_{12}Y(t-2) + \cdots + \beta_{1p}Y(t-p) + \varepsilon_2(t). \tag{2}$$

The regression models introducing each other are as follows:

$$X(t) = [\alpha_1 X(t-1) + \cdots + \alpha_p X(t-p)] + [\delta_1 Y(t-1) + \cdots + \delta_p Y(t-p)] + \varepsilon_3(t) \tag{3}$$

$$Y(t) = [\beta_1 Y(t-1) + \cdots + \beta_p Y(t-p)] + [\gamma_1 X(t-1) + \cdots + \gamma_p X(t-p)] + \varepsilon_4(t). \tag{4}$$

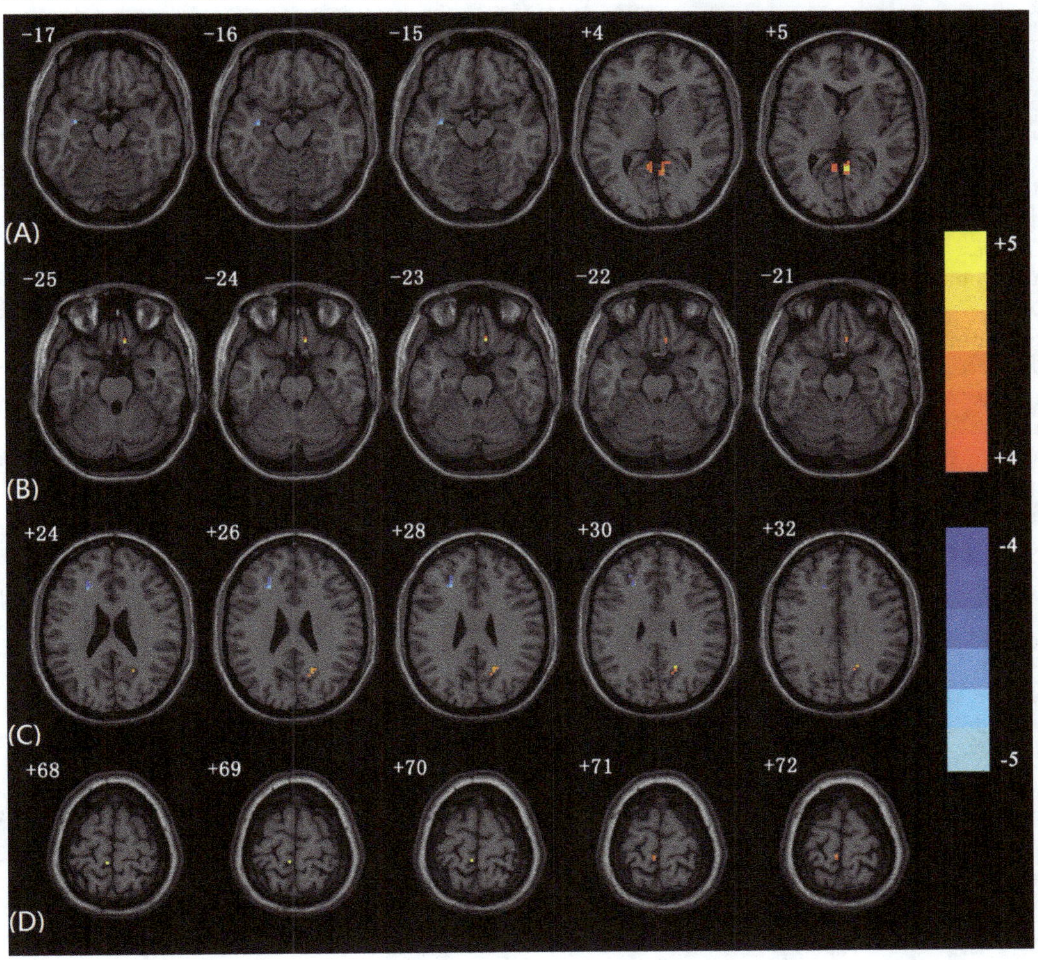

FIGURE 1 | Significantly altered EC in AMs compared to HCs using voxel-wise EC analysis. The color scale represents T-values. **(A)** Altered EC from PVC.L to other brain regions in AMs compared to HCs. **(B)** Altered EC from other brain regions to PVC.L in AMs compared to HCs. **(C)** Altered EC from PVC.R to other brain regions in AMs compared to HCs. **(D)** Altered EC from other brain regions to PVC.R in AMs compared to HCs (In each subgraph, only the slices with obvious differences are presented; the subgraphs including slices without significant differences EC are provided in **Supplementary Figure 1**).

where $\varepsilon_i(t) i = 1, 2, 3, 4$ represent prediction residual; α_{1p}, β_{1p}, α_p, β_p, δ_p, and γ_p represent the regression coefficients of the models; and p is the order of the model.

If the signed-path coefficient $\delta_1, \delta_2, \cdots \delta_p$ is significantly larger or smaller than zero, then $Y(t)$ significantly Granger cause $X(t)$ and vice versa, if the signed-path coefficient $\gamma_1, \gamma_2, \cdots \gamma_p$ is significantly larger or smaller than zero, then $X(t)$ significantly Granger causes $Y(t)$. The positive/negative signed-path coefficients indicate that the activity in one brain region could, respectively, predict the increased/decreased brain activity in another brain region, which may mean excitation/inhibition effects (Zang et al., 2012). The signed-path coefficient value is the value of EC, and the absolute value of EC is expressed by k in this study.

Statistical Analysis of EC

Considering the fact that completely using the data-driven method to calculate EC in a voxel-wise manner will greatly increase the amount of calculation and the difficulty of analysis (for a subject, the EC value should be calculated within more than 100,000 voxels), we use a combination of prior knowledge and data-driven method to calculate EC value. (1) As the PVC is an important brain region for visual information transmission, we selected bilateral PVC as two seed regions to analyze their EC with other brain regions, and compared EC changes between the AMS and the HCs at the group level. (2) Combining the significantly non-zero EC in the HCs (if the HCs is assumed as baseline) and the distribution of visual pathways, we selected 12 regions of interest (ROIs) to analyze the altered EC of these ROIs in amblyopia compared with the HCs. The analysis steps are as follows.

(1) We selected the bilateral PVC as two seed regions each with a radius of 8 mm representing left PVC (PVC.L) and right PVC (PVC.R), respectively. (2) For each subject, the average time series of fMRI data in the seed region of the PVC.L was extracted and calculated its EC with the time series of other brain regions in a voxel-wise manner, which is abbreviated as PVC.L voxel-wise EC. In the same way, we obtained EC between PVC.R and other brain regions, which is abbreviated as PVC.R voxel-wise EC. We called this step voxel-wise EC. (3) We performed a two-sample t-test ($P < 0.001$, AlphaSim correction) on the results of voxel-wise EC to analyze the differences in EC between AMs and HCs (the results are shown in section "Results of Significantly Altered EC Between the Two Groups Using Voxel-Wise EC"). (4) We performed a one-sample t-test ($P < 0.05$, AlphaSim correction) on the results of voxel-wise EC in the HCs. Combining the results and the distribution of visual pathways, we selected 12 brain regions (MNI coordinates: brain region peak, radius: 8 mm) with significantly altered voxel-wise EC as ROIs. (5) For each subject, the average time series of fMRI data in each ROI was extracted and its EC was calculated with the average time series of the other ROIs in an ROI-wise manner. We called this step ROI-wise EC. (6) Then, we performed a one-sample t-test ($P < 0.05$) on the results of ROI-wise EC in the AMs and HCs, respectively (the results are shown in section "EC Network Within the Groups Using ROI-Wise EC") (7). Last, we performed a two-sample t-test ($P < 0.05$) on the results of ROI-wise EC to analyze the altered EC network between the AMs and HCs (the results are shown in section "Comparisons of EC Networks Between the Two Groups Using ROI-Wise EC").

TABLE 2 | Voxel coordinates with the significant EC value between the two groups using voxel-wise EC.

Direction of EC	Brain area	BA	Peak strength	MNI coordinates		
				x	*y*	*z*
From the PVC.L	HIP.L	20	−4.442	−33	−6	−18
	LING.L	18	4.7339	−9	−51	3
	LING.R	30	6.0667	6	−54	6
	PCUN.R	23	4.3513	18	−57	27
To the PVC.L	REC.R	11	5.4256	9	27	−24
From the PVC.R	MFG.L	10	−4.4512	−30	60	15
	IFG.L	45	−4.5183	−33	42	12
	PUCN.R	23	4.7004	18	−57	30
	MFG.L	48	−4.9637	−24	27	27
	MFG.L	32	−5.3912	−15	24	36
To the PVC.R	PCL.L	4	4.7662	−6	−36	69

BA, Brodmann's area; MNI, Montreal Neurological Institute; PVC.L, left primary visual cortex; PVC.R, right primary visual cortex; HIP.L, left hippocampus; LING.L, left lingual gyrus; LING.R, right lingual gyrus; PCUN.R, right precuneus; MFG.L, left middle frontal gyrus; MFG.R, right middle frontal gyrus; REC.R, right gyrus rectus; IFG.L, left inferior frontal gyrus; PCL.L, left paracentral lobule.

TABLE 3 | Information on the ROIs.

ROI	MNI coordinates			ROI	MNI coordinates		
	x	*y*	*z*		*x*	*y*	*z*
CAL.L	−12	−72	9	CAL.R	15	−103	3
ACG	6	36	15	PCG	3	−57	9
IFG.L	−36	33	−3	IFG.R	36	33	−3
STG.L	−57	−30	21	STG.R	57	−30	21
FFG.L	−21	−93	−21	FFG.R	21	−93	−21
LING.L	−18	−57	0	LING.R	18	−57	0

ROI, region of interest; MNI, Montreal Neurological Institute; CAL.L, left calcarine fissure; CAL.R, right calcarine fissure; ACG, anterior cingulate gyrus; PCG, posterior cingulate gyrus; IFG.L, left inferior frontal gyrus; IFG.R, right inferior frontal gyrus; STG.L, left superior temporal gyrus; STG.R, right superior temporal gyrus; FFG.L, left fusiform gyrus; FFG.R, right fusiform gyrus; LING.L, left lingual gyrus; LING.R, right lingual gyrus.

RESULTS

Results of Significantly Altered EC Between the Two Groups Using Voxel-Wise EC

Compared with the HCs, the AMs showed significantly decreased EC from the left PVC to the left hippocampus. Increased EC was found from the left PVC to the left lingual, right lingual, and right precuneus. Amblyopia showed increased EC from the right gyrus rectus to the left PVC (**Figure 1** and **Table 2**). Some individual results of voxel-wise EC are provided in **Supplementary Figures 2–5**.

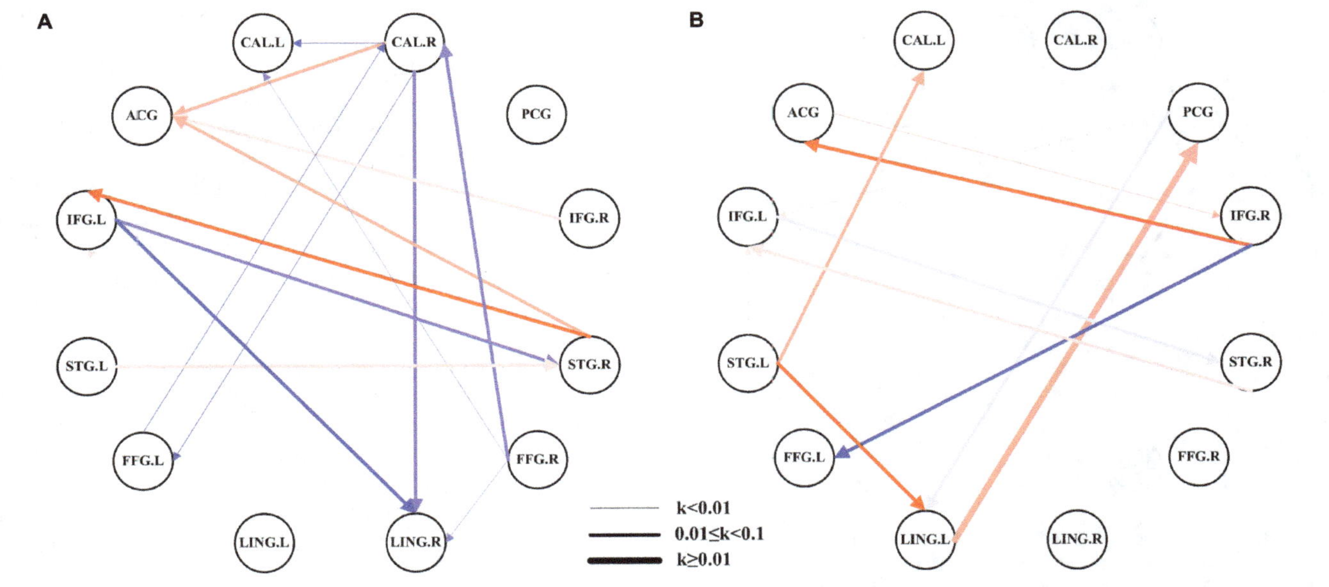

FIGURE 2 | EC network within the groups using ROI-wise EC. **(A)** EC network of ROIs in patients with amblyopia. **(B)** EC network of ROIs in the HCs. The color shades represent significance of EC ($0 < P < 0.015$, $0.015 \leq P \leq 0.03$, and $0.03 < P \leq 0.05$); red represents excitation, blue represents inhibition, and the arrow indicates the direction of connection. The thickness of the line represents the connection strength (weak: $k < 0.01$, medium: $0.01 \leq k < 0.1$, strong: $k \geq 0.1$). CAL.L, left calcarine fissure; CAL.R, right calcarine fissure; ACG, anterior cingulate gyrus; PCG, posterior cingulate gyrus; IFG.L, left inferior frontal gyrus; IFG.R, right inferior frontal gyrus; STG.L, left superior temporal gyrus; STG.R, right superior temporal gyrus; FFG.L, left fusiform gyrus; FFG.R, right fusiform gyrus; LING.L, left lingual gyrus; LING.R, right lingual gyrus.

The AMs showed significantly decreased EC from the right PVC to several brain regions, including the left middle frontal gyrus and left inferior frontal gyrus. Increased EC was found from the right PVC to the right precuneus. The AMs showed increased EC from the left paracentral lobule to the right PVC.

EC in ROIs

According to the EC results in the HCs and the distribution of visual pathways, 12 ROIs (**Table 3**) were selected to construct the EC network.

EC Network Within the Groups Using ROI-Wise EC

The network of the AMs had 15 pairs of substantial EC (**Figure 2A**), while the HCs had 11 pairs (**Figure 2B**). This figure showed considerable differences in the networks between patients with amblyopia and HCs. Most of the EC between ROIs in HCs were excitation, while the patients with amblyopia showed more inhibition. The connectivity of most brain regions was significantly weakened, and some brain effects were lost in patients with amblyopia, such as the EC between the left lingual gyrus and the posterior cingulate gyrus and between the right inferior frontal gyrus and left fusiform gyrus were lost. Besides, the patients with amblyopia also showed significantly altered EC between some brain regions, especially the EC between the right calcarine fissure and some brain regions, which both were inhibited. Some individual results of ROI-wise EC are provided in **Supplementary Tables 1–4**.

Comparisons of EC Networks Between the Two Groups Using ROI-Wise EC

Compared with the HCs, we found significantly altered EC between the two networks in the AMs (**Figure 3**). The AMs showed reduced EC from the left calcarine fissure, posterior cingulate gyrus, left lingual gyrus, right lingual gyrus, and right fusiform gyrus to the right calcarine fissure, and from the right inferior frontal gyrus and right lingual gyrus to the left superior temporal gyrus. The AMs also showed significantly increased EC from the right lingual gyrus to the anterior cingulate gyrus and from the right calcarine fissure to the posterior cingulate gyrus.

DISCUSSION

To our knowledge, this work is the first to examine the altered EC of children and young adults with unilateral amblyopia under resting conditions. We found decreased EC in patients with amblyopia by using GCA.

The Altered EC of Voxel-Wise EC Analysis

We found significantly decreased EC between the left/right of PVC and the left middle frontal gyrus/left inferior frontal gyrus in amblyopia. Both the middle frontal gyrus and inferior frontal gyrus belong to the prefrontal cortex, which plays a significant role in the perception, memory, and regulation of visual information (Majaj et al., 2007). The primate visual

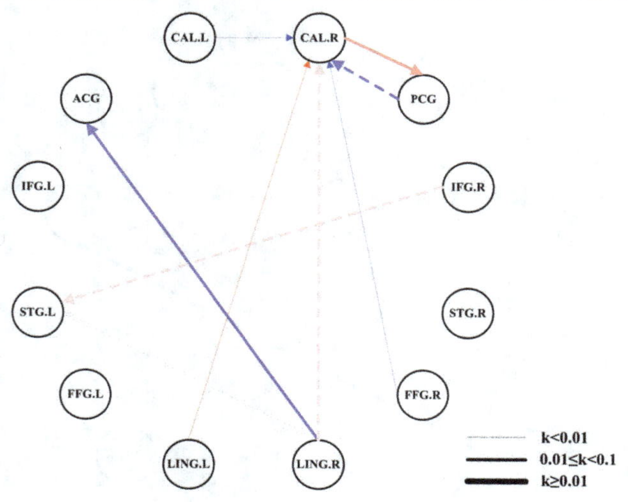

FIGURE 3 | Comparisons of EC networks between the two groups using ROI-wise EC. The color shades represent significance of EC ($0 < P < 0.015$, $0.015 \leq P \leq 0.03$, and $0.03 < P \leq 0.05$); red represents excitation, blue represents inhibition, and the arrow indicates the direction of connection. The dotted line indicated a significantly reduced EC in patients with amblyopia. The solid line indicated a significantly increased EC in patients with amblyopia. The thickness of the line represents the connection strength (weak: $k < 0.01$, medium: $0.01 \leq k < 0.1$, strong: $k \geq 0.1$). CAL.L, left calcarine fissure; CAL.R, right calcarine fissure; ACG, anterior cingulate gyrus; PCG, posterior cingulate gyrus; IFG.L, left inferior frontal gyrus; IFG.R, right inferior frontal gyrus; STG.L, left superior temporal gyrus; STG.R, right superior temporal gyrus; FFG.L, left fusiform gyrus; FFG.R, right fusiform gyrus; LING.L, left lingual gyrus; LING.R, right lingual gyrus.

system mainly includes the dorsal and ventral pathways. The ventral pathway deals with conscious perception, and the dorsal pathway processes visual information and guides action without accompanying conscious knowledge (Fang and He, 2005). The PVC and prefrontal cortex could be considered as the two ends of the bidirectional (feedforward and feedback pathway) visual pathway. The bidirectional decreased EC between the PVC and prefrontal cortex may indicate that amblyopia altered the visual feedforward and feedback pathway. Ding et al. (2013) also found an FC alteration between the frontal lobe and the PVC in anisometropic amblyopia. Their results conformed to the studies of our EC. Besides, the causal relationship between the PVC and the frontal lobe might contribute to the further study of the neurological mechanism.

We also found decreased EC from the PVC.L to the left hippocampus in patients with amblyopia. The hippocampus is located in the inner region of the temporal lobe and forms part of the limbic system. It plays a significant role in the central nervous system, situational memory, regulation, and learning (Ranganath et al., 2004). Decreased EC may indicate the decreased information transfer to the left hippocampus, but to our knowledge, we found no report about the correlation between hippocampus and amblyopia.

For the feedforward direction from the PVC, we found significantly increased EC from the PVC.L to the left lingual gyrus, right lingual gyrus, and right precuneus, and from PVC.R to the right precuneus in amblyopia. The increased EC may reflect that for the left eye amblyopia, the brain function associated with the left eye may be suppressed, while the brain function associated with the right healthy eye may be increased to form a near-normal visual perception, which may increase the EC associated with the right healthy eye, showing the compensatory plasticity (Lazzouni and Lepore, 2014). Huang and Zhou (2017) found that the ReHo in the lingual gyrus of amblyopia increased. Liang et al. (2016) found that children with amblyopia mainly exhibit increased ALFF in the right precuneus. The EC analysis is consistent with the findings of these studies.

For the feedback direction to PVC, we found significantly increased EC from the right gyrus rectus to the PVC.L and from the left paracentral lobule to the PVC.R. The right gyrus rectus is located at the medial most margin of the inferior surface of the frontal lobe, and it plays an important role in the optic chiasm (Smith et al., 2017). The left paracentral lobule is on the medial surface of the hemisphere and is the continuation of the precentral and postcentral gyrus. The postcentral gyrus is an important brain area of somatosensory function (Ebeling and Steinmetz, 1995). Lin et al. (2012) found increased ReHo in the left paracentral lobule in patients with anisometropic amblyopia. The EC analysis is consistent with the finding of this study. The increased EC from the left paracentral lobule to PVC.R may indicate compensatory plasticity in amblyopia.

The Altered EC of ROI-Wise EC Analysis

Comparing EC network differences between the two groups, we found significantly reduced EC from the left calcarine fissure, posterior cingulate gyrus, left lingual gyrus, right lingual gyrus, and right fusiform gyrus to the right calcarine fissure in amblyopia. The calcarine sulcus is where the PVC (V1) is concentrated, and the PVC receives the nerve impulses from the optic nerves and then transmits information to two primary pathways, called the ventral stream and the dorsal stream (Bitar et al., 2016). The significantly reduced EC to the right calcarine fissure may indicate that amblyopia may correlate to the reduced feedback of visual information transmission. These results are consistent with the findings of the following researches. Ding et al. (2013) found significantly decreased FC of the PVC and lingual gyrus, the conjunction area of the posterior cingulate cortex, and the precuneus in mixed (anisometropic and strabismic) amblyopia. Huang et al. (2016) using ReHo examined subjects with strabismic amblyopia and found increased ReHo values in the fusiform gyrus, right lingual gyrus, and bilateral cingulate gyrus.

We also found reduced EC from the right inferior frontal gyrus and right lingual gyrus to the left superior temporal gyrus. In a recent study, David Pitcher (Pitcher and Ungerleider, 2020) found evidence for a third visual pathway specialized for social perception, which begins in the PVC (V1) and projects into the posterior banks of the superior temporal sulcus, so the reduced EC to the left superior temporal gyrus indicates that amblyopia may correlate with the feedforward of the third visual pathway. The results are consistent with the findings of the alteration of ReHo (Lin et al., 2012) and the ALFF (Tang et al., 2017) in the left superior temporal gyrus.

Amblyopia had significantly increased EC from the right lingual gyrus/right calcarine fissure to the anterior cingulate gyrus/posterior cingulate gyrus, which belongs to the cingulate gyrus, and this may be due to the visual compensatory mechanism of children and young adults with monocular amblyopia.

The present study has several limitations. (1) The main limitation of our study was the sample size. Given the difficulty of recruitment and the poor controllability of the test data of children's test subjects, the actual number of subjects studied in the experiment was small, which may reduce the reliability of the statistical results. The patients also all possessed left eye amblyopia. If another group of subjects with right eye amblyopia is added, then the comparative analysis will be comprehensive. In a further study, a stringent threshold for exploratory analysis can be used. (2) In the ROI-wise EC analysis, we selected ROIs based on the analysis of control data and the distribution of visual pathways, which may lead to a bias toward finding between-group differences, and we will conduct a comprehensive analysis by including the AMs in a future study.

CONCLUSION

We investigated the brain function causality of children and young adults with unilateral amblyopia through a comparative analysis of rs-fMRI data. The bidirectional decreased EC between the PVC and prefrontal cortex may indicate that amblyopia altered the visual feedforward and feedback pathway. The decreased effective connectivities in ROIs network are most feedback from other visual-related regions to the right calcarine fissure. It may indicate that amblyopia has an imbalanced relationship with the feedforward and the feedback visual pathway, and it may have a greater relevance with the feedback pathway. The significantly decreased EC to the left superior temporal gyrus in the regions of interest network indicates that amblyopia may correlate with the feedforward of the third visual pathway.

AUTHOR CONTRIBUTIONS

PD: methodology, conceptualization, formal analysis, funding acquisition, investigation, project administration, supervision, validation, writing—original draft, and writing—review and editing. XZ: methodology, software, conceptualization, data curation, formal analysis, visualization, investigation, writing—original draft, and writing—review and editing. YO, TX, ZC, YW, and JZ: formal analysis and investigation. BZ: investigation and project administration. XW: data curation, funding acquisition, investigation, resources, and validation. MX: data curation, funding acquisition, resources, supervision, and writing—review and editing. All authors contributed to the article and approved the submitted version.

ACKNOWLEDGMENTS

We would like to thank all subjects who participated in this study.

REFERENCES

Bitar, A. W., Mansour, M. M., and Chehab, A. (2016). "Algorithmic Optimizations in the HMAX Model Targeted for Efficient Object Recognition," in *Computer Vision, Imaging and Computer Graphics Theory and Applications*. VISIGRAPP 2015. *Communications in Computer and Information Science*, Vol. 598, ed. J. Braz (Cham: Springer), doi: 10.1007/978-3-319-29971-6_20

Brown, H. D., Woodall, R. L., Kitching, R. E., Baseler, H. A., and Morland, A. B. (2016). Using magnetic resonance imaging to assess visual deficits: a review. *Ophthal. Physiol. Optics* 36, 240–265. doi: 10.1111/opo.12293

Chen, P., Xie, Q., Wu, X., Huang, H., Lv, W., Chen, L., et al. (2018). Abnormal effective connectivity of the anterior forebrain regions in disorders of consciousness. *Neurosci. Bull.* 34, 647–658. doi: 10.1007/s12264-018-0250-6

Dai, P., Zhang, J., Wu, J., Chen, Z., Zou, B., Wu, Y., et al. (2019). Altered spontaneous brain activity of children with unilateral amblyopia: a resting state fMRI study. *Neural. Plast.* 2019:3681430. doi: 10.1155/2019/3681430

Ding, K., Liu, Y., Yan, X., Lin, X., and Jiang, T. (2013). Altered functional connectivity of the primary visual cortex in subjects with amblyopia. *Neural. Plast.* 2013:612086. doi: 10.1155/2013/612086

Ebeling, U., and Steinmetz, H. (1995). Anatomy of the parietal lobe: mapping the individual pattern. *Acta Neurochirurg.* 136, 8–11. doi: 10.1007/BF01411428

Fang, F., and He, S. (2005). Cortical responses to invisible objects in the human dorsal and ventral pathways. *Nat. Neurosci.* 8, 1380–1385. doi: 10.1038/nn1537

Granger, C. W. (1969). Investigating causal relations by econometric models and cross-spectral methods. *Economet. J. Econom. Soc.* 1969, 424–438. doi: 10.2307/1912791

Granger, C. W. (2001). *Essays in econometrics: collected papers of Clive WJ Granger*, Vol. 32. Cambridge, MA: Cambridge University Press.

Guo, L., Tao, J., Xia, F., Yang, Z., Ma, X., and Hua, R. (2016). In vivo optical imaging of amblyopia: Digital subtraction autofluorescence and split-spectrum amplitude-decorrelation angiography. *Lasers Surg. Med.* 48, 660–667. doi: 10.1002/lsm.22520

Hofmann, D., and Straube, T. (2019). Resting-state fMRI effective connectivity between the bed nucleus of the stria terminalis and amygdala nuclei. *Hum. Brain Map.* 40, 2723–2735. doi: 10.1002/hbm.24555

Holmes, J. M., and Clarke, M. P. (2006). Amblyopia. *Lancet* 367, 1343–1351. doi: 10.1016/S0140-6736(06)68581-4

Huang, X., Li, S. H., Zhou, F. Q., Zhang, Y., Zhong, Y. L., Cai, F. Q., et al. (2016). Altered intrinsic regional brain spontaneous activity in patients with comitant strabismus: a resting-state functional MRI study. *Neuropsychiatr. Dis. Treat.* 12:1303. doi: 10.2147/NDT.S105478

Huang, Y., Feng, L., and Zhou, Y. (2017). Reduced response cluster size in early visual areas explains the acuity deficit in amblyopia. *Neuroreport* 28, 397–403. doi: 10.1097/WNR.0000000000000767

Huang, Y., and Zhou, Y. (2017). Research on spontaneous activity in adult anisometropic amblyopia with regional homogeneity. *Material. Sci. Eng.* 207:012008. doi: 10.1088/1757-899X/207/1/012008

Jiao, Q., Lu, G., Zhang, Z., Zhong, Y., Wang, Z., Guo, Y., et al. (2011). Granger causal influence predicts BOLD activity levels in the default mode network. *Hum. Brain Map.* 32, 154–161. doi: 10.1002/hbm.21065

Lazzouni, L., and Lepore, F. (2014). Compensatory plasticity: time matters. *Front. Hum. Neurosci.* 8:340. doi: 10.3389/fnhum.2014.00340

Li, C., Cheng, L., Yu, Q., Xie, B., and Wang, J. (2012). Relationship of visual cortex function and visual acuity in anisometropic amblyopic children. *Internat. J. Med. Sci.* 9:115. doi: 10.7150/ijms.9.115

Li, X., Li, X., Mullen, K. T., Thompson, B., and Hess, R. F. (2011). Effective connectivity anomalies in human amblyopia. *Neuroimage* 54, 505–516. doi: 10.1016/j.neuroimage.2010.07.053

Liang, M., Xie, B., Yang, H., Yu, L., Yin, X., Wei, L., et al. (2016). Distinct patterns of spontaneous brain activity between children and adults with anisometropic amblyopia: a resting-state fMRI study. *Graefe's Archiv. Clin. Exp. Ophthalmol.* 254, 569–576. doi: 10.1007/s00417-015-3117-9

Lin, X., Ding, K., Liu, Y., Yan, X., Song, S., and Jiang, T. (2012). Altered spontaneous activity in anisometropic amblyopia subjects: revealed by resting-state FMRI. *PLoS One* 7:e43373. doi: 10.1371/journal.pone.0043373

Liu, D., Duan, S., Zhou, C., Wei, P., Chen, L., Yin, X., et al. (2018). Altered brain functional hubs and connectivity in type 2 diabetes mellitus patients: a resting-state fMRI study. *Front. Aging Neurosci.* 10:55. doi: 10.3389/fnagi.2018.00055

Lu, Z., Huang, Y., Lu, Q., Feng, L., Nguchu, B. A., Wang, Y., et al. (2019). Abnormal intra-network architecture in extra-striate cortices in amblyopia: a resting state fMRI study. *Eye Vision* 6, 1–8. doi: 10.1186/s40662-019-0145-2

Ma, L., Steinberg, J. L., Bjork, J. M., Keyser-Marcus, L., Vassileva, J., Zhu, M., et al. (2018). Fronto-striatal effective connectivity of working memory in adults with cannabis use disorder. *Psychiatr. Res. Neuroimag.* 278, 21–34. doi: 10.1016/j.pscychresns.2018.05.010

Majaj, N. J., Carandini, M., and Movshon, J. A. (2007). Motion integration by neurons in macaque MT is local, not global. *J. Neurosci.* 27, 366–370. doi: 10.1523/JNEUROSCI.3183-06.2007

Mendola, J. D., Lam, J., Rosenstein, M., Lewis, L. B., and Shmuel, A. (2018). Partial correlation analysis reveals abnormal retinotopically organized functional connectivity of visual areas in amblyopia. *NeuroImage Clin.* 18, 192–201. doi: 10.1016/j.nicl.2018.01.022

Min, Y. L., Su, T., Shu, Y. Q., Liu, W. F., Chen, L. L., Shi, W. Q., et al. (2018). Altered spontaneous brain activity patterns in strabismus with amblyopia patients using amplitude of low-frequency fluctuation: a resting-state fMRI study. *Neuropsychiatr. Dis. Treat.* 14:2351. doi: 10.2147/NDT.S171462

Ning, Y., Zheng, R., Li, K., Zhang, Y., Lyu, D., Jia, H., et al. (2018). The altered Granger causality connection among pain-related brain networks in migraine. *Medicine* 97:102. doi: 10.1097/MD.0000000000010102

Ohta, M., Nakataki, M., Takeda, T., Numata, S., Tominaga, T., Kameoka, N., et al. (2018). Structural equation modeling approach between salience network dysfunction, depressed mood, and subjective quality of life in schizophrenia: an ICA resting-state fMRI study. *Neuropsychiatr. Dis. Treat.* 14:1585. doi: 10.2147/NDT.S163132

Park, H. J., Pae, C., Friston, K., Jang, C., Razi, A., Zeidman, P., et al. (2017). Hierarchical dynamic causal modeling of resting-state fMRI reveals longitudinal changes in effective connectivity in the motor system after thalamotomy for essential tremor. *Front. Neurol.* 8:346. doi: 10.3389/fneur.2017.00346

Pitcher, D., and Ungerleider, L. G. (2020). Evidence for a third visual pathway specialized for social perception. *Trends Cogn Sci.* 2020:006. doi: 10.1016/j.tics.2020.11.006

Ranganath, C., Cohen, M. X., Dam, C., and D'Esposito, M. (2004). Inferior temporal, prefrontal, and hippocampal contributions to visual working memory maintenance and associative memory retrieval. *J. Neurosci.* 24, 3917–3925. doi: 10.1523/JNEUROSCI.5053-03.2004

Roper-Hall, G. (2007). Current concepts of amblyopia: a neuro-ophthalmology perspective. *Am. Orthop. J.* 57, 2–12. doi: 10.3368/aoj.57.1.2

Sharaev, M. G., Zavyalova, V. V., Ushakov, V. L., Kartashov, S. I., and Velichkovsky, B. M. (2016). Effective connectivity within the default mode network: dynamic causal modeling of resting-state fMRI data. *Front. Hum. Neurosci.* 10:14. doi: 10.3389/fnhum.2016.00014

Shi, Y., Liu, W., Liu, R., Zeng, Y., Wu, L., Huang, S., et al. (2019). Investigation of the emotional network in depression after stroke: A study of multivariate Granger causality analysis of fMRI data. *J. Affect. Dis.* 249, 35–44. doi: 10.1016/j.jad.2019.02.020

Smith, J., Jack, M. M., Peterson, J. C., and Chamoun, R. B. (2017). Herniated gyrus rectus causing idiopathic compression of the optic chiasm. *Clin. Neurol. Neurosurg.* 153, 79–81. doi: 10.1016/j.clineuro.2016.12.010

Song, X. W., Dong, Z. Y., Long, X. Y., Li, S. F., Zuo, X. N., Zhu, C. Z., et al. (2011). REST: a toolkit for resting-state functional magnetic resonance imaging data processing. *PLoS One* 6:e25031. doi: 10.1371/journal.pone.0025031

Stephan, K. E., and Friston, K. J. (2010). Analyzing effective connectivity with functional magnetic resonance imaging. *Wiley Interdiscip. Rev. Cogn. Sci.* 1, 446–459. doi: 10.1002/wcs.58

Tailor, V., Bossi, M., Greenwood, J. A., and Dahlmann-Noor, A. (2016). Childhood amblyopia: current management and new trends. *Br. Med. Bull.* 119, 75–86. doi: 10.1093/bmb/ldw030

Tang, A., Chen, T., Zhang, J., Gong, Q., and Liu, L. (2017). Abnormal spontaneous brain activity in patients with anisometropic amblyopia using resting-state functional magnetic resonance imaging. *J. Pediatr. Ophthalmol. Strab.* 54, 303–310. doi: 10.3928/01913913-20170320-05

Wang, J., Hu, L., Li, W., Xian, J., Ai, L., and He, H. (2014). Alternations of functional connectivity in amblyopia patients: a resting-state fMRI study. *Biomed. Appl. Mole. Struct. Funct. Imag.* 9038:903809. doi: 10.1117/12.2043424

Wang, T., Chen, N., Zhan, W., Liu, J., Zhang, J., Liu, Q., et al. (2016). Altered effective connectivity of posterior thalamus in migraine with cutaneous allodynia: a resting-state fMRI study with granger causality analysis. *J. Headache Pain* 17, 1–11. doi: 10.1186/s10194-016-0610-4

Wu, Y., and Liu, L. Q. (2017). Research advances on cortical functional and structural deficits of amblyopia. *Chinese J. Ophthalmol.* 53, 392–395. doi: 10.3760/cma.j.issn.0412-4081.2017.05.015

Yan, C. G., Wang, X. D., Zuo, X. N., and Zang, Y. F. (2016). DPABI: data processing & analysis for (resting-state) brain imaging. *Neuroinformatics* 14, 339–351. doi: 10.1007/s12021-016-9299-4

Yang, X., Lu, L., Li, Q., Huang, X., Gong, Q., and Liu, L. (2019). Altered spontaneous brain activity in patients with strabismic amblyopia: A resting-state fMRI study using regional homogeneity analysis. *Experimental and therapeutic medicine* 18, 3877–3884. doi: 10.3892/etm.2019.8038

Zang, Z. X., Yan, C. G., Dong, Z. Y., Huang, J., and Zang, Y. F. (2012). Granger causality analysis implementation on MATLAB: a graphic user interface toolkit for fMRI data processing. *J. Neurosci. Methods* 203, 418–426. doi: 10.1016/j.jneumeth.2011.10.006

Zhou, Z., Jing, B., Wang, H., and Xia, H. (2015). Research on resting state f MRI of strabismus amblyopia children based on functional connectivity algorithms. *Beijing Biomed. Eng.* 2015:05.

4

Simulating Macular Degeneration to Investigate Activities of Daily Living

Anne Macnamara [1], Celia Chen [2], Victor R. Schinazi [3,4], Dimitrios Saredakis [1] and Tobias Loetscher [1]*

[1] Cognitive Ageing and Impairment Neurosciences Laboratory, UniSA Justice & Society, University of South Australia, Adelaide, SA, Australia, [2] College of Medicine and Public Health, Flinders Medical Centre, Flinders University, Adelaide, SA, Australia, [3] Department of Psychology, Faculty of Society & Design, Bond University, Gold Coast, QLD, Australia, [4] Future Health Technologies, Singapore-ETH Centre, Campus for Research Excellence and Technological Enterprise (CREATE), Singapore, Singapore

***Correspondence:**
Anne Macnamara
anne.macnamara@mymail.unisa.edu.au

Purpose: Investigating difficulties during activities of daily living is a fundamental first step for the development of vision-related intervention and rehabilitation strategies. One way to do this is through visual impairment simulations. The aim of this review is to synthesize and assess the types of simulation methods that have been used to simulate age-related macular degeneration (AMD) in normally sighted participants, during activities of daily living (e.g., reading, cleaning, and cooking).

Methods: We conducted a systematic literature search in five databases and a critical analysis of the advantages and disadvantages of various AMD simulation methods (following PRISMA guidelines). The review focuses on the suitability of each method for investigating activities of daily living, an assessment of clinical validation procedures, and an evaluation of the adaptation periods for participants.

Results: Nineteen studies met the criteria for inclusion. Contact lenses, computer manipulations, gaze contingent displays, and simulation glasses were the main forms of AMD simulation identified. The use of validation and adaptation procedures were reported in approximately two-thirds and half of studies, respectively.

Conclusions: Synthesis of the methodology demonstrated that the choice of simulation has been, and should continue to be, guided by the nature of the study. While simulations may never completely replicate vision loss experienced during AMD, consistency in simulation methodology is critical for generating realistic behavioral responses under vision impairment simulation and limiting the influence of confounding factors. Researchers could also come to a consensus regarding the length and form of adaptation by exploring what is an adequate amount of time and type of training required to acclimatize participants to vision impairment simulations.

Keywords: age-related macular degeneration, vision impairment, simulation, activities of daily living, rehabilitation

INTRODUCTION

Age-related macular degeneration (AMD) is a leading cause of visual impairments, that affects ~200 million people globally (Wong et al., 2014; Jonas et al., 2017), and continues to rise due to the aging population (Velez-Montoya et al., 2014). The vision loss experienced by AMD patients can manifest as a blur, distortion, different colors, or darkness (Taylor et al., 2018a). Vision loss due to non-neovascular AMD can be managed with the support of rehabilitation (Hooper et al., 2008), visual aids (Morrice et al., 2017), or environmental adaptions (Brunnström et al., 2004), but in severe cases of exudative AMD there may be irreversible central vision loss (Jonas et al., 2017). As vision declines, those with AMD report increasing difficulties engaging in activities of daily living (ADL), such as reading, cleaning, and cooking (Bennion et al., 2012; Taylor et al., 2016). Recently, there has been increasing interest into the extent to which AMD affects ADL and quality of life (Jelin et al., 2019; Broadhead et al., 2020; Zult et al., 2020). Characterizing these practical difficulties is an important step in adopting intervention strategies and facilitating positive change for visually impaired individuals.

Previous research has identified difficulties in ADL based upon self-reports from visually impaired patients (Scilley et al., 2002; Walker et al., 2006; Desrosiers et al., 2009). However, directly measuring task performance (e.g., reading, writing, collecting groceries) may be more useful than self-reports because it offers clinicians and researchers an objective assessment of the impact of the visual disability (Culham et al., 2004; Varadaraj et al., 2018; Wittich et al., 2018). Testing visually impaired patients for research purposes can sometimes be challenging because of safety, practical, or availability reasons. In addition, interactive experiments can burden the participants, since visually impaired populations are more likely to have multiple physical and mental comorbidities (Court et al., 2014). Here, it may also be difficult to isolate the effects of visual impairment from the impact of coexisting impairments (e.g., cognitive decline; Wood et al., 2010). One approach to avoid these challenges is to simulate vision loss in normally sighted populations.

Simulation experiments have provided insights into people's behaviors and capabilities with visual impairments (Wood et al., 2010; Lehsing et al., 2019). These experiments have also been used as models for diagnostic visual assessments (de Haan et al., 2020), pilot experiments prior to testing in actual patients (Hwang et al., 2018), and as educational tools for the wider community (Juniat et al., 2019). Critically, simulations can contribute to understanding the effects of eye conditions without subjecting a person to potential risks. For example, Foster et al. (2014) simulated cataracts via goggles on younger adults to examine safety aspects of negotiating stairs on older adults with cataracts. They found that highlighting stair edges with tread increased heel clearance placement and improved safety. Likewise, to assess street-crossing behaviors, participants were positioned on the curb of a street and asked to judge when it would be safe to cross, under normal, and simulated central vision loss conditions (Almutleb and Hassan, 2020). The judgements were similar for both conditions, leading researchers to conclude that eccentric viewing can modulate safety judgements, even with central vision deficits.

Effective simulations of visual conditions can also assist in understanding the effects of eye conditions in order to help develop rehabilitation strategies. Simulation studies have allowed researchers to investigate the manner in which adaptive visual strategies (e.g., pseudofovea) can compensate for vision loss (Barraza-Bernal et al., 2018). Oculomotor adaptations play a fundamental role in visually impaired people learning to use their peripheral vision to reengage with vision-dependent activities (Walsh and Liu, 2014). For example, participants under a central scotoma simulation completed reading tasks after training sessions to induce a preferred retinal locus (Barraza-Bernal et al., 2017). Reading performance significantly improved after each training session, indicating that the task became easier for participants as their ability to use their peripheral vision developed (Barraza-Bernal et al., 2017).

Despite these findings, it still remains unclear what constitutes an "effective simulation." This could include validation, which refers to the process of determining whether the simulation is an accurate representation of a visual impairment. Valid simulations can be clinically ascertained through mechanisms such as visual acuity or visual field testing. Ensuring that simulations are as realistic as possible is essential when educating others about visual impairments, especially when making practical recommendations.

Effectively constructed simulations may also consider adaptation periods, the time provided to adjust to a simulation before performance is measured. Since AMD is a progressive disease (Taylor et al., 2016; Jonas et al., 2017), patients will typically lose sight over the course of years, allowing them a longer time to adapt to their changing eye condition. This change in vision is in sharp contrast to the immediate loss of vision experienced during a simulation.

Previous research has been critical of simulations of vision loss and blindness. Researchers have suggested that some simulations may be ineffective because they focus on temporary immediate loss of sight (i.e., putting on a blindfold) as opposed to the long-term realities of being blind (Silverman, 2015; Schinazi et al., 2016). Visually impaired patients would likely develop appropriate behavioral and cognitive compensatory strategies over time (Riazi et al., 2013; Rai et al., 2019). In comparison, a normally sighted person's responses under simulation may be exaggerated due to this lack of adjustment. Consequently, a fair and effectively designed simulation study would allow time for normally sighted participants to acclimatize to a simulation (e.g., training sessions, practice trials) prior to measurement (Aguilar and Castet, 2017). While an adaptation period will never replicate the slow progression of vision loss, providing an adequate adaptation period may at least limit confounding behaviors and stressors exhibited as a result of a sudden deprivation of sight. Adaptation to central vision loss has been investigated previously (Kwon et al., 2013; Walsh and Liu, 2014), but to our knowledge, there are no clear guidelines for the suitable length and form of adaptation periods before testing.

The purpose of this paper is to review studies assessing performance in ADL under an AMD simulation in normally sighted people. The importance of investigating specific simulations (e.g., AMD), as opposed to generalized blur simulations, is because the impact on everyday life may vary in response to the condition's predominant manifestation (e.g., AMD affects central vision while glaucoma affects peripheral vision). Synthesizing this literature is intended to provide an overview on the different types of simulation procedures and their suitability for investigating ADL. Investigating the behavioral challenges of ADL (without exposing actual AMD patients to possible psychological and physical harm) is an important step in adopting intervention strategies and facilitating positive change for visually impaired individuals.

METHODS

A systematic search was conducted to identify studies simulating AMD. The review was registered on Open Science Framework (https://osf.io/xkymc). Five electronic databases (Embase Classic + Embase, Ovid Emcare, Ovid MEDLINE® All, Ovid Nursing Database, and PsycINFO) were simultaneously searched via Ovid, on 25th September 2020. A combination of search terms was employed: ("Macular degeneration" OR "Central vision loss" OR "Central scotoma") AND ("Simulat*" OR "Replicat*" OR "Imitat*" OR "Emulat*"). A subsequent updated search was conducted on 30th Match 2021. Preferred Reporting Items for Systematic Reviews and Meta-Analyses (PRISMA) was followed.

Eligible studies were required to be published in English, contain more than five participants (i.e., not case studies), and were original research published in a peer reviewed journal (i.e., no review articles, no conference abstracts). The key criterion was to include studies that simulated AMD within a group of normally sighted people. Studies were excluded if participants had, or have had a history of, any visual impairment, implant, or visual prosthetic. Of primary interest were the methods from the included studies. Descriptions of the AMD simulations (i.e., type and characteristics, validation, and adaptation procedures), the structure of the experiments, and outcome measures were also examined.

Given that symptoms of AMD, specifically central vision loss and central scotomas, can also be indicators of other visual impairments, the screening process was strict in determining the overall purpose of each simulation experiment. As such, articles needed to have cogent reasoning that the purpose of any central vision loss or central scotoma simulation was to primarily mimic AMD, not another condition (e.g., cataracts). However, studies replicating "macular degeneration" were also included because not all researchers use the "age-related" terminology (Copolillo et al., 2017). Articles that were not explicitly related to AMD or macular degeneration were excluded.

Considering our specific interest in AMD's impact on ADL, there were additional restrictions regarding outcome measures. Specifically, studies were excluded if their main focus was on oculomotor behavior (eye movements) and/or vision assessments. Simulation research of this nature is highly informative about fixation and saccade patterns, and the implications of these patterns for the development of a preferred retinal locus or eccentric fixation (Kwon et al., 2013; Costela et al., 2020). However, studies like these do not directly collect data on performance-based measures (e.g., sorting medications) of everyday activities that can immediately inform researchers about the struggles of living with AMD.

Covidence systematic review management software was used to screen the articles (Covidence Systematic Review Software, 2020). Title and abstract screening were conducted by a single reviewer and, followed by two independent reviewers (AM and DS) completing a full text screening. If a consensus could not be reached on a study, a third independent reviewer settled the dispute (TL). Reference lists of the final full texts were screened, via a snowballing strategy, to locate additional studies.

The quality of the included studies was assessed using the Joanna Briggs Critical Appraisal Tools for Quasi-Experimental Studies (Tufanaru et al., 2020). This purpose of these tools are to evaluate the possibility of bias in each study's design, conduct and analysis. Two independent researchers (AM and DS) appraised the methodological quality of the included studies, using a designated checklist of nine criteria. The studies were classed on their risk of bias, depending on the percentage of criteria met (i.e., low, moderate, and high risk = > 70%, 50–69%, and < 49% criteria, respectively). Cohen's Kappa was calculated to examine the consistency of the independent appraisals.

RESULTS

Our database search identified 1,786 publications (see **Figure 1** for screening flowchart), with an additional record identified through alternative sources (e.g., reference list searching). Nineteen studies met the inclusion criteria in the final synthesis post-screening. The demographic information, study descriptions, measures, key findings, and risks of bias are presented in **Table 1**.

A further 16 studies were identified through our search that primarily measured outcomes relating to eye movements, oculomotor behavior, and vision assessments through AMD simulations. However, these studies were beyond the scope our review, which was intended to examine the role of simulation research on investigating ADL performance affected by AMD.

Critical Appraisal

The reviewers agreed that of the 19 relevant studies, they were generally of moderate methodological quality. The individual assessment of quality originally yielded a moderate level of agreement ($k = 0.48$) prior to discussions and final agreement. The methodological assessment revealed a number of threats to the internal validities for the studies. Also, ~16% of appraisal responses were "unclear." This occurred when the publications did not report enough to make a sound judgement about the methodology. See Appendix A (**Supplementary Material**) for the agreed methodological quality assessments for each individual study.

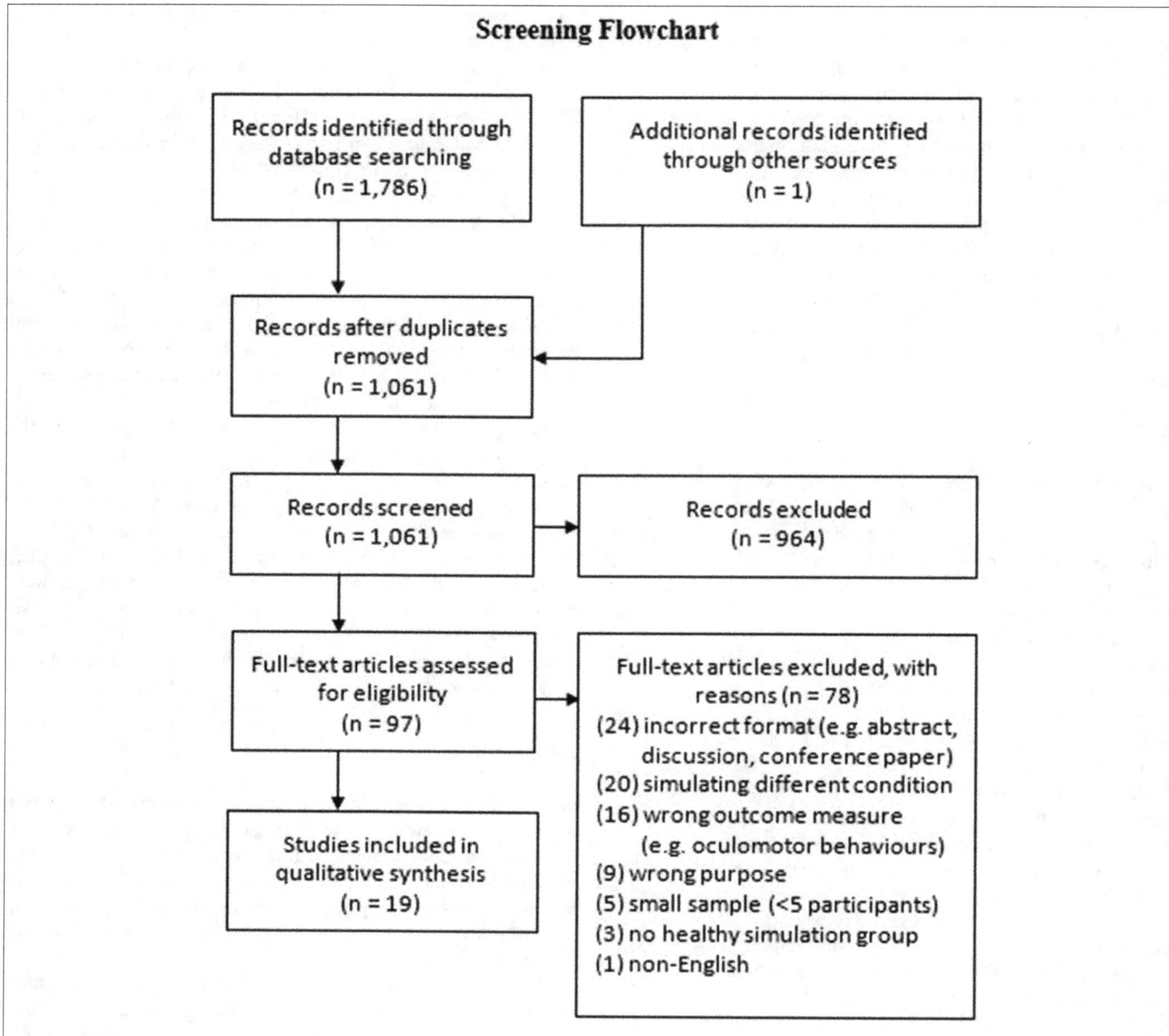

FIGURE 1 | Screening flowchart for studies simulating age-related macular degeneration.

Age-Related Macular Degeneration Simulation Methods

Methods for simulating AMD can be organized into four main categories (see **Table 2**) with researchers employing contact lenses, computer manipulations, gaze contingent displays, or simulation glasses.

Contact Lenses

Contact lenses simulate vision loss through varying opacity levels to replicate AMD characteristics (Czoski-Murray et al., 2009; Almutleb and Hassan, 2020). Because contact lenses are placed directly in the eye and capable of following eye movements, researchers can manipulate them to reflect individualized simulation specifications that mimic different stages of AMD.

Computer Manipulations

The simulation of AMD via a computer has no direct impact on vision itself. Instead, it presents an end-result representation of what people with visual impairments experience.

Gaze Contingent

A gaze contingent simulation is the only method that allows the location of a manufactured scotoma to be continuously realigned in response to a gaze fixation (Aguilar and Castet, 2017; Wu et al., 2018). Due to eye-tracking technology, these simulations can calibrate with a person's pupil. When the person alters their gaze, the simulated scotoma moves to the central region of that new visual field.

Glasses

There is great variability in simulation glasses available for visual impairment research. Basic goggles can be self-manufactured to mimic AMD symptoms (e.g., scotoma) using materials such as paint or tape (Zagar and Baggarly, 2010; Ho et al., 2019). Alternatively, simulation glasses can be bought online which are already designed to reflect diminished visual acuity (Connect Solutions Group, 2020). Augmented and virtual reality glasses are more advanced and have the combined benefit of being able to immerse the user into situations that simulate visual impairments while also incorporating gaze-contingent eye-tracking software (Jin et al., 2005; Wu et al., 2018; Jones et al., 2020).

Other Methods

Researchers can also develop their own techniques to simulate visual impairment. For example, Wensveen et al. (1995) stuck circular gray film of varying scotoma sizes to a computer screen for participants to read around.

Validation and Adaptation Procedures

In terms of validation, approximately two-thirds of the studies report information on how the AMD simulations were validated and half of the studies detail procedures how normally sighted participants were adapted to the simulation.

Validation

The simulations in 12 studies were authenticated using a variety of clinical and computer modeling techniques (see **Table 2**). Only two studies attempted clinical validation techniques (e.g., perimetry and tangent screens; Klee et al., 2018; Almutleb and Hassan, 2020). Perimetry and tangent screens are both clinical visual field tests, administered during the diagnosis, and observation of AMD, which can expose the degree of central and peripheral vision loss (Phipps et al., 2004; Acton et al., 2012). The AMD computer manipulations were validated based upon previously developed blurring formulas (Marmor and Marmor, 2010; Krishnan and Bedell, 2018). This includes a computer model that was developed to reformat images relative to the degree of eccentricity (e.g., 5°) and a blur algorithm that simulates symptoms of macular disease created based upon experimental pixilation's of Snellen letters (see Marmor and Marmor, 2010 for more information). Finally, for computer gaze-contingent simulations, studies reported no standardized validation procedures, but rather the removal of trial blocks with calibration errors $< 1°$ (Kwon et al., 2012; Bernard et al., 2016; Aguilar and Castet, 2017; Gupta et al., 2018; Wu et al., 2018; de Boer et al., 2021).

Adaptation

As specified in **Table 2**, nine studies offered their participants training sessions or allowed them to practice the experiment whilst under simulation (Czoski-Murray et al., 2009; Kwon et al., 2012; Bernard et al., 2016; Aguilar and Castet, 2017; Gupta et al., 2018; Krishnan et al., 2019; Almutleb and Hassan, 2020; de Boer et al., 2021). For example, Bernard et al. (2016) provided participants with an hour adaptation session to become accustomed to reading with an artificial scotoma before reading speed was measured. In one study, without training sessions or practice, participants were simply instructed to spend a few minutes looking around their immediate environment whilst wearing simulation glasses (Ho et al., 2019). The remaining studies did not provide additional information to indicate that participants adapted to the simulation prior to testing.

DISCUSSION

Comparison of Simulation Methods, Validation, and Adaptation Procedures

There are a series of benefits and drawbacks to each simulation method (summarized in **Table 3**), which future researchers need to weigh up when designing their own research. For example, in terms of accuracy, gaze contingent simulations may arguably create scotomas that produce the most realistic AMD experience because of the continual realignment of central vision loss in response to changes in eye movements (Aguilar and Castet, 2017). There has been criticism that contact lenses are not capable of emulating the same level of scotoma characteristics (Butt et al., 2015), although newer contact lens designs have attempted to address these limitations (Klee et al., 2018). While still not as precise as gaze contingent paradigms, contact lenses at least retain the advantage of moving together with the eye. In contrast, simulation glasses do not have the level of gaze precision that the former techniques create. Scotomas depicted on most glasses are fixed and will not realign in response to eye movements. Normally sighted participants adopting glasses may simply become accustomed to the simulated characteristics of AMD (e.g., black paint on glasses; Zagar and Baggarly, 2010) and develop strategies (i.e., participants tilting their heads) to look around an artificial blur.

Furthermore, in contrast to gaze contingent paradigms that create unique scotomas for each person, the computer manipulated images are the same for all participants. This approach does not necessarily subvert the quality of computer manipulations given that the descriptions of the methods in each of the papers are based upon standardized formulas reflecting AMD characteristics (Lane et al., 2019). But behavior or performance measured using this method is likely to lack realism. A normally sighted participant assessing a manipulated image will not need to engage in the same compensatory strategies (i.e., using a preferred retinal locus) that people with AMD will do to perform the same task (e.g., judging facial expressions). This limitation is acknowledged by researchers (Irons et al., 2014), who suggest that computer simulations provide practical piloting opportunities prior to testing in patient populations.

Regarding mobility, the gaze-contingent and computer manipulations have previously been limited in the range of ADL that can be investigated. Eye-tracking software used in this research context has typically been computer-based,

TABLE 1 | Age-related macular degeneration simulation studies.

Studies	Demographic			Study description	Tool/Test measure	Result/Finding	Risk of bias
	N	Age (M)	Sex (F/M)				
Aguilar and Castet (2017)	10	24.3	5 / 5	Computer sentence reading task	Comfort rating scale; reading speed	More comfortable using Electronic Vision Enhancement Systems than CCTV ($p > 0.05$) No difference in reading speeds between device groups ($p < 0.05$)	Moderate
Almutleb and Hassan (2020)	24	27.0	NS	Street crossing judgement task	Visual acuity (ETDRS and Evans chart); cognitive and health assessments (MMSE, TMT, and SF-36); street crossing judgment scale; street crossing habits scale	No difference in street crossing judgements (accuracy and reliability) between normal and simulated vision ($p = 0.35$ and $p = 0.09$) No correlation between street crossing judgements (accuracy and reliability) and scotoma size ($p = 0.83$ and $p = 0.95$)	Moderate
Bernard et al. (2007)	7	23 – 43	NS	Computer sentence reading task	Reading speed	Reading speed decreases as scotoma size increases (6° = 84 wpm and 10° = 72 wpm) Reading speed improves as interline spacing increases (6°: $p = 0.007$ and 10°: $p = 0.004$)	Moderate
Copolillo et al. (2017)	10	69	5/5	Walking (indoors and outdoors); stair climbing; carrying laundry and groceries	Center of mass (postural changes); performance speed	More postural changes for activities under simulated vision than normal vision ($p < 0.05$ for all except laundry) More stabilization strategies for activities under simulated vision than normal vision ($p < 0.05$ for all except sway and therapist assist) Slower performance on activities under simulated vision than normal vision ($p < 0.05$)	Low
Czoski-Murray et al. (2009)	105	32	NS	Walking; reading a newspaper, book, and food label; watching TV	Visual acuity (ETDRS and Pelli-Robson chart); health assessment (Health Utilities Index 3, patient time trade-off, and VF-14); performance self-rating scale	Patient time-trade off declined by severity of the vision simulation lens ($p < 0.001$) Visual function scores declined as participants unable to perform tasks ($p < 0.001$)	High
de Boer et al. (2021)	24	23	15 / 9	Computer emotion identification task	Accuracy	Emotional recognition better when vision intact instead of degraded vision ($p \leq 0.01$)	Low
Gupta et al. (2018)	13	NS	NS	Computer sentence reading task	Reading speed	Reading speed decreases as scotoma size increases ($p < 0.05$) Low vision device remapping increases reading speed around scotomas (exp 1: 4° [$p > 0.1$] and 8° [$p < 0.05$]; exp 2: 4° [$p > 0.1$], 8° [$p > 0.05$] and 16° [$p < 0.01$]; exp 3: 8°, 12°, and 16° [all $p < 0.01$])	Moderate
Ho et al. (2019)	19	18 – 74	NS	Computer face identity, letter acuity, and sentence reading task	Judgement accuracy; response time; letter acuity (ETDRS and Landolt C); reading speed	Letter acuity improved with reduced pixel size Reading speed slower under simulated vision than normal vision Face recognition slower under simulated vision than normal vision	High
Irons et al. (2014)	31	18 – 36	19 / 12	Computer facial dissimilarity and memory task	Judgement accuracy; response time	Facial dissimilarity and discrimination decreased as blur levels increased ($p = 0.02$ and $p < 0.001$) Memory performance (accuracy and speed) decreased as blur levels increased (new: $p < 0.001$ and $p = 0.02$; old: $p < 0.001$ and <	Moderate

TABLE 1 | Continued

Studies	Demographic			Study description	Tool/Test measure	Result/Finding	Risk of bias
	N	Age (M)	Sex (F/M)				
Juniat et al. (2019)	252	NS	NS	Making Tea and filling medicine box	Errors; self-reported difficulty scale	More errors for filling dosette box (0.7) than making tea (0.34) Higher difficulty rating for dosette box (3.23/4) than making tea (2.63/4)	High
Klee et al. (2018)	10	27 – 43	3 / 7	Computer letter and pictogram perception tasks	Accuracy	More correct letters (10 and 20°: $p = 0.01$) and pictograms (10° and 20°: $p = 0.001$) with 5× magnification than 3× magnification	Moderate
Krishnan et al. (2019)	18	Y: 24 – 36 O: 55 – 73	NS	Computer sentence reading task	Reading speed	Reading speed decreases with increasing micro-scotoma density ($p < 0.0001$)	Moderate
Kwon et al. (2012)	55	Y: 18 – 30 O: 55 – 88	28 / 27	Computer target identification task	Response time; accuracy; image preference survey	Visual enhancement improved response time for older participants ($p < 0.05$ for all except high enhancement) but not younger participants ($p > 0.05$) No difference in accuracy by vision enhancement group ($p > 0.05$) Younger participants responded faster and more accurately than older participants	Moderate
Lane et al. (2019)	74	Y: 20.6 O: 73.3	56 / 18	Computer emotional expression task	Judgement accuracy	Emotion expression accuracy decreases as blur levels increase ($p < 0.001$) Older participants have less accuracy than younger participants ($p = 0.001$) Caricaturing increased expression recognition accuracy ($p < 0.001$)	Moderate
McKone et al. (2018)	20	19.0	15 / 5	Computer facial identity task	Perception rating scale	Caricaturing increased dissimilarity perception ($p < 0.01$) Perception improves with increased caricaturing ($p < 0.05$)	Low
Rousek and Hallbeck (2011)	50	18 – 30	25 / 25	Hospital wayfinding task	Task performance; speed; Wayfinding survey	Wayfinding experience better during normal vision than simulated vision ($p = 0.005$) Faster task completion during normal vision than simulated vision ($p < 0.001$)	Moderate
Wensveen et al. (1995)	8	Y: 18 – 24 O: 62 – 78	NS	Computer word reading task	Reading speed; accuracy	Reading rates decrease as scotoma size increases (Exp 1: $p < 0.0001$ and exp 2: $p < 0.0002$) No reading rate differences for older and younger participants ($p > 0.05$) Remapping improves reading rates ($p < 0.01$)	Moderate
Wu et al. (2018)	41	18 – 31	23 / 18	Street crossing judgement task	Visual acuity (Snellen chart); street crossing judgements and behaviors (gap thresholds, curb delays, crossing times)	Street crossing judgements (gap threshold and curb delay) longer as scotoma size increases ($p < 0.05$ for all except 10°/20° scotoma curb delay) No difference in crossing times between groups ($p > 0.05$)	Low
Zagar and Baggarly (2010)	100	20+	66 / 34	Read pill bottle, patient leaflets, and sort medications	Symptom experience rating scale	Decreased peripheral and central vision, and blurred central vision under simulated vision ($p < 0.0001$)	Moderate

NS, not specified; Y, younger adults; O, older adults; wpm, words per minute.
Significance level: $p \leq 0.05$.

TABLE 2 | Age-related macular degeneration simulation methods.

Type	Studies	Apparatus	Simulation description	Validation procedure	Adaptation procedure
Contact lenses	Almutleb and Hassan (2020)	Soft opaque lens	2.8, 3.0, and 3.2 mm diameter opacity	Tangent screen	Practice task (no time specified)
	Czoski-Murray et al. (2009)	Soft opaque lens	Different sizes black dots	Pilot trials	Practice task (no time specified)
	Klee et al. (2018)	Opaque lens with adjustable adaption device	7.25° dark scotoma	Perimetry	No reported information
Computer manipulation	Irons et al. (2014)	Image manipulation	0°, 10°, 20°, and 30° Gaussian Kernel blur filter	Formula*	No reported information
	Krishnan et al. (2019)	Computer generated	2.8°, 5.5°, 8.3°... 16.6° micro-scotomas	Procedure†	Practice task (15 min)
	Lane et al. (2019)	Image manipulation	0°, 50°, and 70° Gaussian Kernel blur filter	Formula*	No reported information
	McKone et al. (2018)	Image manipulation	0°, 20°, and 30° Gaussian Kernel blur filter	Formula*	No reported information
Gaze contingent	Aguilar and Castet (2017)	EyeLink eye tracker	10° gray square scotoma	Calibration (error <1°)	Training session (1 h)
	Bernard et al. (2007)	EyeLink eye tracker	6 and 10° textured and blank square scotoma	Calibration (error <1°)	Practice task (1 h)
	de Boer et al. (2021)	EyeLink eye track	17° × 11.5° semi-circle blurred scotoma	Calibration (error <1°)	Practice trials (no time specified)
	Gupta et al. (2018)‡	Tobii TX 300 eye tracker	4°, 8°, and 16° white circle scotoma	Calibration (error <1°)	Practice trials (no time specified)
	Kwon et al. (2012)	EyeLink eye tracker	10° gray circle scotoma	Calibration (error <1°)	Practice trials (no time specified)
	Wensveen et al. (1995)‡	SRI dual Purkinje eye tracker	2°, 4°, and 8° gray, opaque circle scotoma	No reported information	No reported information
Glasses	Copolillo et al. (2017)	Goggles	20/400 macular degeneration	No reported information	No reported information
	Gupta et al. (2018)‡	Sensics zSight and Oculus DK2 head mounted device/Arrington Research Viewpoint and SMI DK2 Upgrade eye tracker respectively	4°, 8°, and 16° white circle scotoma	Calibration (error <1°)	No practice trials
	Ho et al. (2019)	ODG R-7 augmented reality	20° black opaque tape scotoma	No reported information	Free exploration (few minutes)
	Juniat et al. (2019)	Sim Specs	Age-related macular degeneration	No reported information	No reported information
	Rousek and Hallbeck (2011)	Goggles	20/400 macular degeneration	No reported information	No reported information
	Wu et al. (2018)	NVisor SX60 head mounted device/gaze contingent Arrington eye tracker	10° (20°) and 20° (40°) black circle absolute scotoma (relative blur surrounding scotoma)	Calibration (error <1°)	No reported information
	Zagar and Baggarly (2010)	Goggles	1/2 inch crescent moon black paint; ≤20/70 macular degeneration	No reported information	No reported information
Other	Wensveen et al. (1995)‡	Material fixed to computer screen	2°, 4°, and 8° gray, opaque, circle film scotoma	No reported information	No reported information

*See Marmor and Marmor (2010) for previously established formula.

†See Krishnan and Bedell (2018) for computer generated procedure.

‡Wensveen et al. (1995) and Gupta et al. (2018) used two methods to simulate age-related macular degeneration.

TABLE 3 | Advantages and disadvantages of simulation methods.

Type	Advantages	Disadvantages
Contact lenses	Any activity of daily living can be tested (mobility friendly) Individual customization Clinical validation possible	Semi-invasive Infection risk, possible eye irritations Circumventing simulation possible (i.e., seeing past occlusion) Potentially expensive (single use product)
Computer manipulation	Pre-validated (formula based) Limited expense (reusable) Non-invasive	No mobility (limited activities of daily living) Clinical validation not possible Unrealistic visual scanning and compensatory strategies
Gaze contingent	Reasonable accuracy and realism Individual customization Limited expense (reusable) Non-invasive	Limited mobility and activities of daily living (i.e., virtual/augmented reality glasses possible) Clinical validation not possible
Glasses	Any activity of daily living (mobility friendly) Limited expense (depending on product, i.e., homemade) Non-invasive Clinical validation possible	Circumventing simulation possible (i.e., tilting head) Potentially expensive (depending on product, i.e., virtual/augmented reality glasses) Health concerns (i.e., motion sickness)
Other	Limited expense (home-made) Non-invasive	No mobility (limited activities of daily living) Clinical validation not possible

which means the simulations have naturally given precedence to investigations on stationary behaviors (e.g., reading, facial recognition; Wensveen et al., 1995; Bernard et al., 2016; Aguilar and Castet, 2017; Gupta et al., 2018; Krishnan et al., 2019). Comparatively, contact lenses and glasses are hands free and have allowed the wearer to move around and engage in tasks unimpeded (e.g., walking and carrying laundry; Czoski-Murray et al., 2009; Copolillo et al., 2017). However, with advances in augmented and virtual reality, normally sighted participants can now wear head mounted devices with eye-tracking capabilities (Wu et al., 2018). This means that the benefits of mobility and gaze precision are combined into a single set of simulation glasses. Therefore, future research may evolve to showcase a more diverse range of ADL under gaze-contingent AMD simulations.

Another factor to consider when conducting research is the health and safety of participants. Simulation contact lenses are semi-invasive and participants may not be comfortable inserting them on their eyes. The risks to participants' sight if inserted incorrectly may dissuade participants from taking part in experiments. There are also risks associated with hygiene, as contact lenses can cause corneal infections (Robertson and Cavanagh, 2008). They should not be shared, and therefore could become a costly simulation approach.

The use of augmented and virtual reality simulation glasses may also lead to unwanted side effects (Saredakis et al., 2020). Participants wearing head mounted devices in vision impairment research have reported headaches, nausea, motion sickness (Wu et al., 2018; Deemer et al., 2019; Lorenzini et al., 2019). Such side-effects might result in participants withdrawing from studies or may negatively impact test performance. It may even be challenging to distinguish the outcome effects of the AMD simulation from side-effects of wearing the glasses. Research and technological communities are aware of the limitations of head mounted devices, and efforts to address these issues during the development of newer devices have shown promising results (e.g., less adverse sickness symptomology; Kourtesis et al., 2019). Therefore, the use of augmented and virtual reality glasses as a simulation method in the future may have fewer negative implications on participants' health.

In terms of validation, the use of clinical visual field tests allows the results of a normally sighted person under AMD simulation to be compared with those of a patient with AMD. If the results indicate that a simulation blurs 10° of the visual field, researchers can use this information to conclude whether or not the simulated vision creates an equivalent disruption to central vision as with AMD. However, less direct methods have been used to validate simulations in instances where using clinical diagnostic methods could have been difficult (e.g., the computer manipulations). While the Marmor and Marmor (2010) blur formula to generate AMD images may not be considered a typical validation procedure, adhering to a formula like this is a clever approach for standardizing images that would otherwise be challenging to quantify clinically.

Similarly, gaze-contingent scotomas generated by computers pose barriers for clinical validation. While simulation contact lenses or glasses can be physically worn by participants whilst undertaking a visual field test, computer gaze-contingent simulations cannot. Therefore, researchers rely on the removal of trial blocks with calibration errors (Kwon et al., 2012; Gupta et al., 2018). Since scotomas move with the eye, this technique affords, at a minimum, computer based gaze-contingent simulations a high standard of gaze precision and realism. A visual discrimination task in which foveal processing is tested has been posited to validate gaze-contingent simulations (Geringswald et al., 2013). This method validates simulations based upon the premise that a gaze-contingent scotoma should impair behavioral responses in the same manner that AMD would (Geringswald et al., 2013). More simulation studies should attempt this method in addition to calibration checks.

Virtual visual field tests are another validation process that was not utilized by the studies in this review. Virtual visual field tests can be administered via head mounted glasses, without the assistance of a technician or ophthalmologist, which makes them more accessible than traditional clinical measures. Indeed, there is evidence that the results of virtual visual field tests correlate with that of standard clinical examinations (Wroblewski et al., 2014; Tsapakis et al., 2017). For the AMD simulations, virtual visual field tests could have been administered for contact lens and augmented or virtual reality glasses.

Regardless of whichever validation process is utilized, the importance of validation cannot be underscored. Especially because it is not unusual for researchers to create the simulations themselves. While there might be standard methods employed to manufacture the computer manipulations (i.e., blurring formulas), AMD simulations have also been created by adding paint or tape to glasses (Zagar and Baggarly, 2010; Ho et al., 2019). The consequences of not validating a simulation accurately can have serious real world ramifications. Butt et al. (2015) uncovered such a case when they reassessed a contact lens simulation used by the National Institute for Health and Care Excellence (NICE) for economic evaluations. They found that the contact lenses did not create the reported central scotoma, with the result that the severity of AMD health effects was underestimated with the lenses (Butt et al., 2015). This of real concern if medical professionals and policy makers rely on results derived from poorly validated simulations to justify financial or health care decisions.

Regarding adaptation, it is useful in providing normally sighted participants with the opportunity to adapt to an AMD simulation prior to data collection. Coping strategies, such as relying on different sensory cues or strategically planning alternative behaviors, can be employed by visually impaired people (Riazi et al., 2013; Rai et al., 2019). While those with AMD will have had more time (i.e., months or years) to finesse coping strategies, adaptation periods can still grant normally sighted participants the chance to start mentally strategizing their behavioral adjustments. In experiments of this nature, acknowledging the effect of practice and experience is important in designing a fair comparison. There could be substantial learning effects between the initial moment when participants start a simulation and their performance after a few minutes. Even if the simulation does not exactly replicate vision loss, an adaptation period might be the difference between evaluating an immediate behavior triggered by the reduction in sight and evaluating a more realistic parameter.

Inversely, an adaptation period might also induce unwanted compensatory strategies. For example, during training sessions participants may inadvertently learn ways to circumvent the intended simulation by tilting their heads or squinting (e.g., glasses with opaque lenses). Even when the perceptual deficits of AMD are simulated reasonably realistically and validated, this does not guarantee that normally sighted participants will engage in the same oculomotor behavior as in patients. Participants cannot be compelled to use their peripheral vision rather than evasion techniques. Researchers should prepare for the possibility that normally sighted participants may learn ways to overcome the planned visual deficiencies. Adaptation could therefore be utilized as a method of excluding participants unaffected by vision loss simulations. In one study participants were instructed to centrally fixate on a target while wearing opaque simulation contact lenses, prior to testing (Almutleb and Hassan, 2020). This could have been because people have different resting pupil sizes; therefore, if a participants' pupil was larger than the contact lens occlusion, the participant might have been able to see around the simulated scotoma. In this particular example, four participants were excluded from the study because central fixation was not disrupted as intended (Almutleb and Hassan, 2020). If the researchers had not administered this check, the study may have revealed inaccurate results. The identification of participants seeing pass the simulation is an important reminder that opaque lenses do not always work as intended.

In terms of the length of adaptation periods, researchers have yet to come up with a standard that can be applied in future studies. Studies examining oculomotor strategies have differed in their approaches to inducing a preferred retinal locus in normally sighted participants; training sessions have been conducted over the course of hours, days, or weeks (Kwon et al., 2013; Costela et al., 2020; Maniglia et al., 2020; Prahalad and Coates, 2020). This demonstrates a lack of consistency in how long is considered suitable to reasonable compensate for central vision loss. Within this review, some studies do not specify the length of time while others exposed participants to AMD simulations from a few minutes to up to an hour prior to testing (Aguilar and Castet, 2017; Ho et al., 2019; Krishnan et al., 2019). The few minutes of free visual exploration, offered by Ho et al. (2019), may be preferable to no adaptation time. However, there could be limits to what is learnt regarding practical behavioral changes without specifically guided instructions. Of the other studies which offered adaptation periods, they all included dedicated training or practice with the task. Even though the form of training differed, at least there is a general understanding that training under a simulation is a valuable component of simulation studies. Still, a guideline which offered recommendations on adaptation could help answer questions as to what is the ideal (or minimum) duration and form of training that participants require to acclimatize to vision loss? It is critical to find an answer so that researchers can confidently distinguish that task performance is the direct outcome of any visual simulation. Without adequate adaptation, studies may be confounded by practice effects, as participants initial behavior under simulation may differ from their subsequent behavior by the end of an experiment.

Another consideration to explore is the age of the participants. The average demographic of normally sighted participants in this review is younger adults (see **Table 1**). This is not reflective of the average age group (i.e., 45–85 years of age) affected by AMD (Jonas et al., 2017). Yet, the recruitment of younger participants is not unusual for all types of simulation studies (Wood et al., 2012; Hwang et al., 2018). In this review, four studies compared younger and older normally sighted adults under simulation (Wensveen et al., 1995; Kwon et al., 2012; Krishnan et al., 2019; Lane et al., 2019). They found significantly decreased performance for both age groups under simulation, but comparatively worse performance for the older adults. A caveat in impairment simulation studies using younger participants may be that the degree to which AMD affects behavior is underestimated. Moreover, in terms of adaptation, if younger participants are performing better than older adults, then it may be possible that they are also adapting to the visual impairment simulations at a faster rate. As such, it is worth exploring whether age affects the required length of adaptation. Researchers could then account for this when interpreting their results in the future and determining adaptation periods.

What Can We Learn From Simulations?

In this review, many researchers constructed experiments in which task performance was directly compared using normal vision and simulated AMD vision. The studies routinely found significant negative effects under simulation (e.g., slower speed, reduced accuracy) on the respective measured outcomes (see **Table 1**; Copolillo et al., 2017; Gupta et al., 2018; Lane et al., 2019). For instance, reading focused simulation studies found an expected decrease in reading performance (Wensveen et al., 1995; Gupta et al., 2018; Krishnan et al., 2019), whilst facial recognition studies showed the typical decline in face and emotional perception as simulation of AMD worsens (Irons et al., 2014; McKone et al., 2018; Lane et al., 2019; de Boer et al., 2021). These findings are not surprising as they correspond with similar research findings in AMD populations (Taylor et al., 2018b; Varadaraj et al., 2018). The consistency in the findings implies sufficient AMD simulation accuracy.

Thus, from one viewpoint, it could be concluded that simulation studies are relatively redundant. Instead of offering novel insights into visual impairments, many simulation studies merely confirm findings that can also be established directly from visually impaired participants. However, a unique advantage of AMD simulations is that they allow researchers to control the presentation of symptomology (e.g., size, shape, color, and location of a scotoma). This is not possible when using a clinical population. As AMD is a degenerative eye condition, how ADL are impacted may change as AMD progresses from the non-neovascular to exudative stages. Therefore, the ability to easily alter a scotoma's severity (e.g., 4°, 8°, and 16° scotoma) is a useful manipulation to realistically assess ADL. Significant changes in behavior have been reported in response to different AMD simulation conditions (Wensveen et al., 1995; Krishnan et al., 2019). For example, Wu et al. (2018) found that as the size of a simulated scotoma increased, participants would wait for longer gaps in traffic before deciding to cross a road. This suggests that judging risk is inversely related to the degree of visual decline. An inference such as this can be established quicker by altering an AMD simulation as opposed to recruiting multiple AMD participant groups at different stages of visual decline.

The convenience of control has also been advantageous during investigations into adaptive strategies to loss of central vision (e.g., preferred retinal locus; Barraza-Bernal et al., 2018). This phenomenon may occur if the fovea is damaged during AMD progression (Costela et al., 2020). While not analyzed within this review, simulation research has significantly contributed to our understanding of how a preferred retinal locus can be induced, relocated, or sustained (Kwon et al., 2013; Barraza-Bernal et al., 2017). This knowledge has since been repurposed as a rehabilitative technique to train those with AMD to regain visual ability. Therefore, in the context of studying vision and oculomotor patterns, simulation methods are undoubtably valuable. We acknowledge that by limiting the outcome measures to performance-based measures of ADL, our review may be limited by not examining the benefits that eye movement studies have provided to the visually impaired community.

There is also much that can be learnt from people with AMD on how to improve visual impairment simulations. When patients with AMD were interviewed about their visual loss experience, their descriptions contradicted many widely held beliefs about what AMD looks like (Taylor et al., 2018a). For example, a large proportion of patients reported "missing parts" of their vision, rather than the standard depiction of a central black spot (Taylor et al., 2018a). Many of the studies in this review even portrayed AMD using darkened areas (see **Table 2**). These portrayals are not inherently false, because some patients do experience black or gray distortions, but it is important to dispel overexaggerated misconceptions. In the future, more researchers could generate AMD simulations by adopting blank scotomas, instead of colored scotomas, to account for patients reporting "missing parts" (Bernard et al., 2007; Macedo et al., 2008).

While clinical validation should be standard practice, feedback from patients can be used to generate and confirm if simulations accurately reflect the deficits they experience (Crabb et al., 2013). One study attempted this by recruiting a group of AMD patients who were visually impaired in just one eye (Denniss and Astle, 2018). The researchers presented images portraying AMD to the participants' unafflicted eye until the depiction of AMD on the picture was an indistinguishable match to that of their afflicted eye (Denniss and Astle, 2018). This method affords researchers an unquestionable representation of AMD that can then be used as a foundation for simulations (although it should still be noted that AMD manifests uniquely for each patient). In general, involving patient populations ensures that from research to clinical care, the perspective and lived experience of being visually impaired is always considered (Dean et al., 2017).

Ensuring authentic simulations is additionally vital when educating the wider community about visual impairments. Simulations have long been utilized in the medical field as a teaching tool to cultivate empathy for patients (Bunn and Terpstra, 2009; Dyer et al., 2018). Simulations allow medical professionals, family members, and the broader community, to metaphorically, "walk in someone else's shoes." One study found that after completing simple tasks (e.g., making tea) under an AMD simulation, medical students realized how they take their vision for granted and suggested workplace changes to it easier for visually impaired patients

(Juniat et al., 2019). This type of self-awareness would be particularly beneficial for family members, who historically become the primary caregiver for their visually impaired family members. Taking care of impaired family members can be a large burden, leading to significant strain on relationships and even depression for the carer (Kuriakose et al., 2017). Ideally, a greater understanding of the difficulties that visually impaired individuals endure may engender more understanding from these individuals to facilitate help with ADL.

In terms of the future of simulation research into ADL's, there is still more that can be explored about the extent to which AMD affects everyday life. At present, there is no comprehensive scale, that can be used by clinicians, that incorporates visual function (e.g., near vision) into how a person performs in their ADL. Of the 19 studies identified in this review, there were more publications on reading alone than physical tasks (e.g., walking, making tea, carrying laundry). This systematic review identifies the need for a unified scale for visual function that incorporates the visual acuity and visual field deficit, as well as a functional scale such as Extended Disability Status Scale (for multiple sclerosis) or Modified Rankins' scale for stroke that incorporate both the static and kinetic tasks to assess independence (Pacific Vision Foundation, 1999). There is no doubt that loss of central vision negatively impacts reading ability (Hamade et al., 2016; Varadaraj et al., 2018), therefore more studies are needed in order to determine the effect of AMD on other daily activities.

There is also potential to broaden the range of outcomes measured. As illustrated in **Table 1**, studies primarily assessed task performance (e.g., response time, accuracy, errors). Task performance is highly informative of a person's objective ability to complete an activity, but it does not consider the emotional experience of the person whilst completing the task (and the extent to which these emotions affect the completing of the task). Since it is well-established that AMD negatively affects mental health (e.g., anxiety, depression; Williams et al., 1998; Bennion et al., 2012; Cimarolli et al., 2015; Taylor et al., 2016), future studies could examine additional psychological metrics on top of behavioral measures. Although, researchers would need to interpret these findings with caution as the psychological profile of a person experiencing AMD under a short-term simulation may never replicate a patient who lives with AMD every day. Finally, a person with chronic AMD may develop compensatory strategies such as eccentric fixation and preferred retinal locus. As mentioned, these have not been assessed in the 19 studies examined. But repeating ADL performance with AMD simulations may allow further study on these compensatory mechanisms.

CONCLUSION

In summary, simulation studies can initiate and complement research into ADL for AMD in a controlled manner. But it is critical to be aware that all simulations have limitations, and none can completely replicate the visual impairments experienced by people living with AMD. As discussed, this is a potential problem when simulations are utilized for economic evaluations. However, for some experimental studies, a simulation that underestimates the true effects of vision loss may not necessarily render the entire simulation useless. For example, if a simulation that underestimates AMD severity can still cause participants to struggle completing an ADL, it suggests that the ADL is likely to be even more difficult for a person with AMD. The use of a specific simulation method will always depend on the nature of the study and ADL under investigation. It can be that some tasks lend themselves to simulation glasses (e.g., wayfinding) whilst others to computer-based gaze-contingent scotomas (e.g., reading). Therefore, the choice of simulation should be considered with the constraints of an experiment task in mind. Accordingly, the validation approach then needs to be suitable for the type of simulation method. A combination of clinical techniques and feedback from AMD patients may be needed to ensure that simulations are as realistic as possible. Regarding adaptation, this field of research would benefit from clear guidelines about what is a reasonable length of time and training type needed to acclimate to vision impairment simulations. Future studies could address this by examining the consistency or progression of task performance after varying adaptation lengths and forms.

AUTHOR CONTRIBUTIONS

AM and TL conceptualized the review. AM and DS completed the screening and quality assessment. AM wrote the first draft of the manuscript. AM, CC, VS, DS, and TL contributed to subsequent drafting and the final version of the manuscript. All authors contributed to the article and approved the submitted version.

REFERENCES

Acton, J. H., Gibson, J. M., and Cubbidge, R. P. (2012). Quantification of visual field loss in age-related macular degeneration. *PLoS ONE* 7:e39944. doi: 10.1371/journal.pone.0039944

Aguilar, C., and Castet, E. (2017). Evaluation of a gaze-controlled vision enhancement system for reading in visually impaired people. *PLoS ONE* 12:e0174910. doi: 10.1371/journal.pone.0174910

Almutleb, E. S., and Hassan, S. E. (2020). The effect of simulated central field loss on street-crossing decision-making in young adult pedestrians. *Optom. Vis. Sci.* 97, 229–238. doi: 10.1097/OPX.0000000000001502

Barraza-Bernal, M. J., Rifai, K., and Wahl, S. (2017). A preferred retinal location of fixation can be induced when systematic stimulus relocations are applied. *J. Vis.* 17:11. doi: 10.1167/17.2.11

Barraza-Bernal, M. J., Rifai, K., and Wahl, S. (2018). The retinal locus of fixation in simulations of progressing central scotomas. *J. Vis.* 18:7. doi: 10.1167/18.1.7

Bennion, A. E., Shaw, R. L., and Gibson, J. M. (2012). What do we know about the experience of age related macular degeneration? A systematic review and meta-synthesis of qualitative research. *Soc. Sci. Med.* 75, 976–985. doi: 10.1016/j.socscimed.2012.04.023

Bernard, J. B., Aguilar, C., and Castet, E. (2016). A new font, specifically designed for peripheral vision, improves peripheral letter and word recognition, but not eye-mediated reading performance. *PLoS ONE* 11:e0152506. doi: 10.1371/journal.pone.0152506

Bernard, J. B., Scherlen, A. C., and Castet, E. (2007). Page mode reading with simulated scotomas: a modest effect of interline spacing on reading speed. *Vis. Res.* 47, 3447–3459. doi: 10.1016/j.visres.2007.10.005

Broadhead, G. K., Hong, T., Grigg, J. R., McCluskey, P., Schlub, T. E., Spooner, K., et al. (2020). Does functional assessment predict everyday visual functioning? Visual function testing and quality of life in mild/moderate age-related macular degeneration. *Int. Ophthalmol.* 40, 3241–3249. doi: 10.1007/s10792-020-01508-z

Brunnström, G., Sörensen, S., Alsterstad, K., and Sjöstrand, J. (2004). Quality of light and quality of life–the effect of lighting adaptation among people with low vision. *Ophthalmic. Physiol. Opt.* 24, 274–280. doi: 10.1111/j.1475-1313.2004.00192.x

Bunn, W., and Terpstra, J. (2009). Cultivating empathy for the mentally ill using simulated auditory hallucinations. *Acad. Psychiatry* 33, 457–460. doi: 10.1176/appi.ap.33.6.457

Butt, T., Crossland, M. D., West, P., Orr, S. W., and Rubin, G. S. (2015). Simulation contact lenses for AMD health state utility values in NICE appraisals: a different reality. *Br. J. Ophthalmol.* 99, 540–544. doi: 10.1136/bjophthalmol-2014-305802

Cimarolli, V. R., Casten, R. J., Rovner, B. W., Heyl, V., Sörensen, S., and Horowitz, A. (2015). Anxiety and depression in patients with advanced macular degeneration: current perspectives. *Clin. Ophthalmol.* 10, 55–63. doi: 10.2147/OPTH.S80489

Connect Solutions Group (2020). *Sim Specs*. Connect Design. Available online at: https://connecttodesign.co.uk/sim-specs/ (accessed July 17, 2020).

Copolillo, A., Christopher, A., and Lyons, A. (2017). Effects of simulated low vision on postural adjustment to changes in center of mass in older adults. *Occup. Ther. Health. Care* 31, 115–125. doi: 10.1080/07380577.2016.1278295

Costela, F. M., Reeves, S. M., and Woods, R. L. (2020). Orientation of the preferred retinal locus (PRL) is maintained following changes in simulated scotoma size. *J. Vis.* 20:25. doi: 10.1167/jov.20.7.25

Court, H., McLean, G., Guthrie, B., Mercer, S. W., and Smith, D. J. (2014). Visual impairment is associated with physical and mental comorbidities in older adults: a cross-sectional study. *BMC. Med.* 12:181. doi: 10.1186/s12916-014-0181-7

Covidence Systematic Review Software (2020). *Veritas Health Innovation*. Melbourne, VIC. Available online at: https://www.covidence.org (accessed September 25, 2020).

Crabb, D. P., Smith, N. D., Glen, F. C., Burton, R., and Garway-Heath, D. F. (2013). How does glaucoma look? Patient perception of visual field loss. *Ophthalmology* 120, 1120–1126. doi: 10.1016/j.ophtha.2012.11.043

Culham, L. E., Chabra, A., and Rubin, G. S. (2004). Clinical performance of electronic, head-mounted, low-vision devices. *Ophthalmic. Physiol. Opt.* 24, 281–290. doi: 10.1111/j.1475-1313.2004.00193.x

Czoski-Murray, C., Carlton, J., Brazier, J., Young, T., Papo, N. L., and Kang, H. K. (2009). Valuing condition-specific health states using simulation contact lenses. *Val. Health* 12, 793–799. doi: 10.1111/j.1524-4733.2009.00527.x

de Boer, M. J., Jürgens, T., Cornelissen, F. W., and Başkent, D. (2021). Degraded visual and auditory input individually impair audiovisual emotion recognition from speech-like stimuli, but no evidence for an exacerbated effect from combined degradation. *Vis. Res.* 180, 51–62. doi: 10.1016/j.visres.2020.12.002

de Haan, G. A., Tucha, O., and Heutink, J. (2020). Effects of low visual acuity on neuropsychological test scores: a simulation study. *Clin. Neuropsychol.* 34, 140–157. doi: 10.1080/13854046.2019.1596315

Dean, S., Mathers, J. M., Calvert, M., Kyte, D. G., Conroy, D., Folkard, A., et al. (2017). "The patient is speaking": discovering the patient voice in ophthalmology. *Br. J. Ophthalmol.* 101, 700–708. doi: 10.1136/bjophthalmol-2016-309955

Deemer, A. D., Swenor, B. K., Fujiwara, K., Deremeik, J. T., Ross, N. C., Natale, D. M., et al. (2019). Preliminary evaluation of two digital image processing strategies for head-mounted magnification for low vision patients. *Transl. Vis. Sci. Technol.* 8 23. doi: 10.1167/tvst.8.1.23

Denniss, J., and Astle, A. T. (2018). Modified images reflecting effects of age-related macular degeneration on perception of everyday scenes. *Clin. Exp. Optom.* 101, 686–691. doi: 10.1111/cxo.12672

Desrosiers, J., Wanet-Defalque, M. C., Témisjian, K., Gresset, J., Dubois, M. F., Renaud, J., et al. (2009). Participation in daily activities and social roles of older adults with visual impairment. *Disabil. Rehabil.* 31, 1227–1234. doi: 10.1080/09638280802532456

Dyer, E., Swartzlander, B. J., and Gugliucci, M. R. (2018). Using virtual reality in medical education to teach empathy. *J. Med. Libr. Assoc.* 106, 498–500. doi: 10.5195/jmla.2018.518

Foster, R. J., Hotchkiss, J., Buckley, J. G., and Elliott, D. B. (2014). Safety on stairs: influence of a tread edge highlighter and its position. *Exp. Gerontol.* 55, 152–158. doi: 10.1016/j.exger.2014.04.009

Geringswald, F., Baumgartner, F. J., and Pollmann, S. (2013). A behavioral task for the validation of a gaze-contingent simulated scotoma. *Behav. Res. Methods* 45, 1313–1321. doi: 10.3758/s13428-013-0321-6

Gupta, A., Mesik, J., Engel, S. A., Smith, R., Schatza, M., Calabrese, A., et al. (2018). Beneficial effects of spatial remapping for reading with simulated central field loss. *Invest. Ophthalmol. Vis. Sci.* 59, 1105–1112. doi: 10.1167/iovs.16-21404

Hamade, N., Hodge, W. G., Rakibuz-Zaman, M., and Malvankar-Mehta, M. S. (2016). The effects of low-vision rehabilitation on reading speed and depression in age related macular degeneration: a meta-analysis. *PLoS ONE* 11:e0159254. doi: 10.1371/journal.pone.0159254

Ho, E., Boffa, J., and Palanker, D. (2019). Performance of complex visual tasks using simulated prosthetic vision via augmented-reality glasses. *J. Vis.* 19:22. doi: 10.1167/19.13.22

Hooper, P., Jutai, J. W., Strong, G., and Russell-Minda, E. (2008). Age-related macular degeneration and low-vision rehabilitation: a systematic review. *Can. J. Ophthalmol.* 43, 180–187. doi: 10.3129/i08-001

Hwang, A. D., Tuccar-Burak, M., Goldstein, R., and Peli, E. (2018). Impact of oncoming headlight glare with cataracts: a pilot study. *Front. Psychol.* 9:164. doi: 10.3389/fpsyg.2018.00164

Irons, J., McKone, E., Dumbleton, R., Barnes, N., He, X., Provis, J., et al. (2014). A new theoretical approach to improving face recognition in disorders of central vision: face caricaturing. *J. Vis.* 14:12. doi: 10.1167/14.2.12

Jelin, E., Wisløff, T., Jørstad, Ø. K., Heiberg, T., and Moe, M. C. (2019). Patient-reported outcome measures in the management of neovascular age-related macular degeneration: a 1-year prospective study. *BMJ. Open. Ophthalmol.* 4:e000353. doi: 10.1136/bmjophth-2019-000353

Jin, B., Ai, Z., and Rasmussen, M. (2005). Simulation of eye disease in virtual reality. *Conf. Proc. IEEE. Eng. Med. Biol. Soc.* 2005, 5128–5131. doi: 10.1109/IEMBS.2005.1615631

Jonas, J. B., Cheung, C. M. G., and Panda-Jonas, S. (2017). Updates on the epidemiology of age-related macular degeneration. *Asia. Pac. J. Ophthalmol.* 6, 493–497. doi: 10.22608/APO.2017251

Jones, P. R., Somoskeöy, T., Chow-Wing-Bom, H., and Crabb, D. P. (2020). Seeing other perspectives: evaluating the use of virtual and augmented reality to simulate visual impairments (OpenVisSim). *NPJ. Digit. Med.* 3:32. doi: 10.1038/s41746-020-0242-6

Juniat, V., Bourkiza, R., Das, A., Das-Bhaumik, R., Founti, P., Yeo, C., et al. (2019). Understanding visual impairment and its impact on patients: a simulation-based training in undergraduate medical education. *J. Med. Educ. Curric Dev.* 6, 1–7. doi: 10.1177/2382120519843854

Klee, S., Link, D., Sinzinger, S., and Haueisen, J. (2018). Scotoma simulation in healthy subjects. *Optom. Vis. Sci.* 95, 1120–1128. doi: 10.1097/OPX.0000000000001310

Kourtesis, P., Collina, S., Doumas, L. A. A., and MacPherson, S. E. (2019). Technological competence is a pre-condition for effective implementation of virtual reality head mounted displays in human neuroscience: a technological review and meta-analysis. *Front. Hum. Neurosci.* 13:342. doi: 10.3389/fnhum.2019.00342

Krishnan, A. K., and Bedell, H. E. (2018). Functional changes at the preferred retinal locus in subjects with bilateral central vision loss. *Graefes Arch. Clin. Exp. Ophthalmol.* 256, 29–37. doi: 10.1007/s00417-017-3818-3

Krishnan, A. K., Queener, H. M., Stevenson, S. B., Benoit, J. S., and Bedell, H. E. (2019). Impact of simulated micro-scotomas on reading performance in central and peripheral retina. *Exp. Eye Res.* 183, 9–19. doi: 10.1016/j.exer.2018.06.027

Kuriakose, R. K., Khan, Z., Almeida, D. R. P., and Braich, P. S. (2017). Depression and burden among the caregivers of visually impaired patients: a systematic review. *Int. Ophthalmol.* 37, 767–777. doi: 10.1007/s10792-016-0296-2

Kwon, M., Nandy, A. S., and Tjan, B. S. (2013). Rapid and persistent adaptability of human oculomotor control in response to simulated central vision loss. *Curr. Biol.* 23, 1663–1669. doi: 10.1016/j.cub.2013.06.056

Kwon, M., Ramachandra, C., Satgunam, P., Mel, B. W., Peli, E., and Tjan, B. S. (2012). Contour enhancement benefits older adults with simulated central field loss. *Optom. Vis. Sci.* 89, 1374–1384. doi: 10.1097/OPX.0b013e3182678e52

Lane, J., Robbins, R. A., Rohan, E. M. F., Crookes, K., Essex, R. W., Maddess, T., et al. (2019). Caricaturing can improve facial expression recognition in low-resolution images and age-related macular degeneration. *J. Vis.* 19:18. doi: 10.1167/19.6.18

Lehsing, C., Ruch, F., Kölsch, F. M., Dyszak, G. N., Haag, C., Feldstein, I. T., et al. (2019). Effects of simulated mild vision loss on gaze, driving and interaction behaviors in pedestrian crossing situations. *Accid. Anal. Prev.* 125, 138–151. doi: 10.1016/j.aap.2019.01.026

Lorenzini, M. C., Hämäläinen, A. M., and Wittich, W. (2019). Factors related to the use of a head-mounted display for individuals with low vision. *Disabil. Rehabil.* 1–15. doi: 10.1080/09638288.2019.1704892

Macedo, A. F., Crossland, M. D., and Rubin, G. S. (2008). The effect of retinal image slip on peripheral visual acuity. *J. Vis.* 8, 1–11. doi: 10.1167/8.14.16

Maniglia, M., Jogin, R., Visscher, K. M., and Seitz, A. R. (2020). We don't all look the same; detailed examination of peripheral looking strategies after simulated central vision loss. *J. Vis.* 20:5. doi: 10.1167/jov.20.13.5

Marmor, D. J., and Marmor, M. F. (2010). Simulating vision with and without macular disease. *Arch. Ophthalmol.* 128, 117–125. doi: 10.1001/archophthalmol.2009.366

McKone, E., Robbins, R. A., He, X., and Barnes, N. (2018). Caricaturing faces to improve identity recognition in low vision simulations: how effective is current-generation automatic assignment of landmark points?. *PLoS ONE* 13:e0204361. doi: 10.1371/journal.pone.0204361

Morrice, E., Johnson, A. P., Marinier, J. A., and Wittich, W. (2017). Assessment of the Apple iPad as a low-vision reading aid. *Eye* 31, 865–871. doi: 10.1038/eye.2016.309

Pacific Vision Foundation (1999). *GUIDE for the Evaluation of VISUAL Impairment.* Available online at: http://pp.centramerica.com/pp/bancofotos/328-6099.pdf (accessed April 15, 2021).

Phipps, J. A., Dang, T. M., Vingrys, A. J., and Guymer, R. H. (2004). Flicker perimetry losses in age-related macular degeneration. *Invest. Ophthalmol. Vis. Sci.* 45, 3355–3360. doi: 10.1167/iovs.04-0253

Prahalad, K. S., and Coates, D. R. (2020). Asymmetries of reading eye movements in simulated central vision loss. *Vis. Res.* 171, 1–10. doi: 10.1016/j.visres.2020.03.006

Rai, P., Rohatgi, J., and Dhaliwal, U. (2019). Coping strategy in persons with low vision or blindness - an exploratory study. *Indian J. Ophthalmol.* 67, 669–676. doi: 10.4103/ijo.IJO_1655_18

Riazi, A., Boon, M. Y., Dain, S. J., and Bridge, C. (2013). Coping strategies may not be reflected by simulated performance-based measures of functional ability [Las estrategias de defensa podrían no estar reflejadas por las mediciones basadas en la ejecución simulada de la capacidad funcional]. *J. Optom.* 6, 101–108. doi: 10.1016/j.optom.2012.08.001

Robertson, D. M., and Cavanagh, H. D. (2008). The clinical and cellular basis of contact lens-related corneal infections: a review. *Clin. Ophthalmol.* 2, 907–917. doi: 10.2147/opth.s3249

Rousek, J. B., and Hallbeck, M. S. (2011). The use of simulated visual impairment to identify hospital design elements that contribute to wayfinding difficulties. *Int. J. Ind. Ergon.* 41, 447–458. doi: 10.1016/j.ergon.2011.05.002

Saredakis, D., Szpak, A., Birckhead, B., Keage, H. A. D., Rizzo, A., and Loetscher, T. (2020). Factors associated with virtual reality sickness in head-mounted displays: a systematic review and meta-analysis. *Front. Hum. Neurosci.* 14:96. doi: 10.3389/fnhum.2020.00096

Schinazi, V. R., Thrash, T., and Chebat, D. R. (2016). Spatial navigation by congenitally blind individuals. *Wiley Interdiscip. Rev. Cogn. Sci.* 7, 37–58. doi: 10.1002/wcs.1375

Scilley, K., Jackson, G. R., Cideciyan, A. V., Maguire, M. G., Jacobson, S. G., and Owsley, C. (2002). Early age-related maculopathy and self-reported visual difficulty in daily life. *Ophthalmology* 109, 1235–1242. doi: 10.1016/s0161-6420(02)01060-6

Silverman, A. M. (2015). The perils of playing blind: problems with blindness simulation and a better way to teach about blindness. *J. Blind. Innov. Res.* 5. doi: 10.5241/5-81

Taylor, D. J., Edwards, L. A., Binns, A. M., and Crabb, D. P. (2018a). Seeing it differently: self-reported description of vision loss in dry age-related macular degeneration. *Ophthalmic. Physiol. Opt.* 38, 98–105. doi: 10.1111/opo.12419

Taylor, D. J., Hobby, A. E., Binns, A. M., and Crabb, D. P. (2016). How does age-related macular degeneration affect real-world visual ability and quality of life? A systematic review. *BMJ Open.* 6:e011504. doi: 10.1136/bmjopen-2016-011504

Taylor, D. J., Smith, N. D., Binns, A. M., and Crabb, D. P. (2018b). The effect of non-neovascular age-related macular degeneration on face recognition performance. *Graefes Arch. Clin. Exp. Ophthalmol.* 256, 815–821. doi: 10.1007/s00417-017-3879-3

Tsapakis, S., Papaconstantinou, D., Diagourtas, A., Droutsas, K., Andreanos, K., Moschos, M. M., et al. (2017). Visual field examination method using virtual reality glasses compared with the Humphrey perimeter. *Clin. Ophthalmol.* 11, 1431–1443. doi: 10.2147/OPTH.S131160

Tufanaru, C., Munn, Z., Aromataris, E., Campbell, J., and Hopp, L. (2020). "Chapter 3: systematic reviews of effectiveness," in *JBI Manual for Evidence Synthesis*, eds E. Aromataris and Z. Munn (JBI). Available online at: https://synthesismanual.jbi.global

Varadaraj, V., Lesche, S., Ramulu, P. Y., and Swenor, B. K. (2018). Reading speed and reading comprehension in age-related macular degeneration. *Am. J. Ophthalmol.* 186, 138–143. doi: 10.1016/j.ajo.2017.11.026

Velez-Montoya, R., Oliver, S. C., Olson, J. L., Fine, S. L., Quiroz-Mercado, H., and Mandava, N. (2014). Current knowledge and trends in age-related macular degeneration: genetics, epidemiology, and prevention. *Retina* 34, 423–441. doi: 10.1097/IAE.0000000000000036

Walker, J. G., Anstey, K. J., and Lord, S. R. (2006). Psychological distress and visual functioning in relation to vision-related disability in older individuals with cataracts. *Br. J. Health. Psychol.* 11, 303–317. doi: 10.1348/135910705X68681

Walsh, D. V., and Liu, L. (2014). Adaptation to a simulated central scotoma during visual search training. *Vis. Res.* 96, 75–86. doi: 10.1016/j.visres.2014.01.005

Wensveen, J. M., Bedell, H. E., and Loshin, D. S. (1995). Reading rates with artificial central scotomata with and without spatial remapping of print. *Optom. Vis. Sci.* 72, 100–114. doi: 10.1097/00006324-199502000-00009

Williams, R. A., Brody, B. L., Thomas, R. G., Kaplan, R. M., and Brown, S. I. (1998). The psychosocial impact of macular degeneration. *Arch. Ophthalmol.* 116, 514–520. doi: 10.1001/archopht.116.4.514

Wittich, W., Lorenzini, M. C., Markowitz, S. N., Tolentino, M., Gartner, S. A., Goldstein, J. E., et al. (2018). The effect of a head-mounted low vision device on visual function. *Optom. Vis. Sci.* 95, 774–784. doi: 10.1097/OPX.0000000000001262

Wong, W. L., Su, X., Li, X., Cheung, C. M. G., Klein, R., Cheng, C. Y., et al. (2014). Global prevalence of age-related macular degeneration and disease burden projection for 2020 and 2040: a systematic review and meta-analysis. *Lancet. Glob. Health* 2, e106–e116. doi: 10.1016/S2214-109X(13)70145-1

Wood, J., Chaparro, A., Anstey, K., Lacherez, P., Chidgey, A., Eisemann, J., et al. (2010). Simulated visual impairment leads to cognitive slowing in older adults. *Optom. Vis. Sci.* 87, 1037–1043. doi: 10.1097/OPX.0b013e3181fe64d7

Wood, J. M., Tyrrell, R. A., Chaparro, A., Marszalek, R. P., Carberry, T. P., and Chu, B. S. (2012). Even moderate visual impairments degrade drivers' ability to see pedestrians at night. *Invest. Ophthalmol. Vis. Sci.* 53, 2586–2592. doi: 10.1167/iovs.11-9083

Wroblewski, D., Francis, B. A., Sadun, A., Vakili, G., and Chopra, V. (2014). Testing of visual field with virtual reality goggles in manual and visual grasp modes. *Biomed. Res. Int.* 2014:206082. doi: 10.1155/2014/206082

Wu, H., Ashmead, D. H., Adams, H., and Bodenheimer, B. (2018). Using virtual reality to assess the street crossing behavior of pedestrians with simulated macular degeneration at a roundabout. *Front. ICT* 5:27. doi: 10.3389/fict.2018.00027

Zagar, M., and Baggarly, S. (2010). Low vision simulator goggles in pharmacy education. *Am. J. Pharm. Educ.* 74:83. doi: 10.5688/aj740583

Zult, T., Smith, L., Stringer, C., and Pardhan, S. (2020). Levels of self-reported and objective physical activity in individuals with age-related macular degeneration. *BMC Public Health* 20:1144. doi: 10.1186/s12889-020-09255-7

5

Documentation of the Development of Various Visuomotor Responses in Typically Reared Kittens and those Reared with Early Selected Visual Exposure by use of a New Procedure

Katelyn MacNeill[†], Amber Myatt, Kevin R. Duffy and Donald E. Mitchell[*]

Department of Psychology and Neuroscience, Dalhousie University, Halifax, NS, Canada

***Correspondence:**
Donald E. Mitchell
d.e.mitchell@dal.ca*

A new procedure was used to study the development of gaze (responses to moving targets or laser spots in normal kittens, those that had been reared in total darkness to 6 weeks of age, and others that received a period of monocular deprivation (MD). Gaze responses were observed to all stimuli in normal kittens at between 25–30 days of age and striking responses occurred on the same day or the next. Despite slow acquisition of spatial vision in the dark reared kittens over 3 months, they were able to follow and even strike at moving visual stimuli within a day of their initial exposure to light. By contrast, for a week following a period of MD, kittens showed no gaze or striking responses to moving stimuli when using their previously deprived eye. The very different profiles of acquisition of visuomotor skills and spatial vision in visually deprived kittens point to a dissociation between the neuronal populations that support these functions.

Keywords: visual deprivation, gaze, following, striking, visuomotor, visual acuity, vision

INTRODUCTION

Discovery of the widespread anatomical and physiological changes observed in the central visual pathways of kittens and monkeys that had received abnormal visual exposure in early postnatal life led naturally to many studies of the consequences for visual function. For the most part, the focus of these studies was placed on the consequences of early selected visual deprivation for visual perceptual abilities linked primarily to neural functioning of the geniculostriate visual pathway. Possible consequences of early visual deprivation for visuomotor behavior received far less attention. Early studies of the effects of monocular and binocular visual deprivation in kittens (Wiesel and Hubel, 1963, 1965) remarked upon the severe consequences for general visuomotor behavior but two later studies (Van Hof-Van Duin, 1976; Vital-Durand et al., 1976) reported that cats reared for extended periods from birth in total darkness to at least 4 months of age were able to move their gaze (combined head and eye movement) to follow moving objects within a day or so. This result was particularly surprising because the dark-reared cats appeared otherwise totally blind in terms of their general behavior. By contrast, assessment of spatial vision such as captured by measurement of visual acuity revealed a very slow recovery that is measured in months and is proportional to the length of prior visual deprivation (Timney et al., 1978; Mitchell, 1988).

In this study we deployed a new method to test longitudinally the development of various visuomotor abilities in normal kittens as well as the recovery of such abilities in kittens dark reared from birth to 6 weeks of age. Preliminary observations were also made on kittens following a period of early monocular deprivation. As with techniques devised to monitor fast changes in spatial vision in normal or selectively visually deprived kittens during development (Mitchell et al., 1976, 1977), methods to monitor longitudinal changes in visuomotor abilities must require little training to be effective. Many existing methods to monitor visually guided behavior frequently require months of training (e.g., Fabre-Thorpe et al., 1984). The method employed here was informed by observations and methodologies that are in widespread use for behavioral studies of rodents (Walsh and Cummings, 1976). In addition to providing new information of the development of following and striking responses to moving solid objects and laser spots in normal kittens, we confirmed and extended previous reports of the fast emergence of gaze responses in dark- reared kittens following their initial exposure to light at a time when tests of visual acuity on the jumping stand indicated that they had no spatial vision. By contrast, following a much shorter period of monocular deprivation, no gaze responses were observed for at least a week following the period of deprivation when the kittens used their previously deprived eye.

MATERIALS AND METHODS

Subjects

Four purpose-bred litters of kittens (*Felis domestica*) from a cat-breeding colony at Dalhousie University served as subjects for this study. The rearing history of all 10 animals is summarized in **Table 1**. The Dalhousie Committee on Laboratory Animals, in accordance with regulations of the Canadian Council on Animal Care, approved the breeding, rearing and behavioral testing protocols employed for this study. Five kittens from the first litter were assigned to two rearing conditions, a group of 3 kittens that were dark-reared to 6 weeks of age (C114, C115, and C116) and two others that received daily periods of exposure to light (C117 and C118). The latter kittens wore collars around their neck so that from P10 they could be identified in the darkroom and removed with their mother into an illuminated room for 1 h each day over a week. At P17 the daily period of light exposure for these kittens was increased gradually to 2 h and at P33 was increased to 3 h. At 6 weeks, all littermates, including the 3 kittens that hitherto had been dark-reared, were moved permanently with their mother to a regular colony room that was illuminated on a 12:12 h light/dark cycle. The second litter yielded only a single kitten (C119) that was reared with its mother under normal colony lighting conditions from the day of birth. A third litter of 3 kittens born in 2010 was dark-reared from birth to 6 weeks of age and provided data on the recovery of visual acuity with subsequent exposure to light. The remaining data for this paper was obtained from two kittens (C479 and C480) from a litter of 5 born in 2020. These two kittens were reared normally until P30 at which age they received a 3 week period of monocular deprivation by eyelid suture that was followed by either a 7 day period of binocular exposure (C479) or a 10 day period of reverse occlusion (C480). Both kittens were then employed in a separate electrophysiological study.

TABLE 1 | Information concerning the litter composition, gender and rearing history of the 11 animals of the study.

Animal ID.	Gender	Visual experience
Litter 1		
C114	F	DR: P0-P42; LR P42-
C115	F	DR: P0-P42; LR P42-
C116	M	DR: P0-P42; LR P42-
C117	M	DR to P10 then LR 1 h/day P11-17, LR 2 h/day P17-33, LR 3 h/day P33-42
C118.	M	DR to P10 then LR 1 h/day P11-17, LR 2 h/day P17-33, LR 3 h/day P33-42
Litter 2		
C119	M	LR from birth
Litter 3		
C127	M	DR: P0-42
C128	M	DR: P0-P42
C129	M	DR: P0-P42
Litter 4		
C479	F	MD: P30-51; BV: P51-59
C480	F	MD: P31-52; RO P52-62

M, male; F, female; DR, Dark-reared; LR, light-reared; MD, monocular deprivation; BV, binocular visual input; RO, reverse occlusion; P, postnatal day.

Darkroom Facility and Colony Rooms

After being seen by a university veterinarian the first litter was placed within an hour of birth into a darkroom facility that has been described in detail elsewhere (Mitchell, 2013). The facility includes two large interconnected darkrooms, one of which contains a large rearing cage in which kittens and their mother were housed while the other darkroom allowed for cleaning of the first room and for the interchange of clean cages on a regular basis. Both darkrooms were accessed through a series of smaller dark anterooms and hallways separated by a series of entryways and doors. All walls and doors within the darkrooms, surrounding corridors and anterooms were painted black. A large rearing cage (93 cm high, 66.5 cm deep, and 153 cm wide) was used to contain the mother and her kittens. A litter box, dry food and water were available at all times, and cardboard boxes and towels were present for bedding. To entrain a daily circadian rhythm a radio was timed to turn on at 7 am and to turn off at 5 pm, an interval that coincided with the approximate work day of departmental animal care technicians. At 6 weeks of age, the mother and all kittens were relocated to a colony room illuminated with fluorescent lights on a 12:12-h light/dark cycle.

Behavioral Testing Arena

The arena, drawn in schematic fashion in **Figure 1**, was modeled on the design of those used widely for studies of locomotion in rodents and consisted of a robust plywood square enclosure (80 cm × 80 cm) with an open top. Three of the walls (B) were constructed of 1.6 cm thick plywood while the fourth wall (A) consisted of a translucent white plastic screen onto which laser

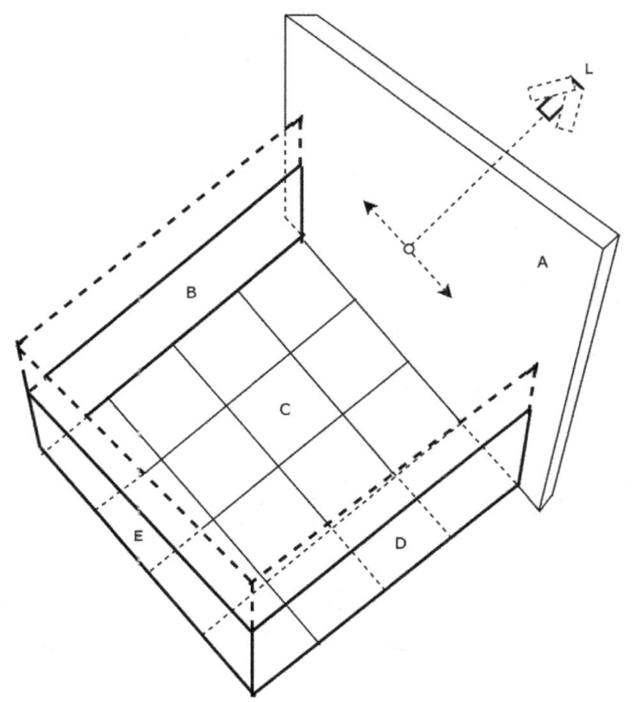

FIGURE 1 | The testing arena. Walls B and C are opaque while wall A is translucent plastic upon which a laser spot could be projected from a laser (L) mounted on a stepping motor and made to move under computer control (L).

light spots could be back-projected. For the youngest animals, the wooden walls were only 41 cm high, but as the animals grew and became more mobile, a second set of walls (shown by dashed lines) of the same dimensions were placed on top of the first to double the height to 82 cm. On the cardboard floor (C) of the enclosure a 4 × 4 grid of squares (20 cm × 20 cm) was drawn to allow quantification of the mobility of the animals. The overall mobility of the animals and their gaze responses to moving stimuli were captured by either a tripod mounted video camera (JVC Everio GZ-MG135) camcorder or more recently by a GoPro camera (G) clamped to one of the wooden walls. It was observed that some kittens followed or struck at a moving laser spot with greater frequency if it was projected onto the floor rather than onto the walls of the arena. Consequently, for these animals the arena was modified by replacing the opaque floor with translucent plastic and raising it above the floor so that the laser spot could be projected from below. In addition to use of a hand-held laser, a small laser and assorted electronic components that included a stepping motor were purchased from a toy store and were configured to be controlled by a Mac iBook in order to project a laser spot onto the translucent floor or wall of the arena. The laser spot could be made to move in either linear or sinusoidal fashion at various speeds along the translucent floor or wall of the arena in response to sawtooth or sinusoidal input signals to the stepping motor that controlled the laser. To introduce some unpredictability, the laser spot could be made to make sudden vertical steps during its horizontal motion. The photograph in **Figure 2** shows the computer-controlled laser and the laser spot projected onto the lower part of the translucent wall of the arena. Because of diffusion by the translucent plastic wall of the arena, the laser spot had an overall diameter of 5 mm with a central bright region that was 2 mm wide.

Behavioral Testing in the Arena

As pioneered with rodents, general locomotive behavior was assessed by counts of the number of gridlines on the floor crossed in a fixed amount of time. These measurements were initiated when kittens were 10–12 days old, at a time when their eyelids had been open for a week or less. With the exception of C479 and C480, all animals were video recorded in the arena for a period of 5 min in order to assess their spontaneous behavior. The video records were viewed later to permit numerical scoring of the number of times the kittens crossed the gridlines on the floor of the enclosure with any paw, the number of episodes of sleeping, sitting, play, grooming, crawling or escape attempts. From 25 to 30 days of age, kittens were placed in the arena for videotaped periods of exposure to moving stimuli that included two light spherical pendulums held on strings (one large 55 mm diameter hollow plastic ball that weighed 7 grams; and one small 28 mm diameter solid wooden ball that weighed 9 grams). In addition, responses were assessed to movement of light spots from either a hand-held laser or else the computer-controlled laser described that were shone on either the walls or floor of the arena. In order to assess the responses to more regular movement of a laser spot, a Mac iBook computer was programmed to control the movement of a small laser attached to a stepping motor (see **Figure 2**). The laser spot was projected onto the translucent screen (A, **Figure 1**) and moved horizontally at controlled speeds according to either a sinusoidal or sawtooth waveform. In order to introduce a degree of unpredictability to the horizontal path of the spot, it could be programmed to suddenly jump in a vertical direction by the superposition of a vertical sawtooth to the horizontal motion.

In response to moving stimuli, normal kittens at a certain age begin to follow the target by changes of gaze which refer to the coordinated head and eye movements that collectively alter the position of the visual axis (Guitton et al., 1984). Cats have a limited oculomotor range of only ± 25 deg, (Stryker and Blakemore, 1972; Guitton et al., 1980) so that gaze movements are often dominated by motion of the head. Analysis of the changes of gaze from analysis of the video records from the video or GoPro cameras that viewed the kittens from above allowed only for monitoring of changes in head position as a proxy for changes of gaze., Plots of the gaze following responses to the various moving stimuli were plotted from a frame by frame analysis of the video records by use of ImageJ software. Separate plots were made of the angular change of position of the stimulus object (pendulum or laser spot) and of the gaze responses with respect to a fixed reference point on the arena. For gaze responses rotation of the head was measured with respect to an imaginary line orthogonal to the line joining the two ears at its midpoint. The plots of gaze following responses were made independently a decade apart by two of the authors (AM and KM). The plots shown in **Figures 6, 7** were made by AM but were very similar

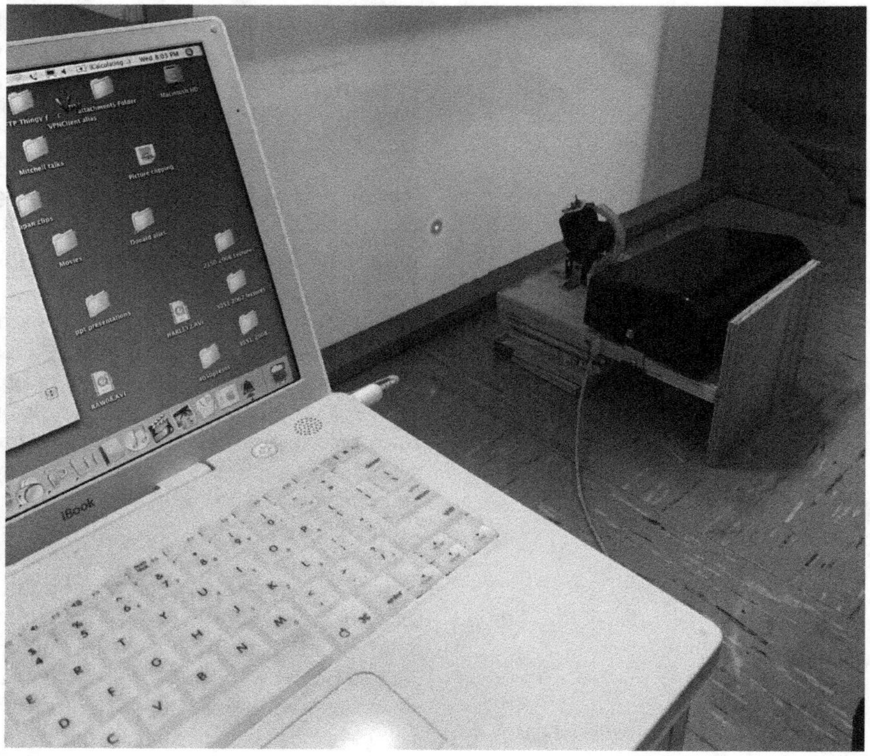

FIGURE 2 | A photograph of the set-up used to project moving laser spots on the wall or floor of the arena. Note the expanded diameter (5 mm) of the laser spot due to scatter by the translucent screen upon which it is projected.

to those made earlier by KM for different episodes of following responses for the same animal and day of light exposure.

The Jumping Stand

Emergence of spatial vision was documented in 5 of the 6 dark-reared kittens by use of a jumping stand and techniques developed and refined in this laboratory over the last 4 decades (Mitchell et al., 1976, 1977; Mitchell, 2013). Upon removal from the darkroom, kittens exhibited few signs of vision apart from those noted when they were tested in the arena. On the jumping stand they appeared blind as they were unable to discriminate an open door (platform) from an adjacent closed door (on which a large vertical square-wave grating with a period of 32 mm was placed) except by use of tactile cues such as use of their whiskers or paws. From a platform located only 1–2 cm above the divider that separated the open from the closed door they reached out very tentatively to either side in an attempt to locate a surface (the closed door) onto which they could step. Once the animals were able to jump onto the closed door from a few centimeters above it, an ability that we define operationally as an open door discrimination (OD) that may reflect only the ability to make discriminations on the basis of luminance, the kittens were tested formally for the ability to discriminate form information in the manner outlined in many previous papers but summarized by Mitchell (2013). This ability was assessed by closing the open door and placing a horizontal grating with the same period as the vertical grating on the adjacent door. Once the animal could jump correctly to the positive (vertical) grating, it was possible to test acuity by a combination of progressive increases in the spatial frequency of the gratings, and by raising the jumping height until discrimination was not possible. Because the animals had been housed in the darkroom since birth, there was no opportunity to familiarize or train the animals on the jumping stand before they were removed to an illuminated colony room at 6 weeks of age. Notwithstanding this delay in training and the slow emergence of visual guided behavior on the jumping stand, animals learned the essential discrimination task between a vertical and a horizontal grating within a day or two following the ability to detect a closed door (OD discrimination). All tests of vision were made binocularly.

RESULTS

Dark-Reared Animals

To set the stage for a description of the results from tests of mobility, visual following, and striking at moving objects, it is important to highlight the slow emergence of spatial vision in the 5 dark-reared animals from which measurements were made.

Development of Grating Visual Acuity

In earlier studies (Timney et al., 1978; Mitchell, 1988) of animals dark-reared for long periods (to 12 months of age) spatial vision was shown to emerge very slowly at a rate that decreased with the length of the deprivation and only in animals deprived to 4 months of age or less did the visual acuity achieve the level of typically reared adults. The results of longitudinal measurements of the acuity of 5 dark-reared animals upon emergence from the darkroom are displayed in **Figure 3**. Different colors are used to depict the data from animals from the two litters with blue used to represent data from C115 and C116 while data from the second litter are shown by orange symbols (C127-129). For 1–2 days after emerging from the dark, animals appeared blind (designated by the letter "B" in **Figure 3**) on the jumping stand because they appeared to employ only tactile cues such as reaching from one side or the other for the closed door with their paws to locate a closed from an adjacent open door on the jumping stand (Mitchell, 2013). The first indication that the kittens were able to locate the closed door by visual cues alone occurred after 1 (C128), 3 (C115, C116, and C129) or 5 (C127) days and was designated as an "open door" discrimination (OD) in **Figure 3**. The mean time (3 days) for this initial sign of vision to emerge on the jumping stand is consistent with data and predictions (5 days) based on an earlier study (Mitchell, 1988; Figure 7). Because this discrimination could in theory be solved by luminance cues alone, the operational indication of the acquisition of spatial vision was assumed to coincide with the ability to discriminate a vertical from a horizontal grating, a task passed on average 2.5 days later, or 5.5 days after animals were first exposed to light. Thereafter the acuity improved very gradually to stabilize at normal age-matched levels after 3 months in the light at about 4 1/2 months of age (**Figure 3**). Comparison of the time course of development of visual acuity in normal kittens (Giffin and Mitchell, 1978; Figure 2) permits an additional perspective to be placed on the slow improvement of the acuity of the dark-reared kittens. After a month in the light, when they were 10 weeks old, the latter kittens had achieved an average acuity of only 1.5 cycles/deg, or nearly one-quarter that of normal kittens of the same age.

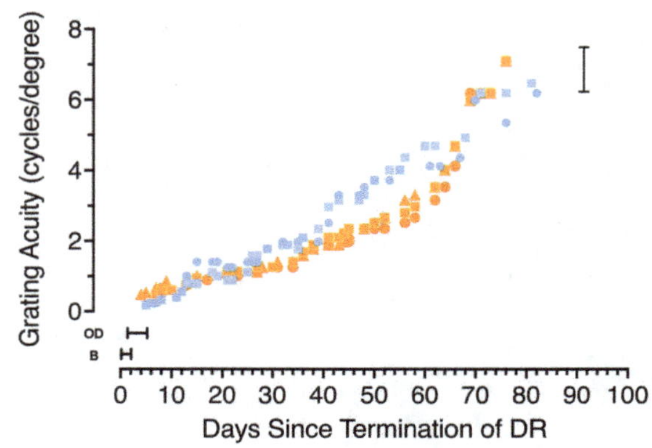

FIGURE 3 | The development of grating acuity in 5 kittens that were reared in total darkness (DR) from birth until 6 weeks of age. Data from the two kittens tested from the first litter are depicted with blue symbols (C115 circles, C116 squares) while orange symbols show data from the second litter (C127 squares, C128 circles and C129 triangles). Periods during which the kittens appeared blind on the jumping stand are indicated by the letter B, while the time during which they were capable of only the ability to discriminate an open from a closed door is indicated by then letters OD. The vertical bracket on the right indicates the range of acuities measured in normal kittens at an equivalent age.

Overall Motility

The mobility of kittens was assessed in terms of the number of line crossings made during a 5-min videotaped period in the arena. **Figure 4** shows the results of these measures for the 3 light-reared kittens and representative data from one (C116) of the dark-reared animals plotted as cumulative frequency distributions as is common in studies with rodents. All kittens began moving around the apparatus slowly and cautiously as a possible consequence of the novelty of the new environment. For more than a week the normal kittens crossed less than 5 lines in 5 min but at about 3 weeks of age. the number of lines crossed each day tripled for two animals who were littermates (C117, C118). By contrast, the activity of the third normal kitten (C119) from another litter was consistently lower and delayed by approximately a week in comparison to the data from the other two. In addition to its origin from another litter, C119 was exposed to light earlier (at birth) in comparison to the other two kittens. The rapid increase in locomotion exhibited by C117 and C118 suggest that this occurred despite their having received only 1–3 h of light exposure each day. Their mobility became more deliberate as they grew accustomed to the arena, at which point play behavior began. Kittens appeared to react to imaginary objects and struck at the lines drawn on the arena floor. By comparison, the dark-reared animals were immediately very active upon their initial exposure to light, although it is important to note that this exposure occurred at an older age (6 weeks). Daily line crossing data was collected from only one dark-reared animal but data from the first 3 days in the light for two others (C114, C115) was almost identical. The high overall motility of the dark-reared animals appeared to reflect their age rather than with the limited amount of light exposure they had received. Interestingly, the normal light-reared animal, C119, that received the greatest daily exposure to light, was less mobile than the other two light-exposed kittens, suggesting that only a short period of light exposure (1–3 h) per day in the period from P10 to P42 may be sufficient for kittens to develop a high degree of mobility.

Visuomotor Responses to Pendulums

Following Behavior

Visuomotor development was tested in terms of the response to pendulums of two different sizes held on nylon or regular strings and swung in front of the kitten's face. The behavior exhibited by kittens during the first 15 s of recorded attention to these stimuli was scored for the time they spent following the stimuli with their head and eyes (gaze), and the amount of time they attempted to strike at them. Only the first 15 s of this behavior was scored since the kittens appeared to engage with the stimuli in bursts of about this length. Cumulative following times (**Figure 5**, top) for the large pendulum as a function of age demonstrated that light-reared kittens began following pendulums at between 25 and 30 days of age, while dark-reared kittens followed either pendulum within a day of their initial exposure to light at 42 days

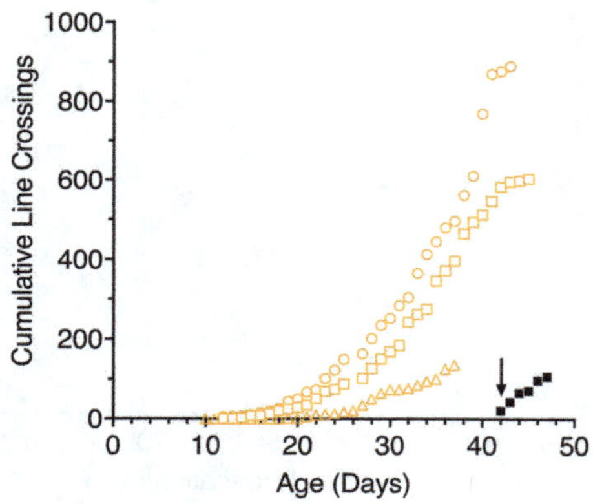

FIGURE 4 | Cumulative line crossings obtained from 5-min trials of 3 light-exposed (open orange symbols: C117 squares, C118 circles, C119 triangles) and a representative dark-reared kitten (C116, filled black symbols) as a function of age. The arrow indicates when the dark reared kitten was first exposed to an illuminated environment.

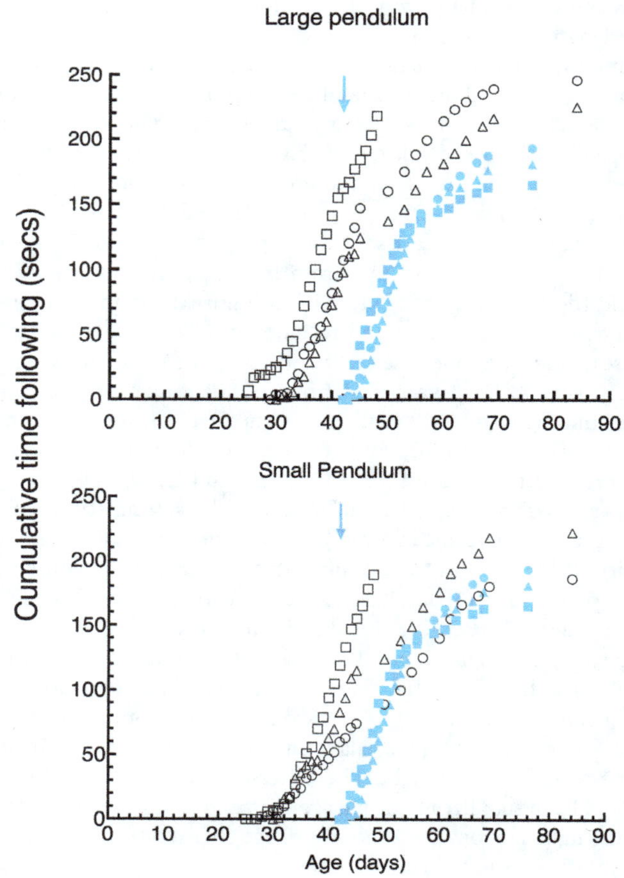

FIGURE 5 | Cumulative gaze- following behavior in daily 15 s episodes as a function of age for large (top) and small (bottom) pendulum swinging pendulums. Data are displayed for 3 light- exposed (open black symbols: C117 triangles, C118 circles, C119 squares) and 3 dark-reared (blue filled symbols: C114 triangles, C115 circles, C116 squares) kittens. The blue arrows indicate the age of the dark-reared kittens when they were first exposed to light.

of age. While the overall following behavior of the 3 light-reared animals was similar, the kitten that received the longest daily visual exposure (C119) began following the large pendulum earlier (by 4 days) than did the others. Interestingly, the initial responses of the 3 light-reared kittens to the small pendulum (**Figure 4**, bottom) began at the same age (at ~ 30 days of age). Thereafter the daily amount of gaze following increased rapidly in the next 10 days followed by a slower increase to reach an asymptote at about 70 days of age. Despite differences between the amount of daily light exposure received by the 3 light-reared kittens, the acquisition of gaze following behavior followed a closely similar path for all animals, a result that suggests that only short periods of light each day (1–3 h) was sufficient for normal development of following behavior.

Undoubtedly. the most remarkable result was the fast emergence of gaze following responses to the pendulums by the 3 dark-reared kittens that began in the first 2 days of exposure to light at a time when they exhibited no sign of spatial vision on the jumping stand (**Figure 3**) an ability that was not achieved for on average 5.5 days following their introduction to light. Furthermore, the subsequent pattern of following behavior was remarkably similar to the progression observed in light reared kittens following emergence of this behavior albeit at a younger age.

A more detailed description of the following behavior of the dark-reared kittens is provided by analysis of the accuracy of the gaze responses obtained through frame by frame analysis of the video records. Representative results from analysis of the video records of the gaze responses to motion of the large pendulum for one dark-reared kitten (C114) made on its second day in the light are shown in **Figure 6**. The blue symbols show plots of the gaze responses to motion of the pendulum which is indicated by the gray symbols. Even though following responses to the pendulum at that stage were quite infrequent, the few gaze responses that did occur were quite accurate in terms of their amplitude and speed, albeit with a slight temporal delay. Results from a littermate (C115) made after an extra day in the light are displayed in **Figure 7** and exhibit a somewhat longer delay and reduced amplitude of the gaze movements with respect to the motion of the pendulum. These following responses occurred at a time when C115 was designated as blind on the jumping stand. The following responses observed in the first few days in the light were somewhat variable as a possible reflection of fluctuation in the degree of engagement with the stimuli after several repetitions of the regular pendulum arc of motion.

Striking Behavior

Large variability was observed between the kittens in their striking behavior, especially for the large pendulum and one kitten (C115) responded only to the small pendulum. All kittens struck at the smaller pendulum first, possibly because they may have been intimidated by the larger one. Because of the much larger variability of striking observed among animals with the large pendulum, striking behavior of all kittens is displayed in

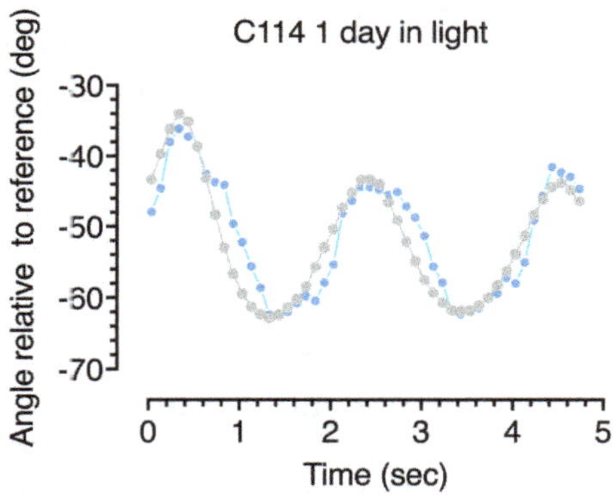

FIGURE 6 | Gaze following responses (blue symbols) to a swinging large pendulum (gray symbols) for a 6-week dark-reared kitten (C114) made on the second day of exposure to light.

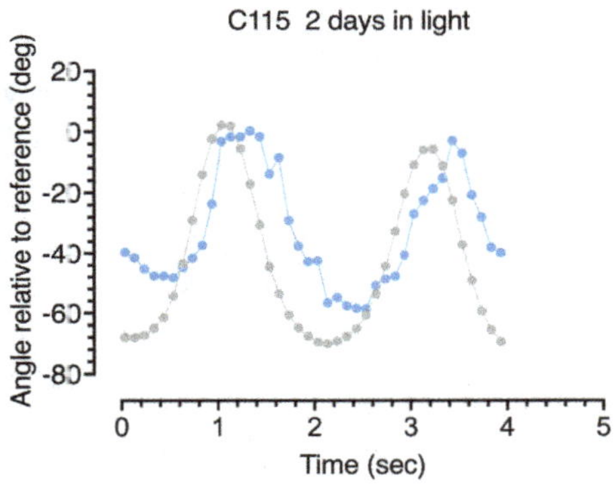

FIGURE 7 | Gaze following responses (blue symbols) to a swinging large pendulum (gray symbols) for a 6-week dark-reared kitten (C115) made on the third day of exposure to light.

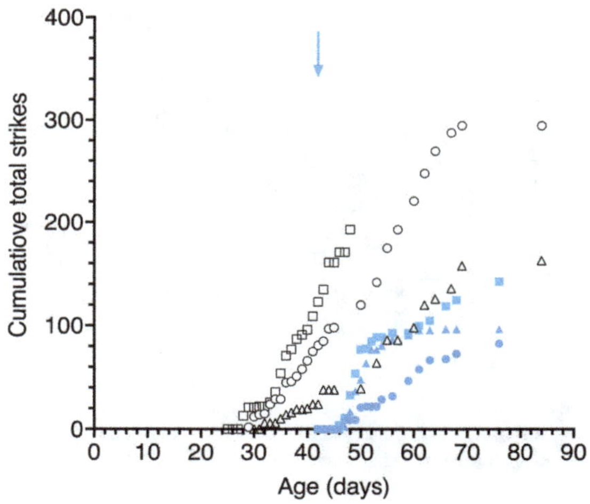

FIGURE 8 | Cumulative total strikes to the swinging small pendulum in daily 15 s episodes as a function of age. Data are displayed for 3 light- exposed (open black symbols: C117 triangles, C118 circles, C119 squares) and 3 dark-reared kittens (blue filled symbols: C114 triangles, C115 circles, C116 squares). The blue arrow indicates the age of the dark-reared kittens when they were first exposed to light.

Figure 8 for only the small pendulum. Although the dark-reared kittens followed the small pendulum after 1–3 days in the light, striking responses occurred on average 2 days later. Light reared kittens struck at the small pendulum on the same or the next day (C117) as their following responses were first observed.

Responses to Moving Laser Spots

Robust following gaze responses were observed to moving laser spots (**Figure 9**) with a similar time course of development as that observed with moving pendulums (**Figure 5**). However, a comparison of the ordinates of **Figure 9** with **Figure 5** reveals that all animals consistently followed pendulums for longer than laser spots, a possible reflection of a preference for following solid objects by kittens in the age-range tested. As with pendulums, the dark-reared animals followed moving laser spots almost immediately after exposure to light. Another consistent observation was that kittens preferred the movement of hand-held lasers as compared to spots moved under computer control. A likely explanation for this preference was the regularity of the linear or sinusoidal motion of the latter as opposed to the unpredictable movements of the hand-held laser.

With the exception of C118 for whom initial strikes to both stimuli occurred at the same age, all kittens stuck at moving laser spots 1 to 3 days earlier than they did at moving pendulums. This preference may arise from the small size of the laser spot (5 mm dia.) which may have made it less intimidating than even the moving solid small pendulum (28 mm dia.). Although detailed analysis of the trajectory and accuracy of the striking responses of the dark reared kittens to either laser spots or pendulums were not made because of the slow video frame rate employed, it was apparent that this merits further study as the nature of these responses changed with exposure to light. At first the striking responses were slow and tentative and appeared to be stereotypical as they appeared directed toward a target at a constant distance from the animal irrespective of its actual distance. These observations confirmed those made earlier by Vital-Durand et al. (1976).

Monocularly Deprived Animals

Preliminary observations were made on two kittens of their visuomotor responses to moving pendulums or laser spots in the days surrounding termination of a 3-week period of monocular deprivation that began at P30. Data on visual following and striking at the stimuli were collected in the first minute after the kitten was placed in the arena. Before termination of the period of MD, the visuomotor responses of both kittens reflected the ability of the non-deprived eye. However, after the period of MD, one animal (C480) was reverse occluded so that it was forced to exclusively employ its formerly deprived eye. By contrast, C479 had both eyes open after the period of MD so that tests of the visual abilities of the formerly deprived eye were made with a hard opaque contact lens placed on the cornea of the fellow eye (Mitchell, 1988). Whereas the kittens actively followed and struck

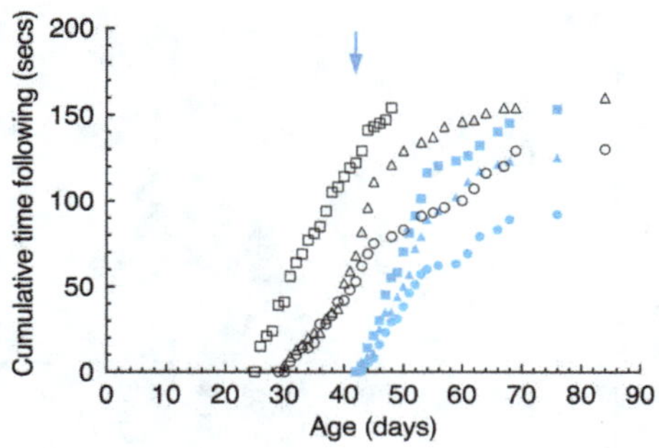

FIGURE 9 | Cumulative gaze following behavior of a moving laser spot in daily 15 s episodes as a function of age. Data are displayed for 3 light-exposed (open black symbols: C117 triangles, C118 circles, C119 squares) and 3 dark-reared kittens (blue filled symbols: C114 triangles, C115 circles, C116 squares). The blue arrow indicates the age of the dark-reared kittens when they were first introduced to light (at P42 days). The blue arrows indicate the age of the dark-reared kittens when they were first exposed to light.

at the pendulum for about 50 s of the 1 min of exposure to the moving pendulum using the non-deprived eye on the day before the end of the period of MD, in the next 6 days using the formerly deprived eye they only followed the pendulum if it was dragged across the floor of the arena to provide an auditory cue to its changing location. Once lifted above the floor, the kittens appeared unable to follow the pendulum at all. On the seventh day one kitten (C479) followed the pendulum for 5 s and struck at it 4 times when using the formerly deprived eye. Because these two kittens participated in another experiment it was not possible to follow any possible further recovery. This very preliminary result suggests that a 3-week period of monocular deprivation had a far greater impact on gaze following and striking than did a much longer period of dark-rearing.

DISCUSSION

This study was designed as a preliminary exploration of the use of a simple arena to allow longitudinal recording of changes in visuomotor behavior in normal kittens as well as in kittens that had experienced two forms of selected early visual deprivation. In addition to documenting increases in general locomotion in normal kittens from 10–12 days of age, changes in their reaction to visual stimuli in terms of gaze following and striking responses were studied from about 25 days of age. Normal kittens showed a regular increase in locomotion in the arena beginning at about 3 weeks of age, and approached an asymptotic level at about 6 weeks. Within the small sample there was evidence of considerable variability in both the onset and the rate of increase of motility. Dark reared kittens showed a high degree of motility on immediate introduction to light which the limited data suggested increased subsequently at a rate similar to that of normal kittens once they became mobile in the arena at about 3 weeks of age.

Several salient points emerged from studies of the responses of normal kittens to moving solid objects (pendulums) or laser spots. First, gaze following movements to the pendulums and to laser spots began at between 25 and 30 days of age followed by a rapid and steady increase to an asymptotic level at about 70 days. On any day, normal kittens followed pendulums for longer than for laser spots, indicating a possible preference for solid objects. Second, striking responses to pendulums with their paws began on or within a day of initiation of gaze responses. Kittens struck at the small pendulum more than they did to the large pendulum and one kittens did not strike at the latter at all. Third, striking responses to moving laser spots began either on the same day or as much as 3 days earlier than strikes to pendulums.

Study of the two groups of selectively visually deprived kittens in the arena revealed some important differences between the immediate consequences of the two forms of deprivation on visuomotor behavior. Whereas monocular deprivation had a profound effect on motility as well as on the following and striking responses to moving stimuli when kittens were forced to use their deprived eye, the consequences of a period of darkness (binocular visual deprivation) were far less. A very salient finding of this study was the almost immediate acquisition of gaze following movements of the head and eyes to moving stimuli of the dark-reared kittens on first exposure to light that were accompanied by an equally fast emergence of striking responses. The fast emergence of visuomotor responses stood in clear contrast to the very slow recovery of spatial acuity in the same animals over many months This divergence was especially apparent in the first few days after emergence from the darkroom at which time on the jumping stand kittens could only find a closed door by use of tactile cues and appeared incapable of jumping at all to a visual stimulus. For several more days, even after they were able to step or jump from a few centimeters above the stimuli, they were unable to discriminate a vertical from a horizontal grating suggesting that they may possess only the ability to make luminance discriminations. By contrast, gaze following behavior in the dark reared kittens was evident immediately upon exposure to light with a very similar time course to the maturation of such behavior in light-reared kittens once it began at 25–30 days of age, suggesting that the maturation of this behavior in dark-reared kittens was triggered immediately upon their introduction to light. A similar conclusion was reached by Van Hof-Van Duin (1976) on the basis of an array of different tests.

The rapid emergence of responses to moving stimuli in the dark-reared kittens suggests that neurons and pathways involved in the analysis of motion for visuomotor responses may mature fast and be partially or completely immune to disruption by early binocular visual deprivation. Evidence accumulated over decades (Schneider, 1969; Goodale and Milner, 1992) suggests that the analysis of motion and the execution of motor action toward stimuli in space are processed in a separate processing stream to that involved in the analysis of spatial form. In humans, non-human primates and cats (Lomber et al., 1996), these are identified, respectively, as the parietal and temporal cortical processing streams. In addition, initial orienting toward the visual stimuli and the gaze responses to their movement suggests involvement of the superior colliculus. Neural structures of the temporal visual pathway that are known to be involved in the analysis of fine spatial detail, are extremely vulnerable to disruption by early visual deprivation (Mitchell and Maurer, 2022) which would explain the more severe and protracted deficits in spatial acuity. Although less is known of the effects of visual deprivation on either the superior colliculus or the parietal processing stream in the cat, there is some evidence to suggest that the effects of deprivation may differ for the two cortical visual processing streams. For example, the profile of the sensitive period of vulnerability to the effects of early monocular deprivation in the cat lateral suprasylvian cortex is shorter than that for the visual cortex (Jones et al., 1984). In contrast to cells in the primary visual cortex, cells of the lateral suprasylvian cortex appear to be functionally specialized for motion processing and in general the development of the stimulus response properties of these cells begins earlier and proceeds faster than the stimulus selectivity of cells in the primary visual cortex (Price et al., 1988).

With respect to the profound effects of monocular deprivation on the visuomotor responses of C479 and C480, it has been known for some time that this form of deprivation exerts substantial effects on the response properties of cells in the superficial layers of the superior colliculus (Hoffmann and Sherman, 1974) and in addition, promotes substantial shifts of ocular dominance in the lateral suprasylvian cortex (Jones et al., 1984) to favor the non-deprived eye. Thus, the known effects of monocular deprivation on the superior colliculus and on the parietal visual pathway provide a ready explanation for the substantial loss of visuomotor responses when the monocularly deprived kittens viewed stimuli with their deprived eye. By contrast, the smaller deficits observed with dark-reared kittens suggest that cells in either the superior colliculus or in the lateral suprasylvian cortical areas may not have been effected by this form of early visual deprivation.

Future studies with the methodology employed here must include the ability to manipulate the speed of the visual targets whether they be solid objects or moving laser spots as anecdotal observations suggested that kittens made gaze movements more frequently to stimuli moved slowly and with a certain degree of unpredictability to their path. Such tweaks to the methodology would facilitate study of the temporal characteristics of the following and striking responses to solid stimuli and to laser spots at different times following early visual deprivation. In particular it will be of interest to determine how the strike trajectory and accuracy of these responses evolves with time during recovery. Relevant to this work were observations made many years ago on kittens reared without sight of their limbs (Hein and Held, 1967) of a gradual evolution of visual placing responses with time into elicited versus guided components.

AUTHOR CONTRIBUTIONS

KM, DM, and KD collected the data. KM and AM analyzed the data. DM and KD contributed in concepts and writing of the manuscript. All authors contributed to the article and approved the submitted version.

ACKNOWLEDGMENTS

Much of the research described here formed part of the (Hons) thesis of KM.

REFERENCES

Fabre-Thorpe, M , Viéard, A., Fuzellier, A. J., and Buser, P. (1984). Visually guided movements in the cat: a test using a randomly moving target. *Behav. Brain Res.* 11, 11–19. doi: 10.1016/0166-4328(84)90004-4

Giffin, F., and Mitchell, D. E. (1978). The rate of recovery of vision after early monocular deprivation in kittens. *J. Physiol.* 274, 511–537. doi: 10.1113/jphysiol.1978.sp012164

Goodale, M. A., and Milner, A. D. (1992). Separate visual pathways for perception and action. *Trends Neurosci.* 15, 20–25. doi: 10.1016/0166-2236(92)90344-8

Guitton, D., Crommelinck, M., and Roucoux, A. (1980). Stimulation of the superior colliculi in the alert cat. I. Eye movements and neck EMG activity evoked when the head is restrained. *Exp. Brain Res.* 39, 63–73. doi: 10.1007/BF00237070

Guitton, D., Douglas, R. M., and Volle, M. (1984). Eye-head coordination in cats. *J. Neurophysiol.* 52, 1030–1050. doi: 10.1152/jn.1984.52.6.1030

Hein, A., and Held, R. (1967). Dissociation of the visual placing responses into elicited and guided components. *Science* 158, 390–392. doi: 10.1126/science.158.3799.390

Hoffmann, K. P., and Sherman, S. M. (1974). Effects of early monocular deprivation on visual input to cat superior colliculus. *J. Neurophysiol.* 37, 1276–1286. doi: 10.1152/jn.1974.37.6.1276

Jones, K. R., Spear, P. D., and Tong, L. (1984). Critical periods for effects of monocular deprivation: differences between striate and extrastriate cortex. *J. Neurosci.* 4, 2543–2552. doi: 10.1523/JNEUROSCI.04-10-02543.1984

Lomber, S. G., Payne, B. R., Cornwell, P., and Long, K. D. (1996). Perceptual and cognitive visual functions of parietal and temporal cortices in the cat. *Cereb. Cortex* 6, 673–695. doi: 10.1093/cercor/6.5.673

Mitchell, D. E. (1988). The extent of visual recovery from early monocular or binocular visual deprivation in kittens. *J. Physiol.* 395, 639–660. doi: 10.1113/jphysiol.1988.sp016939

Mitchell, D. E. (2013). A shot in the dark: the use of darkness to investigate visual development and as a therapy for amblyopia. *Clin. Exp. Optom.* 96, 363–372. doi: 10.1111/cxo.12084

Mitchell, D. E., Giffin, F., and Timney, B. (1977). A behavioural technique for the rapid assessment of the visual capabilities of kittens. *Perception* 6, 181–193. doi: 10.1068/p060181

Mitchell, D. E., Giffin, F., Wilkinson, F., Anderson, R., and Smith, M. L. (1976). Visual resolution in young kittens. *Vis. Res.* 16, 363–366. doi: 10.1016/0042-6989(76)90197-8

Mitchell, D. E., and Maurer, D. (2022). Critical periods in vision revisited. *Ann. Rev. Vis.* 8. (in press).

Price, D. J., Zumbroich, T. J., and Blakemore, C. (1988). Development of stimulus selectivity and functional organization in the suprasylvian visual cortex of the cat. *Proc. R. Sot. Lond. Biol.* 233, 123–163. doi: 10.1098/rspb.1988.0015

Schneider, G. E. (1969). Two visual systems. *Science* 163, 895–902. doi: 10.1126/science.163.3870.895

Stryker, M. P., and Blakemore, C. (1972). Saccadic and disjunctive eye movements in cats. *Vis. Res.* 12, 2005–2013.

Timney, B., Mitchell, D. E., and Giffin, F. (1978). The development of vision in cats after extended periods of dark-rearing. *Exp. Brain Res.* 31, 547–560. doi: 10.1007/BF00239811

Van Hof-Van Duin, J. (1976). Development of visuomotor behavior in normal and dark-reared cats. *Brain Res.* 104, 233–241.

Vital-Durand, F., Putkonen, P. T. S., and Jeannerod, M. (1976). Motion detection and optokinetic responses in dark-reared kittens. *Vis. Res.* 14, 141–142. doi: 10.1016/0042-6989(74)90130-8

Walsh, R. N., and Cummings, R. A. (1976). The open field test: a critical review. *Psychol. Bull.* 83, 482–504. doi: 10.1037/0033-2909.83.3.482

6

Age-Related Deficits in Binocular Vision are Associated with Poorer Inhibitory Control in Healthy Older Adults

*Grace Lin, Raghda Al Ani and Ewa Niechwiej-Szwedo**

Department of Kinesiology, University of Waterloo, Waterloo, ON, Canada

***Correspondence:**
Ewa Niechwiej-Szwedo
eniechwi@uwaterloo.ca;
eniechwiej@uwaterloo.ca

A robust association between reduced visual acuity and cognitive function in older adults has been revealed in large population studies. The aim of this work was to assess the relation between stereoacuity, a key aspect of binocular vision, and inhibitory control, an important component of executive functions. Inhibition was tested using the antisaccade task in older adults with normal or reduced stereopsis (study 1), and in young adults with transiently reduced stereopsis (study 2). Older adults with reduced stereopsis made significantly more errors on the antisaccade task in comparison to those with normal stereopsis. Specifically, there was a significant correlation between stereoacuity and antisaccade errors ($r = 0.27$, $p = 0.019$). In contrast, there were no significant differences in antisaccade errors between the normal and reduced stereopsis conditions in the young group. Altogether, results suggest that the association between poorer stereopsis and lower inhibitory control in older adults might arise due to central nervous system impairment that affects the processing of binocular disparity and antisaccades. These results add to a growing body of literature, which highlights the interdependence of sensory and cognitive decline in older adults.

Keywords: aging, stereopsis, executive functions, eye movements, antisaccade error rate

INTRODUCTION

Aging is associated with reduced physical strength, visual and hearing impairments, poorer memory, and lower scores on cognitive tests. These age-related changes were first documented in separate studies (Thompson, 2009; Owsley, 2011; Whitson et al., 2018); however, accumulating research has revealed a robust relation between visual and hearing deficits and lower performance on cognitive tests (Anstey et al., 2001b; Lin et al., 2004; Tay et al., 2006; Ong et al., 2012; Spierer et al., 2016; Chen et al., 2017; Ward et al., 2018). Previous studies that found a correlation between visual function and cognition focused on testing acuity and contrast sensitivity. Stereoacuity is an important aspect of binocular visual function that is often reduced in older adults (Wright and Wormald, 1992; Leat et al., 2013). However, the association between stereoacuity and cognitive function in older individuals has not been assessed to date. Therefore, the purpose of this study was to examine the relation between stereoacuity and one aspect of executive functions, namely, inhibitory control.

Evidence from large cross-sectional and longitudinal studies indicates that aging is associated with an increase in covariation between visual impairment and reduced cognitive function (Li and Lindenberger, 2002; Zheng et al., 2018). Specifically, the relation between vision and cognition is not significant in young or middle-aged adults, but it emerges in older adults (Baltes and Lindenberger, 1997). The association was first revealed in a large cohort of individuals aged 70–103 years, where visual acuity explained 41% of variance in intellectual functioning (Lindenberger and Baltes, 1994). These findings were subsequently confirmed and extended by the Australian longitudinal study of aging (ALSA), which included a cohort of 894 adults (70–98 years old) (Anstey et al., 2001a). Results showed that 78% of the age-related variance in cognition was shared with vision and hearing function. A robust relation between sensory and cognitive function persisted even when the cognitive assessment was performed using a test designed for people with low vision (Spierer et al., 2016). Importantly, inducing poor visual acuity experimentally in middle-aged adults was not associated with reduced performance on cognitive tests (Lindenberger et al., 2001). Overall, the research supports a robust correlation between visual impairment and poorer cognitive function in older individuals. Acuity has been the most commonly used measure to assess vision, and contrast sensitivity was used in one study (Ward et al., 2018). To date, no studies have examined the association between other aspects of visual function, such as binocular vision, and cognitive performance in older adults.

Binocular vision requires the ability to process inputs from both eyes. The two components of binocular function are stereopsis and ocular vergence, which are elicited by binocular disparity and provide relative and absolute depth cues (Howard and Rogers, 2002). Binocular viewing is associated with improved performance on many everyday tasks (Jones and Lee, 1981; Melmoth and Grant, 2006; Blake and Wilson, 2011).Processing of binocular disparity involves a distributed cortical network lateralized to the right, including the occipital, temporal, and partial areas (Nishida et al., 2001; Fortin et al., 2002; Koh et al., 2008), as well as the prefrontal cortex (Gulyas and Roland, 1994). Aging is associated with reduced binocular visual function (Leat et al., 2013). Notably, stereoacuity deteriorates more with age compared to high contrast visual acuity (Haegerstrom-Portnoy, 2005), and fewer than 30% of individuals 70–79 years old have normal stereoacuity thresholds (Zaroff et al., 2003). Age-related reduction in stereoacuity could arise due to changes in ocular alignment (i.e., phoria or tropia due to extraocular muscle weakness), reduced acuity in one or both eyes from cataracts or age-related macular degeneration, or changes in the central nervous system pathways involved in the processing of binocular disparity. In addition, studies have shown that individuals with neurodegenerative disorders, such as Alzheimer's disease (Mittenberg et al., 1994), Parkinson's disease (Koh et al., 2013), or glaucoma (Gupta et al., 2006), tend to have lower stereopsis. Although the association between binocular vision and cognitive function has not been examined in older persons without a diagnosed neurological disorder, a recent study revealed that poorer binocular function due to convergence insufficiency was correlated with lower inhibitory control in a cohort of young adults (Daniel and Kapoula, 2016).

Inhibition is an important aspect of executive functions, which is mediated by the prefrontal cortex (Langenecker et al., 2004; Tiego et al., 2018). The antisaccade oculomotor test has been used extensively to assess inhibitory control (Munoz and Everling, 2004). When performing an antisaccade, participants are instructed to look away from a target presented in the periphery, which requires inhibiting a reflexive saccade and remapping the saccade-related neural activity to the contralateral hemisphere. Importantly, this oculomotor test allows inhibition to be measured without relying on other visual (i.e., color vision, acuity) or cognitive (i.e., reading) processes, which can limit performance when using other clinical tests to evaluate inhibitory control (van Boxtel et al., 2001).

Inhibition of reflexive eye movements relies on an extensive neural network, which includes the frontoparietal areas, such as the dorsal lateral prefrontal cortex and the supplementary frontal eye fields, as well as the parietal eye fields (Ford et al., 2005; Brown et al., 2007). Research shows that inhibitory control, measured by the number of directional errors where participants fail to inhibit a reflexive saccade and look toward the target, matures over the first two decades of life, and the frequency of errors begins to rise again slowly in healthy middle-aged adults between 30 and 40 years old (Coe and Munoz, 2017). Extensive research reveals that aging is associated with a greater frequency of directional errors and increased latency of correct antisaccades (Olincy et al., 1997; Munoz et al., 1998; Butler et al., 1999; Peltsch et al., 2011; Noiret et al., 2017; Fernandez-Ruiz et al., 2018), suggesting that inhibitory control declines progressively with age in healthy older adults. Neuroimaging studies indicate that these age-related behavioral changes are correlated with a shift of neural activation from posterior to frontal areas, such that activity in visual and parietal areas is reduced while frontal activation is increased (Raemaekers et al., 2006; Alichniewicz et al., 2013).

To summarize, inhibitory control is a key component of executive functions, therefore, it is important to elucidate a better understanding of the influential individual variables associated with lower inhibition, particularly in older individuals. At present, a relationship between one aspect of binocular function (i.e., convergence insufficiency) and inhibitory control has been revealed in young adults (Daniel and Kapoula, 2016). However, little is known about the association between binocular visual function and inhibition in older adults. Therefore, the current study consisted of two experiments which sought to assess the relation between inhibitory control and one aspect of binocular vision, namely stereoacuity. Older adults with normal or reduced stereopsis were tested in experiment 1. It was hypothesized that older individuals with poorer stereopsis will have a greater number of errors on the antisaccade task and a longer latency for correct antisaccades. A second experiment was conducted with young adults with normal binocular vision to assess whether experimentally induced transient reduction of stereopsis affects inhibitory control. Results from this experiment provide insight into the mechanism underlying the correlation between reduced stereopsis and inhibition. Specifically, if transiently induced poor stereopsis is not associated with inhibitory control in younger adults, then the effects seen in older adults are more likely due to central nervous system changes affecting both binocular processing and inhibition rather than just a peripheral reduction in stereoacuity.

MATERIALS AND METHODS

Experiment 1

Participants

A sample of convenience consisting of 94 community dwelling older adults (>66 years old) were recruited from the University of Waterloo Research and Aging Pool database. Nine participants were excluded from the study because of visual impairment due to age-related macular degeneration, glaucoma, or a scheduled cataract surgery. The Montreal Cognitive Assessment (MoCA) was used to assess general cognitive function and to ensure that participants scored within the normal range, which was considered as a score of 26 or greater (Nasreddine et al., 2005). Ten participants scored below 26 and were therefore excluded from the study. The final sample included 75 participants (M = 75.45 years of age, SD = 5.71): 59 females (age: 74.37 ± 5.19 years; education: 15.59 ± 2.79 years) and 16 males (age: 79.44 SD 5.97 years; education: 16.44 ± 3.41 years). The mean number of years of education was 15.77 (SD 2.92; range 12–26 years).

Procedure

The study protocol received ethics clearance through the Research Ethics Committee in accordance with the Declaration of Helsinki. All participants provided written consent. Testing was performed in a quiet, well-lit room. The study protocol included assessment of visual acuity and stereoacuity, which were performed under standard illumination. Participants wore their prescription spectacles during the assessment. Binocular and monocular visual acuities were tested at a 6 m distance using the Bailey-Lovie acuity chart. Visual acuity was defined as the lowest line for which at least three of the five optotypes were reported correctly. Stereoacuity was examined using the Randot Circles Stereotest (Stereo Optical Co. Inc.), which was administered according to the manual. The stereoacuity threshold was determined as the smallest disparity that was reported correctly. Participants were placed into one of two groups based on the results of the Randot test: stereo normal (stereoacuity threshold of 50 arc sec or better) or stereo reduced (stereoacuity threshold worse than 50 arc sec). Demographics and results from the vision tests for the two groups are shown in **Table 1**. A Wilcoxon two-sample test was performed to assess differences between groups. A significant difference was revealed between the groups, indicating that the stereo reduced group was on average older by 2.6 years.

Next, participants completed two oculomotor tasks: prosaccades and antisaccades, which were performed in separate blocks. The task and stimuli were designed following the recommendation outlined by Antoniades et al. (2013). Participants were seated at a distance of 80 cm away from a computer monitor (19 inch ViewSonic CRT monitor; resolution of 1,024 × 768 pixels; refresh rate of 85 Hz) with their chin placed in a chinrest. A video-based eye-tracker (EyeLink II; SR Research, Ontario, Canada) was used to record eye position at a sampling frequency of 250 Hz. The eye-tracker was calibrated using a 5-point calibration method. Validation of eye tracking was performed after the calibration, where the validation acceptance criterion was set at <1° error to ensure reliability.

The experimental protocol was created using the Experiment Builder software (ver. 1.8; SR Research, Ontario, Canada). At the initiation of each trial, participants focused their gaze on a black fixation cross (stimulus size 0.25°) shown at the midline at eye level and presented for a duration ranging between 1,500 and 2,250 ms. When the cross disappeared, a peripheral target (stimulus size 0.25°) was shown (step paradigm) at ±10° to the left or right of the fixation for 2,000 ms. In the prosaccade experimental condition, participants were instructed to look at the stimulus as quickly as possible. Participants completed one block of 50 trials in the prosaccade task. There was one block of antisaccade trials where participants were asked to look away from the target. Instructions were provided verbally, as well as on the computer monitor at the beginning of the pro and antisaccade block of trials. Directional errors were expected in the antisaccade task; therefore, 60 trials were conducted. The oculomotor tests were completed in 15 min.

Data Analysis

Eye movement data were analyzed offline using the eyetracker's Data Viewer software (ver 1.8; SR Research, Ontario, Canada). Eye position data from each trial for both eyes were plotted and visually inspected. The eye which provided less noisy tracking results was selected for analysis. Trials were excluded if a blink or loss of eye tracking occurred within 100 ms prior to or 500 ms following target presentation. These criteria resulted in rejection of 8.5% of trials in the prosaccade task, and 8.6% of trials in the antisaccade task. Saccades were detected using the algorithm implemented in Data Viewer: 30°/s velocity threshold, and 8,000°/s^2 acceleration threshold. The main outcome measure for the prosaccade task was saccade latency, which reflects speed of processing. For the antisaccade task, the main measures were directional error, which indicates difficulty in inhibiting a reflexive response, and latency of saccades made in the correct direction (i.e., away from the target).

Analysis of covariance (ANCOVA) was used to test for differences in inhibitory control between the groups (stereo normal and stereo reduced). Age was entered as a covariate because the stereo normal group was on average 2.6 years younger compared to the stereo reduced group. Although the interocular difference (IOD) was not significantly different between the groups, IOD was also entered as a covariate because larger IOD has been associated with reduced stereoacuity in previous studies (Lam et al., 1996). Statistical analyses were conducted using the Statistical Analysis System (SAS) Studio, ver. 3.5 Enterprise Edition (SAS Institute Inc., Cary, NC, United States).

Experiment 2

Participants

Twelve healthy young adults were recruited (8 females; age: 24.1 years *SD* = 6.8). All participants provided written consent prior to testing. Participants had normal or corrected to normal visual acuity ($\leq$0.0 logMAR) and stereoacuity ($<$50 arc sec).

Procedure

The same testing protocol was used as described in experiment 1. Participants completed one block of the prosaccade task and two blocks of the antisaccade task (one block with normal stereopsis, and one block with reduced stereopsis), which were randomized between participants. One of the antisaccade blocks was performed under normal viewing condition. Stereoacuity was reduced experimentally in the other antisaccade block using a convex lens, which was placed in front of the left eye. This manipulation reduces stereopsis because the retinal images are discordant (Melmoth et al., 2007; Niechwiej-Szwedo et al., 2012). The lenses used in the current experiment ranged between 2.25 and 3.50 prism diopters. Each participant was assessed prior to the experiment to determine which lens power should be used to increase the individual's stereoacuity threshold to 200 arc sec.

RESULTS

Experiment 1

Average binocular visual acuity, IOD, and stereoacuity thresholds for stereo normal and stereo reduced groups are reported in **Table 1**. Results from the Wilcoxon two sample test showed that acuity and IOD were not significantly different between the two groups. Average stereoacuity in the stereo normal group was 35.76 arc sec (*SD* = 11.39, *Mdn* = 30, *range* = 20–50). Three participants in the stereo reduced group had no measurable stereopsis, and the average stereoacuity for the remaining participants with measurable stereopsis was 126.06 arc sec (*SD* = 85.40, *Mdn* = 100, *range* = 70–400).

Results from a univariate analysis for the full cohort showed that mean prosaccade latency was 237 ms (*SD* = 43), which was in the range of slow regular latency saccades (i.e., 181–400 ms). Short latency saccades in the range of express saccades (i.e., 80–139 ms) were found on 3.7% of prosaccade trials, and 1.5% of antisaccade trials. Average antisaccade latency on correct trials was 370 ms (*SD* = 85). Overall, directional errors were found on 31% of antisaccade trials (*SD* = 18), and the average error latency on antisaccade trials was 249 ms (*SD* = 67), which was comparable to prosaccade latency.

Next, analysis was conducted to assess the influence of stereopsis on inhibitory control. Results from the ANCOVA adjusted for age and IOD revealed a significantly greater percent of directional errors in the antisaccade task in the stereo reduced group (36.92%, *SD* = 20.24) compared to the stereo normal group [25.99%, *SD* = 14.67; $F_{(1, 71)}$ = 5.20, *p* = 0.026; **Figure 1A**]. **Figure 2** shows the percentage of errors plotted for individuals in each group as a function of age, illustrating that individuals with reduced stereopsis were more likely to have more errors on the antisaccade task regardless of age. Additional Spearman correlation analysis was conduced to assess the strength of association between stereopsis and antisaccade error. Results showed a moderate correlation, *r*(74) = 0.27, *p* = 0.019, 95% CI [0.05–0.47]. The magnitude of correlation did not change after adjusting for age and IOD, *r*(71) = 0.27, *p* = 0.018.

There were no statistically significant differences between the groups with normal and reduced stereopsis for antisaccade latency [$F_{(1, 71)}$ = 0.88, *p* = 0.350; **Figure 1B**] or prosaccade latency [$F_{(1, 71)}$ = 0.11, *p* = 0.745; **Figure 1C**]. Average antisaccade latency was 359 ms (*SD* = 87) for the stereo normal group and 382 ms (*SD* = 82) for the stereo reduced group. Average prosaccade latency was 234 ms (*SD* = 34) for the stereo normal group and 241 ms (*SD* = 50) for the stereo reduced group. Additional analysis was conducted to assess whether the frequency of short latency (i.e., express) saccades was different between the groups with normal and reduced stereopsis. Express saccades occurred on 148 trials in the prosaccade task, with the majority (66%) occurring in the stereo normal group. Similarly, express saccades occurred on 74 trials in the antisaccades task with the majority (69%) occurring in the stereo normal group.

Experiment 2

The aim of this experiment was to examine the effect of transiently reduced stereopsis on inhibitory control. As expected, the average latency of prosaccades was shorter (172 ms, *SD* = 24) in comparison to antisaccades, and there was no significant difference [$t_{(11)}$ = -1.03; *p* = 0.325] between the two antisaccade conditions (stereo normal: 246 ms, *SD* = 34; stereo reduced: 252 ms, *SD* = 34). There was also no significant difference in the percentage of directional errors between the conditions where stereoacuity was normal (14.54%, *SD* = 16.20 and transiently reduced (15.69%, *SD* = 16.11; $t_{(11)}$ = -0.54; *p* = 0.601; **Figure 1A**).

TABLE 1 | Demographics and visual function characteristics (mean ± SD) for participants with normal stereoacuity and reduced stereoacuity.

	Normal stereoacuity (*n* = 39; 31 females) (threshold ≤ 50 arc sec)	Reduced stereoacuity (*n* = 36; 28 females) (threshold > 50 arc sec)	Wilcoxon test; *p*-value
Age (years)	74.20 ± 5.57	76.80 ± 5.64	*Z* = 2.13; *p* = 0.033
Stereoacuity (arc sec)	35.76 ± 11.39	*182.22 ± 205.80	*Z* = 7.49; *p* < 0.001
Best corrected binocular visual acuity (logMAR)	0.05 ± 0.10	0.08 ± 0.09	*Z* = 1.19; *p* = 0.231
Interocular acuity difference (logMAR)	0.07 ± 0.06	0.14 ± 0.19	*Z* = 0.72; *p* = 0.470

**Participants with no measurable stereopsis were assigned a score of 800 arc sec.*

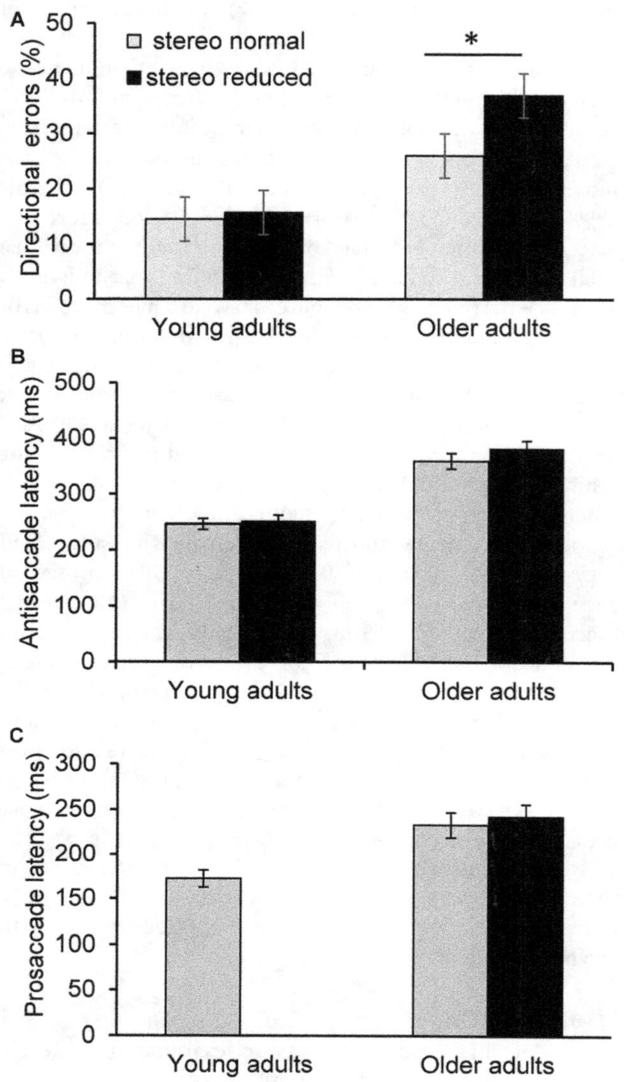

FIGURE 1 | Saccade latency and error measures across task conditions. Error bars represent ± 1 standard error. Average percent of directional errors in the antisaccade task in young and older adults as a function to stereoacuity **(A)**. Older adults with reduced stereopsis exhibited significantly more errors ($p < 0.05$). In contrast, there was no significant difference in antisaccade errors between the stereo normal condition and when stereopsis was transiently reduced in young adults. There was no significant difference in antisaccade latency **(B)** or prosaccade latency **(C)** between the stereo conditions in the older or younger group. Prosaccade latency was not assessed as a function of reduced stereoacuity in the younger adults in Experiment 2. *$p < 0.05$.

DISCUSSION

The primary goal of the current study was to assess the association between stereoacuity and inhibitory control in a cohort of healthy, community-dwelling older adults. A secondary goal was to determine if a transient reduction in stereoacuity affects inhibitory control in young adults. Results showed that older adults with reduced stereopsis exhibited a greater percentage of directional errors on the antisaccade task, which indicates poorer inhibitory control. This is the first study to report such an association, which extends the current knowledge about the interdependence of visual and executive functions in older individuals. Importantly, such correlation was not found when younger adults with experimentally induced poor stereopsis performed the antisaccade task. Therefore, it is unlikely that stereopsis is directly influencing inhibitory control. Instead, the association revealed in the current study could be indicative of a common age-related disruption in neural function that affects both the processing of binocular disparity and other aspects of executive function, specifically, inhibition.

A robust relation between sensory impairments and cognition has been reported in older individuals in large population studies (Anstey et al., 2001b; Li and Lindenberger, 2002; Ong et al., 2012; Zheng et al., 2018). Binocular visual acuity has been the most frequently used measure in previous studies, and the association with cognition was shown for both distance and near acuity. Because the current study sought to assess the relation between stereopsis and inhibition, only participants with relatively good binocular visual acuity, which was at least 0.3 logMAR (i.e., Snellen 20/40), were included. Consistent with previous studies (Zaroff et al., 2003; Haegerstrom-Portnoy, 2005), stereoacuity was significantly reduced in 48% of our cohort. As hypothesized, results revealed an association between stereopsis and inhibitory control, manifested as increased number of errors on the antisaccade task, which remained significant after controlling for age and interocular acuity difference. This indicates that individuals with poorer stereoacuity experienced greater difficulty inhibiting reflexive eye movements. In contrast, the latency of the correct antisaccades was not different between the groups with normal or reduced stereoacuity. Thus, antisaccade errors rather than latency appear to be a more sensitive marker of executive dysfunction. These findings are consistent with the results from studies conducted with adults with a history of concussion, which demonstrated that brain injury is associated with persistent errors on the antisaccade task even in cases when antisaccade latency is normal (Mani et al., 2018). The fact that stereopsis was correlated with inhibitory control in individuals with relatively good visual acuity suggests that stereoacuity may be a more sensitive test than acuity that could help to identify individuals with lower executive function. The cohort tested in the current study consisted of individuals with normal cognitive function, according to the MoCA test. However, it is possible that some individuals with poorer stereopsis might be at a greater risk of developing cognitive deficits, and this remains to be tested in longitudinal studies.

Stereopsis is one of the key measures of binocular vision and requires the ability to process inputs from both eyes. Stereoacuity deficits may arise due to optical factors that reduce acuity and contrast sensitivity (e.g., cataracts), photoreceptor degeneration, ocular muscle weakness that affects vergence control, or neural processing of binocular disparity. The results from our second experiment showed that a transient reduction in stereopsis is not associated with antisaccade errors, which suggests that optical image blur is not sufficient to impair inhibitory control. Thus,

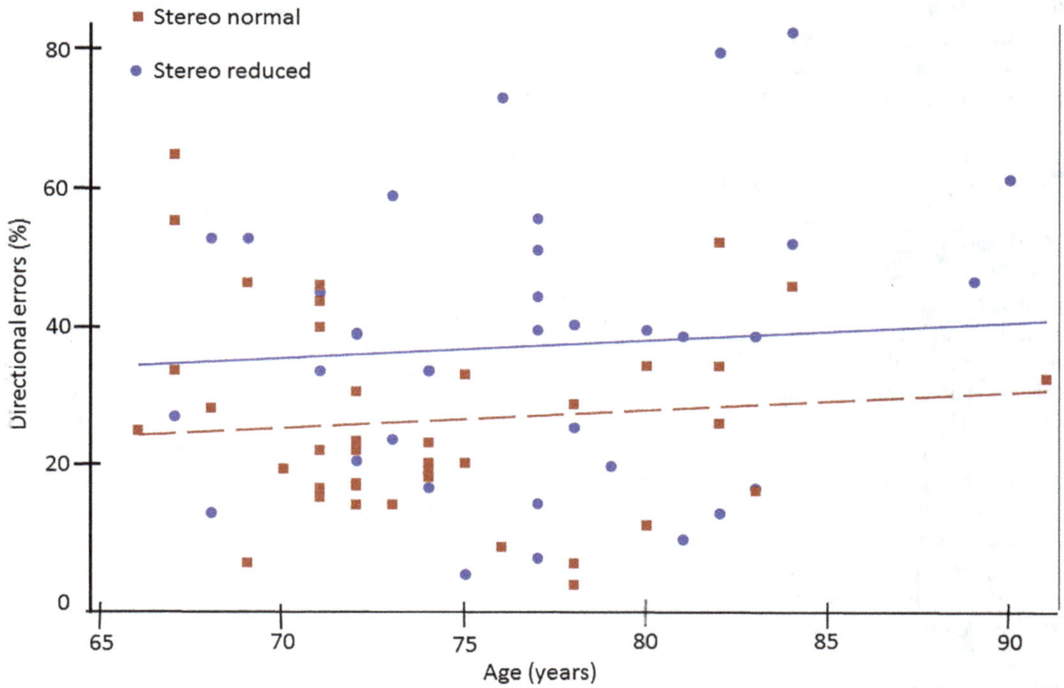

FIGURE 2 | Percent of directional errors in the antisaccade task plotted as a function of age for older adults with normal (squares) and reduced (circles) stereoacuity. Individuals with normal stereoacuity made significantly fewer directional errors compared to individuals with reduced stereoacuity ($p < 0.05$).

it is more likely that the deficits in stereopsis and inhibition in older adults arise due to a disruption in central nervous system processing that affects both of these functions.

Stereoscopic processing and the antisaccade task engage distributed neural networks, including extrastriate visual, parietal and prefrontal areas (Ford et al., 2005; Brown et al., 2007). Aging is associated with structural and functional changes in cortical networks, including reduced grey matter volume, white matter atrophy (Fjell et al., 2009; Liu et al., 2017), and compensatory activation patterns (Fernandez-Ruiz et al., 2018). Recent studies also highlight the relation between disruption in white matter tracts and age-related decline in sensorimotor and cognitive processing (Fling et al., 2011; Kohama et al., 2012). For example, microstructural changes in the corpus callosum have been found in apparently healthy older adults (Fan et al., 2019), and these changes have been linked with lower performance on various cognitive tasks (Sullivan et al., 2010; Wong et al., 2017; Halliday et al., 2019). It is possible that widespread disruption of white matter, including the corpus callosum, could lead to both reduced stereopsis and inhibitory processing because efficient performance of both tasks relies on activation of distributed cortical networks within and between the hemispheres. Specifically, processing of crossed disparities presented at midline stimulates the temporal part of each retina, and these inputs are first processed in different hemispheres. Thus, the splenium of the corpus callosum is involved in stereoscopic processing of small stimuli with crossed disparities presented at midline (Bridge, 2016). On the other hand, neuroimaging studies show that the antisaccade task activates an extensive frontoparietal network (Munoz and Everling, 2004; Ford et al., 2005), and improved selection and inhibition performance is associated with white matter integrity between these regions (Thakkar et al., 2016; Jarvstad and Gilchrist, 2019). Interestingly, fractional anisotropy, a measure of white matter integrity was correlated positively with saccade latency and lower behavioral cost of inhibition (Jarvstad and Gilchrist, 2019). Thus, lower white matter integrity may be contributing to poorer inhibition in our study. To summarize, deficits in stereoscopic processing and lower inhibitory control on the antisaccade task may arise due to a widespread age-related changes in white matter connectivity; however, imaging studies are needed to test this hypothesis directly.

The underlying mechanism to explain the relation between vision and cognitive function remains to be established. However, several hypotheses have been proposed (reviewed in: Li and Lindenberger, 2002). First, the sensory loss consequence hypothesis suggests that visual impairment leads to fewer social interactions and less cognitive stimulation, which is a risk factor for cognitive decline. Second, the resource allocation hypothesis speculates that individuals with sensory impairments require more neural resources to detect and discriminate sensory inputs, which leaves limited neural resources for cognitive processing. These two hypotheses postulate a causal relationship where deteriorating sensory function eventually leads to cognitive decline. Finally, the third hypothesis proposes a common cause for sensory and cognitive impairment. Although the current study cannot differentiate between these hypotheses, our results and interpretation are more consistent with the third hypothesis. Specifically, our results showed an association between a visual test (i.e., stereopsis) and a measure of executive function in the older cohort, but given the results of the second experiment, it is unlikely that reduced stereopsis directly leads to antisaccade errors. Instead, it is more likely that age-related microstructural and functional changes of the central nervous system could lead to a decrease in both sensory and cognitive function.

Our results provide new insight into the association between visual and cognitive function; however, it is important to acknowledge some limitations. First, the recruited participants included mainly women, while men represented less than a third of the cohort. Therefore, caution should be exercised when generalizing the results. Second, stereoacuity was assessed using a single clinical test which measures local stereopsis. Different clinical tests can be used to measure other components of stereopsis, such as global stereopsis. Research shows that local and global stereopsis rely on different neural networks (Ptito et al., 1991); thus, assessment of these different components of stereopsis could provide additional insight into the association with cognitive function in older individuals. Finally, individuals diagnosed with macular degeneration, glaucoma, or scheduled cataract surgery were excluded from the current study. However, these ocular disorders progress slowly, and it is possible that our cohort included individuals who had reduced stereopsis resulting from these conditions but were not yet formally diagnosed. In order to gain a fuller understanding into the relation between stereoacuity and cognitive function, future studies should include a more comprehensive assessment of visual and oculomotor function in order to stratify participants according to the underlying cause of stereopsis impairment.

In conclusion, this is the first study to reveal that reduced stereoacuity is correlated with poorer inhibitory control. This exploratory study cannot definitively reveal the nature of this association; however, it is possible that the deficits in processing of binocular disparity and inhibitory control are both due to a common impairment of neural function. Results from the current study have implications for future research investigating the interdependence of vision and cognitive function. Specifically, acuity has been the most commonly used measure of visual function in large population studies examining its relation to cognition. However, future studies should consider adding a stereoacuity assessment, which seems to be more closely associated with executive dysfunction. The findings from the current study improve our understanding of the nature of the interaction between sensory and executive functions, and this knowledge could be used to develop better diagnostic and prognostic tools to monitor older individuals at risk of cognitive decline.

AUTHOR CONTRIBUTIONS

GL and RA collected the data. GL, RA, and EN-S performed the data analysis. GL wrote the first draft. All authors contributed to the conception and design of the study, contributed to the manuscript revision, read and approved the submitted version.

REFERENCES

Alichniewicz, K., Brunner, F., Klünemann, H., and Greenlee, M. (2013). Neural correlates of saccadic inhibition in healthy elderly and patients with amnestic mild cognitive impairment [Internet]. *Front. Psychol.* 4:467.

Anstey, K., Luszcz, M., and Sanchez, L. (2001a). A reevaluation of the common factor theory of shared variance among age, sensory function, and cognitive function in older adults. *J. Gerontol. Ser. B* 56, 3–11.

Anstey, K., Luszcz, M., and Sanchez, L. (2001b). Two-year decline in vision but not hearing is associated with memory decline in very old adults in a population-based sample. *Gerontology* 47, 289–293. doi: 10.1159/000052814

Antoniades, C., Ettinger, U., Gaymard, B., Gilchrist, I., Kristjánsson, A., Kennard, C., et al. (2013). An internationally standardised antisaccade protocol. *Vision Res. [Internet]* 84, 1–5. doi: 10.1016/j.visres.2013.02.007

Baltes, P. B., and Lindenberger, U. (1997). Emergence of a powerful connection between sensory and cognitive functions across the adult life span: A new window to the study of cognitive aging? *Psychol. Aging* 12, 12–21. doi: 10.1037/0882-7974.12.1.12

Blake, R., and Wilson, H. R. (2011). Binocular vision. *Vision Res.* 51, 754–770.

Bridge, H. (2016). Effects of cortical damage on binocular depth perception. *Philos. Trans. R. Soc. B* 371:20150254. doi: 10.1098/rstb.2015.0254

Brown, M. R. G., Vilis, T., and Everling, S. (2007). Frontoparietal activation with preparation for antisaccades. *J. Neurophysiol.* 98, 1751–1762. doi: 10.1152/jn.00460.2007

Butler, K. M., Zacks, R. T., and Henderson, J. M. (1999). Suppression of reflexive saccades in younger and older adults: age comparisons on an antisaccade task. *Mem. Cognit. [Internet]* 27, 584–591. doi: 10.3758/bf03211552

Chen, S. P., Bhattacharya, J., and Pershing, S. (2017). Association of vision loss with cognition in older adults. *JAMA Ophthalmol. [Internet]* 135, 963–970. doi: 10.1001/jamaophthalmol.2017.2838

Coe, B., and Munoz, D. (2017). Mechanisms of saccade suppression revealed in the anti-saccade task. *Philos. Trans. R. Soc. B Biol. Sci. [Internet]* 372:20160192. doi: 10.1098/rstb.2016.0192

Daniel, F., and Kapoula, Z. (2016). Binocular vision and the Stroop test. *Optom. Vis. Sci.* 93, 194–208. doi: 10.1097/opx.0000000000000774

Ettinger, U., ffytche, D. H., Kumari, V., Kathmann, N., Reuter, B., Zelaya, F., et al. (2007). Decomposing the neural correlates of antisaccade eye movements using event-related fMRI. *Cereb. Cortex [Internet]* 18, 1148–1159. doi: 10.1093/cercor/bhm147

Fan, Q., Tian, Q., Ohringer, N. A., Nummenmaa, A., Witzel, T., Tobyne, S. M., et al. (2019). Age-related alterations in axonal microstructure in the corpus callosum measured by high-gradient diffusion MRI. *Neuroimage* 191, 325–336. doi: 10.1016/j.neuroimage.2019.02.036

Fernandez-Ruiz, J., Peltsch, A., Alahyane, N., Brien, D. C., Coe, B. C., Garcia, A., et al. (2018). Age related prefrontal compensatory mechanisms for inhibitory control in the antisaccade task. *Neuroimage* 165, 92–101. doi: 10.1016/j.neuroimage.2017.10.001

Fjell, A. M., Walhovd, K. B., Fennema-Notestine, C., McEvoy, L. K., Hagler, D. J., Holland, D., et al. (2009). One-year brain atrophy evident in healthy aging. *J. Neurosci.* 29, 15223–15231. doi: 10.1523/jneurosci.3252-09.2009

Fling, B. W., Peltier, S. J., Bo, J., Welsh, R. C., and Seidler, R. D. (2011). Age differences in interhemispheric interactions: Callosal structure, physiological function, and behavior. *Front. Neurosci.* 5:38.

Ford, K. A., Goltz, H. C., Brown, M. R. G., and Everling, S. (2005). Neural processes associated with antisaccade task performance investigated with event-related FMRI. *J. Neurophysiol.* 94, 429–440. doi: 10.1152/jn.00471.2004

Fortin, A., Ptito, A., Faubert, J., and Ptito, M. (2002). Cortical areas mediating stereopsis in the human brain: a PET study. *Neuroreport* 13, 895–898. doi: 10.1097/00001756-200205070-00032

Gulyas, B., and Roland, P. E. (1994). Binocular disparity discrimination in human cerebral cortex: functional anatomy by positron emission tomography. *Proc. Natl. Acad. Sci. U.S.A.* 91, 1239–1243. doi: 10.1073/pnas.91.4.1239

Gupta, N., Krishnadev, N., Hamstra, S. J., and Yücel, Y. H. (2006). Depth perception deficits in glaucoma suspects. *Br. J. Ophthalmol.* 90, 979–981. doi: 10.1136/bjo.2006.091025

Haegerstrom-Portnoy, G. (2005). The Glenn A. Fry award lecture 2003: vision in elders–summary of findings of the SKI study. *Optometry Vis. Sci.* 82, 87–93. doi: 10.1097/01.opx.0000153162.05903.4c

Halliday, D. W. R., Gawryluk, J. R., Garcia-Barrera, M. A., and MacDonald, S. W. S. (2019). White matter integrity is associated with intraindividual variability in neuropsychological test performance in healthy older adults. *Front. Hum. Neurosci.* 13:352.

Howard, I. P., and Rogers, B. (2002). *Seeing in Depth.* Toronto: Porteus.

Jarvstad, A., and Gilchrist, I. D. (2019). Cognitive control of saccadic selection and inhibition from within the core cortical saccadic network. *J. Neurosci.* 39, 2497–2508.

Jones, R. K., and Lee, D. N. (1981). Why two eyes are better than one: the two views of binocular vision. *J. Exp. Psychol. Hum. Percept. Perform.* 7, 30–40. doi: 10.1037/0096-1523.7.1.30

Koh, S.-B., Kim, B.-J., Lee, J., Suh, S., Kim, T.-K., and Kim, S.-H. (2008). Stereopsis and color vision impairment in patients with right extrastriate cerebral lesions. *Eur. Neurol.* 60, 174–178. doi: 10.1159/000148244

Koh, S.-B., Suh, S.-I., Kim, S.-H., and Kim, J. H. (2013). Stereopsis and extrastriate cortical atrophy in Parkinson's disease: a voxel-based morphometric study. *Neuroreport* 24, 229–232. doi: 10.1097/wnr.0b013e32835edbc5

Kohama, S. G., Rosene, D. L., and Sherman, L. S. (2012). Age-related changes in human and non-human primate white matter: From myelination disturbances to cognitive decline. *Age (Omaha)* 34, 1093–1110. doi: 10.1007/s11357-011-9357-7

Lam, A. K., Chau, A. S., Lam, W. Y., Leung, G. Y., and Man, B. S. (1996). Effect of naturally occurring visual acuity differences between two eyes in stereoacuity. *Ophthalmic Physiol. Opt.* 16, 189–195. doi: 10.1016/0275-5408(95)00034-8

Langenecker, S. A., Nielson, K. A., and Rao, S. M. (2004). fMRI of healthy older adults during Stroop interference. *Neuroimage* 21, 192–200. doi: 10.1016/j.neuroimage.2003.08.027

Leat, S. J., Chan, L. L., Maharaj, P. D., Hrynchak, P. K., Mittelstaedt, A., Machan, C. M., et al. (2013). Binocular vision and eye movement disorders in older adults. *Invest. Ophthalmol. Vis. Sci.* 54, 3798–3805. doi: 10.1167/iovs.12-11582

Li, K. Z. H., and Lindenberger, U. (2002). Relations between aging sensory/sensorimotor and cognitive functions. *Neurosci. Biobehav. Rev.* 26, 777–783. doi: 10.1016/s0149-7634(02)00073-8

Lin, M. Y., Gutierrez, P. R., Stone, K. L., Yaffe, K., Ensrud, K. E., Fink, H. A., et al. (2004). Vision impairment and combined vision and hearing impairment predict cognitive and functional decline in older women. *J. Am. Geriatr. Soc.* 52, 1996–2002. doi: 10.1111/j.1532-5415.2004.52554.x

Lindenberger, U., and Baltes, P. B. (1994). Sensory functioning and intelligence in old age: a strong connection. *Psychol. Aging* 9, 339–355. doi: 10.1037/0882-7974.9.3.339

Lindenberger, U., Scherer, H., and Baltes, P. B. (2001). The strong connection between sensory and cognitive performance in old age: not due to sensory acuity reductions operating during cognitive assessment. *Psychol. Aging* 16, 196–205. doi: 10.1037/0882-7974.16.2.196

Liu, H., Yang, Y., Xia, Y., Zhu, W., Leak, R. K., Wei, Z., et al. (2017). Aging of cerebral white matter. *Ageing Res. Rev.* 34, 64–76.

Mani, R., Asper, L., and Khuu, S. K. (2018). Deficits in saccades and smooth-pursuit eye movements in adults with traumatic brain injury: a systematic review and meta-analysis *Brain Inj.* 32, 1315–1336. doi: 10.1080/02699052.2018.1483030

Melmoth, D. R., and Grant, S. (2006). Advantages of binocular vision for the control of reaching and grasping. *Exp. Brain Res.* 171, 371–388. doi: 10.1007/s00221-005-0273-x

Melmoth, D. R., Storoni, M., Todd, G., Finlay, A. L., and Grant, S. (2007). Dissociation between vergence and binocular disparity cues in the control of prehension. *Exp. Brain Res.* 183, 283–298. doi: 10.1007/s00221-007-1041-x

Mittenberg, W., Malloy, M., Petrick, J., and Knee, K. (1994). Impaired depth perception discriminates Alzheimer's dementia from aging and major depression. *Arch. Clin. Neuropsychol.* 9, 71–79. doi: 10.1016/0887-6177(94)90015-9

Munoz, D. P., Broughton, J. R., Goldring, J. E., and Armstrong, I. T. (1998). Age-related performance of human subjects on saccadic eye movement tasks. *Exp. Brain Res.* 121, 391–400. doi: 10.1007/s002210050473

Munoz, D. P., and Everling, S. (2004). Look away: the anti-saccade task and the voluntary control of eye movement. *Nat. Rev. Neurosci.* 5, 218–228. doi: 10.1038/nrn1345

Nasreddine, Z. S., Phillips, N. A., Bédirian, V., Charbonneau, S., Whitehead, V., Collin, I., et al. (2005). The montreal cognitive assessment, MoCA: a brief screening tool for mild cognitive impairment. *J. Am. Geriatr. Soc.* 53, 695–699. doi: 10.1111/j.1532-5415.2005.53221.x

Niechwiej-Szwedo, E., Kennedy, S. A., Colpa, L., Chandrakumar, M., Goltz, H. C., and Wong, A. M. F. (2012). Effects of induced monocular blur versus anisometropic amblyopia on saccades, reaching, and eye-hand coordination. *Investig. Ophthalmol. Vis. Sci.* 53, 4354–4362. doi: 10.1167/iovs.12-9855

Nishida, Y., Hayashi, O., Iwami, T., Kimura, M., Kani, K., Ito, R., et al. (2001). Stereopsis-processing regions in the human parieto-occipital cortex. *Neuroreport* 12, 2259–2263. doi: 10.1097/00001756-200107200-00043

Noiret, N., Vigneron, B., Diogo, M., Vandel, P., and Laurent, E. (2017). Saccadic eye movements: what do they tell us about aging cognition? *Neuropsychol. Dev. Cogn. B Aging Neuropsychol. Cogn.* 24, 575–599. doi: 10.1080/13825585.2016.1237613

Olincy, A., Ross, R. G., Youngd, D. A., and Freedman, R. (1997). Age diminishes performance on an antisaccade eye movement task. *Neurobiol. Aging* 18, 483–489. doi: 10.1016/s0197-4580(97)00109-7

Ong, S. Y., Cheung, C. Y., Li, X., Lamoureux, E. L., Ikram, M. K., Ding, J., et al. (2012). Visual impairment, age-related eye diseases, and cognitive function: The Singapore Malay eye study. *JAMA Ophthalmol.* 130, 895–900.

Owsley, C. (2011). Aging and vision. *Vision Res.* 51, 1610–1622. doi: 10.1016/j.visres.2010.10.020

Peltsch, A., Hemraj, A., Garcia, A., and Munoz, D. P. (2011). Age-related trends in saccade characteristics among the elderly. *Neurobiol. Aging* 32, 669–679. doi: 10.1016/j.neurobiolaging.2009.04.001

Ptito, A., Zatorre, R. J., Larson, W. L., and Tosoni, C. (1991). Stereopsis after unilateral anterior temporal lobectomy. Dissociation between local and global measures. *Brain* 114(Pt 3), 1323–1333.

Raemaekers, M., Vink, M., van den Heuvel, M. P., Kahn, R. S., and Ramsey, N. F. (2006). Effects of aging on BOLD fMRI during prosaccades and antisaccades. *J. Cogn. Neurosci.* 18, 594–603. doi: 10.1162/jocn.2006.18.4.594

Spierer, O., Fischer, N., Barak, A., and Belkin, M. (2016). Correlation between vision and cognitive function in the elderly: a cross-sectional study. *Medicine (Baltimore)* 95:e2423. doi: 10.1097/md.0000000000002423

Sullivan, E. V., Rohlfing, T., and Pfefferbaum, A. (2010). Quantitative fiber tracking of lateral and interhemispheric white matter systems in normal aging: relations to timed performance. *Neurobiol. Aging* 31, 464–481. doi: 10.1016/j.neurobiolaging.2008.04.007

Tay, T., Wang, J. J., Kifley, A., Lindley, R., Newall, P., and Mitchell, P. (2006). Sensory and cognitive association in older persons: findings from an older Australian population. *Gerontology* 52, 386–394. doi: 10.1159/000095129

Thakkar, K. N., van den Heiligenberg, F. M. Z., Kahn, R. S., and Neggers, S. F. W. (2016). Speed of saccade execution and inhibition associated with fractional anisotropy in distinct fronto-frontal and fronto-striatal white matter pathways. *Hum. Brain Mapp.* 37, 2811–2822. doi: 10.1002/hbm.23209

Thompson, L. V. (2009). Age-related muscle dysfunction. *Exp. Gerontol.* 44, 106–111. doi: 10.1016/j.exger.2008.05.003

Tiego, J., Testa, R., Bellgrove, M., Pantelis, C., and Whittle, S. (2018). A hierarchical model of inhibitory control. *Front. Psychol.* 9:1339.

Ting, W. K., Schweizer, T. A., Topolovec-Vranic, J., and Cusimano, M. D. (2016). Antisaccadic eye movements are correlated with corpus callosum white matter mean diffusivity, stroop performance, and symptom burden in mild traumatic brain injury and concussion. *Front. Neurol.* 6:271.

van Boxtel, M. P., ten Tusscher, M. P., Metsemakers, J. F., Willems, B., and Jolles, J. (2001). Visual determinants of reduced performance on the Stroop color-word test in normal aging individuals. *J. Clin. Exp. Neuropsychol.* 23, 620–627.

Ward, M. E., Gelfand, J. M., Lui, L.-Y., Ou, Y., Green, A. J., Stone, K., et al. (2018). Reduced contrast sensitivity among older women is associated with increased risk of cognitive impairment. *Ann. Neurol.* 83, 730–738. doi: 10.1002/ana.25196

Whitson, H. E., Cronin-Golomb, A., Cruickshanks, K. J., Gilmore, G. C., Owsley, C., Peelle, J. E., et al. (2018). American geriatrics society and national institute on aging bench-to-bedside conference: Sensory impairment and cognitive decline in older adults. *J. Am. Geriatr. Soc. [Internet]* 66, 2052–2058.

Wong, N. M. L., Ma, E. P.-W., and Lee, T. M. C. (2017). The integrity of the corpus callosum mitigates the impact of blood pressure on the ventral attention network and information processing speed in healthy adults. *Front. Aging Neurosci.* 9:108.

Wright, L. A., and Wormald, R. P. (1992). Stereopsis and ageing. *Eye* 6(Pt 5), 473–476. doi: 10.1038/eye.1992.100

Zaroff, C. M., Knutelska, M., and Frumkes, T. E. (2003). Variation in stereoacuity: normative description, fixation disparity, and the roles of aging and gender. *Invest. Ophthalmol. Vis. Sci.* 44, 891–900. doi: 10.1167/iovs.02-0361

Zheng, D. D., Swenor, B., Christ, S. L., West, S. K., Lam, B. L., and Lee, D. J. (2018). Longitudinal associations between visual impairment and cognitive functioning: The salisbury eye evaluation study. *JAMA Ophthalmol.* 136, 989–995. doi: 10.1001/jamaophthalmol.2018.2493

7

Temporal Characteristics of Visual Processing in Amblyopia

Xia Hu[1], Yi Qin[1], Xiaoxiao Ying[1], Junli Yuan[1], Rong Cui[2], Xiaowei Ruan[1], Xianghang He[1,3], Zhong-Lin Lu[4,5,6], Fan Lu[1] and Fang Hou[1]**

[1] School of Ophthalmology & Optometry and Eye Hospital, Wenzhou Medical University, Wenzhou, China, [2] Biosysen Ltd., Shenzhen, China, [3] Fuzhou Aier Eye Hospital, Fuzhou, China, [4] Division of Arts and Sciences, NYU Shanghai, Shanghai, China, [5] Department of Psychology, Center for Neural Science, New York University, New York, NY, United States, [6] NYU-ECNU Institute of Brain and Cognitive Science, NYU Shanghai, Shanghai, China

***Correspondence:**
Fan Lu
lufan62@mail.eye.ac.cn
Fang Hou
houf@mail.eye.ac.cn

Purpose: Amblyopia affects not only spatial vision but also temporal vision. In this study, we aim to investigate temporal processing deficits in amblyopia.

Methods: Twenty amblyopic patients (age: 27.0 ± 5.53 years, 15 males), and 25 normal observers (age: 25.6 ± 4.03 years, 15 males) were recruited in this study. Contrast thresholds in an orientation discrimination task in five target-mask stimulus onset asynchronies (SOA) conditions (16.7 ms, 33.4 ms, 50.0 ms, 83.4 ms, and ∞/no noise) were measured. An elaborated perceptual template model (ePTM) was fit to the behavioral data to derive the temporal profile of visual processing for each participant.

Results: There were significant threshold differences between the amblyopic and normal eyes [$F(1,43) = 10.6$, $p = 0.002$] and a significant group × SOA interaction [$F(2.75,118) = 4.98$, $p = 0.004$], suggesting different temporal processing between the two groups. The ePTM fitted the data well (χ^2 test, all $ps > 0.50$). Compared to the normal eye, the amblyopic eye had a lower template gain ($p = 0.046$), and a temporal window with lower peak and broader width (all $ps < 0.05$). No significant correlation was found between the observed temporal deficits and visual acuity in amblyopia ($ps > 0.50$). Similar results were found in the anisometropic amblyopia subgroup. No significant difference was found between the fellow eyes of the monocular amblyopia and the normal eyes.

Conclusion: Amblyopia is less efficient in processing dynamic visual stimuli. The temporal deficits in amblyopia, represented by a flattened temporal window, are likely independent of spatial vision deficits.

Keywords: amblyopia, contrast threshold, perceptual template model, temporal deficits, external noise, temporal window

INTRODUCTION

Amblyopia, also called "lazy eye," is a developmental disorder of the visual system caused by abnormal visual experience during early life (Kiorpes, 2019). It is one of the most common causes of vision loss in children, affecting approximately 2–5% of children worldwide (Webber and Wood, 2005; Wang et al., 2011; Tailor et al., 2016; Faghihi et al., 2017). Amblyopia can induce structural and functional changes in the visual pathways, which are commonly believed to begin at the level of the primary visual cortex (V1) (Kiorpes, 2019). Typically, patients with amblyopia exhibit deficits including reduced spatial contrast sensitivity (Hess and Howell, 1977; Kosovicheva et al., 2019), loss of stereopsis (Giaschi et al., 2013; Levi et al., 2015), reduced grating and Vernier acuity (Levi and Klein, 1982, 1985; Birch and Swanson, 2000), spatial distortions (Barrett et al., 2003; Piano et al., 2015), deficits in spatial localization (Hess and Holliday, 1992), and spatial localization deficit (Hess and Holliday, 1992). Amblyopia also accompanied temporal deficits, such as reduced temporal contrast sensitivity (Levi and Harwerth, 1977; Wesson and Loop, 1982; Kosovicheva et al., 2019), higher flicker fusion frequency (Miles, 1949; Manny and Levi, 1982), as well as deficits in local and global motion (Simmers et al., 2003, 2006; Ho et al., 2005; Ho and Giaschi, 2006, 2007). Moreover, accumulating evidences suggested that the temporal deficit could be independent from the spatial deficit in amblyopia (Kiorpes et al., 2006; Huang et al., 2012; Tao et al., 2019).

Extracting ecologically relevant information in a complex environment is essential for humans. The perceptual system must quickly pick up the signal-of-interest buried in the often noisy spatiotemporal input. In the spatial domain, many studies have shown that the amblyopic visual system is susceptible to the disturbance of irrelevant spatial information. External noise analysis provided a powerful tool to separate the observer's ability from her intrinsic noise (Lu and Dosher, 1998, 2008, 2013; Pelli and Farell, 1999). External noise studies on amblyopia revealed that, in addition to the larger internal noise due to a shift in spatial scale of visual processing, the amblyopic eye exhibited lower processing efficiency, suggesting that it was more difficult for amblyopes to exclude external noise in the spatial domain (Wang et al., 1998; Pelli et al., 2004; Xu et al., 2006). The lower processing efficiency has been conceptualized as a "poor spatial template" of amblyopia in a perceptual template model analysis (Xu et al., 2006). By investigating the performance of amblyopic patients in the detection and position identification tasks of a bar-like stimulus using the classification image technique (Eckstein and Ahumada, 2002), Levi and Klein (2003) also concluded that the loss of efficiency in amblyopia could be partially attributed to a poor spatial template. Other studies have also found that the amblyopic visual system had a larger interaction zone in which performance on the central target is impaired by flanking stimuli (Hess et al., 2001; Levi et al., 2002).

On the other hand, how amblyopia affects patients' ability to extract signal in dynamic visual stimuli has not been well understood. Bonneh et al. (2007) found that, in a digit identification task with the rapid serial visual presentation (RSVP) task, the size threshold difference between the fast (5 Hz) and slow (2.5 Hz) conditions was much greater in the strabismic amblyopia group than the normal group, and the threshold difference was independent of visual acuity. Their results suggest that it was more difficult for the strabismic amblyopes to identify the target embedded in a temporally crowded RSVP stream. By measuring the effect of metacontrast masking as a function of stimulus onset asynchrony (SOA) in the amblyopic and normal observers, Tytla and Steinbach (1984) found that the range of SOA for inducing masking effects with the same masks was wider in amblyopic than normal vision. Although the authors suggested that the amblyopic eye was worse in discounting distractors in time, the metacontrast mask effect was measured with a ring stimulus surrounding the target and may reflect abnormal spatial interaction in amblyopia.

In order to investigate how amblyopia affects visual processing in the temporal domain, we measured the contrast thresholds of amblyopic and normal observers in an orientation identification task with external noise masks under multiple target-mask SOA conditions, and without external noise masks. By systematically manipulating the SOA of the external noise masks relative to the target, we quantified masking effects at different SOA conditions and used the results to infer how processing efficiency changes as a function of time based on the perceptual template model (PTM) (Lu and Dosher, 1999, 2008). The original PTM has been applied in studying the spatial template in amblyopia (Xu et al., 2006). The elaborated PTM (ePTM) with additional parameters describing the temporal profile of visual processing has been used to study effect of attention (Lu et al., 2004) and aging (He et al., 2020). Here, we adopted the ePTM (Lu and Dosher, 1999, 2008; Lu et al., 2004; Hou et al., 2014) to fit the trial-by-trial response data for each observer. The temporal profile of the perceptual template was estimated based on the best fitting model parameters and compared between the amblyopic and normal groups.

MATERIALS AND METHODS

Participants

Twenty amblyopic patients (age: 27.0 ± 5.53 years; 15 males), and 25 age-matched normal observers (age: 25.6 ± 4.03 years, 15 males) participated in the study. All participants went through detailed ophthalmological examinations. The observers in the normal group had normal or corrected-to-normal vision (visual acuity, VA $\leq$ 0.0 logMAR). Eye dominance was determined with the hole-in-card method for the normal group. Among the 20 amblyopic participants, there were 16 participants with monocular amblyopia (A1 – A16) and four with binocular amblyopia (A17 – A20). These participants could also be classified as anisometropic amblyope (A1 – A13, A18 – A20, n = 16), combined strabismic-anisometropic amblyope (combined with anisometropia, A14 – A15, n = 2), and deprivation amblyope (A16 – A17, n = 2). The detailed clinical information of all amblyopic participants was listed in **Supplementary Table 1**.

All observers were naive about the purpose of the study and provided written informed consent. Most of the amblyopic observers had the experience of psychophysical experiments before. The study adhered to the tenets of the Declaration of Helsinki and was approved by the institutional review board of human subject research of the Eye Hospital, Wenzhou Medical University.

Apparatus

The experiment was conducted in a dimly lighted room. We used customized programs to present visual stimuli and collect responses from the observers. The programs used in the experiment were coded in MATLAB (The MathWorks Inc., Natick, MA, United States) with Psychtoolbox extensions (Kleiner et al., 2007), and run on a HP ProDesk 680 G2 MT computer (Hewlett-Packard, Palo Alto, CA, United States). Stimuli were displayed on a gamma-corrected Sony Multiscan G520 CRT display (Sony Corp., Tokyo, Japan) with a mean luminance of 44.6 cd/m2. The resolution of the display was 800 × 600 pixels and the refresh rate was 120 Hz. The viewing distance was 1.44 m, at which each pixel subtended 0.01 degrees. A chin rest was used to minimize head movement during the experiment. Observers viewed the stimuli monocularly with their best correction (if any). The non-tested eye was occluded by an opaque patch.

Stimuli

The stimulus in each trial consisted of a sequence of 17 image frames. Each image frame lasted two display refresh cycles (16.7 ms) (**Figure 1**). The image in the ninth frame was the target, a Gabor oriented +45° or −45° from vertical with a center spatial frequency of 1 cycle per degree (cpd). The size of the Gabor was 300 × 300 pixels. The standard deviation of the Gaussian window was the same as the wavelength of the Gabor.

The external noise masks were white noise images, in which the contrast of each pixel was independently sampled from a Gaussian distribution with a mean of 0 and a standard deviation of 0.333. The size of the external noise images was also 300 × 300 pixels. The size of each noise element was 10 × 10 pixels, which was one-fifth of the wavelength of the signal stimuli. All signal and external noise frames were centered at fixation. The external noise frames were always symmetric around the signal frame. For simplicity of description, the frames in the sequence were numbered from −8 to 8, with the signal frame at 0. Four external noise configurations were used: external noise images occurred in ±1, ±2, ±3 ∼±4, or ±5 ∼±8 frames, which in the rest of the article are noted as SOA 16.7 ms, 33.4 ms, 50.0 ms, and 83.4 ms, respectively (**Figure 1**). There was also a condition with no noise mask (SOA ∞, **Figure 1**).

The remaining frames in the 17-frame sequence other than those of signal or external noise were filled with blank frames with background luminance. The same temporal configurations were also used in Lu et al. (2004) and He et al. (2020).

Design

The quick forced-choice method (Lesmes et al., 2015) targeted at three different performance levels (percentage correct = 65, 75, and 85%, respectively) was used to measure contrast thresholds. Data collected at three different performance levels are necessary to constrain the non-linearities in the PTM (Lu and Dosher, 1999, 2008). Trials of the five temporal masking conditions were interleaved randomly with equal number of trials in each test session. Each test session consisted of 750 trials and lasted about 40 min. The two eyes of amblyopic patients were measured separately. Because no significant difference between the two eyes of normal observers was found in our previous study (He et al., 2020), only the dominant eye of the normal observer was tested. Each observer was given a practice session of about 75 trials before the experiment started.

Procedure

Each trial began with a brief tone. At the same time, a fixation crosshair was presented in the center of the screen and lasted 250 ms. A blank screen (125 ms) with background luminance followed. Then the 17-frame (16.7 × 17 = 283.9 ms) stimulus sequence was presented and ended with another blank frame. Observers were instructed to indicate whether the Gabor stimulus was oriented to the left or to the right from vertical by pressing the left or right arrow key on the keyboard. Auditory feedback was provided after each correct response. A new trial started 500 ms after the response was made.

Analysis

We first calculated the contrast threshold in different SOA conditions for each observer. The raw response data were pooled across performance levels in each condition and fit with the Weibull function using a maximum likelihood procedure (Watson, 1979). The threshold from the best fitting model was used to analyze masking effects. To quantitatively estimate the characteristics of temporal processing, the ePTM (Lu et al., 2004) was fit to the data (see "The Model" section below).

Repeated measures ANOVA and t-test were used to compare the thresholds and parameters between the amblyopic and normal groups. Degrees of freedom were corrected using Greenhouse-Geisser estimates of sphericity in the case of violation of sphericity. Comparisons were made between the amblyopic eyes (AE, $n = 20$) and normal eyes (NE, $n = 25$), the amblyopic eyes of the anisometropic amblyopia subgroup (AAE, $n = 16$) and the NE, as well as the fellow eyes of the monocular amblyopia subgroup (FE, $n = 16$) and the NE. Please note the AAE were a subset of the AE. For binocular amblyopic observers, the weaker eye (with worse VA) was used as the amblyopic eye except observer A19. The left eye of A19 was used as the amblyopic eye because the data from his weaker (right) eye was excluded based on the result from the ePTM analysis – the full width at half maximum (FWHM) of the temporal window of A19's weaker eye exceeded two standard deviations from the means of the amblyopic group.

The Model

To characterize the temporal properties of visual processing in the amblyopic and normal groups, we adopted the ePTM (Lu et al., 2004) to analyze the behavioral data and to derive the temporal processing profile. The key idea of the ePTM is that masking effects at different SOA conditions represent the relative impacts of the external noise mask, and can be used to infer the temporal profile of the template, which has different weights W_t at different time t (from −8 to 8) for the 17-frame stimuli (**Figure 2**). The external noise masks were presented at ±1, ±2, ±3 ∼±4, or ±5 ∼±8 frames symmetrically around the signal frame. That is to say, we can

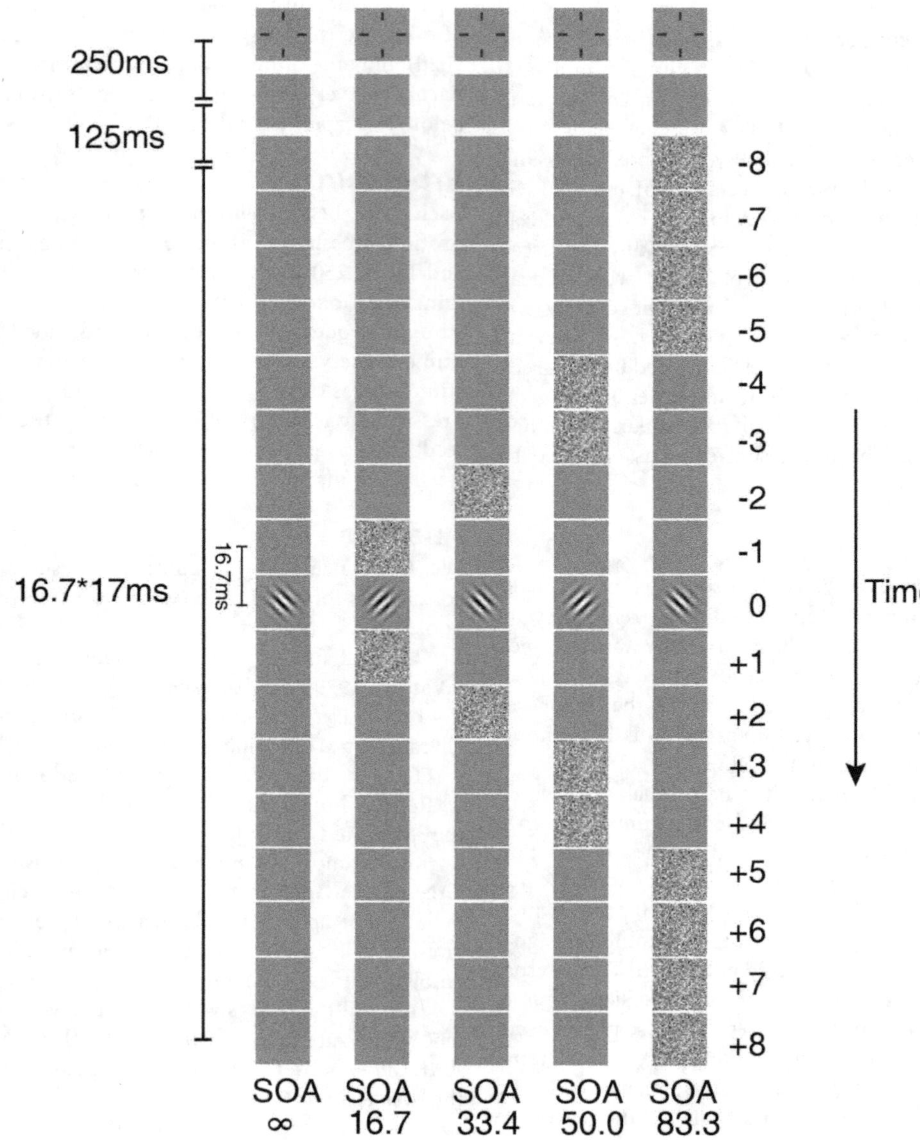

FIGURE 1 | Temporal configurations of the five masking conditions in the experiment. In condition SOA ∞, only the Gabor target was presented. In the other four conditions, the external noise masks were presented symmetrically around the target.

only obtain the average weight in the multi-frame external noise conditions.

$$W_t = \begin{cases} W_{16.7}, \; if\; t = -1,\; 1, \\ W_{33.4}, \; if\; t = -2,\; 2, \\ W_{50.0}, \; if\; t = -4, -3,\; 3,\; 4, \\ W_{83.4}, \; if\; t = -8, -7, -6, -5,\; 5,\; 6, 7, 8. \end{cases} \tag{1}$$

Because the total gain of the perceptual template to external noise is normalized to 1.0 in the PTM (Lu and Dosher, 1999), the weights of the perceptual temporal window satisfies the constraint:

$$\sum_{t=-8}^{8} W_t^2 = 1. \tag{2a}$$

It can also be written as:

$$\sum_{i=1}^{4} F_i W_i^2 = 1. \tag{2b}$$

where F_i = 2, 2, 4, and 8, F_i represents the number of frames, i = 1, 2, 3, and 4 corresponds to condition SOA 16.7 ms, 33.4 ms, 50.0 ms, and 83.4 ms, respectively. For external noise images each with rms contrast σ, the total variance of external noise in a given temporal configuration is:

$$N_{ext}^2 = \sum_{t=-8}^{8} (W_t \sigma_t)^2 = \sum_{i=1}^{4} F_i (W_i \sigma)^2 . \tag{3}$$

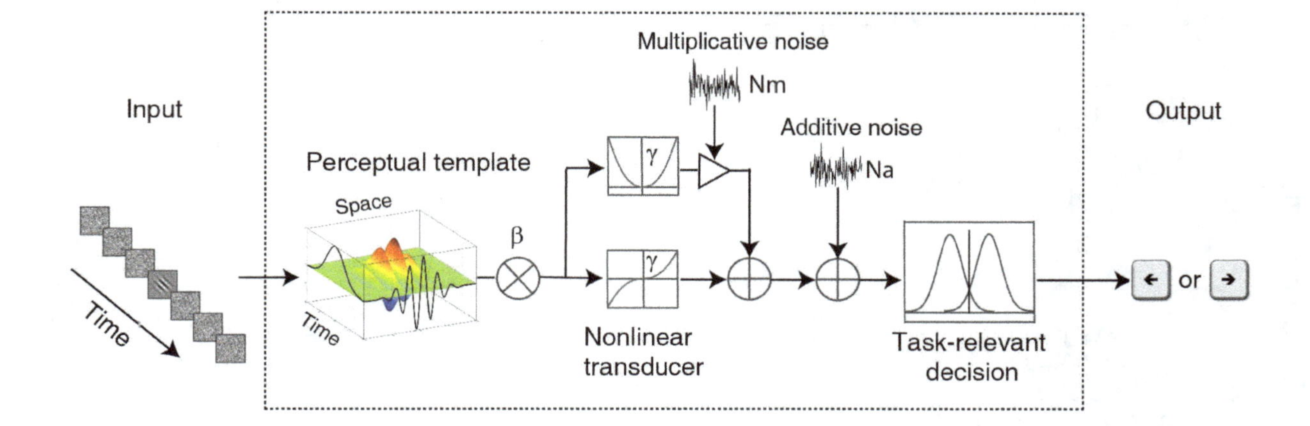

FIGURE 2 | A diagram of the elaborated perceptual template model (ePTM). The visual information first passes through a perceptual template. The perceptual template has a total signal gain of β. It also has different weight at different time. After the template matching, the information goes through a non-linear transducer with an exponent of γ, then gets contaminated by an internal additive noise *Na* and a multiplicative noise *Nm*, and finally is sent to the decision unit. The temporal weights at different SOAs can be inferred from the masking effects at different target-mask SOA conditions.

where $\sigma_t = c$, when the external noise frames were presented and $\sigma_t = 0$, when there was no mask (**Figure 1**).

Combine the equation 3 with the original PTM (Lu and Dosher, 1999, 2008), we have:

$$d' = \frac{(\beta c)^{\gamma}}{\sqrt{\left((\beta c)^{2\gamma} + (\sum_{t=-8}^{8} (W_t \sigma_t)^2)^{\gamma}\right) Nm^2 + Na^2}}. \quad (4)$$

where *Na*, *Nm*, β, and γ represent additive internal noise, multiplicative noise, overall gain of the perceptual template, and non-linear transducer function of the system, respectively (Lu and Dosher, 1999, 2008).

The probability of making a correct response in a trial can be derived from the *d'* equation for each observer (Hacker and Ratcliff, 1979):

$$P(c) = \int_{-\infty}^{+\infty} \phi\left(x - d'(c)\right) \Phi^{m-1}(x)\, dx. \quad (5)$$

where, $m = 2$ for the 2-alternative forced orientation identification task, and, $\phi()$ and $\Phi()$ are the probability density and cumulative probability density functions of a standard normal distribution, respectively. The ePTM had seven free parameters: Na, Nm, β, γ, $W_{16.7}$, $W_{33.4}$, and $W_{50.0}$. Weight $W_{83.4}$ was calculated from equation 2 based on the values of the other three weights. The model was fit to raw response data in each trial for each observer using a maximum likelihood procedure.

RESULTS

Contrast Thresholds in Amblyopia

In **Figure 3A**, the average contrast thresholds of the AE and NE are plotted as functions of SOA. A two-way repeated measures ANOVA with factors of group and SOA was conducted. Both factors group and SOA were found to have significant effects on threshold [group: $F(1,43) = 10.6$, $p = 0.002$; SOA: $F(2.75,118) = 597$, $p = 3.20 \times 10^{-69}$]. The contrast thresholds were higher in the AE than the NE. There was also a significant interaction between the two factors [$F(2.75,118) = 4.98$, $p = 0.004$]. It indicated that the pattern of the masking effect over different SOAs was different between the AE and NE.

Similar analysis was applied to the subgroup of the patients with anisometropic amblyopia. The average contrast thresholds of the AAE are plotted against SOA, along with that of the NE in **Figure 3B**. A two-way repeated measures ANOVA showed that both group and SOA had significant effects [group: $F(1,39) = 8.14$, $p = 0.007$; SOA: $F(2.72,106) = 544$, $p = 2.42 \times 10^{-62}$]. The patients with anisometropic amblyopia had higher contrast thresholds than the normal participants. The interaction between group and SOA was also significant [$F(2.72,106) = 4.77, p = 0.005$].

The data from the fellow eyes of the subgroup of patients with monocular amblyopia was also analyzed. The average contrast thresholds of the FE and the NE are plotted as functions of SOA in **Figure 3C**. There was no significant difference in threshold between the groups [$F(1,39) = 0.003, p = 0.96$]. The group × SOA interaction was not significant [$F(2.91,13.6) = 0.90$, $p = 0.44$]. The fellow eyes of the patients with monocular amblyopia had comparable contrast thresholds as the normal eyes.

The Results of Model Fitting

The ePTM provided good fits to the raw response data for all participants (χ^2 test, all $ps > 0.50$). We first looked at the internal additive noise *Na* and template gain β of the best fitting ePTM (**Figure 4**). There was a marginally significant difference in *Na* between the AE and NE [-3.40 ± 1.03 vs. -4.03 ± 1.17, $t(43) = 1.89$, $p = 0.066$]. There was also a marginally significant difference in *Na* between the AAE and NE [-3.40 ± 0.98 vs. -4.03 ± 1.17, $t(39) = 1.81$, $p = 0.078$]. No significant *Na* difference was found between the FE and

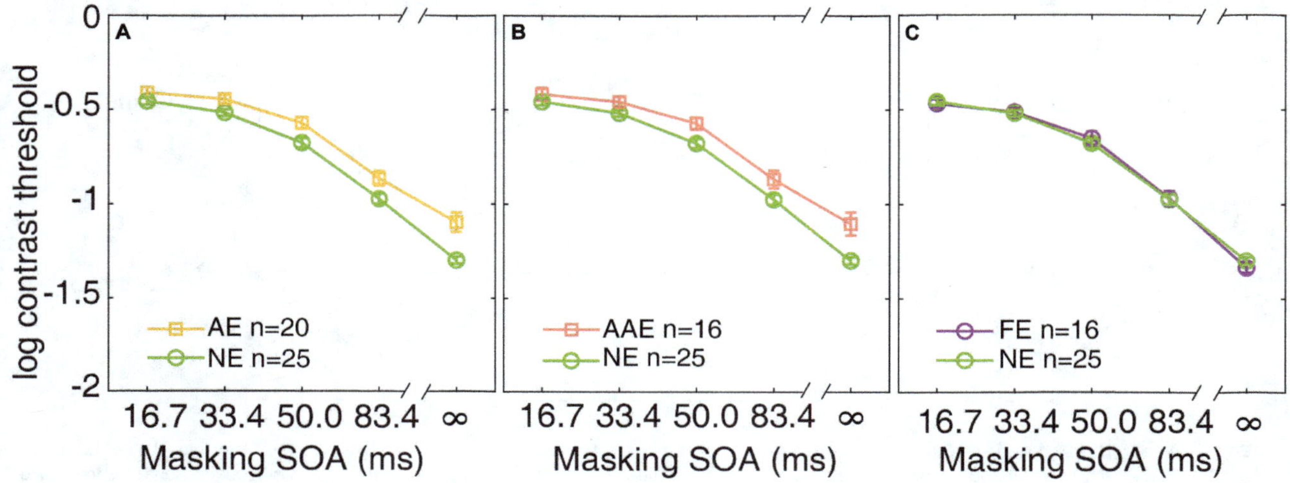

FIGURE 3 | Average contrast thresholds as a function of SOA are shown for the AE **(A)**, the AAE **(B)**, and the FE **(C)**. The average contrast thresholds of the NE are also plotted in each panel for comparison. Yellow: AE. Pink: AAE. Purple: FE. Green: NE. Error bars represent ±1 standard error.

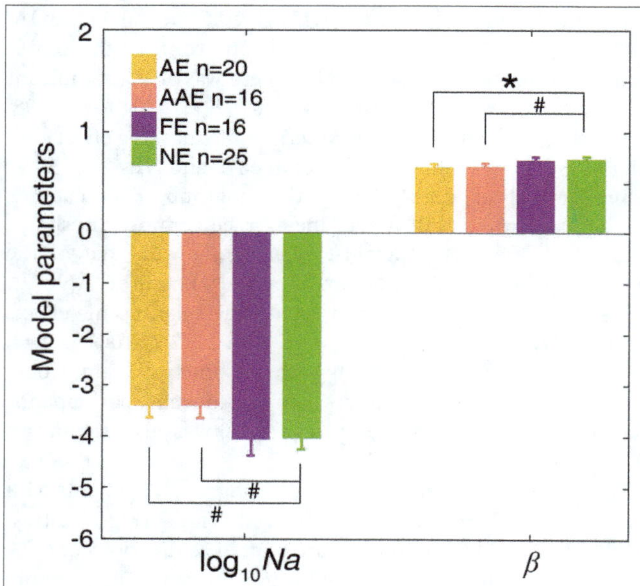

FIGURE 4 | The average *Na* (in log10 units) and β of the best-fitting ePTM. Yellow: AE. Pink: AAE. Purple: FE. Green: NE. Error bars represent ±1 standard error. *: $p < 0.05$. #: $0.05 < p < 0.1$.

NE [$t(39) = -0.062$, $p = 0.95$]. The template gain β in the AE was significantly smaller than that in the NE [0.65 ± 0.13 vs. 0.73 ± 0.13, $t(43) = -2.06$, $p = 0.046$]. The β in the AAE was marginally smaller than that in the NE [0.66 ± 0.13 vs. 0.73 ± 0.13, $t(39) = -1.74$, $p = 0.090$]. There was no significant β difference between the FE and NE [$t(39) = -0.28$, $p = 0.78$]. No significant difference in the multiplicative noise *Nm*, or the non-linear exponent γ was found in any comparisons (all *ps* > 0.10).

Change in Temporal Window

The temporal weights $W_{16.7}$, $W_{33.4}$, $W_{50.0}$, and $W_{83.4}$ of the AE, FE, and NE were derived from the best fitting ePTM. The temporal weights W_t over the range (−8 to 8 frames) can be derived from $W_{16.7}$, $W_{33.4}$, $W_{50.0}$, and $W_{83.4}$ based on equation 1. The average temporal profile of the AE, AAE, and FE are plotted as functions of time in **Figures 5A–C**, respectively. The unit of the abscissa has been converted into the actual time (ms). The average temporal profile of the NE is also plotted in each panel.

A repeated measures ANOVA was applied to the weights at different SOAs. The effect of group was not significant [$F(1,43) = 0.13$, $p = 0.72$]. There was a significant effect of SOA [$F(2.13,91.5) = 1068$, $p = 2.31 \times 10^{-65}$]. There was also a significant interaction between group and SOA [$F(2.13,91.5) = 3.29$, $p = 0.039$], suggesting that the temporal profiles were different between the AE and NE. *Post-hoc* analysis showed that the temporal weight at SOA 16.7 ms was significantly lower in the AE group than in the NE group [one-tailed, $t(41.0) = -2.41$, $p = 0.010$. **Figure 5A**], the temporal weight at SOA 50.0 ms was higher in the AE group than in the NE group [one-tailed, $t(43) = 2.12$, $p = 0.020$]. There was no significant weight difference at SOA 33.4 and 83.4 ms (all *ps* > 0.20).

We then compared the temporal weights between the AAE and NE. Similarly, there was no significant weight difference between the two groups [$F(1,39) = 0.013$, $p = 0.91$]. There was a significant effect of SOA [$F(2.16,84.1) = 984$, $p = 2.90 \times 10^{-60}$]. There was also a significant interaction between group and SOA [$F(2.16,84.1) = 3.05$, $p = 0.032$]. The temporal weight at SOA 16.7 ms was significantly lower in the AAE than in the NE group [one-tailed, $t(39) = -2.32$, $p = 0.013$], the temporal weight at SOA 50.0 ms was higher in the AE than in the NE [one-tailed, $t(39) = 1.99$, $p = 0.027$]. There was no significant weight difference at SOA 33.4 and 83.4 ms (all *ps* > 0.20).

When comparing the weights between the FE and NE, an ANOVA revealed that only SOA had significant effect

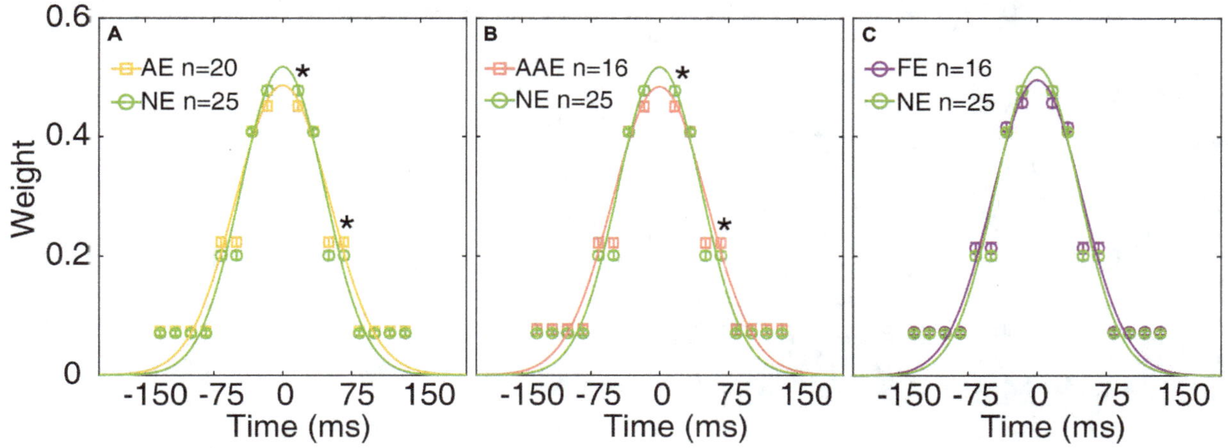

FIGURE 5 | The average temporal weights of the best-fitting ePTM of the AE (yellow), AAE (pink), and FE (purple) are plotted as functions of time in **(A–C)**, respectively. The average temporal profile of the NE (green) is also plotted in each panel. *Error bar*: ±1 standard error. *: $p < 0.05$. The continuous curves are the best-fitting Gaussians.

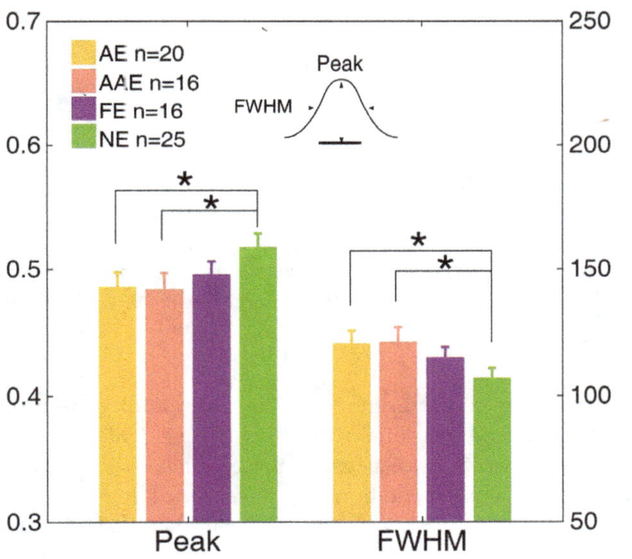

FIGURE 6 | The peak and full width at half maximum (FWHM) of the temporal window of the AE (yellow), AAE (pink), FE (purple), and NE (green). The left *y*-axis shows the peak and the right *y*-axis shows the FWHM. *Error bar*: ±1 standard error. *: $p < 0.05$.

[$F(2.05,79.9) = 1154$, $p = 4.08 \times 10^{-60}$]. No significant weight difference was found between the FE and NE [$F(1,39) = 1.18$, $p = 0.29$]. The interaction between group and SOA was not significant [$F(2.05,79.9) = 1.90$, $p = 0.16$].

The temporal weight decreased as the external noise mask was presented further (in time) away from the onset of the target, thus the temporal profile was termed as the "temporal window." A Gaussian function, $g(t) = peak \cdot \exp\left(-\left(\frac{t^2}{2\sigma^2}\right)\right)$, was fit to W_t to quantify the shape of the temporal window. The residual of each data point was weighted to make sure that the data derived in each external noise condition contributed equally to the entire fitting. The peak amplitude and full width at half maximum (FWHM), computed as $2\sqrt{2\ln(2)}\sigma$, were derived for each observer (**Figure 6**).

The peak and FWHM of the AE, AAE, and FE are shown in **Figure 6**. The peak amplitude of the AE was significantly lower than that of the NE [0.49 ± 0.051 vs. 0.52 ± 0.044, $t(43) = -2.24$, $p = 0.030$]. The FWHM of the AE was significantly greater than that of the NE [120 ± 22.1 ms vs. 107 ± 15.7 ms, $t(43) = 2.39$, $p = 0.020$]. The peak amplitude of the AAE was significantly lower than that of the NE [0.48 ± 0.050 vs. 0.52 ± 0.044, $t(39) = -2.25$, $p = 0.031$]. The FWHM of the AAE was significantly greater than that of the NE [121 ± 22.6 ms vs. 107 ± 15.7 ms, $t(39) = 2.38$, $p = 0.022$]. No significant peak or FWHM difference was found between the FE and NE (all $ps > 0.10$).

The Relationship Between the Temporal Window and Spatial Vision

We also investigated the relationship between the temporal window and spatial vision using correlation analysis of the AE. The peak and FWHM of the temporal window are plotted against the visual acuity of the AE in **Figures 7A,B**, respectively. Neither the correlation between the peak and visual acuity ($r = 0.061$, $p = 0.80$), nor that between the FWHM and visual acuity ($r = -0.064$, $p = 0.79$) was significant. In **Figures 7C,D**, the peak and FWHM are plotted against the thresholds of SOA ∞ (no noise condition) for the AE. Neither correlation was significant (all $ps > 0.60$). The results indicated that the temporal deficit in amblyopia was likely independent of spatial vision.

DISCUSSION

Using an orientation identification task with external noise masks in various target-mask SOA conditions, we measured the contrast thresholds of amblyopic and normal observers. The contrast

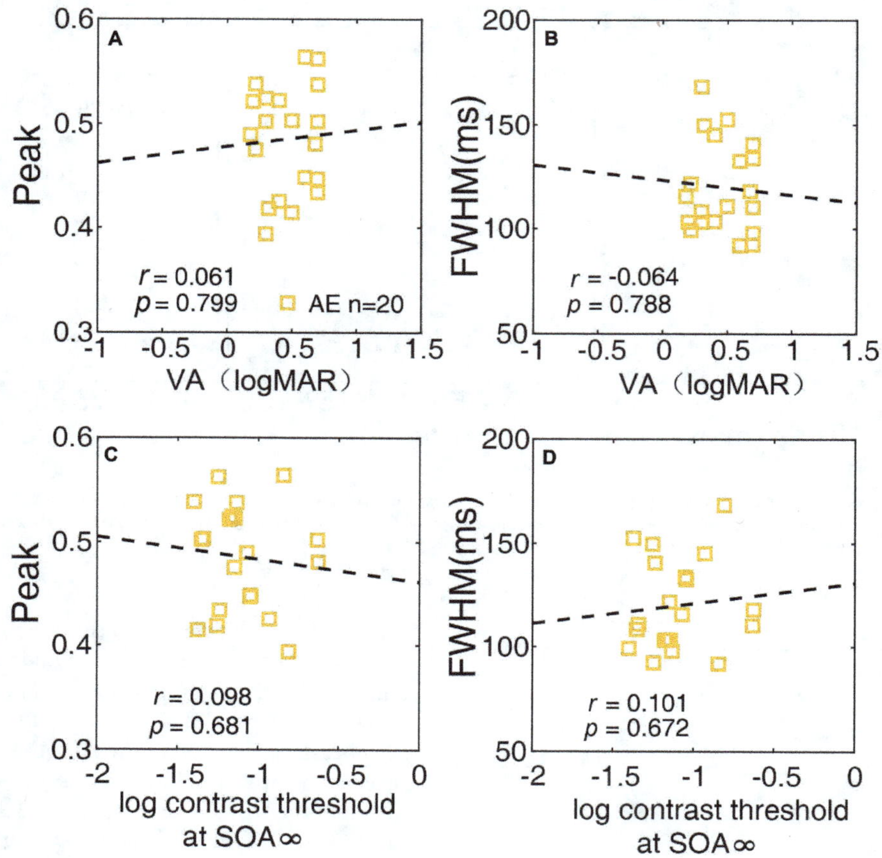

FIGURE 7 | The relationship between the peak of the temporal window and VA **(A)**, between the width (FWHM) of the temporal window and VA **(B)**, between the peak of the temporal and contrast threshold at SOA ∞ **(C)**, and between the width (FWHM) of the temporal window and contrast threshold at SOA ∞ **(D)** of the AE are plotted.

thresholds of the amblyopic eyes were higher than that of the normal eyes. A significant interaction between group and SOA was found, indicating that the pattern of masking effect in the amblyopic eyes was different from that in the normal eyes. By fitting the ePTM to the trial-by-trial data, we derived several parameters of the observer model. The additive noise of the amblyopic eyes was marginally higher than that of the normal eyes, and the template gain of the amblyopic eyes was significantly lower than the normal eyes. A further analysis of the weight parameters of the temporal window revealed that the amblyopic eyes had a flatter (lower peak and broader width) temporal window than the normal eyes. No significant difference was found between the shape of the temporal window and spatial vision of the amblyopic eyes. Additional analysis showed that the anisometropic amblyopic eyes had similar temporal deficits. However, we did not observe any difference in the contrast threshold or temporal window between the fellow eyes of the patients with monocular amblyopia and the normal eyes.

The different patterns of the masking effects between the AE and NE (**Figure 3A**), as evidenced by the significant interaction between the group and SOA in ANOVA, indicated that the masking effect (computed as the threshold elevation) of the AE was smaller than that in the NE. This result did not mean that the AE tolerated the noise better than the NE. This is because the threshold difference between the external noise condition and the no noise condition was determined jointly by the internal additive noise and the template efficiency (external noise exclusion) (Lu and Dosher, 1999, 2008). The counterintuitive result was due to the marginally increased internal additive noise and significantly decreased template efficiency as revealed by the ePTM. Our result was consistent with that reported in Xu et al. (2006). As shown in their Figures 2, 3, the threshold difference between high noise and no noise conditions was smaller in the amblyopic eyes than that in the normal eyes. They also found that the amblyopic patient had an increased internal additive noise and a defective template.

The decreased template gain indicated that it was difficult for amblyopia to exclude external noise and therefore a lower processing efficiency in amblyopia (Wang et al., 1998; Pelli et al., 2004; Xu et al., 2006). By systematically manipulating the SOA of the noise masks, we can estimate the temporal profile of the perceptual template (temporal window), which represents how the processing efficiency of the visual template varies in time. We found that the temporal window of the amblyopic visual processing was flattened relative to the normal one. It should be noted that the temporal window applies to both signal and noise. If the temporal window is flat, it means the processing efficiency at small SOA (i.e., 16.7 ms) is low – it is true that the template excluded more external noises, but it also attenuated more signals. Moreover, the broader extent of the temporal window also implies that the amblyopic eyes are not properly tuned to the timing of signal thus have more difficulties in processing dynamic visual information, even at low spatial frequencies. Taken together, our finding combined with the previous studies in spatial domain suggests the amblyopia has an impaired spatio-temporal template.

Amblyopia is commonly associated with strabismus or anisometropia in early life. Apart from the oculomotor difference, it has been shown that the pattern of visual deficits were different between strabismic and anisometropic amblyopes (McKee et al., 2003). Using a RSVP digit identification task, Bonneh et al. (2007) found that strabismic amblyopes showed a significant VA reduction in the fast RSVP condition. However, the anisometropic amblyopes and normal observers did not show any significant VA difference between the fast and slow conditions. In our study, with a more quantitative approach, we found that anisometropic amblyopia had a temporal window with lower peak and broader width, indicating that anisometropic amblyopia also led to temporal deficits. Although there were not enough strabismic participants in the current experiment for us to draw any concrete conclusion on how the temporal window in strabismic amblyopia was affected, we performed some preliminary analyses based on the data from the two combined strabismic-anisometropic amblyopes. Similar to the anisometropic eye, the combined strabismic- anisometropic eyes showed significantly different results compared to the normal eyes. No significant difference between the combined strabismic-anisometropic and anisometropic eyes was found. The detailed result was described in the **Supplementary Material**: Preliminary Results in Strabismic Amblyopia. It is possible that the temporal deficits in anisometropic amblyopia are less severe than those in strabismic amblyopia. Future studies are necessary to evaluate whether subtypes of amblyopia have different temporal processing deficits.

The defective temporal window in amblyopia could be due to the deficits in low level visual processing. In an animal study, Kiorpes et al. (2006) measured sensitivity to visual motion in random dot displays for strabismic and anisometropic amblyopic monkeys. They found that amblyopic losses in motion sensitivity were not correlated with losses in spatial contrast sensitivity, and also found a specific impairment for detecting long temporal offsets, revealing a deficit in spatiotemporal integration in amblyopia which cannot be explained by the lower spatial resolution of amblyopic vision. Similarity, in human studies, Spang and Fahle (2009) used a time-based figure–ground segregation task and demonstrated that the temporal resolution of the amblyopic eye was reduced. Huang et al. (2012) and Tao et al. (2019) found that the temporal synchrony sensitivity of amblyopic eyes was higher than that of the fellow eyes, which was uncorrelated with the visual acuity, suggesting that amblyopes have a low-level temporal processing deficit in the fovea.

Some studies have suggested that abnormal visual experience during the developmental critical period in amblyopia could also affect higher level of cortical areas (Popple and Levi, 2008; Farzin and Norcia, 2011; Perdziak et al., 2018). Popple and Levi (2008) found that, when viewing displays with their amblyopic eyes, observers had a shallower attentional blink 200 ms after the first target, compared with the preferred eye, depending on the depth of amblyopia, and made more wrong responses consisting of non-distractor letters, when the distractors and targets were confusable. These findings may be the result of an altered time course of attention in amblyopia. Bonneh et al. (2007) also suggested that their findings reflected a lower attentional resolution, i.e., the ability to isolate successive stimuli in time. Farzin and Norcia (2011) measured the response time and accuracy of amblyopes in a variant of the Eriksen flanker task. They found a selective deficit in visual decision making when individuals with amblyopia used either the amblyopic or non-amblyopic (dominant) eye. Thus the defective temporal window found in this study could also be due to abnormalities in higher cortical areas.

Taken together, our results showed that amblyopia had temporal processing deficits captured by a flattened temporal window of visual processing, and the deficits were independent of spatial vision. How temporal deficits interact with spatial deficits, and how they affect the quality of life of amblyopic patients remain to be investigated in future studies.

AUTHOR CONTRIBUTIONS

FH, FL, Z-LL, and RC conceived the experiments. XHu, YQ, XY, and JY performed the experiments. XHu, XR, YQ, XY, JY, and XHe analyzed the data and interpreted the data. XHu, FL, Z-LL, and FH wrote the manuscript. All authors contributed to manuscript revision, read and approved the submitted version.

REFERENCES

Barrett, B. T., Pacey, I. E., Bradley, A., Thibos, L. N., and Morrill, P. (2003). Nonveridical visual perception in human amblyopia. *Invest. Ophthalmol. Vis. Sci.* 44, 1555–1567. doi: 10.1167/iovs.02-0515

Birch, E. E., and Swanson, W. H. (2000). Hyperacuity deficits in anisometropic and strabismic amblyopes with known ages of onset. *Vision Res.* 40, 1035–1040. doi: 10.1016/s0042-6989(00)00011-0

Bonneh, Y. S., Sagi, D., and Polat, U. (2007). Spatial and temporal crowding in amblyopia. *Vision Res.* 47, 1950–1962. doi: 10.1016/j.visres.2007.02.015

Eckstein, M. P., and Ahumada, A. J. Jr. (2002). Classification images: a tool to analyze visual strategies. *J. Vis.* 2, i–i. doi: 10.1167/2.1.i

Faghihi, M., Hashemi, H., Nabovati, P., Saatchi, M., Yekta, A., Rafati, S., et al. (2017). The prevalence of amblyopia and its determinants in a population-based study. *Strabismus* 25, 176–183. doi: 10.1080/09273972.2017.1391849

Farzin, F., and Norcia, A. M. (2011). Impaired visual decision-making in individuals with amblyopia. *J. Vis* 11:10.1167/11.14.66. doi: 10.1167/11.14.6

Giaschi, D., Lo, R., Narasimhan, S., Lyons, C., and Wilcox, L. M. (2013). Sparing of coarse stereopsis in stereodeficient children with a history of amblyopia. *J Vis* 13:17. doi: 10.1167/13.10.17

Hacker, M., and Ratcliff, R. (1979). A revised table of d' for M-alternative forced choice. *Percept. Psychophys.* 26, 168–170. doi: 10.3758/bf03208311

He, X., Shen, M., Cui, R., Zheng, H., Ruan, X., Lu, Z.-L., et al. (2020). The temporal window of visual processing in aging. *Invest. Ophthalmol. Vis. Sci.* 61, 60–60. doi: 10.1167/iovs.61.5.60

Hess, R. F., Dakin, S. C., Tewfik, M., and Brown, B. (2001). Contour interaction in amblyopia: scale selection. *Vision Res.* 41, 2285–2296. doi: 10.1016/S0042-6989(01)00099-2

Hess, R. F., and Holliday, I. E. (1992). The spatial localization deficit in amblyopia. *Vision Res.* 32, 1319–1339. doi: 10.1016/0042-6989(92)90225-8

Hess, R. F., and Howell, E. R. (1977). The threshold contrast sensitivity function in strabismic amblyopia: evidence for a two type classification. *Vision Res.* 17, 1049–1055. doi: 10.1016/0042-6989(77)90009-8

Ho, C. S., and Giaschi, D. E. (2006). Deficient maximum motion displacement in amblyopia. *Vision Res.* 46, 4595–4603. doi: 10.1016/j.visres.2006.09.025

Ho, C. S., and Giaschi, D. E. (2007). Stereopsis-dependent deficits in maximum motion displacement in strabismic and anisometropic amblyopia. *Vision Res.* 47, 2778–2785. doi: 10.1016/j.visres.2007.07.008

Ho, C. S., Giaschi, D. E., Boden, C., Dougherty, R., Cline, R., and Lyons, C. (2005). Deficient motion perception in the fellow eye of amblyopic children. *Vision Res.* 45, 1615–1627. doi: 10.1016/j.visres.2004.12.009

Hou, F., Lu, Z. L., and Huang, C. B. (2014). The external noise normalized gain profile of spatial vision. *J. Vis.* 14:9. doi: 10.1167/14.13.9

Huang, P. C., Li, J., Deng, D., Yu, M., and Hess, R. F. (2012). Temporal synchrony deficits in amblyopia. *Invest. Ophthalmol. Vis. Sci.* 53, 8325–8332. doi: 10.1167/iovs.12-10835

Kiorpes, L. (2019). Understanding the development of amblyopia using macaque monkey models. *Proc. Natl. Acad. Sci.U.S.A.* 116:26217. doi: 10.1073/pnas.1902285116

Kiorpes, L., Tang, C., and Movshon, J. A. (2006). Sensitivity to visual motion in amblyopic macaque monkeys. *Vis. Neurosci.* 23, 247–256. doi: 10.1017/s0952523806232097

Kleiner, M., Brainard, D. H., Pelli, D., Ingling, A., Murray, R., and Broussard, C. (2007). What's new in Psychtoolbox-3. *Perception* 36, 1–16. doi: 10.1068/v070821

Kosovicheva, A., Ferreira, A., Vera-Diaz, F. A., and Bex, P. J. (2019). Effects of temporal frequency on binocular deficits in amblyopia. *Vision Res.* 163, 52–62. doi: 10.1016/j.visres.2019.08.004

Lesmes, L. A., Lu, Z. L., Baek, J., Tran, N., Dosher, B. A., and Albright, T. D. (2015). Developing Bayesian adaptive methods for estimating sensitivity thresholds (d') in Yes-No and forced-choice tasks. *Front. Psychol.* 6:1070. doi: 10.3389/fpsyg.2015.01070

Levi, D. M., Hariharan, S., and Klein, S. A. (2002). Suppressive and facilitatory spatial interactions in amblyopic vision. *Vision Res.* 42, 1379–1394. doi: 10.1016/S0042-6989(02)00061-5

Levi, D. M., and Harwerth, R. S. (1977). Spatio-temporal interactions in anisometropic and strabismic amblyopia. *Invest. Ophthalmol. Vis. Sci.* 16, 90–95.

Levi, D. M., and Klein, S. (1982). Hyperacuity and amblyopia. *Nature* 298, 268–270. doi: 10.1038/298268a0

Levi, D. M., and Klein, S. A. (1985). Vernier acuity, crowding and amblyopia. *Vision Res.* 25, 979–991. doi: 10.1016/0042-6989(85)90208-1

Levi, D. M., and Klein, S. A. (2003). Noise provides some new signals about the spatial vision of amblyopes. *J. Neurosci.* 23:2522. doi: 10.1523/JNEUROSCI.23-07-02522.2003

Levi, D. M., Knill, D. C., and Bavelier, D. (2015). Stereopsis and amblyopia: a mini-review. *Vision Res.* 114, 17–30. doi: 10.1016/j.visres.2015.01.002

Lu, Z.-L., and Dosher, B. (2013). *Visual Psychophysics: From Laboratory to Theory.* Cambridge, MA: The MIT Press, doi: 10.7551/mitpress/9780262019453.001.0001

Lu, Z. L., and Dosher, B. A. (1998). External noise distinguishes attention mechanisms. *Vision Res.* 38, 1183–1198. doi 10.1016/s0042-6989(97)00273-3

Lu, Z. L., and Dosher, B. A. (1999). Characterizing human perceptual inefficiencies with equivalent internal noise. *J. Opt. Soc. Am. A Opt. Image Sci. Vis.* 16, 764–778. doi: 10.1364/josaa.16.000764

Lu, Z. L., and Dosher, B. A. (2008). Characterizing observers using external noise and observer models: assessing internal representations with external noise. *Psychol. Rev.* 115, 44–82. doi: 10.1037/0033-295X.115.1.44

Lu, Z. L., Jeon, S. T., and Dosher, B. A. (2004). Temporal tuning characteristics of the perceptual template and endogenous cuing of spatial attention. *Vision Res.* 44, 1333–1350. doi: 10.1016/j.visres.2003.12.017

Manny, R. E., and Levi, D. M. (1982). Psychophysical investigations of the temporal modulation sensitivity function in amblyopia: uniform field flicker. *Invest. Ophthalmol. Vis. Sci.* 22, 515–524.

McKee, S. P., Levi, D. M., and Movshon, J. A. (2003). The pattern of visual deficits in amblyopia. *J. Vis.* 3, 380–405. doi: 10.1167/3.5.5

Miles, P. W. (1949). Flicker fusion frequency in amblyopia ex anopsia*. *Am. J. Ophthalmol.* 32, 225–231. doi 10.1016/s0002-9394(14)78377-1

Pelli, D. G., and Farell, B. (1999). Why use noise? *J. Opt. Soc. Am. A Opt. Image Sci. Vis.* 16, 647–653. doi: 10.1364/josaa.16.000647

Pelli, D. G., Levin, D. M., and Chung, S. T. L. (2004). Using visual noise to characterize amblyopic letter identification. *J. Vis.* 4, 904–920. doi: 10.1167/4.10.6

Perdziak, M., Witkowska, D., Gryncewicz, W., and Ober, J. (2018). Strabismic amblyopia affects decision processes preceding saccadic response. *Biocybern. Biomed. Eng.* 38, 190–199. doi: 10.1016/j.bbe.2017.12.003

Piano, M. E., Bex, P. J., and Simmers, A. J. (2015). Perceptual visual distortions in adult amblyopia and their relationship to clinical features. *Invest. Ophthalmol. Vis. Sci.* 56, 5533–5542. doi: 10.1167/iovs.15-17071

Popple, A. V., and Levi, D. M. (2008). The attentional blink in amblyopia. *J. Vis.* 8, 12–12. doi: 10.1167/8.13.12

Simmers, A. J., Ledgeway, T., Hess, R. F., and Mcgraw, P. V. (2003). Deficits to global motion processing in human amblyopia. *Vision Res.* 43, 729–738. doi: 10.1016/s0042-6989(02)00684-3

Simmers, A. J., Ledgeway, T., Mansouri, B., Hutchinson, C. V., and Hess, R. F. (2006). The extent of the dorsal extra-striate deficit in amblyopia. *Vision Res.* 46, 2571–2580. doi: 10.1016/j.visres.2006.01.009

Spang, K., and Fahle, M. (2009). Impaired temporal, not just spatial, resolution in amblyopia. *Invest. Ophthalmol. Vis. Sci.* 50, 5207–5212. doi: 10.1167/iovs.07-1604

Tailor, V., Bossi, M., Greenwood, J. A., and Dahlmann-Noor, A. (2016). Childhood amblyopia: current management and new trends. *Br. Med. Bull.* 119, 75–86. doi: 10.1093/bmb/ldw030

Tao, C., Wu, Y., Gong, L., Chen, S., Mao, Y., Chen, Y., et al. (2019). Abnormal monocular and dichoptic temporal synchrony in adults with amblyopia. *Invest. Ophthalmol. Vis. Sci.* 60, 4858–4864. doi: 10.1167/iovs.19-27893

Tytla, M. E., and Steinbach, M. J. (1984). Metacontrast masking in amblyopia. *Can. J. Psychol.* 38, 369–385. doi: 10.1037/h0080858

Wang, H., Levi, D. M., and Klein, S. A. (1998). Spatial uncertainty and sampling efficiency in amblyopic position acuity. *Vision Res.* 38, 1239–1251. doi: 10.1016/S0042-6989(97)00278-2

Wang, Y., Liang, Y. B., Sun, L. P., Duan, X. R., Yuan, R. Z., Wong, T. Y., et al. (2011). Prevalence and causes of amblyopia in a rural adult population of Chinese. *Ophthalmology* 118, 279–283. doi: 10.1016/j.ophtha.2010.05.026

Watson, A. B. (1979). Probability summation over time. *Vision Res.* 19, 515–522. doi: 10.1016/0042-6989(79)90136-6

Webber, A. L., and Wood, J. (2005). Amblyopia: prevalence, natural history, functional effects and treatment. *Clin. Exp. Optom.* 88, 365–375. doi: 10.1111/j.1444-0938.2005.tb05102.x

Wesson, M. D., and Loop, M. S. (1982). Temporal contrast sensitivity in amblyopia. *Invest. Ophthalmol. Vis. Sci.* 22, 98–102.

Xu, P., Lu, Z. L., Qiu, Z., and Zhou, Y. (2006). Identify mechanisms of amblyopia in Gabor orientation identification with external noise. *Vision Res.* 46, 3748–3760. doi: 10.1016/j.visres.2006.06.013

8

Longitudinal Rehabilitation of Binocular Function in Adolescent Intermittent Exotropia after Successful Corrective Surgery

*Tingting Peng[1], Meiping Xu[1], Fuhao Zheng[1], Junxiao Zhang[1], Shuang Chen[1], Jiangtao Lou[1], Chunxiao Wang[1], Yuwen Wang[1] and Xinping Yu[1,2]**

[1] *The Eye Hospital, School of Ophthalmology and Optometry, Wenzhou Medical University, Wenzhou, China,* [2] *State Key Laboratory of Ophthalmology, Zhongshan Ophthalmic Center, Sun Yat-sen University, Guangzhou, China*

Correspondence:
Xinping Yu
yu-xinping@163.com

Purpose: To study the longitudinal rehabilitation of binocular visual function in adolescent intermittent exotropia (IXT) after successful surgery and compare the results with those of a normal population. The role of binocular function in ocular alignment stability was also evaluated postoperatively.

Methods: In this prospective study, 30 adolescents with IXT successfully corrected after 1 month were followed for 12 months, and 30 children with normal vision were enrolled as controls. Stereopsis, the fusional vergence amplitude, sensory fusion, and accommodative flexibility were measured to assess binocular function at baseline and 6 and 12 months postoperatively. The controls were tested once when they were enrolled in the study.

Results: The deviation was −32.00 ± 8.60 prism diopters (PD) at distance fixation and −36.0 ± 9.10 PD at near fixation preoperatively with an average correction of 28.53 ± 3.79 PD and 30.67 ± 1.34 PD at 1 month postoperatively. Distance stereoacuity and near stereoacuity improved from 1 to 12 months postoperatively (p = 0.025 and p = 0.041, respectively). Compared with the controls, the fusional convergence reserve at distance (p = 0.025) and near (p = 0.033) fixations and fusion reserve ratio at distance (p = 0.000) and near (p = 0.000) fixations remained subnormal, whereas sensory fusion (p = 0.237), distance stereopsis (p = 0.120), and the fusional divergence amplitude at a distance (p = 0.168) were normal. However, no significant correlations were found between binocular functions at 1 month postoperatively and the postoperative drift.

Conclusion: Binocular function significantly improved from before to after successful corrective surgery and continued to improve from 1 to 12 months postoperatively in adolescents with IXT. No significant correlations were found between binocular functions at 1 month postoperatively and ocular alignment stability.

Keywords: intermittent exotropia, strabismus surgery, binocular function, rehabilitation, ocular alignment

INTRODUCTION

Intermittent exotropia (IXT) is the most common form of exotropia in children and adolescents. The prevalence of IXT is approximately 1% in Western countries (Hutchinson, 2001) and approximately 3% in teenagers in China (Pan et al., 2016). IXT is characterized by intermittent fusion when the eyes experience proper ocular alignment in the early stage of strabismus, leading to the development of binocularity and stereopsis; patients with IXT possess the potential to regain normal binocular functions after treatment (Donahue, 2007). Surgical treatment is critical for IXT (Jie et al., 2010; Yu et al., 2016) in children and adolescents. Binocular functions (e.g., stereopsis, sensory fusion, and motor fusion) improve after surgery (O'Neal et al., 1995; Yildirim et al., 1999; Wu et al., 2006; Adams et al., 2008; Sharma et al., 2008; Feng X. et al., 2015; Pineles et al., 2015; Wu Y. et al., 2020). Feng X. et al. (2015) found that stereopsis and sensory fusion improved from 2 to 6 weeks postoperatively, whereas binocular fusion and alignment were not evaluated over longer periods. Distance stereoacuity improved in individuals with IXT at 6 weeks (Adams et al., 2008) and 1 year after successful surgery (Yildirim et al., 1999; Wu et al., 2006). Sharma et al. (2008) found an increase in fusional vergence and both near and distance stereoacuities 6 months after surgery in individuals with IXT. However, these studies performed only one follow-up after surgery. Longitudinal rehabilitation in binocular function after successful surgery as well as their associations with ocular alignment drift were not evaluated. The longitudinal recovery of binocular function in IXT patients after successful surgery should be evaluated extensively.

The high recurrence rate after surgery reduces the benefits of corrective surgery in IXT patients. The specific factors for recurrence or drift after surgery in IXT have not yet been established. However, factors, such as the surgical procedure, age at surgery, angle of deviation, and preoperative binocular functions, have been studied previously (Pineles et al., 2010; Lee et al., 2018; Mohan and Sharma, 2020; Repka et al., 2020). Postoperative binocular function was not related to postoperative ocular alignment stability in our retrospective study (Wu Y. et al., 2020). An adequate understanding of the recovery of binocular function after successful surgery may help identify the factors associated with the recurrence of IXT after surgery.

Based on these findings, we designed a prospective study to evaluate the longitudinal rehabilitation of binocular visual function (e.g., sensory fusion, stereoacuity, fusional vergence amplitude, amplitude of accommodation, accommodative flexibility) after successful surgery to compare the results with those of a normal population and to determine whether binocular function is involved in the stability of ocular alignment postoperatively.

SUBJECTS AND METHODS

This prospective case–control study was approved by the Ethics Committee of the Eye Hospital of Wenzhou Medical University and was performed in accordance with the Declaration of Helsinki.

Subjects

Thirty patients aged 7–17 years with IXT successfully corrected for 1 month after surgery and 30 asymptomatic age- and sex-matched controls were recruited from the Eye Hospital of Wenzhou Medical University from July 2019 to September 2019. Only patients with basic IXT (Donahue et al., 2019) preoperatively were included in the study. The definition of successful motor alignment is orthotropia, X(T) $\leq$ 10 prism diopters (PD) and E(T) $\leq$ 5 PD in the primary position at distance and near fixations (Kim and Choi, 2016; Donahue et al., 2019). Patients were excluded if any of the following conditions were encountered: diplopia at 1 month after surgery, vertical deviation $\geq$ 5 PD, dissociated vertical deviation (DVD), oblique muscle dysfunction, an A or V pattern, eye movement restricted in one direction, a congenital cranial nerve abnormality, a history of extraocular muscle surgery or botulinum toxin injection treatment, amblyopia ($\geq$2 lines interocular difference on Snellen's vision chart), anisometropia (a spherical or cylindrical difference $\geq$ 2.0 diopters), or a history of binocular vision therapy pre- or postoperatively.

Data Collection

The following data were recorded for each patient: name, sex, age, age at the time of surgery, best-corrected visual acuity (BCVA), eye movements (EOM), preoperative and postoperative angle of deviation and binocular functions, including sensory (sensory fusion, stereoacuity) and motor function (fusional vergency amplitude, amplitude of accommodation, and accommodative flexibility).

The angle of deviation was measured using the prism and alternate cover test (PACT) at 33 cm for near and 6 m for distance fixations. The deviation of tropia was measured using the simultaneous prism and cover test (SPCT) at 33 cm for near fixation and 6 m for distance fixation (Donahue et al., 2019).

Sensory fusion was tested using the Worth 4-dot test at distance and near fixations. Patients who detected four dots were considered to have fusion, those who saw five dots were considered diplopic, and those who saw two or three dots were considered to have suppression. Subjects who saw 2 or 3 dots at distance fixation and 4 dots at near fixation were defined as having peripheral fusion (Yildirim et al., 1999; Feng X. et al., 2015).

Near stereoacuity was assessed using TNO stereopsis tests at 40 cm (Laméris Ootech B.V., Nieuwegein, Netherlands), ranging from 15 to 480 s of arc (arcsec) (Wu Y. et al., 2020). Distance stereoacuity was assessed using the Distance Randot Stereotest (DRS, American Stereo Optical Company) at 3 m, ranging from 63 to 400 arcsec (Wang et al., 2010). Stereoacuity was recorded as "nil" if the patient could not pass the largest disparity (Hatt et al., 2008). The stereopsis examination was performed before any other examination that required binocular fusion to be broken.

The fusional vergence amplitude was measured using a horizontal prism bar, and an accommodative target was used first at distance fixation (3 m) and then at near fixation (1/3 m) (Sharma et al., 2008; Hatt et al., 2011) with base-in (BI) for negative vergence and base-out (BO) for positive vergence. Negative fusional vergence was measured before positive vergence to prevent bias caused by the prismatic demand of positive fusional vergence. To determine the fusional convergence break point (convergence reserve), the magnitude of prism was gradually increased from 1 PD until diplopia appeared with no subsequent recovery of motor fusion or one eye drifted outwards when control was lost. If the patient could still perform fusion up to the maximum prism volume of 45^{Δ}, the break point was recorded as 45^{Δ} for statistical analysis (Hatt et al., 2011). If a patient could not perform fusion, both the break point and recovery point were recorded as 0. The total fusional convergence amplitude (Hatt et al., 2011) was the sum of the individual deviation angle and convergence reserve. The fusion reserve ratio (Hatt et al., 2011) was calculated as the fusional convergence reserve divided by the angle of deviation measured using the PACT (e.g., fusional convergence reserve = 20; angle of deviation = 10; fusion reserve ratio = 2).

For the near point of convergence (NPC), the patient looked at an accommodative target located 40 cm away, and the examiner gradually moved the target toward the patient's eyes until the patient reported that the target had become two targets. The distance between the break point and parallel point of the patient's lateral canthus was measured.

The amplitude of accommodation (AMP) was measured using the negative lens method, and the right eye's data were used for analysis.

Binocular accommodative flexibility (BAF) was measured by reading the "E" visual acuity chart at 40 cm in sequence with a ± 2.00 D reverse lens within 1 min (García et al., 2000; Wick et al., 2002). Positive and negative counts comprise one cycle. The measurement starts with the positive lens, and the number of cycles that occur within 1 min is recorded.

All the tests were performed after appropriate refractive correction. Each of these tests was performed at 1, 6, and 12 months postoperatively. Two patients were lost to follow-up at 6 months after surgery. The controls were tested once when they were enrolled in the study.

Statistical Analysis

Postoperative drift was defined as the change in ocular alignment from the 1-month follow-up to the final follow-up. The Friedman test was used to compare the angle of deviation, stereoacuity, and fusional vergence amplitude (1, 6, and 12 months). The Wilcoxon signed-rank test was used to compare rehabilitation between 1 and 12 months postoperatively, and the Mann–Whitney U test was used to compare IXT patients and controls. The sensory fusion status at each time point (1, 6, and 12 months) was evaluated using chi-squared test or Fisher's exact test. Additionally, we evaluated the relationships between postoperative binocular functions and postoperative drift using Spearman's correlation coefficient.

RESULTS

Thirty cases and 30 age- and sex-matched controls were included. A summary of the subjects' demographics and clinical characteristics is provided in **Table 1**. The deviations at both distance and near fixations decreased significantly from preoperatively to 1 month postoperatively ($p < 0.001$), sensory fusion improved ($p = 0.009$), and distance stereoacuity improved ($p = 0.026$); however, near stereoacuity did not recover significantly ($p = 0.657$).

Postoperative Drift

Figure 1A shows that the eye position steadily drifted outwards. The mean exodrift at distance fixation was 1.53 ± 7.19 PD from postoperative month 1 to postoperative month 6 and 2.67 ± 9.38 PD from postoperative month 6 to postoperative month 12 ($p = 0.338$), and the mean exodrift values at near fixation were 2.00 ± 9.83 PD and 2.97 ± 11.62 PD, respectively ($p = 0.459$). No relationship was found between the preoperative deviation and postoperative drift at distance or near fixations [$rs = 0.352$ ($p = 0.056$) and $rs = 0.048$ ($p = 0.802$), respectively]. The greater was the amount of preoperative deviation, the greater was the postoperative drift at a distance. However, the difference was not statistically significant.

Binocular Functions After Surgery

Sensory Fusion

No significant differences were found in sensory fusion between 1 and 12 months postoperatively ($p = 0.601$) or between the patient and control groups ($p = 0.117$ and $p = 0.237$, respectively).

Stereoacuity

The patients' median value of distance stereoacuity improved from 3.18 (range, 1.8–4.0) at 1 month postoperatively to 2.77 (range, 1.8–4) at 12 months postoperatively ($p = 0.025$), and the values did not significantly differ from those of the controls ($p = 0.120$). The patients' median value of near stereoacuity improved from 2.20 (range, 1.7–2.98) at 1 month postoperatively to 2.03 (range, 1.48–2.68) at 12 months postoperatively ($p = 0.041$), which was still poorer than that of the controls ($p = 0.017$). Distance stereoacuity before and after surgery (1 month and 12 months postoperatively) did not significantly differ [$rs = 0.308$ ($p = 0.098$) and $rs = 0.210$ ($p = 0.266$), respectively], whereas near stereoacuity was significantly different [$rs = 0.492$ ($p = 0.006$) and $rs = 0.547$ ($p = 0.002$), respectively]. These results demonstrated that the better was preoperative near stereoacuity, the better was the postoperative recovery.

Fusional Vergence Amplitude

The patients' median fusional vergence amplitudes, total fusional convergence amplitudes, and fusion reserve ratio at distance or near fixation improved at the three follow-ups (**Figure 1B–E**). However, the number of distance and near BO break points in the IXT group at the final visit was still worse than that in the controls ($p = 0.025$ and $p = 0.033$, respectively). The number of BI break points in the IXT group at the final visit at distance fixation was similar to that of the controls, whereas the number at near fixation exceeded that of the controls ($p = 0.168$ and $p = 0.003$, respectively). The distance and near-total fusional convergence amplitudes in the IXT group were similar to those of the

TABLE 1 | Demographics and clinical characteristics of the patients with IXT and normal controls.

Characteristic	IXT patients				Normal controls
	Preoperatively	1 month postoperatively	6 months postoperatively	12 months postoperatively	
Sex: female, male	–	11, 19	11, 17	11, 19	10, 20
Age (years)	–	10.87 ± 2.40	–	–	9.90 ± 2.06
SE of the right eye (D)	–	−2.20 ± 2.38	−2.11 ± 2.13	−2.48 ± 2.37	−0.97 ± 1.33
SE of the left eye (D)	–	−2.00 ± 2.39	−1.67 ± 2.05	−1.90 ± 2.77	−0.87 ± 1.20
Sensory fusion (fusion, peripheral fusion, no fusion)	15, 9, 6	26, 3, 1	27, 1, 0	27, 3, 0	30, 0, 0
Distance stereoacuity (log arcsec)	3.55 ± 0.77	3.18 ± 0.97	2.79 ± 0.88	2.77 ± 0.85	2.33 ± 0.63
Near stereoacuity (log arcsec)	2.24 ± 0.44	2.20 ± 0.34	2.06 ± 0.34	2.03 ± 0.35	1.98 ± 0.29
Distance deviation (PD)	-32.0 ± 8.60	−3.47 ± 4.81	−5.36 ± 6.63	−7.67 ± 7.70	−0.23 ± 0.57
Near deviation (PD)	−36.0 ± 9.10	−5.33 ± 7.76	−7.86 ± 8.29	−10.30 ± 9.87	−2.27 ± 3.04
Distance base-out	–	15.43 ± 13.78	15.50 ± 11.89	18.70 ± 15.14	23.70 ± 9.90
Distance base-in	–	6.14 ± 4.47	7.68 ± 5.02	10.23 ± 5.58	8.67 ± 2.37
Near base-out	–	21.43 ± 15.39	22.14 ± 11.14	24.67 ± 14.48	32.37 ± 9.29
Near base-in	–	9.86 ± 6.41	11.89 ± 6.93	17.07 ± 8.28	11.90 ± 3.97
NPC (cm)	–	4.00 ± 4.21	6.13 ± 4.61	4.13 ± 4.53	2.25 ± 2.88
Binocular accommodative flexibility (BAF)	–	9.67 ± 4.30	11.64 ± 3.97	12.38 ± 3.45	9.03 ± 3.34
AMP (D)	–	8.83 ± 3.26	8.33 ± 2.47	8.18 ± 2.16	7.37 ± 2.16

D, diopters. PD, prism diopters.
The angle of deviation was measured using the PACT. Base-out and base-in were the break points. Two patients were lost to follow-up 6 months postoperatively. AMP, the right eye's amplitude of accommodation.

controls at the final visit ($p = 0.619$ and $p = 0.935$, respectively). The fusion reserve ratio at 12 months postoperatively differed significantly between the patient and control groups at both distance ($p = 0.000$) and near ($p = 0.000$) fixation.

Binocular Accommodative Flexibility

The patients' median amount of BAF improved from 9.67 (range, 0–19) at 1 month postoperatively to 12.38 (range, 3–20) at 12 months postoperatively. The magnitude of improvement significantly differed at these three follow-ups ($p = 0.021$). The amount of BAF in the IXT group at 1 month postoperatively was not significantly different from that of the controls ($p = 0.533$) and was better than that in the controls at 12 months postoperatively ($p = 0.001$).

Accommodative Amplitude

The patients' median accommodative amplitude in the right eye improved from 8.43 ± 3.81 at 1 month postoperatively to 8.64 ± 3.67 at 12 months postoperatively ($p = 0.700$), which was not significantly different from that of the controls (7.37 ± 2.16, $p = 0.689$ and $p = 0.791$, respectively).

Relationship Between Postoperative Binocular Functions and Postoperative Drift

Relationship Between Stereoacuity and Postoperative Drift

Figures 2A,B show that the relationships between 1-month postoperative stereoacuity and postoperative drift for distance and near fixation were not significant [$rs = 0.106$ ($p = 0.579$) and $rs = 0.143$ ($p = 0.450$), respectively].

Relationship Between the Fusional Vergence Amplitude and Postoperative Drift

No significant correlations were found between the angle of postoperative drift and fusional vergence amplitudes at 1 month postoperatively for distance or near fixation in IXT patients (**Figure 2**).

Classification of the IXT Group Into the Orthophoria/Heterophoria Group and Small Residual Manifest Angle Group

By combining the measurements of the Worth 4-dot test and simultaneous prism and cover test (SPCT) at 1 month after surgery, the IXT group was divided into the orthophoria/heterophoria group (26 cases) and small residual manifest angle group (three cases with suppression and one case with diplopia). All four patients in the residual manifest group recovered normal single vision and motor function at the 12-month postoperative visit. Ocular alignment became better controlled to heterophoria at 12 months postoperatively. The other three cases in the orthophoria/heterophoria group exhibited reduced binocular vision functions and exodrifted significantly during the follow-up at 12 months postoperatively; thus, the operation was not successful in these patients.

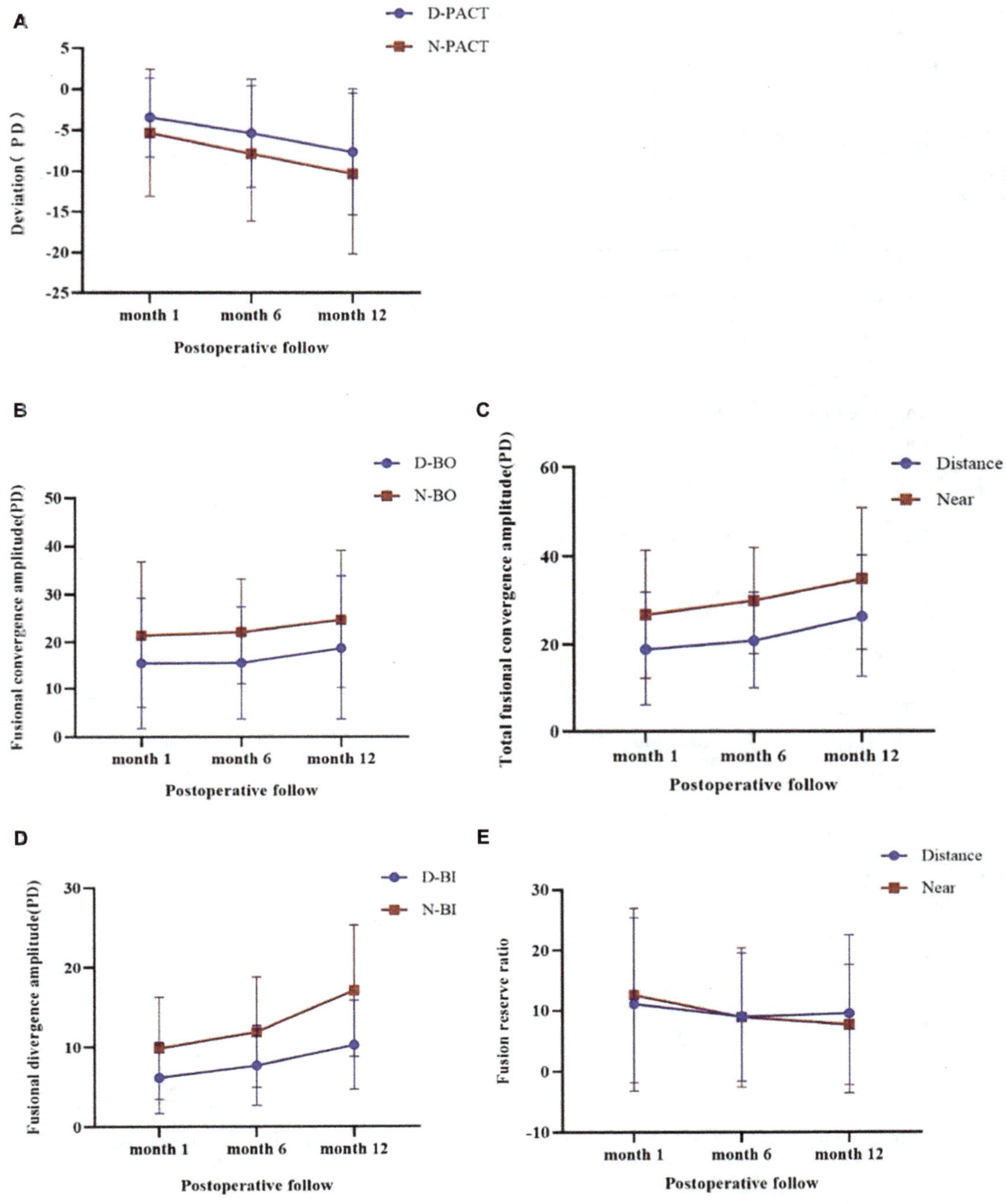

FIGURE 1 | Changes in the eye position and fusional vergence amplitude during the three follow-ups after surgery and using the Friedman test. A negative value indicates an exodrift. **(A)** Shows that the eye position steadily drifts outwards for distance and near fixations ($p < 0.001$). **(B)** Shows that the BO break point leads to different recoveries in distance and near fixations ($p = 0.045$ and $p = 0.000$, respectively). **(C)** Shows that the total fusional convergence amplitude has different recoveries in distance and near fixations ($p = 0.169$ and $p = 0.000$, respectively). **(D)** Shows that the BI break point has different increases in distance and near fixations ($p < 0.001$). **(E)** Shows that the fusion reserve ratio worsens in distance and near fixations ($p = 0.001$ and $p < 0.001$, respectively).

DISCUSSION

To our best knowledge, this is the first longitudinal study to evaluate the rehabilitation of binocular function in IXT after successful corrective surgery. Our results showed that most patients recovered binocular vision function after successful surgery, and the highest recovery rate was noted from postoperative months 1 to 6. This rate improved steadily over the next 6 months. Although the patients recovered binocular functions after strabismus surgery,

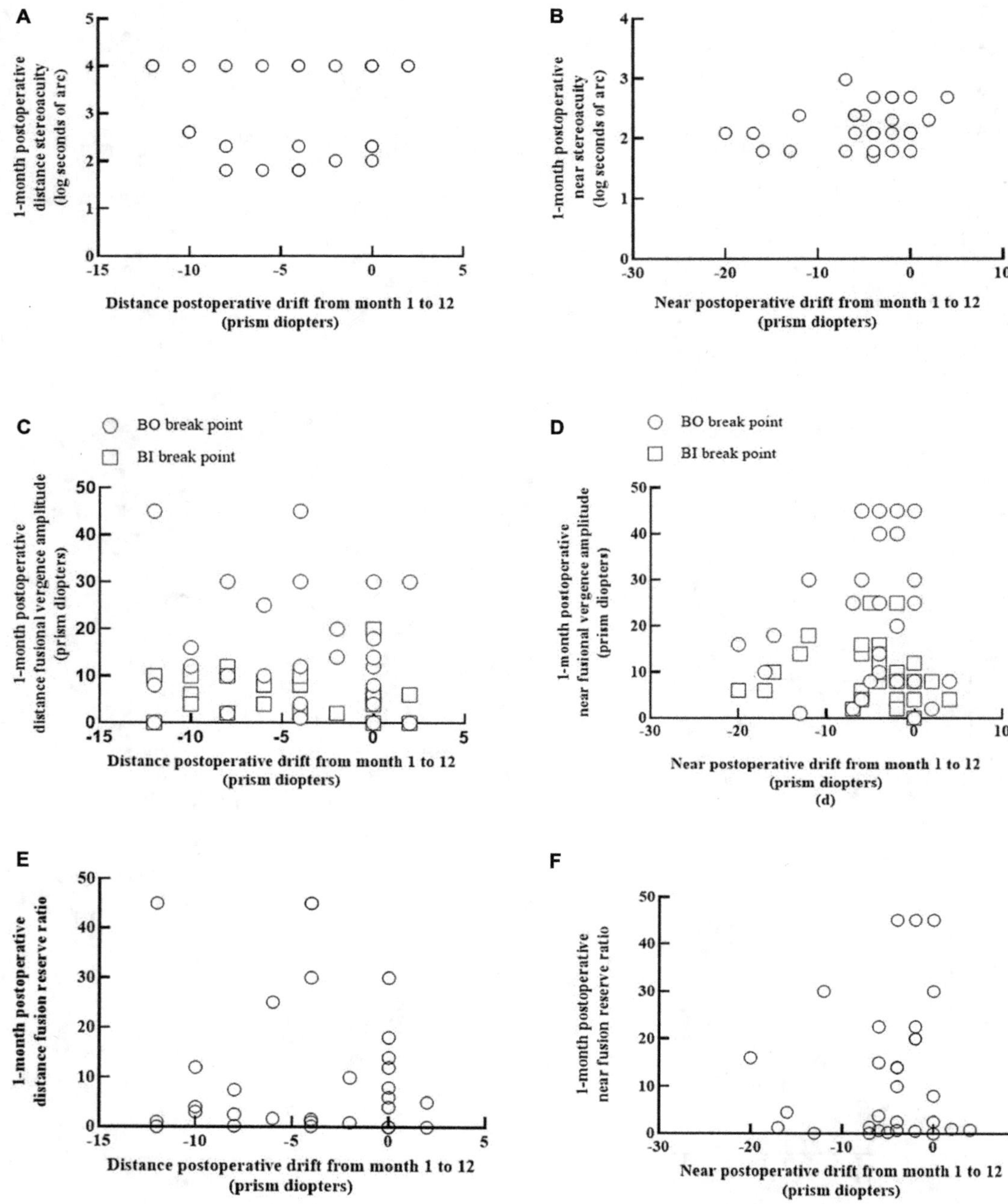

FIGURE 2 | Relationships between postoperative binocular functions and postoperative drift at distance and near fixations. Each panel shows the data from 30 patients. The positive values indicate esodrift, and the negative values indicate exodrift. **(A,B)** Show the relationship between 1-month postoperative stereoacuity and the postoperative drift from months 1 to 12 for distance and near fixations [$rs = 0.106$ ($p = 0.579$) and $rs = 0.143$ ($p = 0.450$), respectively]. **(C,D)** Show the relationship between the convergence and divergence amplitude and postoperative drift at distance fixation (BO: $rs = -0.115$, $p = 0.546$; BI: $rs = -0.336$, $p = 0.075$) and at near fixation (BO: $rs = 0.031$, $p = 0.870$; BI: $rs = -0.268$, $p = 0.159$). **(E,F)** Show that the relationships between the 1-month postoperative fusion reserve ratio and postoperative drift from months 1 to 12 were not significant for distance or near fixation [$rs = 0.003$ ($p = 0.987$) and $rs = 0.110$ ($p = 0.564$), respectively].

some functions (i.e., near stereopsis, fusional convergence reserve, and the fusion reserve ratio) were still subnormal compared with those in controls. Few previous studies have evaluated the effects of postoperative binocular visual functions on the long-term stability of postoperative ocular alignment. Our study findings indicated no significant correlation between postoperative drift and postoperative binocular functions, suggesting that postoperative binocular functions may not be involved in the stability of postoperative ocular alignment.

Stereoacuity is typically considered an important indicator of the severity of IXT and is used to determine surgical indications, particularly for distance stereopsis (Stathacopoulos et al., 1993; von Noorden and Campos, 2002; Holmes et al., 2007). The degree of recovery of stereopsis in IXT was inconsistent. O'Neal and associates (O'Neal et al., 1995) demonstrated that even with excellent postoperative alignment, the distance stereoacuity, particularly in the random dot test, does not recover fully. Notably, the age range of the subjects in that study was large, ranging from 5 to 87 years. Sharma et al. (2008) found that the mean distance stereoacuity of patients at 6 months postoperatively became similar to that of normal subjects. Our study also confirmed that distance stereopsis improved to the same level as that of the normal controls at the 6- or 12-month follow-up. Adams et al. (2008) and Feng X. et al. (2015) found that near stereoacuity remained essentially unchanged following surgery. However, it should be noted that the subjects were assessed 6 weeks postoperatively and were not compared with controls. We found that near stereoacuity remained poorer in the patients at the last follow-up compared with that in the controls; however, it improved after surgery. Our results are consistent with those reported by Sharma et al. (2008), who found that even at 6 months postoperatively, the mean level of near stereopsis was still poor compared with that of control subjects.

The fusional vergence amplitude reflects a patient's ability to "control" a latent or intermittent deviation in IXT (von Noorden and Campos, 2002; Adams et al., 2008) or a patient's ability to maintain phoria in childhood X(T) (Wakayama et al., 2018). Kushner and Morton (1998) and Kushner (1999) found that exotropia becomes more pronounced when fusional convergence is suspended. Few studies have observed the postoperative fusional vergence amplitude and its longitudinal rehabilitation as well as its association with postoperative drift. The IXT group drifted outwards, and the exodeviation increased during the follow-up. As expected, the number of BI break points increased. We also found that the convergence reserve and total convergence amplitude improved in the follow-up period, but the values remained lower than those of the normal controls. This finding indicates that patients' fusional convergence ability may improve after the successful correction of IXT. Sharma et al. (2008) found no significant differences in the fusional vergence amplitude between patients at 6 months postoperatively and normal subjects. However, adult subjects were included in the study, and fusion data were collected after the angle of deviation had been corrected using prisms. Furthermore, Liebermann et al. (2012) believe that common measurement methods may not reveal the true divergence amplitudes. Most IXT patients have normal fusional divergence at near fixation, and approximately half show decreased fusional divergence at distance fixation. Hatt et al. (2011) found that the fusion reserve ratio correlates well with exodeviation control and may be useful in grading the severity of IXT. According to Sheard's criterion, the fusional convergence reserve should be twice the magnitude of the angle of deviation. Moreover, Yam et al. (2013) found that a fusional reserve ratio ≥ 2 was an indicator of good control in patients. However, the postoperative fusional reserve ratio showed a decreasing trend and was not significantly correlated with postoperative drift in this study. The decreasing trend may be related to the change in exodrift after the surgery.

Consistent with most previous studies, we found that sensory fusion improved from before to after the operation (O'Neal et al., 1995; Yildirim et al., 1999; Feng X. et al., 2015; Wu Y. et al., 2020) and remained stable during the follow-up period without a trend of deterioration.

BAF improved at the last follow-up and exceeded that of the normal group, and the accommodative amplitude remained stable during the follow-up period and slightly exceeded that of the normal controls. Ha and his colleagues (Ha et al., 2016) suggested that the rehabilitation of accommodative loads at near fixation increases more in IXT patients than in normal controls, whereas binocular fusion remains consistent. One possible explanation is that disparity is a major driver of accommodation, and extra accommodation is a consequence in IXT patients.

According to Yildirim and her colleagues (Yildirim et al., 1999), better distance stereoacuity and central fusion before surgery are frequently associated with better surgical success in X(T). Beneish and Flanders (1994) found that overcorrection of poor preoperative stereopsis resulted in significant improvements in the surgical success rate and suggested that individuals with poor preoperative stereopsis may have good long-term alignment stability postoperatively. In this study, we found no significant relationship between postoperative stereopsis and postoperative drift. Furthermore, postoperative fusional vergence functions—i.e., fusional convergence reserve, total convergence amplitude, and fusional divergence amplitude—were not associated with postoperative drift and could not predict drift in the follow-up period. Considering the findings of previous studies (Hatt et al., 2008) and our study, other factors may exist in addition to postoperative binocular functions that are involved in postoperative alignment. For example, the surgery method and age at surgery will also affect the long-term stability of ocular alignment postoperatively. In this study, the operations were performed by the same doctor, the surgical procedures were all unilateral recession–resection procedures, and the school-aged children were older than seven years. The factors that interfere with postoperative eye position stability are relatively limited. Previous studies (Feng L. et al., 2015; Zhou et al., 2017; Wu H. et al., 2020) have shown that visual perception disorders occur in IXT patients; sensory imbalance persisted in surgically corrected subjects although they had normal levels of stereopsis (Park and Kim, 2013), and the level of sensory imbalance was subnormal in the follow-up period (Leow et al., 2010).

In the present study, we chose postoperative month 1 as baseline to observe the rehabilitation in binocular visual functions with IXT after surgery and excluded any immediate responses and complications related to surgery (e.g., pain, edema, bleeding, and reactions to anaesthetics). Furthermore, to minimize the influence of other factors, we set strict inclusion criteria (i.e., amblyopia, anisometropia, and vertical deviation). Similarly, we excluded patients with overcorrection (>5 PD) at 1 month postoperatively. Overcorrection is correlated with long-term motor benefits but has potential negative effects on binocular function (Leow et al., 2010; Choi et al., 2011; Park and Kim, 2013).

Our study has limitations. First, the control score plays a vital role in assessing the patients' ability to maintain phoria (Hatt and Gnanaraj, 2013; Wakayama et al., 2018). However, it is unsuitable for patients with IXT after surgery. Second, we included a limited number of patients, and the follow-up time was not sufficiently long. Binocular functions and eye position drift should be assessed in larger study populations and over longer periods. Binocular function measurements can be affected by the testing method—i.e., the fusional convergence reserve in IXT is greater when viewing a stereo target (Cooper, 1993) and reduced during intense light exposure (Campos and Cipolli, 1992). The testing conditions were uniform across all subjects in the present study; thus, there is likely no measurement bias in our results. Finally, we found a tendency of larger deviation before surgery with more drift after surgery, which would also affect the evaluation of the postoperative factors related to the postoperative alignment stability. A stricter definition of deviation before surgery and a larger sample would minimize the effect.

Binocular functions remained poorer in IXT patients at 1 month postoperatively than in the control group and continued to improve from 1 to 12 months. Some parameters of the binocular functions recovered to the same level as those in the normal controls, whereas some remained worse than those in the normal controls. No significant correlations were found between binocular functions after surgery and the stability of the alignment.

AUTHOR CONTRIBUTIONS

MX, FZ, JL, CW, and YW: technical assistance and guidance. JZ and SC: participating in the follow-up and contact patients to collect data. XY: research and academic guidance. All authors contributed to the article and approved the submitted version.

REFERENCES

Adams, W. E., Leske, D. A., Hatt, S. R., Mohney, B. G., Birch, E. E., Weakley, D. R. Jr., et al. (2008). Improvement in distance stereoacuity following surgery for intermittent exotropia. *J. AAPOS* 12, 141–144. doi: 10.1016/j.jaapos.2007.09.015

Beneish, R., and Flanders, M. (1994). The role of stereopsis and early postoperative alignment in long-term surgical results of intermittent exotropia. *Can. J. Ophthalmol.* 29, 119–124.

Campos, E. C., and Cipolli, C. (1992). Binocularity and photophobia in intermittent exotropia. *Percept. Mot. Skills* 74, 1168–1170. doi: 10.2466/pms.1992.74.3c.1168

Choi, J., Kim, S. J., and Yu, Y. S. (2011). Initial postoperative deviation as a predictor of long-term outcome after surgery for intermittent exotropia. *J. AAPOS* 15, 224–229. doi: 10.1016/j.jaapos.2010.12.019

Cooper, J. M. N. (1993). Intermittent exotropia, basic and divergence excess type. *Binocul. Vis. Strabismus Q.* 8, 187–216.

Donahue, S., Chandler, D., Holmes, J., Arthur, B. W., Paysse, E. A., Wallace, D. K., et al. (2019). A Randomized Trial Comparing Bilateral Lateral Rectus Recession versus Unilateral Recess and Resect for Basic-Type Intermittent Exotropia. *Ophthalmology* 126, 305–317. doi: 10.1016/j.ophtha.2018.08.034

Donahue, S. P. (2007). Clinical practice. Pediatric strabismus. *N. Engl. J. Med.* 356, 1040–1047.

Feng, L., Zhou, J., Chen, L., and Hess, R. F. (2015). Sensory eye balance in surgically corrected intermittent exotropes with normal stereopsis. *Sci. Rep.* 5:13075.

Feng, X., Zhang, X., and Jia, Y. (2015). Improvement in fusion and stereopsis following surgery for intermittent exotropia. *J. Pediatr. Ophthalmol. Strabismus* 52, 52–57. doi: 10.3928/01913913-20141230-08

García, A., Cacho, P., Lara, F., and Megías, R. (2000). The relation between accommodative facility and general binocular dysfunction. *Ophthalmic Physiol. Opt.* 20, 98–104. doi: 10.1016/s0275-5408(99)00034-4

Ha, S. G., Jang, S. M., Cho, Y. A., Kim, S. H., Song, J. S., and Suh, Y. W. (2016). Clinical exhibition of increased accommodative loads for binocular fusion in patients with basic intermittent exotropia. *BMC Ophthalmol.* 16:77. doi: 10.1186/s12886-016-0260-y

Hatt, S. R., and Gnanaraj, L. (2013). Interventions for intermittent exotropia. *Cochrane Database Syst. Rev.* 2013:CD003737.

Hatt, S. R., Leske, D. A., Mohney, B. G., Brodsky, M. C., and Holmes, J. M. (2011). Fusional convergence in childhood intermittent exotropia. *Am. J. Ophthalmol.* 152, 314–319. doi: 10.1016/j.ajo.2011.01.042

Hatt, S. R., Mohney, B. G., Leske, D. A., and Holmes, J. M. (2008). Variability of stereoacuity in intermittent exotropia. *Am. J. Ophthalmol.* 145, 556–561. doi: 10.1016/j.ajo.2007.10.028

Holmes, J. M., Birch, E. E., Leske, D. A., Fu, V. L., and Mohney, B. G. (2007). New tests of distance stereoacuity and their role in evaluating intermittent exotropia. *Ophthalmology* 114, 1215–1220. doi: 10.1016/j.ophtha.2006.06.066

Hutchinson, A. K. (2001). Intermittent exotropia. *Ophthalmol. Clin. North Am.* 14, 399–406.

Jie, Y., Xu, Z., He, Y., Wang, N., Wang, J., Lu, W., et al. (2010). A 4 year retrospective survey of strabismus surgery in Tongren Eye Centre Beijing. *Ophthalmic Physiol. Opt.* 30, 310–314. doi: 10.1111/j.1475-1313.2010.00716.x

Kim, H. J., and Choi, D. G. (2016). Clinical analysis of childhood intermittent exotropia with surgical success at postoperative 2 years. *Acta Ophthalmol.* 94, e85–e89.

Kushner, B. J. (1999). Diagnosis and treatment of exotropia with a high accommodation convergence-accommodation ratio. *Arch. Ophthalmol.* 117, 221–224. doi: 10.1001/archopht.117.2.221

Kushner, B. J., and Morton, G. V. (1998). Distance/near differences in intermittent exotropia. *Arch. Ophthalmol.* 116, 478–486. doi: 10.1001/archopht.116.4.478

Lee, H. J., Kim, S. J., and Yu, Y. S. (2018). Long-term Outcomes After Same Amount of Bilateral Rectus Muscle Recession for Intermittent Exotropia With the Same Angle of Deviation. *J. Pediatr. Ophthalmol. Strabismus* 55, 319–325. doi: 10.3928/01913913-20180329-02

Leow, P. L., Ko, S. T., Wu, P. K., and Chan, C. W. (2010). Exotropic drift and ocular alignment after surgical correction for intermittent exotropia. *J. Pediatr. Ophthalmol. Strabismus* 47, 12–16. doi: 10.3928/01913913-20100106-04

Liebermann, L., Hatt, S. R., Leske, D. A., Yamada, T., Mohney, B. G., Brodsky, M. C., et al. (2012). Assessing divergence in children with intermittent exotropia. *Strabismus* 20, 11–16. doi: 10.3109/09273972.2012.655838

Mohan, K., and Sharma, S. K. (2020). Long-term Motor and Sensory Outcomes After Unilateral Lateral Rectus Recession-Medial Rectus Resection for Basic Intermittent Exotropia. *J. Pediatr. Ophthalmol. Strabismus* 57, 326–332. doi: 10.3928/01913913-20200731-01

O'Neal, T. D., Rosenbaum, A. L., and Stathacopoulos, R. A. (1995). Distance stereo acuity improvement in intermittent exotropic patients following strabismus surgery. *J. Pediatr. Ophthalmol. Strabismus* 32, 353–357. discussion 358, doi: 10.3928/0191-3913-19951101-06

Pan, C. W., Zhu, H., Yu, J. J., Ding, H., Bai, J., Chen, J., et al. (2016). Epidemiology of Intermittent Exotropia in Preschool Children in China. *Optom. Vis. Sci.* 93, 57–62. doi: 10.1097/opx.0000000000000754

Park, K. H., and Kim, S. Y. (2013). Clinical characteristics of patients that experience different rates of exodrift after strabismus surgery for intermittent exotropia and the effect of the rate of exodrift on final ocular alignment. *J. AAPOS* 17, 54–58. doi: 10.1016/j.jaapos.2012.10.014

Pineles, S. L., Demer, J. L., Isenberg, S. J., Birch, E. E., and Velez, F. G. (2015). Improvement in binocular summation after strabismus surgery. *JAMA Ophthalmol.* 133, 326–332. doi: 10.1001/jamaophthalmol.2014.5265

Pineles, S. L., Ela-Dalman, N., Zvansky, A. G., Yu, F., and Rosenbaum, A. L. (2010). Long-term results of the surgical management of intermittent exotropia. *J. AAPOS* 14, 298–304. doi: 10.1016/j.jaapos.2010.06.007

Repka, M. X., Chandler, D. L., Holmes, J. M., Donahue, S. P., Hoover, D. L., Mohney, B. G., et al. (2020). The Relationship of Age and Other Baseline Factors to Outcome of Initial Surgery for Intermittent Exotropia. *Am. J. Ophthalmol.* 212, 153–161. doi: 10.1016/j.ajo.2019.12.008

Sharma, P., Saxena, R., Narvekar, M., Gadia, R., and Menon, V. (2008). Evaluation of distance and near stereoacuity and fusional vergence in intermittent exotropia. *Indian J. Ophthalmol.* 56, 121–125. doi: 10.4103/0301-4738.39116

Stathacopoulos, R. A., Rosenbaum, A. L., Zanoni, D., Stager, D. R., McCall, L. C., Ziffer, A. J., et al. (1993). Distance stereoacuity. Assessing control in intermittent exotropia. *Ophthalmology* 100, 495–500.

von Noorden, G. K., and Campos, E. C. (2002). *Binocular Vision and Ocular Motility: Theory and Management of Strabismus. Vol 6th ed.* Missouri: CV Mosby.

Wakayama, A., Seki, Y., Takahashi, R., Umebara, I., Tanabe, F., Abe, K., et al. (2018). Role of fusional convergence amplitude in postoperative phoria maintenance in children with intermittent exotropia. *Jpn. J. Ophthalmol.* 62, 307–314. doi: 10.1007/s10384-018-0585-6

Wang, J., Hatt, S. R., O'Connor, A. R., Drover, J. R., Adams, R., Birch, E. E., et al. (2010). Final version of the Distance Randot Stereotest: normative data, reliability, and validity. *J. AAPOS* 14, 142–146. doi: 10.1016/j.jaapos.2009.12.159

Wick, B., Yothers, T. L., Jiang, B. C., and Morse, S. E. (2002). Clinical testing of accommodative facility: part 1. A critical appraisal of the literature. *Optometry* 73, 11–23.

Wu, H., Li, X., Tang, Y., Xu, Q., Zhang, X., Zhou, L., et al. (2020). Optimal Stereoacuity Reveals More Than Critical Time in Patients With Intermittent Exotropia. *Front. Neurosci.* 14:133. doi: 10.3389/fnins.2020.00133

Wu, H., Sun, J., Xia, X., Xu, L., and Xu, X. (2006). Binocular status after surgery for constant and intermittent exotropia. *Am. J. Ophthalmol.* 142, 822–826. doi: 10.1016/j.ajo.2006.06.045

Wu, Y., Xu, M., Zhang, J., Zhou, J., Wan, M., Dai, Z., et al. (2020). Can Clinical Measures of Postoperative Binocular Function Predict the Long-Term Stability of Postoperative Alignment in Intermittent Exotropia? *J. Ophthalmol.* 2020:7392165.

Yam, J. C., Chong, G. S., Wu, P. K., Wong, U. S., Chan, C. W., and Ko, S. T. (2013). A prospective study of fusional convergence parameters in Chinese patients with intermittent exotropia. *J. AAPOS* 17, 347–351. doi: 10.1016/j.jaapos.2013.03.023

Yildirim, C., Mutlu, F. M., Chen, Y., and Altinsoy, H. I. (1999). Assessment of central and peripheral fusion and near and distance stereoacuity in intermittent exotropic patients before and after strabismus surgery. *Am. J. Ophthalmol.* 128, 222–230.

Yu, X., Ji, Z., Yu, H., Xu, M., and Xu, J. (2016). Exotropia Is the Main Pattern of Childhood Strabismus Surgery in the South of China: a Six-Year Clinical Review. *J. Ophthalmol.* 2016:1489537.

Zhou, J., Wang, Y., Feng, L., Wang, J., and Hess, R. F. (2017). Straightening the Eyes Doesn't Rebalance the Brain. *Front. Hum. Neurosci.* 11:453. doi: 10.3389/fnhum.2017.00453

9

The Integration of Eye Tracking Responses for the Measurement of Contrast Sensitivity

Yijing Zhuang[1†], Li Gu[1†], Jingchang Chen[1†], Zixuan Xu[1], Lily Y. L. Chan[1,2], Lei Feng[1], Qingqing Ye[1], Shenglan Zhang[1], Jin Yuan[1] and Jinrong Li[1*]*

[1] State Key Laboratory of Ophthalmology, Zhongshan Ophthalmic Center, Sun Yat-sen University, Guangzhou, China,
[2] School of Optometry, The Hong Kong Polytechnic University, Hong Kong, China

***Correspondence:**
Jinrong Li
lijingr3@mail.sysu.edu.cn
Jin Yuan
yuanjincornea@126.com

† These authors have contributed equally to this work

Contrast sensitivity (CS) is important when assessing functional vision. However, current techniques for assessing CS are not suitable for young children or non-verbal individuals because they require reliable, subjective perceptual reports. This study explored the feasibility of applying eye tracking technology to quantify CS as a first step toward developing a testing paradigm that will not rely on observers' behavioral or language abilities. Using a within-subject design, 27 healthy young adults completed CS measures for three spatial frequencies with best-corrected vision and lens-induced optical blur. Monocular CS was estimated using a five-alternative, forced-choice grating detection task. Thresholds were measured using eye movement responses and conventional key-press responses. CS measured using eye movements compared well with results obtained using key-press responses [Pearson's $r_{best-corrected} = 0.966$, $P < 0.001$]. Good test–retest variability was evident for the eye-movement-based measures (Pearson's $r = 0.916$, $P < 0.001$) with a coefficient of repeatability of 0.377 log CS across different days. This study provides a proof of concept that eye tracking can be used to automatically record eye gaze positions and accurately quantify human spatial vision. Future work will update this paradigm by incorporating the preferential looking technique into the eye tracking methods, optimizing the CS sampling algorithm and adapting the methodology to broaden its use on infants and non-verbal individuals.

Keywords: contrast sensitivity, eye tracking, preferential-looking, psychophysical, preverbal

INTRODUCTION

Early detection and treatment of vision problems in young children can prevent visual impairment and the development of amblyopia. However, quantitative measurement of visual function, especially spatial vision, in young children is complicated by their immature cognition, attention and communication.

Eye movements can be used as a non-verbal cue to determine thresholds for the detection or discrimination of visual stimuli. With the development of infrared eye tracking technology, a number of techniques for objectively estimating visual function based on eye movements have been described (Schütz et al., 2011). Specifically, the rate of microsaccades has been used to measure visual responses to visual stimuli. As such, visual acuity (VA; Adler and Fliegelman, 1934), contrast sensitivity (CS; Denniss et al., 2018), and convergence angle (Okada et al., 2006) can be estimated from microsaccade rate using an eye tracker. Optokinetic nystagmus (OKN), a series of involuntary ocular movements elicited by moving visual stimuli, has been used as visual feedback to test visual functions (Schor and Levi, 1980; Leguire et al., 1991; Masson et al., 1994; Hyon et al., 2010). Eye tracking techniques have also been used to detect smooth pursuit tracking of moving stimuli to estimate CS (Mooney et al., 2018).

Preferential-looking (PL) exploits the fact that infants have a greater tendency to fixate on a more interesting or salient stimulus than a plain homogeneous field (Fantz, 1963). The PL technique has been used to measure vision in infants and adults with cognitive or speech impairments (Atkinson et al., 1974; Banks and Salapatek, 1978). For example, the Teller acuity cards (McDonald et al., 1985) have a grating printed on one side and a blank region on the opposite side. By subjectively monitoring the infant's gaze behavior, an examiner can identify whether the grating can be discriminated from the blank region. A disadvantage of current PL tests is that they require a high level of skill to determine which stimulus the infant fixates on and rely on the subjective judgment of the testing clinician. Previous knowledge about the tested infant's known or suspected visual disorder could also bias the test results. Eye tracking technology has the potential to remove subjectivity from PL tests and to enable the use of PL without experienced investigators. This study aimed to test the possibility of using an eye-tracker to accurately record eye movements and evaluate the contrast threshold. The study was conducted with a group of healthy adults as a first step toward developing a CS measurement system that combines eye tracking and PL technique for infants and adults with cognitive disabilities.

There are several challenges in designing an integrated eye tracking CS measurement suitable for clinical use. For instance, a fast and precise eye tracking calibration procedure is necessary, and the stimuli have to be positioned appropriately within the visual field for a suitable period of time. In addition, an algorithm for deciding which difficulty level to show on each trial and when to terminate the test is required. An algorithm for identifying gaze position and assessing whether the participant can see the presented optotype is also necessary.

In this study, we developed a novel paradigm to objectively and accurately assess CS using an eye tracking technology to potentially broaden its application on pre-verbal children and others with speech impairments. We used Gabor patches, the standard CS measurement optotype, which were attractive enough for non-verbal children, as the stimuli. Using initial pilot measurements, we determined the appropriate position and duration of stimulus presentation, and the number of trials required for accurate results interpretation. A widely used three-down, one-up staircase procedure that decreased signal contrast by 10% (multiplied the previous value by 0.9) after every three consecutive correct responses and increased signal contrast by 10% after every incorrect response was adopted in estimating contrast thresholds (Huang et al., 2008). Moreover, the five-alternative forced-choice method rather than the traditional two-interval forced-choice method was used in the eye tracking test (elk) which is highly recommended for inexperienced observers, especially in children and within a clinical setting (Jakel and Wichmann, 2006). We anticipated that the fixation points obtained by an eye-tracker would be concentrated in the region of the grating pattern where the observer was able to distinguish the stimuli.

To demonstrate the feasibility of applying today's eye tracking technology to CS measurement, we investigated the consistency between the contrast thresholds obtained from eye movement measurements compared to those using keypress responses. As a first step toward developing a system for use in infants and adults with cognitive or speech impairments, we tested adult participants with normal vision under two conditions: full refractive correction and lens-induced optical blur to simulate a vision defect.

MATERIALS AND METHODS

Participants

A total of 27 healthy subjects, from 19 to 35 years old (mean = 25.4 ± 2.85 years; 10 females) with normal or corrected-to-normal vision and healthy eyes were recruited from The Optometry Clinic of Zhongshan Ophthalmic Center (Guangzhou, China). Nine participants were randomly selected to participate in a repeated test session to verify the repeatability of the experimental results for the eye tracking test on separate days. Ten subjects also repeated the test with optical defocus. They were under-corrected with plus spherical lenses until their VA dropped to logMAR 0.20. The study protocol was approved by the Ethics Committee of Zhongshan Ophthalmic Center of Sun Yat-sen University and adhered to the tenets of the Declaration of Helsinki. All subjects signed informed consents after they were given written and verbal explanations of the nature and purpose of the study.

Apparatus

Visual acuity was measured using the Binoptometer 4P (OCULUS, Germany) and it was used again to determine the correction needed to create a VA drop of logMAR 0.20 under the blur stimulus condition. The stimuli were presented at a viewing distance of 60 cm on a gamma-corrected display (ASUS ROG SWIFT PG278QR), with a uniform background luminance of 52.1 ± 1.30 cd/m^2, resolution of 2,560 × 1,440 pixels, and refresh rate of 165 Hz. A special circuit was used to produce a 14-bit gray-level resolution (Li et al., 2003). Experiments were written in MATLAB (MathWorks Inc. Natick, MA, United States) using elements of the Psychophysics Toolbox (Brainard, 1997). Monocular eye movements were recorded using an Eye-link

1000 Infrared eye tracker (SR Research, Ontario, Canada). Eye movements were streamed to the stimulus computer via a high-speed Ethernet connection and were processed in MATLAB using the Eye-link Toolbox.

Stimuli

A sinusoidal grating detection task, in which the test stimuli randomly appeared in one of four circles, as shown in **Figure 1**, was presented to the participant. The luminance of the four circles was programmed to be homogenous before the test. Michelson contrasts of the sinusoidal gratings were adjusted on each trial by a transformed three-down-one-up staircase (Wetherill and Levitt, 1965) with a proportional step size of 10%, which terminated after 100 trials. Stimulus orientation was varied randomly from 0 to 180 degrees, and the stimuli appeared 25 times in each location. The phase of the Gabor patches was set to zero. The means of the last four staircase reversals were taken as the contrast detection threshold for each spatial frequency (SF) tested [1, 4 and 16 cycle per degree (cpd)].

Procedure

Two experiments were conducted to measure log contrast sensitivity (logCS) by means of eye tracking and conventional perceptual reporting. The order of measurements and spatial frequency presentations was random. Testing was conducted in a dark room. Subjects' heads were stabilized using a chin and forehead rest. An adhesive eye patch was used to occlude the untested eye. Participants were tested with their best refractive correction and in the presence of a positive blur lens that reduced their VA to 0.20 (logMAR).

Eye Tracking Test (Elk)

Each subject underwent a five-point calibration procedure before starting the test session. During the test, the eye tracker was used to record the fixation point while the observer was instructed to stare at the location where they detected the target (a grating pattern) until a break screen was presented. If they could not see any grating patterns within any of the circles, they were instructed to stare at the central blank area of the screen. Fixation on a potential target location for more than 1 s was regarded as a response. In each trial, the stimulus lasted for no more than 6 s, with a one-second break in between trials to allow participants to blink. A fixation point appeared at the center of the display in between each trial to prompt the subject to refixate at the center in order to avoid any misjudgment of the next eye movement. Contrast thresholds were estimated independently for each SF after 100 trials. A longer break time was provided in between each spatial frequency block to minimize visual fatigue.

Conventional Perceptual Report: Behavioral Test (Beh)

In this testing design, observers were instructed to report the perceived location of the stimuli using the four arrow keys on a computer keyboard. Observers were given an option to report "I don't know," upon which the response was regarded as incorrect. If the observer did not respond after 6 s, the

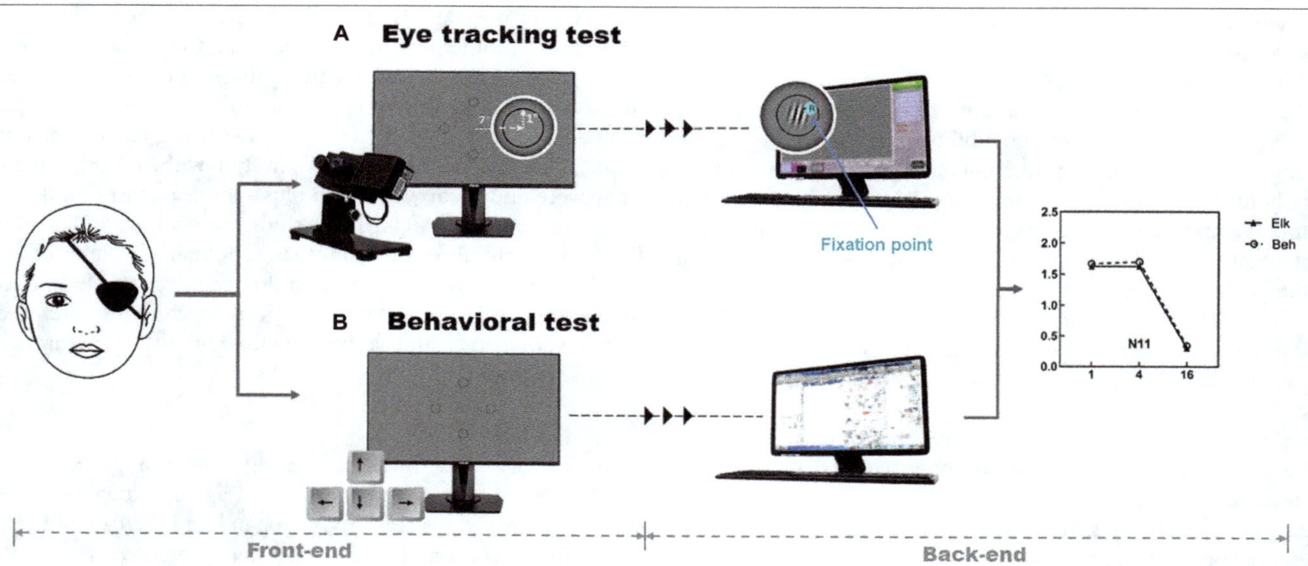

FIGURE 1 | Graphical representation of the study task and procedure. The front-end is the interface on which the subjects performed the test. Monocular CS was estimated via an **(A)** eye tracking test and a conventional psychophysical method [**(B)** Behavioral test], which were both based on a five-alternative forced-choice grating detection task. The task stimuli were the gratings that randomly appeared in one of the four circles, which are equidistant from the tested eye. Each circle had a radius of 1° and were located at the upper, lower, left and right sides, 7° away from the center point of the screen. The observer was instructed to stare at the location where the stimulus appeared and the fixation points recorded by the eye tracker were transmitted to a second monitor. The same task was performed in the Behavioral test using the four arrow keys on a computer keyboard to report perceived location of the stimuli. The examiners observed the subjects' fixation points and key presses on the second monitor (the back-end) and an automated algorithm presented the next stimulus and determined the contrast threshold. Then, the contrast threshold obtained with two methods were compared across spatial frequencies. elk, eye tracking test; beh, behavioral test (conventional perceptual report).

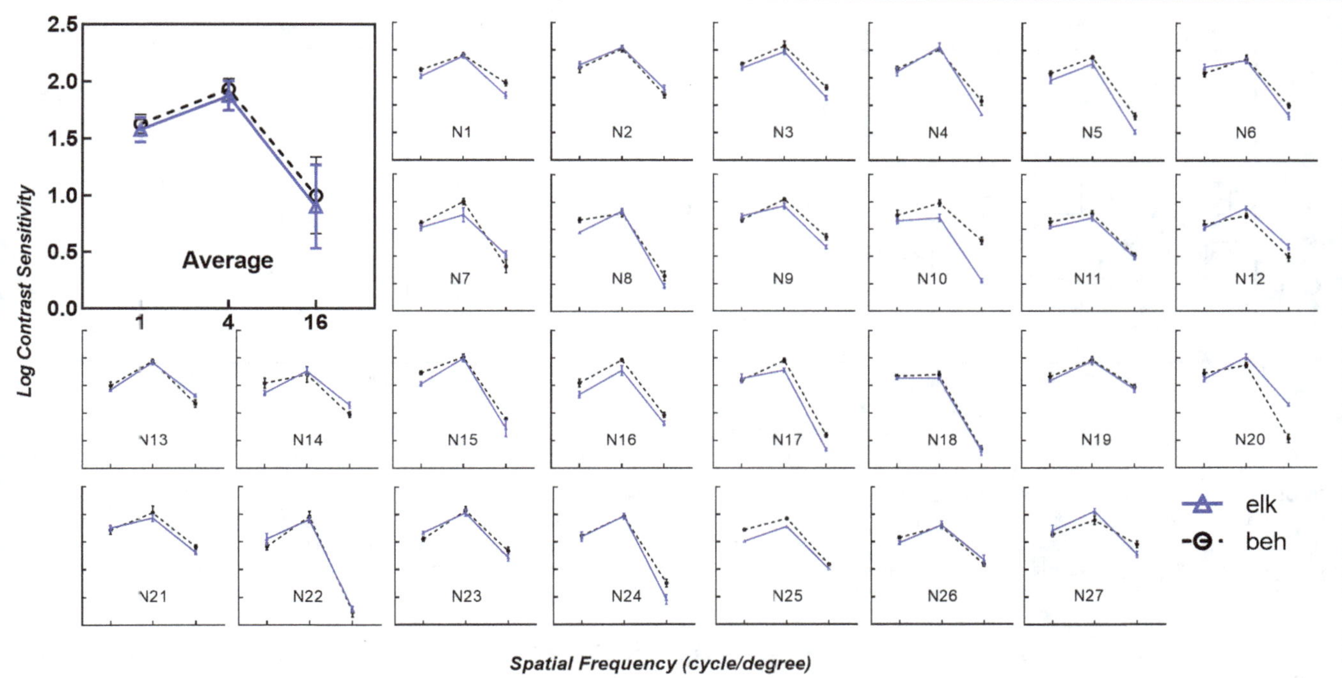

FIGURE 2 | Eye tracking logCS versus behavioral logCS under best-corrected visual acuity (BCVA). The average of all subjects' data for each spatial frequency is shown in the first subplot (Average). The remaining subplots (N1 to N27) depict the logCS from each subject obtained from the eye tracking test (solid blue line with triangles, elk) and perceptual report (dashed black line with circles, beh) under BCVA. Error bars represent the standard deviation across last four reversals under each spatial frequency. The layout is consistent in each subplot, with the horizontal axes representing spatial frequency in log scale and the vertical axes representing log units of CS. In the average subplot, error bars represent the standard deviation across subjects under each spatial frequency. elk, eye tracking test; beh, behavioral test (conventional perceptual report).

program automatically treated this stimulus as a wrong answer and skipped to the next trial.

Data Analysis

Data analyses were performed with SPSS version 25 for Windows (SPSS Inc., IBM, Somers, NY, United States). The normal distribution of data was confirmed using the Shapiro–Wilks test. For the best refractive correction condition, the interaction and main effects of spatial frequency (three frequencies) and measurement type (eye tracking vs. keypress) were tested using a two-way repeated measures ANOVA analysis. The differences in logCS obtained with Elk and Beh at each spatial frequency were further compared with paired *t*-tests (Bonferroni corrected). To assess the relationship between the two measurement types, we computed a Pearson correlation coefficient to indicate the strength and directionality of the linear relationships. The test–retest repeatability of the eye tracking test was determined using a Bland–Altman plot and the Pearson correlation between the first and second logCS measurements. The coefficient of repeatability (CoR) was used to determine the test reliability, where a lower value indicated less variability with repeated measurements; therefore, better reliability. It was calculated by multiplying the within-subject standard deviation values from the test–retest differences (test 2 - test 1) by 1.96. The average difference between test and retest represented the bias.

RESULTS

Comparison of Contrast Sensitivity Measured Using Eye Tracking and Perceptual Report

As shown in **Figure 2**, the contrast thresholds obtained by the eye tracking method (solid blue line) were compared to thresholds measured using the conventional subjective response method (dashed black line). In each subplot, the trend of logCS obtained from the eye tracking method is highly consistent with the conventional CS measure, with the greatest sensitivity at 4 cpd, followed by 1 cpd and 16 cpd. Similar results were noted in the first subplot illustrating the mean logCS of the eye tracking and the behavioral tests based on all participants at each SF.

The box and scatter plots in **Figure 3** show the median logCS measured using the eye tracking and the behavioral methods at each SF. A two-way repeated-measures ANOVA was performed on the logCS obtained using the two methods. Mauchly's sphericity test indicated that for the main effects of measurement type and SF, the assumption of sphericity had been violated, $\chi^2(2) = 33.5$, $P < 0.001$; therefore, degrees of freedom were corrected using Greenhouse-Geisser estimates of sphericity ($\varepsilon = 0.575$). However, for the measurement type by SF interaction effect, sphericity was met as indicated by, $\chi^2(2) = 3.14$, $P = 0.208$. ANOVA showed that the measurement

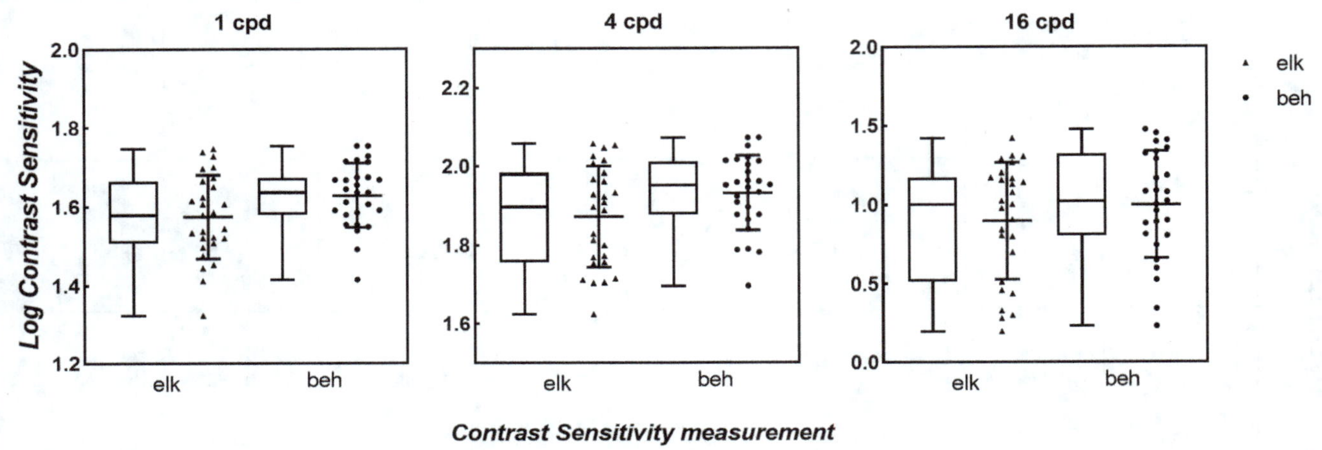

FIGURE 3 | Box and Scatter plots of logCS measured by eye tracking and behavioral tests under BCVA. For each box plot, the middle horizontal lines denote median values of logCS; the top and bottom of each box represent the 25th and 75th percentiles of the data; vertical extending lines and the error bars denote the maximum and the minimum values in each group. For each scatter plot, the middle solid black lines mark the mean of logCS in each SF and the error bars represent ±1 SD. Triangles: logCS of eye tracking method. Circles: logCS of behavioral method. elk, eye tracking test; beh, behavioral test (conventional perceptual report).

type by SF interaction effect was not significant, $F(2,52.0) = 1.39$, $P = 0.257$, while the main effects of both measurement types and SF were significant [$F_{SF}(1,29.9) = 184$, $P < 0.001$, $\eta^2 = 0.874$; $F_{measurement}(1,26.0) = 24.1$, $P < 0.001$, $\eta^2 = 0.481$]. Since our study aimed to evaluate the difference between measurements, a paired t-test was then used to compare the logCS obtained with the two measurements at each SF. A statistically significant difference was present between the two methods at each SF [1cpd: $Mean_{elk} = 1.57 \pm 0.107$, $Mean_{beh} = 1.63 \pm 0.0810$, $Mean_{dif} = 0.0543 \pm 0.103$, $t(2,26.0) = 2.72$, $P_{corrected} = 0.036$; 4cpd: $Mean_{elk} = 1.87 \pm 0.129$, $Mean_{beh} = 1.93 \pm 0.0952$, $Mean_{dif} = 0.0601 \pm 0.105$, $t(2,26.0) = 2.95$, $P_{corrected} = 0.003$; 16cpd: $Mean_{elk} = 0.897 \pm 0.370$, $Mean_{beh} = 1.00 \pm 0.338$, $Mean_{dif} = 0.103 \pm 0.152$, $t(2,26.0) = 3.50$, $P_{corrected} = 0.006$]. CS measured using the conventional perceptual reporting method was slightly higher (better) than CS measured using the eye tracking method at each SF. However, linear correlation (blue solid line in **Figure 4**) shows a strong relationship between logCS measured by the two methods (Pearson's $r = 0.966$, $P < 0.001$). The linear correlation slope between the two methods was 1.03 [95% confidence interval (CI): 0.969–1.09]. Therefore, we can conclude that the eye tracking technology is comparable to the behavioral method for the measurement of CS.

Comparison of Contrast Sensitivity Measured Using Eye Tracking and Perceptual Report With Reduced Visual Acuity

To verify the applicability of eye tracking technology for subjects with altered visual functions, we reduced participant's logMAR VA to 0.20 using optical blur. Data from the eye tracking tests and psychophysical perceptual tests are shown in **Figure 5**, with identical layout and axes to **Figure 2**. As shown in **Figure 5**, the same logCS trend obtained from the two techniques at different spatial frequencies can be observed in each subplot. The logCS of most subjects decreased with increasing spatial frequency.

Figure 6 compares the logCS at different spatial frequencies under best-corrected VA and under-corrected VA using eye tracking. A drop in logCS is noted when observers were tested in an under-corrected viewing condition.

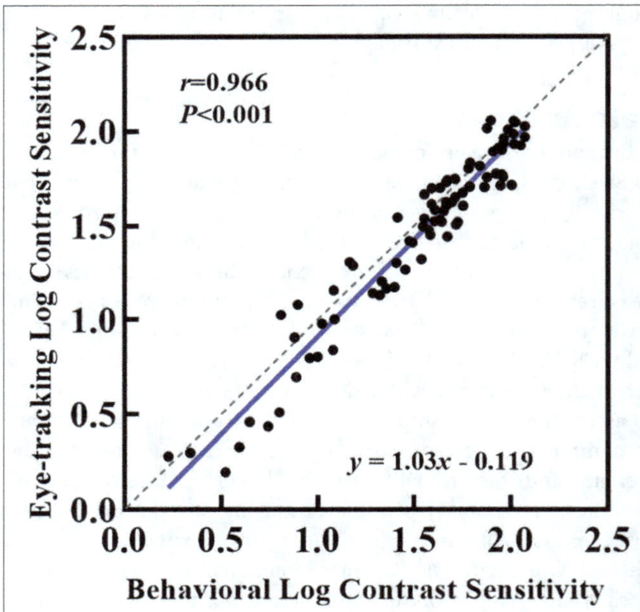

FIGURE 4 | Relationship between logCS estimated from the conventional perceptual and eye tracking report. Each point represents one of the 27 participants who completed eye tracking and behavioral measurements under BCVA. The solid blue line represents the best linear fit to the data.

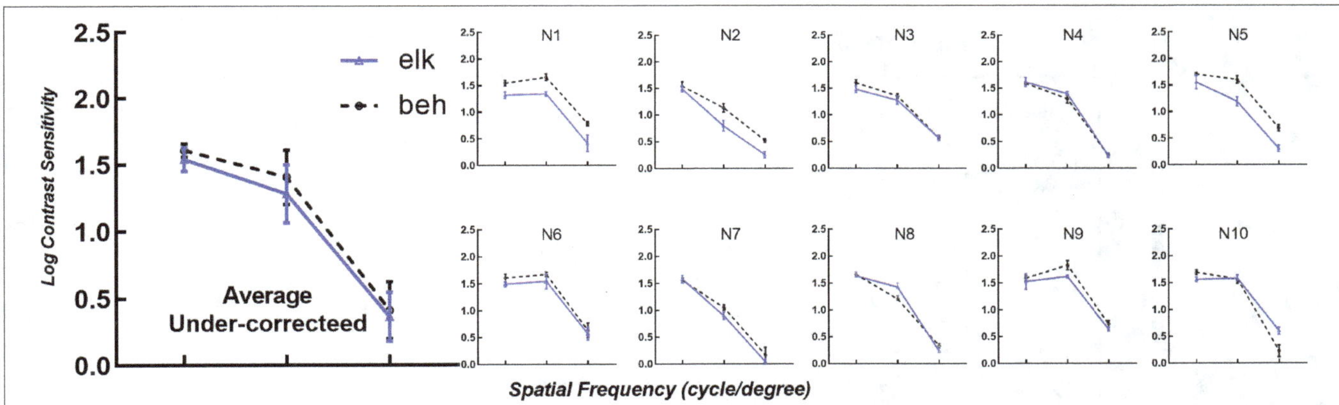

FIGURE 5 | LogCS measured with the two methods with visual acuity reduced to logMAR 0.20. The mean logCS of the eye tracking and behavioral tests of all participants with under-corrected visual acuities for each spatial frequency is shown in the first subplot (Average Under-corrected). The layout and icons are identical to **Figure 2**. elk, eye tracking test; beh, behavioral test (conventional perceptual report).

Repeatability of the Eye Tracking Test

Results of the eye tracking test under the same darkroom conditions on different days are illustrated in **Figure 7**. We calculated the Pearson correlation between logCS measured during the first and second runs, at three different spatial frequencies. The test-retest correlation for the eye tracking method was 0.916, with a slope of 0.893 (95%CI: 0.819–0.962, R^2 = 0.839, **Figure 7A**). **Figure 7B** presents the Bland–Altman CoR and bias of eye tracking method. The CoR value was 0.377 logCS (95%CI: −0.369 to 0.384) and the average test–retest difference (bias) was 0.00710 logCS. Both are much lower than those values obtained from the CS test using Gabor patches in previous studies with CoR values ranging from 0.410 to 0.630 logCS and bias ranging from 0.0500 to 0.120 logCS (Thurman et al., 2016). An outlier can be observed in **Figure 7B**, defined as a test-retest difference exceeding the range expected to contain 95% of the test-retest differences.

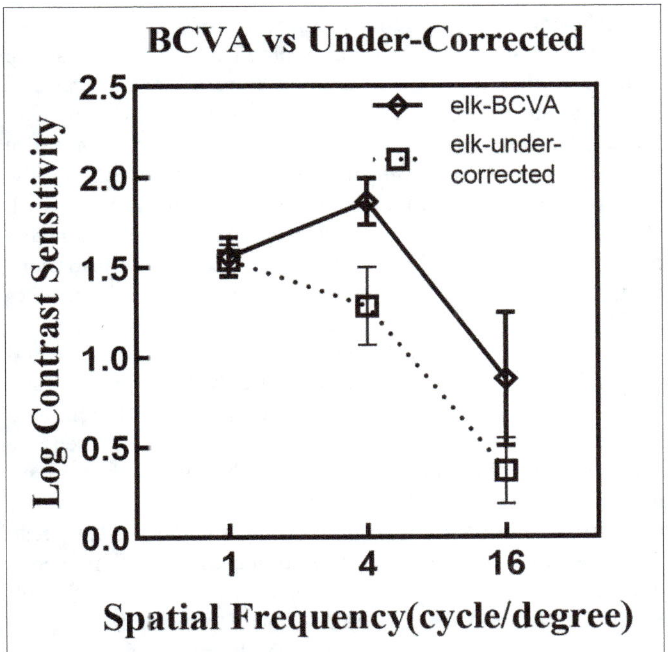

FIGURE 6 | A comparison of the mean logCS at different spatial frequencies under the BCVA (solid line) and under-corrected visual acuity (dotted line) using the eye tracking test. Error bars denote one standard deviation across spatial frequencies. LogCS was significantly reduced at medium and high spatial frequencies, while no distinct difference was noted for the low spatial frequency. BCVA, best-corrected visual acuity; elk, eye tracking test.

DISCUSSION

Visual fixation is spontaneously attracted to more interesting or salient stimuli. This type of spontaneous behavior is termed PL. As such, some contemporary charts designed to test pre-verbal infant's vision utilize spatial grating patterns of varying visibility in order to elicit PL, while the examiner observes the infant's fixation (Brown et al., 2015; Thomas et al., 2021). In this pilot study, we introduced an eye tracker to allow for rapid detection of contrast threshold in adult subjects via a three-down-one-up staircase task starting with low contrast (most difficult level) rather than a trial-by-trial presentation of printed cards. While several challenges in establishing CS measurement using an eye tracker should be addressed, in this study, we proposed point-by-point solutions to challenges encountered, including optimizing calibration, choosing the stimulus, defining the protocol for presenting the stimuli, fixation point judgment, and contrast thresholds.

To verify the feasibility and accuracy of eye tracking technology to test spatial CS, we compared the logCS obtained using the eye tracking format to those from conventional psychophysical perceptual reports. The thresholds measured using perceptual reports were slightly higher than those measured with the eye tracker at each SF. This is most likely caused by fatigue because the eye tracking test usually lasted twice

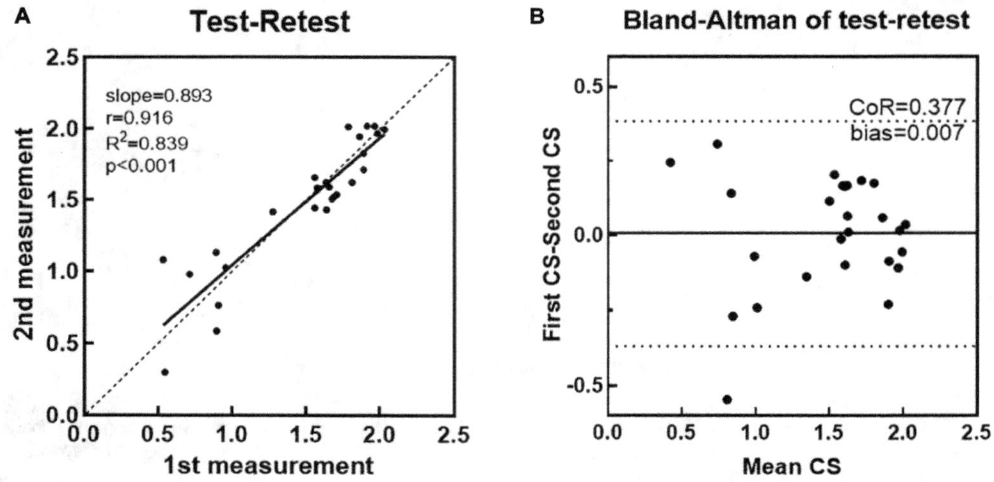

FIGURE 7 | (A) LogCS measured on the second run plotted against those obtained in the first run. The Pearson correlation coefficient (r) between two runs was 0.916. Linear regression was performed to evaluate the test–retest reliability. **(B)** The Bland–Altman plot shows the differences (first CS - second CS) between sensitivity estimates obtained from each eye tracking measure, plotted against their mean (first CS + second CS/2). Each dot represents 1 data point. The central solid line indicates the mean difference (bias) between different measures. Dotted lines indicate the 95% agreement upper and lower limit intervals.

as long as the behavioral test. However, a strong correlation under both best-corrected vision and under-corrected conditions was observed. The logCS results demonstrate sensitivity to an acuity reduction due to under-correction. As Woods and Wood (1995) described, significant loss of CSs at medium and high spatial frequencies were found in refractive blur subjects. Since refractive errors produce an out-of-focus image on the retina, which is equivalent to a low-pass filtered image, the lack of low-frequency components renders them invisible when out of focus (Medina and Howland, 1988). The same results can be observed in the data from our eye tracking tests, which indicate that the eye tracker can precisely record the expected reduction in CS. Moreover, the test–retest repeatability across different days was high. Thus, the eye tracking technology shows a promising application as a reliable objective method for CS assessment within clinical settings.

Our results are in agreement with previous studies that have used eye tracking technology to measure visual function by inducing and quantifying OKN (Schor and Levi, 1980; Leguire et al., 1991; Masson et al., 1994; Hyon et al., 2010) or smooth pursuit tracking of moving stimuli (Mooney et al., 2018). Our work complements these previous studies and provides an alternative paradigm that can be integrated with PL methodology in the future.

However, several cautionary points need to be addressed before the technique can be applied clinically. First, adult subjects were instructed to stare at the location where they detected the target grating, such that, the PL technique was not actually utilized in this pilot study. The feasibility of combining PL technique with an eye tracker for real pre-verbal infants has been previously reported (Vrabič et al., 2021). As such, our subsequent studies will include both pre-verbal infants and pre-literate toddlers in our testing paradigm where we will measure uninstructed response with an eye tracker to test CS. Secondly, it is quite time-consuming as a clinical procedure. In this study, it took subjects approximately 10 min to complete a standard sitting of individual adaptive staircases totaling 100 trials, for each spatial frequency to achieve as many reversals as possible. Visual fatigue associated with prolonged tests resulted in the generally lower logCS with the eye tracking test than those observed with the behavioral test. Moreover, only three SFs were measured for each participant to minimize physical and visual fatigue from distorting the results. Thus, it remains impractical and inadequate to fit the results using a clinical contrast sensitivity function (CSF) plot (Pelli and Bex, 2013). We plan to optimize the testing algorithm by using the quick CSF method. Specifically, the quick CSF uses a computerized Bayesian adaptive framework allowing for direct and quick estimation of several parameters to define a CSF plot (Hou et al., 2010). Such an information-gain testing paradigm is highly efficient and greatly reduces CSF testing time compared with the standard adaptive staircase procedure. Furthermore, the monotonous grating stimuli could be replaced with cartoon patterns filtered with a raised cosine filter and rescaled to different sizes to generate stimuli with different spatial frequencies, so that the paradigm could engage children from different age groups. Lastly, this method might not be suitable for children who are too young to restrain their head movement throughout the testing on a chin rest. A simple and attractive initial calibration interface with free head movement will be more suitable for young children. Although many companies such as Tobii (Tobii Technology) and SMI (SensoMotoric Instruments) offer remote eye tracking (heads free) solutions, they are expensive and remains unsuitable for clinical setting. Sangi et al. (2015) presented offline tools and methods for stabilizing the head based on random facial feature detection to analyze OKN in children. These readily available algorithms and consumer-grade equipment can be adopted in our future optimization model.

This study represents the first step in the development of a paradigm to objectively assess CS via eye-tracking technology, which can be used as a baseline model for a system that can measure visual function in infants and adults with cognitive or speech disabilities. It aimed to develop a testing paradigm that neither depended on observers' cognitive ability nor their language ability. An eye tracker was employed to judge the observer's fixation location. Our results from a group of adults with normal vision and their simulated defocused viewing condition provided a preliminary model, which demonstrated the feasibility and accuracy of our method. Strong agreement was found between the measurements made using the eye tracking test and those made using conventional psychophysical perceptual reports.

AUTHOR CONTRIBUTIONS

JL, JY, YZ, and LG designed the research. YZ, LG, LF, and QY performed the research. YZ and LG analyzed the data and drafted the manuscript. YZ, LG, JC, LC, JL, and JY revised the manuscript. All authors commented on and edited the manuscript, and approved the final version of the manuscript.

REFERENCES

Adler, F. H., and Fliegelman, M. (1934). Influence of fixation on the visual acuity. *Arch. Ophthalmol.* 12, 475–483. doi: 10.1001/archopht.1934.00830170013002

Atkinson, J., Braddick, O., and Braddick, F. (1974). Acuity and contrast sensivity of infant vision. *Nature* 247, 403–404. doi: 10.1038/247403a0

Banks, M. S., and Salapatek, P. (1978). Acuity and contrast sensitivity in 1-, 2-, and 3-month-old human infants. *Invest. Ophthalmol. Vis. Sci.* 17, 361–365.

Brainard, D. H. (1997). The psychophysics toolbox. *Spat. Vis.* 10, 433–436. doi: 10.1163/156856897x00357

Brown, A. M., Lindsey, D. T., Cammenga, J. G., Giannone, P. J., and Stenger, M. R. (2015). The contrast sensitivity of the newborn human infant. *Invest. Ophthalmol. Vis. Sci.* 56, 625–632. doi: 10.1167/iovs.14-14757

Denniss, J., Scholes, C., McGraw, P. V., Nam, S.-H., and Roach, N. W. (2018). Estimation of contrast sensitivity from fixational eye movements. *Invest. Ophthalmol. Vis. Sci.* 59, 5408–5416. doi: 10.1167/iovs.18-24674

Fantz, R. L. (1963). Pattern vision in newborn infants. *Science* 140, 296–297. doi: 10.1126/science.140.3564.296

Hou, F., Huang, C. B., Lesmes, L., Feng, L. X., Tao, L., Zhou, Y. F., et al. (2010). qCSF in clinical application: efficient characterization and classification of contrast sensitivity functions in amblyopia. *Invest. Ophthalmol. Vis. Sci.* 51, 5365–5377. doi: 10.1167/iovs.10-5468

Huang, C.-B., Zhou, Y., and Lu, Z.-L. (2008). Broad bandwidth of perceptual learning in the visual system of adults with anisometropic amblyopia. *Proc. Natl. Acad. Sci. U. S. A.* 105, 4068–4073. doi: 10.1073/pnas.0800824105

Hyon, J. Y., Yeo, H. E., Seo, J.-M., Lee, I. B., Lee, J. H., and Hwang, J.-M. (2010). Objective measurement of distance visual acuity determined by computerized optokinetic nystagmus test. *Invest. Ophthalmol. Vis. Sci.* 51, 752–757. doi: 10.1167/iovs.09-4362

Jakel, F., and Wichmann, F. A. (2006). Spatial four-alternative forced-choice method is the preferred psychophysical method for naive observers. *J. Vis.* 6, 1307–1322. doi: 10.1167/6.11.13

Leguire, L., Zaff, B., Freeman, S., Rogers, G., Bremer, D., and Wali, N. (1991). Contrast sensitivity of optokinetic nystagmus. *Vision Res.* 31, 89–97. doi: 10.1016/0042-6989(91)90076-h

Li, X., Lu, Z.-L., Xu, P., Jin, J., and Zhou, Y. (2003). Generating high gray-level resolution monochrome displays with conventional computer graphics cards and color monitors. *J. Neurosci. Methods* 130, 9–18. doi: 10.1016/s0165-0270(03)00174-2

Masson, G., Mestre, D. R., Blin, O., and Pailhous, J. (1994). Low luminance contrast sensitivity: effects of training on psychophysical and optokinetic nystagmus thresholds in man. *Vision Res.* 34, 1893–1899. doi: 10.1016/0042-6989(94)90313-1

McDonald, M. A., Dobson, V., Sebris, S. L., Baitch, L., Varner, D., and Teller, D. Y. (1985). The acuity card procedure: a rapid test of infant acuity. *Invest. Ophthalmol. Vis. Sci.* 26, 1158–1162.

Medina, A., and Howland, B. (1988). A novel high–frequency visual acuity chart. *Ophthalmic Physiol. Opt.* 8, 14–18. doi: 10.1111/j.1475-1313.1988.tb01076.x

Mooney, S. W., Hill, N. J., Tuzun, M. S., Alam, N. M., Carmel, J. B., and Prusky, G. T. (2018). Curveball: a tool for rapid measurement of contrast sensitivity based on smooth eye movements. *J. Vis.* 18, 7–7. doi: 10.1167/18.12.7

Okada, Y., Ukai, K., Wolffsohn, J. S., Gilmartin, B., Iijima, A., and Bando, T. (2006). Target spatial frequency determines the response to conflicting defocus- and convergence-driven accommodative stimuli. *Vision Res.* 46, 475–484. doi: 10.1016/j.visres.2005.07.014

Pelli, D. G., and Bex, P. (2013). Measuring contrast sensitivity. *Vision Res.* 90, 10–14. doi: 10.1016/j.visres.2013.04.015

Sangi, M., Thompson, B., and Turuwhenua, J. (2015). An optokinetic nystagmus detection method for use with young children. *IEEE J. Transl. Eng. Health Med.* 3, 1–10. doi: 10.1109/jtehm.2015.2410286

Schor, C. M., and Levi, D. M. (1980). Disturbances of small-field horizontal and vertical optokinetic nystagmus in amblyopia. *Invest. Ophthalmol. Vis. Sci.* 19, 668–683.

Schütz, A. C., Braun, D. I., and Gegenfurtner, K. R. (2011). Eye movements and perception: a selective review. *J. Vis.* 11, 9–9.

Thomas, R., Vinekar, A., Mangalesh, S., Mochi, T. B., Sarbajna, P., and Shetty, B. (2021). Evaluating contrast sensitivity in asian indian pre-term infants with and without retinopathy of prematurity. *Transl. Vis. Sci. Technol.* 10, 12–12. doi: 10.1167/tvst.10.4.12

Thurman, S. M., Davey, P. G., McCray, K. L., Paronian, V., and Seitz, A. R. (2016). Predicting individual contrast sensitivity functions from acuity and letter contrast sensitivity measurements. *J. Vis.* 16, 15–15. doi: 10.1167/16.15.15

Vrabič, N., Juroš, B., and Pompe, M. T. (2021). Automated visual acuity evaluation based on preferential looking technique and controlled with remote eye tracking. *Ophthalmic Res.* 64, 389–397. doi: 10.1159/000512395

Wetherill, G., and Levitt, H. (1965). Sequential estimation of points on a psychometric function. *Br. J. Math. Stat. Psychol.* 18, 1–10. doi: 10.1111/j.2044-8317.1965.tb00689.x

Woods, R. L., and Wood, J. M. (1995). The role of contrast sensitivity charts and contrast letter charts in clinical practice. *Clin. Exp. Optom.* 78, 43–57. doi: 10.1111/j.1444-0938.1995.tb00787.x

10

Blur Detection Sensitivity Increases in Children using Orthokeratology

Jingjing Xu[1,2†], Chunwen Tao[1†], Xinjie Mao[1,2], Xin Lu[1], Jinhua Bao[1,2], Björn Drobe[2,3] and Hao Chen[1,2]*

[1] School of Ophthalmology and Optometry, Affiliated Eye Hospital, State Key Laboratory of Ophthalmology, Optometry and Vision Science, Wenzhou Medical University, Wenzhou, China, [2] WEIRC, Wenzhou Medical University-Essilor International Research Center, Wenzhou, China, [3] R&D AMERA, Essilor International, Singapore, Singapore

***Correspondence:**
Hao Chen
chenhao@mail.eye.ac.cn

† These authors have contributed equally to this work*

Purpose: To investigate changes in blur detection sensitivity in children using orthokeratology (Ortho-K) and explore the relationships between blur detection thresholds (BDTs) and aberrations and accommodative function.

Methods: Thirty-two children aged 8–14 years old who underwent Ortho-K treatment participated in and completed this study. Their BDTs, aberrations, and accommodative responses (ARs) were measured before and after a month of Ortho-K treatment. A two forced-choice double-staircase procedure with varying extents of blur in three images (Tumbling Es, Lena, and Street View) was used to measure the BDTs. The participants were required to judge whether the images looked blurry. The BDT of each of the images (BDT_Es, BDT_Lena, and BDT_Street) was the average value of the last three reversals. The accommodative lag was quantified by the difference between the AR and the accommodative demand (AD). Changes in the BDTs, aberrations, and accommodative lags and their relationships were analyzed.

Results: After a month of wearing Ortho-K lenses, the children's BDT_Es and BDT_Lena values decreased, the aberrations increased significantly (for all, $P \leq 0.050$), and the accommodative lag decreased to a certain extent [$T(31) = 2.029$, $P = 0.051$]. Before Ortho-K treatment, higher-order aberrations (HOAs) were related to BDT_Lena ($r = 0.463$, $P = 0.008$) and the accommodative lag was related to BDT_Es ($r = -0.356$, $P = -0.046$). After one month, no significant correlations were found between the BDTs and aberrations or accommodative lags, as well as between the variations of them (for all, $P \geq 0.069$).

Conclusion: Ortho-K treatment increased the children's level of blur detection sensitivity, which may have contributed to their good visual acuity.

Keywords: blur detection sensitivity, orthokeratology, blur adaptation, higher-order aberration, accommodation lag

INTRODUCTION

Orthokeratology (Ortho-K) has been demonstrated to improve naked visual acuity during the day (Swarbrick, 2006; Khan et al., 2016) by reshaping the corneal surface and to slow myopia progression (Swarbrick, 2006; Le et al., 2010; Santodomingo-Rubido et al., 2015, 2017; Wen et al., 2015; Huang et al., 2016; Chen et al., 2018) by changing the peripheral defocusing state

(Queirós et al., 2010; Kang and Swarbrick, 2011; Santodomingo-Rubido et al., 2013). An increasing number of children have been using them in China (Tay et al., 2017), Singapore (Saw et al., 2019), etc., especially for the latter reason.

Although some studies (Queiros et al., 2012; Zhao et al., 2018) have shown that myopic children's quality of life partially improves with good acceptance of Ortho-K (Wen et al., 2015; Li et al., 2016), visual and optical quality in children wearing Ortho-K lenses deteriorate because of the reshaped cornea and the affected tear film (Li et al., 2018). Previous studies have reported that Ortho-K inevitably increases higher-order aberrations (HOAs) and decreases contrast sensitivity (Hiraoka et al., 2008a,b; Gifford et al., 2013; Vincent et al., 2020). Santolaria et al. (2013) reported that people using Ortho-K tend to complain about distortions from car headlights and bright lights at home. Bad visual and optical quality may cause the perception of blur to some extent. However, it is not common for people receiving Ortho-K to complain about blur in the clinic. Hiraoka et al. (2009b) investigated patient satisfaction with visual outcomes using a visual analog scale. The results showed a relatively high level of patient satisfaction following Ortho-K use, which was associated with pretreatment myopic error and posttreatment uncorrected visual acuity.

Blur is a visual signal that triggers the visual feedback mechanism and plays an important role in the emmetropization process (Norton and Siegwart, 1995). It has been shown that people are likely to adapt to blur if it lasts for a certain period of time (Khan et al., 2013). Therefore, we speculated that children with Ortho-K experience a blur adaptation induced by increased aberrations and greater diurnal variations in vision (Queiros et al., 2012; Guo et al., 2018). Blur adaptation is defined as an improvement in visual resolution after exposure to the blur (i.e., defocusing) without a change in the refractive error (Vera-Diaz et al., 2004; Cufflin et al., 2007). After blur adaptation, contrast sensitivity (Pesudovs and Brennan, 1993), blur sensitivity (Cufflin et al., 2007), and sometimes even the accommodative response (AR) (Vera-Diaz et al., 2004) improve. The blur detection threshold (BDT), that is, the amount of detectable blur equivalent to the depth of focus (Jacobs et al., 1989), is closely related to blur sensitivity.

We present a novel hypothesis that Ortho-K provides good naked visual acuity with good satisfaction, partially because children with Ortho-K undergo a blur adaptation. Since the BDT is a good indicator of blur sensitivity, we evaluate the BDT in children before and after Ortho-K treatment to verify whether the deteriorated visual quality changes their blur perception after wearing Ortho-K lenses. Optical physical parameters, such as accommodative lag and ocular aberrations, might explain the changes in the visual feedback mechanism. The relationship between BDTs and visual quality or accommodative function also needs to be clarified.

To the best of our knowledge, no literature has reported the effect of wearing Ortho-K lenses on blur sensitivity. Therefore, this study aimed to evaluate changes in blur detection sensitivity after Ortho-K treatment by measuring the BDT. Moreover, we probed whether this change is related to aberrations or accommodative lag.

MATERIALS AND METHODS

Participants

This clinical study was conducted at the Eye Hospital of Wenzhou Medical University (Wenzhou, China) between May 2016 and October 2017. Forty-three children aged 8–14 years old wore Ortho-K lenses in both eyes, and the right eyes were initially recruited in this study. The spherical equivalent (SE), calculated by adding half of the cylinder (in minus lens notation) to the sphere, ranging from −1.00 diopters (D) to −6.00 D and no more than −0.75 D of astigmatism. None of the participants had records of ocular, systemic, or neurologic diseases or any type of vision dysfunction. In addition, none of the participants had previously undergone Ortho-K treatment or other myopia control treatments. At enrollment, their visual acuity was correctable to 0.00 (logarithm of the minimum angle of resolution (logMAR) visual acuity) or better, and after a month of Ortho-K treatment, their naked visual acuity during the day should have reached 0.00 (logMAR visual acuity) or better. One child was excluded because of excessive follow-up ARs, and ten children did not have ideal naked visual acuity. In total, thirty-two children completed this study. The participants and their guardians were informed of and understood the adverse reactions, and they all signed the informed consent forms. This study followed the tenets of the Declaration of Helsinki and was approved by the Ethics Committee of Wenzhou Medical University.

Procedure

All the Ortho-K lenses used in this study were VST-DESIGN with four-zone reverse geometry rigid contact lenses (Lucid, South Korea), included the base curve, reverse curve, alignment curve, and peripheral curve and were composed of Boston XO material, with an oxygen permeability (DK) of 100×10^{-12} $(cm^2 \times mlO_2)/(s \times ml \times mmHg)$. The lenses had a total diameter of 10.2–10.8 mm, a central zone diameter of 0.6 mm, and a central thickness of 0.23 mm.

The detailed produce is summarized in **Figure 1**. The participants first underwent a series of pre-examinations, including subjective refraction, intraocular pressure, axial length, corneal topography and endothelial cell count analysis. Then, lens fitting was performed and evaluated by experienced doctors with slit-lamp biomicroscopy according to the fluorescence pattern and topography. All of the participants were instructed to regularly follow up 1 day, 1 week, 1 month, and then every 3 months after lens delivery.

After enrollment, the BDTs, aberrations, and ARs of the participants were measured before receiving Ortho-K. Measurements were taken on the right eyes, fully corrected with frames, with the left eyes occluded. After a month, the aberrations, ARs and BDTs of the remaining participants were measured for a second time. For most of the Ortho-K children, their corneal parameters as well as refraction (Li et al., 2018; Queirós et al., 2020), visual quality (Stillitano et al., 2008; Santolaria Sanz et al., 2015), and visual performance including

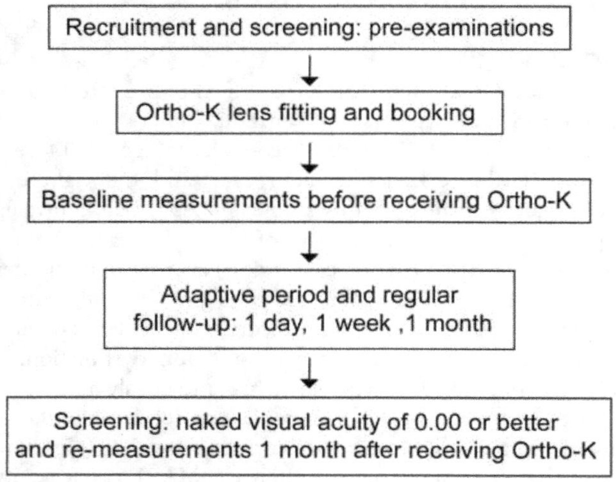

FIGURE 1 | Procedure of this study. Forty-three children who were scheduled to wear Ortho-K lenses had a series of pre-examinations. After lens fitting was performed, the personalized Ortho-K lenses were ordered. The baseline measurements were conducted before they received the Ortho-K lenses. After a month of Ortho-K use, ten children without ideal naked visual acuity were excluded, and the remaining children were measured again. Visual acuity of 0.00 refers to the logMAR visual acuity.

naked visual acuity (Lu et al., 2018; Xia et al., 2019) reached a steady state at one month.

Blur Detection Threshold (BDT)

The testing procedure was designed to be similar to a computer game, easy for children to complete, which was presented on a 19" LCD Monitor (DELL^{TM} P1914S Monitor, 1280 × 1024 pixels, TX, United States). A neutral gray background provided uniform illumination for the test. The environmental luminance was 155 lux. The heads of the participants were stabilized with a chinrest to keep the eyes one meter away from the screen. This distance was chosen to reduce accommodative lag.

The procedure included three images: Tumbling Es, Lena, and Street View (**Figure 2**), with an average luminance of 50.85, 19.41, and 13.24 cd/m^2, respectively. Two hundred pictures with spherical defocus ranging from 0 D ~ 2 D in steps of 0.01 D for each image were obtained by fast Fourier transformation (FFT) based on a pupil radius of 2 mm. The Stiles-Crawford effect (Applegate and Lakshminarayanan, 1993) was considered, with an attenuation factor of r = 0.05 mm^2 and a vertical offset of 0.2 mm.

A double-staircase method was used. The two staircases occurred alternately and in parallel, and the three images also appeared in random order. Images with different blur levels were presented for 1 second. The participants were required to judge whether the image looked blurred by clicking on a "blurred" or a "not blurred" button. The first image in the ascending staircase was the clearest one with 0 D defocus, and the first image in the descending staircase was the most blurred with +2 D defocus. The steps of the staircases were 0.20 D until the first inversion, 0.10 D until the second inversion and 0.05 D from the third inversion onward. The BDT was calculated automatically on the last 3 reversals out of 5 (**Figure 3**).

Accommodative Lag

The AR was obtained with a Grand Seiko WAM-5500 open field infrared autorefractor (Grand Seiko, Hiroshima, Japan). One "Tumbling Es" image, a 4 × 4 array of high-contrast letters (the same image used in the BDT procedure with 0 D defocus) was displayed 1 m away from the target. The AR was measured three times in static mode. The mean value was taken as the AR, and the accommodative lag was calculated based on the following formulas for accommodative demand (AD) and the AR (Gwiazda et al., 1993):

$$\text{Accommodative Demand} = \frac{1/\text{DTE}}{1 - \text{DLE} * \text{LENS} * 2}$$

$$\text{Accommodative Response} = \text{RI}$$

$$\text{Accommodative lag} = \text{AR-AD}$$

where DTE = the distance from the eye to the target (1 m), DLE = the distance from the lens to the eye (0.12 m), LENS = the signed dioptric power of the lens, and RI = the mean value (calculated above) from the values read from the Grand Seiko device.

These equations correct for the effectivity of a spectacle lens placed 12 mm in front of the eye.

Aberrations

The ocular aberrations were measured three times in a dark room with a WASCA wavefront analyzer (Carl Zeiss Meditec, Jena, Germany) through the natural pupil without the use of dilation drugs, and the mean value was used for data analysis. The pupil diameter used for analysis was 5 mm. The total HOAs, trefoil, coma, and spherical aberrations (SA) were used for analysis. The total HOAs were calculated as the root mean square (RMS) of the third- to seventh-order coefficients. The RMS of C_3^{-3} and C_3^{3} and the RMS of C_3^{-1} and C_3^{1} were calculated to represent trefoil and coma, respectively. The SA was equal to C_4^{0}.

Data Analysis

SPSS version 22.0 was used for data analysis. The normality of the data was assessed using the Shapiro-Wilk test before conducting parametric tests. Differences between baseline measurements and remeasurements after one month of Ortho-K were tested using paired Student's t-tests or Wilcoxon signed-rank tests, depending on whether the data were normally distributed. Similarly, correlations between the BDTs and aberrations or accommodative lags, including baseline measurements, remeasurements and their variations, were assessed with Pearson correlation coefficients or Spearman correlation coefficients, depending on whether the data were normally distributed. $P \leq 0.05$ was set as the level of significance.

RESULTS

Thirty-two participants (15 boys and 17 girls), aged 8 to 14 years old (11.05 ± 1.59, mean ± SD), successfully completed the

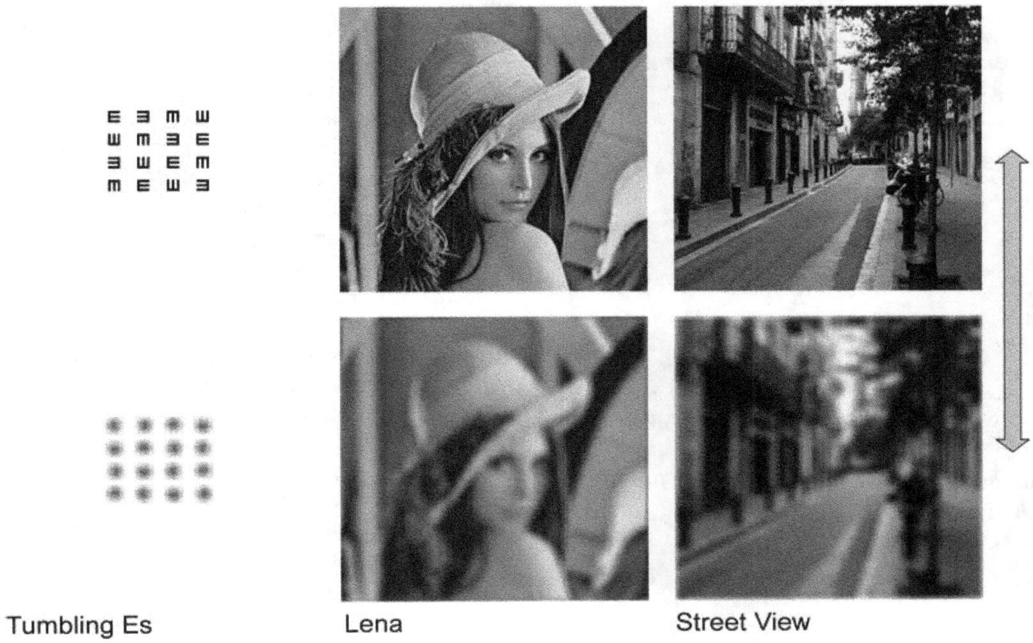

FIGURE 2 | Images used to measure the BDT. Three images with spherical defocus ranging from 0 D ~ 2 D in steps of 0.01 D are included in the procedure. From left to right: Tumbling Es, Lena, and Street View. The defocus degree of the top images is 0 D and that of the bottom images is 2 D.

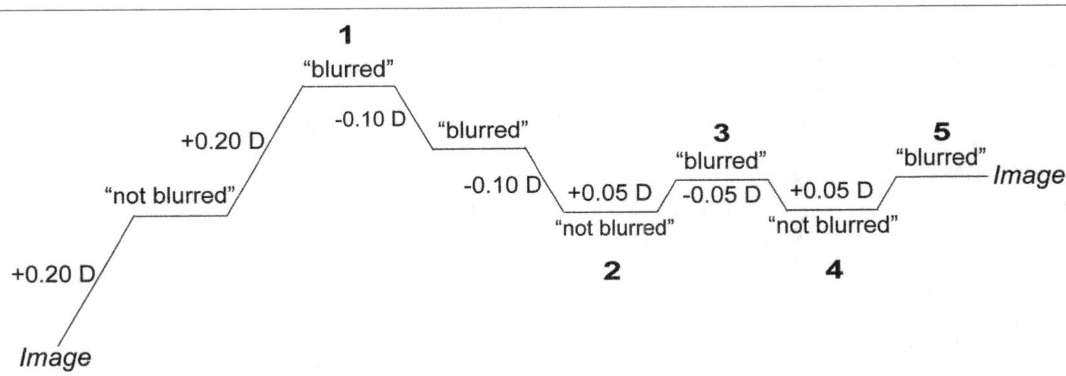

FIGURE 3 | Ascending staircase. The first image in the ascending staircase was the clearest picture with 0 D defocus. The numbers in the figure represent the last five reversals in the procedure, and the BDT is the average value over the last three reversals.

1-month follow-up examinations. The SE at baseline was > -6.00 and < -1.00 D (-3.57 ± 1.23) and ≥ -0.75 and ≤ 0.00 D (-0.19 ± 0.28) with refractive astigmatism. Before Ortho-K treatment, the AD was 0.92 ± 0.03 D, and the AR was 0.52 ± 0.41 D; 1 month after receiving Ortho-K, the AD was 1.00 ± 0 D, and the AR was 0.79 ± 0.42 D. The mean value of the corrected visual acuity was 0.00 ± 0.02 (logMAR) at baseline, and the naked visual acuity after one month of treatment was 0.04 ± 0.05 (logMAR) (Wilcoxon signed-rank test, $Z = -2.982$, $P = 0.003$). There were no complaints from the subjects about wearing the Ortho-K lenses.

BDT_Es and BDT_Lena decreased significantly following treatment ($P \leq 0.040$). The HOAs, trefoil, coma, and SAs increased significantly (all $P \leq 0.050$); accommodative lag decreased from 0.40 ± 0.41 D at baseline to 0.26 ± 0.31 D after 1 month [$T(31) = 2.029$, $P = 0.051$]. In summary, the results showed that after Ortho-K, the BDTs (BDT_Es and BDT_Lena) and the accommodative lags of the participants decreased, while the aberrations increased (**Table 1**).

Before Ortho-K treatment, HOAs were significantly related to BDT_Lena ($r = 0.463$, $P = 0.008$), accommodative lag was related to BDT_Es ($r = -0.356$, $P = -0.046$) (**Figure 4**), and the other possible combinations between aberrations and the BDTs were not significant (all $P \geq 0.051$). After Ortho-K treatment, there were no relationships among accommodative lag, aberrations and the BDTs (all $P \geq 0.069$) (**Figure 4**). The relationships among the variations in accommodative lag, aberrations and BDTs (BDT_Es and BDT_Lena) after Ortho-K treatment were further analyzed,

TABLE 1 | Variations in aberrations, accommodations and BDTs before and one month after Ortho-K treatment.

	N	Before (M ± SD)	After (M ± SD)	T/Z	*P*
BDT_Es (D)	32	0.51 ± 0.14	0.47 ± 0.16	2.146	0.040
BDT_Lena (D)	32	0.65 ± 0.18	0.60 ± 0.16	2.321	0.027
HOAs (μm)	32	0.21 ± 0.09	0.54 ± 0.18	−9.501	< 0.001
Trefoil (μm)	32	0.07 ± 0.04	0.10 ± 0.06	1.963	0.050
Coma (μm)	32	0.13 ± 0.08	0.30 ± 0.18	−5.028	< 0.001
SAs (μm)	32	0.07 ± 0.07	0.35 ± 0.13	4.693	< 0.001
Accommodative lag (D)	32	−0.40 ± 0.41	−0.26 ± 0.31	2.029	0.051

N, number of participants; HOAs, total higher-order aberrations; SAs, spherical aberrations; BDT_ Es, the blur detection threshold for the Tumbling Es image; BDT_Lena, the blur detection threshold for the Lena image; BDT_Street, the blur detection threshold for the Street View image; M ± SD, mean ± standard deviation.

and no significant correlations were found (for all, $P \geq 0.201$) (**Supplementary Figures 1–5**).

DISCUSSION

This is the first study that investigated the effect of Ortho-K on the BDTs and analyzed the correlations among BDTs, aberrations and accommodative lags. To prevent the influence of nonideal visual acuity on BDT evaluation, participants whose naked visual acuity was 0.00 logMAR or better at the one-month follow-up examination were included, and the experiments were all conducted in the morning. These parameters were evaluated before and one month after Ortho-K treatment because the naked visual acuity of the subjects may become worse than 0.00 (LogMAR visual acuity) at a long-term follow-up visit due to myopia progression (Wen et al., 2015; Na and Yoo, 2018). The results showed that the blur detection sensitivity for Es and Lena in the children improved after Ortho-K treatment. Previous studies (Battaglia et al., 2004; Wang et al., 2006; Venkataraman et al., 2015) have indicated that the blur adaptation effect exists only in fovea, therefore more arresting images are a better target for BDT measurement. According to our previous study (Lu et al., 2016), the Es and Lena images are more suitable for measuring the blur adaptation effect.

In this study, aberrations (HOAs, trefoil, coma and SAs) increased significantly, demonstrating that the visual quality in the children worsened after Ortho-K treatment. The HOAs increased from 0.21 ± 0.09 μm to 0.54 ± 0.18 μm, coma increased from 0.13 ± 0.08 μm to 0.30 ± 0.18 μm, and the SAs increased from 0.07 ± 0.07 μm to 0.35 ± 0.13 μm after one month. Our results were consistent with those from previous articles. Lian et al. (2014) found that 30 days after wearing Ortho-K lenses, HOAs increased from 0.27 ± 0.12 μm to 0.69 ± 0.21 μm, coma increased from 0.14 ± 0.10 μm to 0.36 ± 0.26 μm, and SAs increased from 0.06 ± 0.11 μm to 0.44 ± 0.20 μm. The reason for the minor difference is likely the different pupil diameters used for analysis; we used 5 mm diameters, while their study used 6 mm diameters. Analysis with a larger pupil diameter can result in larger aberrations (Wang et al., 2003); therefore, the values in this study were slightly smaller than those of the other study. Indeed, the changes observed in our study and in the study by Lian et al. are similar. Gifford et al. (2013) also reported that ocular HOAs, SAs and coma increased considerately after 7 nights of wearing Ortho-K lenses. Studies have shown that increased HOAs in Ortho-K Children can be induced by changes in the corneal surface and treatment zone decentration (Berntsen et al., 2006; Hiraoka et al., 2009a; Gifford et al., 2013).

Few studies have investigated the blur sensitivity of Ortho-K lens wearers, especially in children. Because of the high correlation between the BDTs and HOAs before Ortho-K treatment, there is reason to believe that the blur detection ability is affected by visual inputs not only from lower-order aberrations such as defocus and astigmatism but also from HOAs. However, after Ortho-K treatment, the HOAs significantly increased, while the BDTs did not increase but significantly decreased. This phenomenon seems to be an unintended variation in which BDTs changed in the opposite direction as the HOAs after Ortho-K, whereas they were positively correlated before Ortho-K. The correlation between the BDTs and HOAs did not exist any more after Ortho-K treatment because HOAs were variously affected by corneal shape, lens parameters, lens location et al. The changes of BDTs induced by HOAs were also individually different. We suggest that the variations in BDTs are due to blur adaptation, which could be induced by blur perception. Labhishetty et al. (2019) found there were no significant differences in BDTs between progressive myopic children and their non-myopic peers, which could be explained by compensation in higher visual processes for poor retinal image quality. Hence, the amount of BDT variations induced by additional blur caused by Ortho-K treatment was small, however, the difference is significant because the measurements are quite repeatable and precise. In present study, BDT_Es decreased by 0.04 D and BDT_Lena decreased by 0.05 D. The value is even higher than that with the blur adaptation effect induced with a plus lens. In our previous study, after blur adaptation with 2-diopter plus lens, BDT_Es decreased by 0.023 D and BDT_Lena decreased by 0.035 D (Lu et al., 2016)). Therefore the same targets were used in this study to evaluate the BDTs.

The markedly increased HOAs (0.21 vs. 0.54 μm) indicate deteriorated visual quality, which could lead to the subjects' blur perception. This unnatural blur may induce blur adaptation in children. The decreased BDTs could be explained as a blur adaptation effect. Several studies have indicated that after blur adaptation, blur sensitivity is significantly improved (Cufflin et al., 2007; Lu et al., 2016). The phenomenon wherein the BDT decreases after blur adaptation was also demonstrated in our previous study (Lu et al., 2016). Mon-Williams et al. indicated that "neural compensation" may be achieved in children after receiving Ortho-K (Mon-Williams et al., 1998). Therefore, the ability to discriminate blur signals in children must have been improved after wearing Ortho-K lenses for 1 month.

Another piece of evidence indicating blur adaptation was the decrease observed in the accommodative lag after Ortho-K treatment in our study. The decrease in the accommodative lag was essentially consistent with but less than the change observed in Han et al. (2018)'study as a result of a smaller AD. Blur is the main signal that drives accommodation. Previous studies have suggested that accommodation is related to blur adaptation. One such study (Vera-Diaz et al., 2004) reported

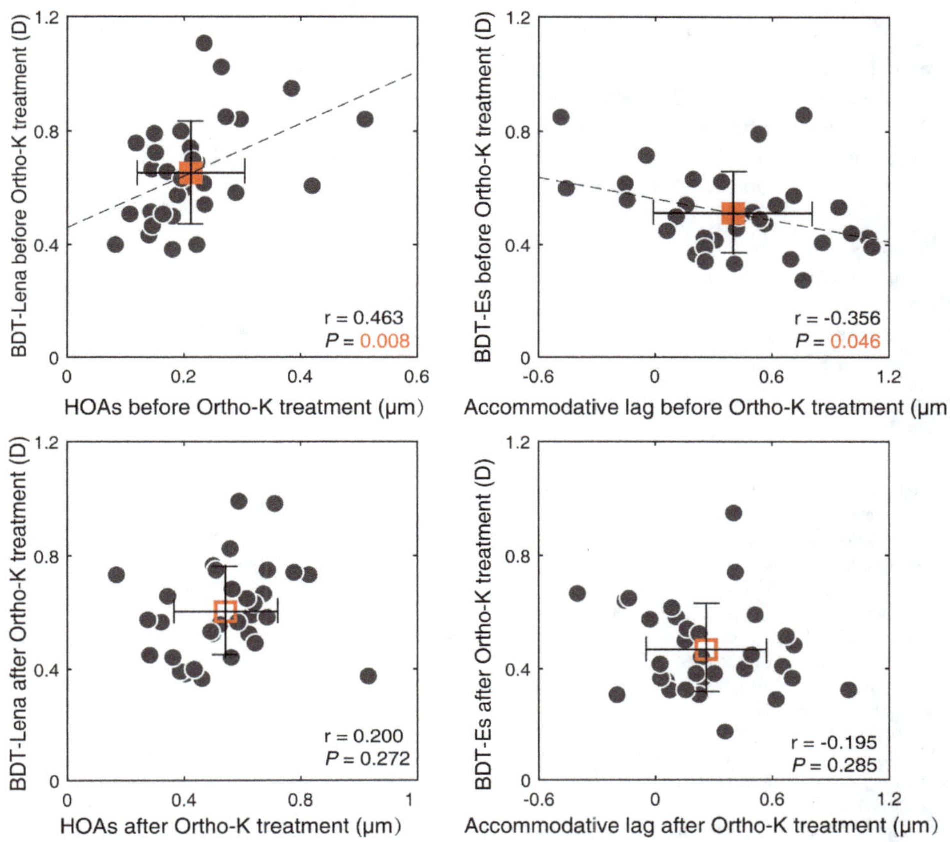

FIGURE 4 | Relationships between BDTs and aberrations and accommodative lag. Two of the BDTs are plotted as a function of aberrations or accommodative lag. Each dot represents the results from one participant. The average of these results is plotted with a square symbol. Red solid square represents pre-treatment, and the hollow one represents post-treatment. The error bars represent the standard deviation. HOAs, total higher-aberrations; BDT_Lena, the blur detection threshold for the Lena image; BDT_Es, the blur detection threshold for Tumbling Es image.

that individuals with myopia showed a significant increase in the near AR (33 cm) after a 3-minute blur adaptation exercise. Le et al. (2010) indicated that blur adaptation in both myopic and emmetropic participants would elevate instability of the AR. The increase in accommodative lag in individuals with myopia or premyopia might be due to the decrease in blur stimuli during near work (Gcss and Wickham, 1995), indicating that blur should be an effective signal for increasing the AR. We speculate that the decreased accommodative lag is induced by blur adaptation, which is caused by the deterioration in visual quality following Ortho-K in children. The presence of similar BDTs in myopic and emmetropic children but a larger accommodative lag in myopic eyes means the low sensitivity to defocus could be compensated by some form of an adjustment in the higher visual processes (i.e., blur adaptation) to preserve or increase the subjective perception (Labhishetty et al., 2019).

In another way, it was indicated (Wang et al., 2018) that the increased coma was highly related to the decentration of orthokeratology lenses. Oshika et al. (2002) found that coma-like aberration and corneal multifocality had significant positive correlations with the magnitude of apparent accommodation in pseudophakic eyes. His group (Hiraoka et al., 2015) reported later that the ocular coma-like aberration and corneal multifocality significantly increased in children undergoing orthokeratology and the change in coma-like aberration was highly associated with the change in corneal multifocality. In this study, the increased coma-like aberration and increased range of focus after orthokeratology treatment also might induce greater accommodative response, that is less accommodative lag, although no correlation was found between HOAs and accommodative lag as well as variations of them (**Supplementary Figure 6**).

Based on the close correlation between the BDTs and HOAs as well as the accommodative lag before Ortho-K treatment and the variable trend after treatment, we speculate that the significantly worsened visual quality could result in blur, leading to a blur adaptation effect and therefore a decrease in the BDTs and accommodative lags. A smaller BDT, which represents higher blur sensitivity, may promote the ability to recognize visual targets, which could explain the subjective sharpness and visual acuity of the children wearing Ortho-K lenses despite their poor visual quality, provided that a large number of lower-order aberrations were excluded. A number of studies have affirmed that blur could induce the emmetropization process and be closely related to myopic progression (Norton and Siegwart, 1995; Read et al., 2010; Chakraborty et al., 2012; Wang et al., 2016; Delshad et al., 2020). We have verified that blur adaptations do exist in children wearing Ortho-K lenses, and the role of blur adaptation in the myopia control effect of Ortho-K needs further study.

In conclusion, this study confirmed that after receiving Ortho-K lenses, aberrations increased, blur sensitivity increased, and the accommodative lag decreased. The correlation among these visual function parameters supports the notion that increased blur sensitivity is related to deteriorated visual quality caused by cornea reshaping by Ortho-K. Children with Ortho-K undergo blur adaptation, contributing to their good visual acuity in the daytime.

AUTHOR CONTRIBUTIONS

HC and JX conceived the experiments. JX and BD determined the experimental methods. CT, XM, and XL performed the experiments. CT and JX analyzed the data and interpreted the data. CT, JX, and JB wrote the manuscript. BD and HC modified the manuscript. All authors contributed to manuscript revision, read and approved the submitted version.

REFERENCES

Applegate, R. A., and Lakshminarayanan, V. (1993). Parametric representation of Stiles-Crawford functions: normal variation of peak location and directionality. *J. Opt. Soc. Am. A* 10, 1611–1623. doi: 10.1364/josaa.10.001611

Battaglia, P. W., Jacobs, R. A., and Aslin, R. N. (2004). Depth-dependent blur adaptation. *Vis. Res.* 44, 113–117. doi: 10.1016/j.visres.2003.09.010

Berntsen, D. A., Mitchell, G. L., and Barr, J. T. (2006). The effect of overnight contact lens corneal reshaping on refractive error-specific quality of life. *Optom. Vis. Sci.* 83, 354–359. doi: 10.1097/01.opx.0000221401.33776.54

Chakraborty, R., Read, S. A., and Collins, M. J. (2012). Monocular myopic defocus and daily changes in axial length and choroidal thickness of human eyes. *Exp. Eye Res.* 103, 47–54. doi: 10.1016/j.exer.2012.08.002

Chen, Z., Zhou, J., Qu, X., Zhou, X., and Xue, F. (2018). Effects of orthokeratology on axial length growth in myopic anisometropes. *Cont. Lens. Anterior. Eye* 41, 263–266. doi: 10.1016/j.clae.2017.10.014

Cufflin, M. P., Mankowska, A., and Mallen, E. A. (2007). Effect of blur adaptation on blur sensitivity and discrimination in emmetropes and myopes. *Invest. Ophthalmol. Vis. Sci.* 48, 2932–2939. doi: 10.1167/iovs.06-0836

Delshad, S., Collins, M. J., Read, S. A., and Vincent, S. J. (2020). The time course of the onset and recovery of axial length changes in response to imposed defocus. *Sci. Rep.* 10:8322. doi: 10.1038/s41598-020-65151-5

Gifford, P., Li, M., Lu, H., Miu, J., Panjaya, M., and Swarbrick, H. A. (2013). Corneal versus ocular aberrations after overnight orthokeratology. *Optom. Vis. Sci.* 90, 439–447. doi: 10.1097/OPX.0b013e31828ec594

Goss, D. A., and Wickham, M. G. (1995). Retinal-image mediated ocular growth as a mechanism for juvenile onset myopia and for emmetropization. A literature review. *Doc. Ophthalmol.* 90, 341–375. doi: 10.1007/bf0126 8122

Guo, H. C., Jin, W. Q., Pan, A. P., Wang, Q. M., Qu, J., and Yu, A. Y. (2018). Changes and diurnal variation of visual quality after orthokeratology in myopic children. *J. Ophthalmol.* 2018:3174826. doi: 10.1155/2018/3174826

Gwiazda, J. E., Thorn, F., Bauer, J., and Held, R. (1993). Myopic children show insufficient accommodative response to blur. *Invest. Ophthalmol. Vis. Sci.* 34:690. doi: 10.1097/00004397-199303320-00025

Han, X., Xu, D., Ge, W., Wang, Z., Li, X., and Liu, W. (2018). A comparison of the effects of orthokeratology lens, medcall lens, and ordinary frame glasses on the accommodative response in myopic children. *Eye Contact Lens* 44, 268–271. doi: 10.1097/icl.0000000000000390

Hiraoka, T., Kakita, T., Okamoto, F., and Oshika, T. (2015). Influence of ocular wavefront aberrations on axial length elongation in myopic children treated with overnight orthokeratology. *Ophthalmology* 122, 93–100. doi: 10.1016/j.ophtha.2014.07.042

Hiraoka, T., Mihashi, T., Okamoto, C., Okamoto, F., Hirohara, Y., and Oshika, T. (2009a). Influence of induced decentered orthokeratology lens on ocular higher-order wavefront aberrations and contrast sensitivity function. *J. Cataract. Refract. Surg.* 35, 1918–1926. doi: 10.1016/j.jcrs.2009.06.018

Hiraoka, T., Okamoto, C., Ishii, Y., Kakita, T., Okamoto, F., and Oshika, T. (2008a). Time course of changes in ocular higher-order aberrations and contrast sensitivity after overnight orthokeratology. *Invest. Ophthalmol. Vis. Sci.* 49, 4314–4320. doi: 10.1167/iovs.07-1586

Hiraoka, T., Okamoto, C., Ishii, Y., Kakita, T., Okamoto, F., Takahashi, H., et al. (2009b). Patient satisfaction and clinical outcomes after overnight orthokeratology. *Optom. Vis Sci.* 86, 875–882. doi: 10.1097/OPX.0b013e3181ae34d5

Hiraoka, T., Okamoto, C., Ishii, Y., Takahira, T., Kakita, T., and Oshika, T. (2008b). Mesopic contrast sensitivity and ocular higher-order aberrations after overnight orthokeratology. *Am. J. Ophthalmol.* 145, 645–655. doi: 10.1016/j.ajo.2007.11.021

Huang, J., Wen, D., Wang, Q., McAlinden, C., Flitcroft, I., Chen, H., et al. (2016). Efficacy comparison of 16 interventions for myopia control in children: a network meta-analysis. *Ophthalmology* 123, 697–708. doi: 10.1016/j.ophtha.2015.11.010

Jacobs, R. J., Smith, G., and Chan, C. D. (1989). Effect of defocus on blur thresholds and on thresholds of perceived change in blur: comparison of source and observer methods. *Optom. Vis. Sci.* 66, 545–553. doi: 10.1097/00006324-198908000-00010

Kang, P., and Swarbrick, H. (2011). Peripheral refraction in myopic children wearing orthokeratology and gas-permeable lenses. *Optom. Vis. Sci.* 88, 476–482. doi: 10.1097/OPX.0b013e31820f16fb

Khan, K. A., Dawson, K., Mankowska, A., Cufflin, M. P., and Mallen, E. A. (2013). The time course of blur adaptation in emmetropes and myopes. *Ophthalmic. Physiol. Opt.* 33, 305–310. doi: 10.1111/opo.12031

Khan, M. A., Gupta, A., Ahluwalia, T. S., Moulick, P. S., Gurunadh, V. S., and Gupta, S. (2016). A prospective interventional study of effect of accelerated orthokeratology on the corneal curvature and refraction among young adults with myopia. *Med. J. Armed. Forces India* 72, 125–130. doi: 10.1016/j.mjafi.2016.02.016

Labhishetty, V., Chakraborty, A., and Bobier, W. R. (2019). Is blur sensitivity altered in children with progressive myopia? *Vis. Res.* 154, 142–153. doi: 10.1016/j.visres.2018.11.002

Le, R., Bao, J., Chen, D., He, J. C., and Lu, F. (2010). The effect of blur adaptation on accommodative response and pupil size during reading. *J. Vis.* 10:1. doi: 10.1167/10.14.1

Li, J., Dong, P., and Liu, H. (2018). Effect of overnight wear orthokeratology lenses on corneal shape and tears. *Eye Contact Lens* 44, 304–307. doi: 10.1097/icl.0000000000000357

Li, S. M., Kang, M. T., Wu, S. S., Liu, L. R., Li, H., Chen, Z., et al. (2016). Efficacy, safety and acceptability of orthokeratology on slowing axial elongation in myopic children by meta-analysis. *Curr. Eye Res.* 41, 600–608. doi: 10.3109/02713683.2015.1050743

Lian, Y., Shen, M., Huang, S., Yuan, Y., Wang, Y., Zhu, D., et al. (2014). Corneal reshaping and wavefront aberrations during overnight orthokeratology. *Eye Contact Lens* 40, 161–168. doi: 10.1097/icl.0000000000000031

Lu, D., Gu, T., Lin, W., Li, N., Gong, B., and Wei, R. (2018). Efficacy of trial fitting and software fitting for orthokeratology lens: one-year follow-up study. *Eye Contact Lens* 44, 339–343. doi: 10.1097/icl.000000000000 0539

Lu, X., Xu, J. J., Drobe, B., Chen, H., and Qu, J. (2016). Influence of blur adaptation on blur detection threshold among myopic adults. *Chin. J. Optom. Ophthalmol. Vis. Sci.* 18, 170–173. doi: 10.3760/cma.j.issn.1674-845X.2016.03.009

Mon-Williams, M., Tresilian, J. R., Strang, N. C., Kochhar, P., and Wann, J. P. (1998). Improving vision: neural compensation for optical defocus. *Proc. Biol. Sci.* 265, 71–77. doi: 10.1098/rspb.1998.0266

Na, M., and Yoo, A. (2018). The effect of orthokeratology on axial length elongation in children with myopia: contralateral comparison study. *Jpn. J. Ophthalmol.* 62, 327–334. doi: 10.1007/s10384-018-0573-x

Norton, T. T., and Siegwart, J. T. Jr. (1995). Animal models of emmetropization: matching axial length to the focal plane. *J. Am. Optom. Assoc.* 66, 405–414.

Oshika, T., Mimura, T., Tanaka, S., Amano, S., Fukuyama, M., Yoshitomi, F., et al. (2002). Apparent accommodation and corneal wavefront aberration in pseudophakic eyes. *Invest. Ophthalmol. Vis. Sci.* 43, 2882–2886.

Pesudovs, K., and Brennan, N. A. (1993). Decreased uncorrected vision after a period of distance fixation with spectacle wear. *Optom. Vis. Sci.* 70, 528–531. doi: 10.1097/00006324-199307000-00002

Queirós, A., González-Méijome, J. M., Jorge, J., Villa-Collar, C., and Gutiérrez, A. R. (2010). Peripheral refraction in myopic patients after orthokeratology. *Optom. Vis. Sci.* 87, 323–329. doi: 10.1097/OPX.0b013e3181d951f7

Queirós, A., Lopes-Ferreira, D., Yeoh, B., Issacs, S., Amorim-De-Sousa, A., Villa-Collar, C., et al. (2020). Refractive, biometric and corneal topographic parameter changes during 12 months of orthokeratology. *Clin. Exp. Optom.* 103, 454–462. doi: 10.1111/cxo.12976

Queiros, A., Villa-Collar, C., Gutierrez, A. R., Jorge, J., and Gonzalez-Meijome, J. M. (2012). Quality of life of myopic subjects with different methods of visual correction using the NEI RQL-42 questionnaire. *Eye Contact Lens* 38, 116–121. doi: 10.1097/ICL.0b013e3182480e97

Read, S. A., Collins, M. J., and Sander, B. P. (2010). Human optical axial length and defocus. *Invest. Ophthalmol. Vis. Sci.* 51, 6262–6269. doi: 10.1167/iovs.10-5457

Santodomingo-Rubido, J., Villa-Collar, C., Gilmartin, B., and Gutiérrez-Ortega, R. (2013). Factors preventing myopia progression with orthokeratology correction. *Optom. Vis. Sci.* 90, 1225–1236. doi: 10.1097/opx.0000000000000034

Santodomingo-Rubido, J., Villa-Collar, C., Gilmartin, B., Gutiérrez-Ortega, R., and Sugimoto, K. (2017). Long-term efficacy of orthokeratology contact lens wear in controlling the progression of childhood myopia. *Curr. Eye Res.* 42, 713–720. doi: 10.1080/02713683.2016.1221979

Santodomingo-Rubido, J., Villa-Collar, C., Gilmartin, B., Gutierrez-Ortega, R., and Suzaki, A. (2015). The effects of entrance pupil centration and coma aberrations on myopic progression following orthokeratology. *Clin. Exp. Optom.* 98, 534–540. doi: 10.1111/cxo.12297

Santolaria, E., Cervino, A., Queiros, A., Brautaset, R., and Gonzalez-Meijome, J. M. (2013). Subjective satisfaction in long-term orthokeratology patients. *Eye Contact Lens* 39, 388–393. doi: 10.1097/ICL.0b013e3182a27777

Santolaria Sanz, E., Cerviño, A., Queiros, A., Villa-Collar, C., Lopes-Ferreira, D., and González-Méijome, J. M. (2015). Short-term changes in light distortion in orthokeratology subjects. *Biomed. Res. Int.* 2015:278425. doi: 10.1155/2015/278425

Saw, S. M., Matsumura, S., and Hoang, Q. V. (2019). Prevention and management of myopia and myopic pathology. *Invest. Ophthalmol. Vis. Sci.* 60, 488–499. doi: 10.1167/iovs.18-25221

Stillitano, I., Schor, P., Lipener, C., and Hofling-Lima, A. L. (2008). Long-term follow-up of orthokeratology corneal reshaping using wavefront aberrometry and contrast sensitivity. *Eye Contact Lens* 34, 140–145. doi: 10.1097/ICL.0b013e318145ab5d

Swarbrick, H. A. (2006). Orthokeratology review and update. *Clin. Exp. Optom.* 89, 124–143. doi: 10.1111/j.1444-0938.2006.00044.x

Tay, S. A., Farzavandi, S., and Tan, D. (2017). Interventions to reduce myopia progression in children. *Strabismus* 25, 23–32. doi: 10.1080/09273972.2016.1276940

Venkataraman, A. P., Winter, S., Unsbo, P., and Lundström, L. (2015). Blur adaptation: contrast sensitivity changes and stimulus extent. *Vis. Res.* 110(Pt A), 100–106. doi: 10.1016/j.visres.2015.03.009

Vera-Diaz, F. A., Gwiazda, J., Thorn, F., and Held, R. (2004). Increased accommodation following adaptation to image blur in myopes. *J. Vis.* 4, 1111–1119. doi: 10.1167/4.12.10

Vincent, S. J., Tan, Q., Ng, A. L. K., Cheng, G. P. M., Woo, V. C. P., and Cho, P. (2020). Higher order aberrations and axial elongation in combined 0.01% atropine with orthokeratology for myopia control. *Ophthalmic. Physiol. Opt.* 40, 728–737. doi: 10.1111/opo.12730

Wang, B., Ciuffreda, K. J., and Vasudevan, B. (2006). Effect of blur adaptation on blur sensitivity in myopes. *Vis. Res.* 46, 3634–3641. doi: 10.1016/j.visres.2006.03.015

Wang, D., Chun, R. K., Liu, M., Lee, R. P., Sun, Y., Zhang, T., et al. (2016). Optical defocus rapidly changes choroidal thickness in school children. *PLoS One* 11:e0161535. doi: 10.1371/journal.pone.0161535

Wang, J., Yang, D., Bi, H., Du, B., Lin, W., Gu, T., et al. (2018). A new method to analyze the relative corneal refractive power and its association to myopic progression control with orthokeratology. *Transl. Vis. Sci. Technol.* 7:17.

Wang, Y., Zhao, K., Jin, Y., Niu, Y., and Zuo, T. (2003). Changes of higher order aberration with various pupil sizes in the myopic eye. *J. Refract. Surg.* 19(2 Suppl.), S270–S274. doi: 10.1067/mpr.2003.47

Wen, D., Huang, J., Chen, H., Bao, F., Savini, G., Calossi, A., et al. (2015). Efficacy and acceptability of orthokeratology for slowing myopic progression in children: a systematic review and meta-analysis. *J. Ophthalmol.* 2015:360806. doi: 10.1155/2015/360806

Xia, R., Su, B., Bi, H., Tang, J., Lin, Z., Zhang, B., et al. (2019). Good visual performance despite reduced optical quality during the first month of orthokeratology lens wear. *Curr. Eye Res.* 45, 440–449. doi: 10.1080/02713683.2019.1668950

Zhao, F., Zhao, G., and Zhao, Z. (2018). Investigation of the effect of orthokeratology lenses on quality of life and behaviors of children. *Eye Contact Lens* 44, 335–338. doi: 10.1097/icl.0000000000000529

11

Feature Counting is Impaired when Shifting Attention between the Eyes in Adults with Amblyopia

Chuan Hou and Gabriela Acevedo Munares*

Smith-Kettlewell Eye Research Institute, San Francisco, CA, United States

Correspondence:
Chuan Hou
chuanhou@ski.org

Background: Feature counting requires rapid shifts of attention in the visual field and reflects higher-level cortical functions. This process is drastically impaired in the amblyopic eye of strabismic amblyopes. In this study, we hypothesized that feature counting performance in anisometropic and strabismic amblyopes is further impaired when shifts in attention is required between the eyes.

Materials and Methods: Through a mirror stereoscope, highly visible Gabor patches were presented to the same eye within a block or randomly presented to the left eye or to the right eye with an equal probability within a block. The task was to report the number of Gabors (3 to 9) as accurately as possible. Counting performance was compared between the amblyopes and the normal-vision observers and between the viewing conditions (shifting attention between the eyes versus maintaining attention in the same eye).

Results: When attention was maintained in the same eye, the amblyopic eye of both anisometropic and strabismic groups undercounted the number of Gabors, but achieved near-perfect performance with their fellow eye, compared to normal-vision observers. In contrast, when shifting attention randomly to the left or to the right eye, the amblyopic eye further undercounted the number of Gabors. Undercounting was also found in the fellow eye of strabismic amblyopes, but was not in the fellow eye of anisometropic amblyopes. Performance in normal-vision observers did not differ between shifting attention between the eyes and maintaining attention in the same eye.

Conclusion: Our data showed that the amblyopic eye of both anisometropic and strabismic amblyopes further undercounted features when shifting attention between the eyes, compared to when maintaining attention in the same eye. This suggests that the ability to quickly redirect attention, particularly under interocular suppression, is impaired in amblyopia. The fellow eye of strabismic amblyopes also undercounted features when shifting attention between the eyes. However, such fellow eye abnormality was not found in anisometropic amblyopes, suggesting that different patterns of visual deficits are associated with amblyopia of different etiologies. The inability to count multiple features accurately reflects dysfunctions of high-level cortices in the amblyopic brain.

Keywords: amblyopia, strabismus, selective attention, feature counting, interocular suppression

INTRODUCTION

Amblyopia, the leading cause of monocular vision loss worldwide, is a neurodevelopmental disorder of vision, affecting about 3% of the population (Holmes and Clarke, 2006). Amblyopia is commonly caused by misaligned eyes (strabismus), chronic optical blur due to unequal refractive error in the two eyes (anisometropia), or a mixture of both during early childhood. In addition to visual acuity loss in one eye and reduced stereopsis, individuals with amblyopia also exhibit diverse deficits, including deficits in illusory contour perception (Popple and Levi, 2000; Hou et al., 2014), contour integration (Hess et al., 1997; Kovacs et al., 2000; Chandna et al., 2001; Kozma and Kiorpes, 2003), global motion sensitivity (Simmers et al., 2003; Ho and Giaschi, 2006, 2007, 2009; Hou et al., 2008), object enumeration (Sharma et al., 2000; Li R. W. et al., 2011), attentional blink (Popple and Levi, 2008), object tracking (Ho et al., 2006; Tripathy and Levi, 2008), and decision making (Farzin and Norcia, 2011).

The diverse perceptual deficits in amblyopia described above are commonly reported in studies using tasks requiring high-level cortical functions. Therefore, such deficits are commonly considered as evidence of high-level cortical dysfunction in the amblyopic brain. For instance, Sharma et al. (2000) reported that the amblyopic eye of strabismic amblyopes is unable to count features accurately as the eyes of normal-vision observers, but the non-amblyopic fellow eye achieves near-perfect counting performance as the normal-vision eye (Li J. et al., 2011). The authors argue that the inability to count features accurately is due to high-level cortical dysfunction, but not due to the well-established limitations of low-level processing in the amblyopic visual system (Levi and Klein, 1985, 1986; Smith et al., 1997; Kiorpes et al., 1998). This is because their experiments ruled out low-level processing factors such as feature visibility, crowding, positional jitter, and abnormal temporal integration. Studies have also reported that feature counting requires rapid shifts of attention in the visual field (Egeth et al., 2008; Anobile et al., 2012). When the number of features to be enumerated is small ($N < 5$) and briefly presented, rapid, error-free performance is achieved through a process known as subitizing, which is thought to be "pre-attentive." In contrast, when the number of features to be enumerated is larger than 4, performance is slow and subject to error (Balakrishnan and Ashby, 1992; Pylyshyn, 1994; Trick and Pylyshyn, 1994), as well as dependent on the higher visual pathways, in particular the parietal cortex (Sathian et al., 1999; Nieder et al., 2006; Nieder and Dehaene, 2009), a region known to be involved in visual attention (Bressler et al., 2008). Therefore, Sharma et al. (2000) suggests that the finding of inability to count multiple features are likely due to attention deficits from the visual input of the amblyopic eye. Indeed, a number of studies have also reported attention deficits in amblyopia, including attentional blink (Popple and Levi, 2008), object tracking (Ho et al., 2006; Tripathy and Levi, 2008; Ho and Giaschi, 2009; Secen et al., 2011; Chow et al., 2018), conjunctive visual search (Tsirlin et al., 2018), line bisection task (Thiel and Sireteanu, 2009) and feature counting under dichoptic viewing (Wong-Kee-You et al., 2020).

Behaviorally measured attention deficits in amblyopia are consistent with our previous EEG-source imaging study (Hou et al., 2016), in which we found that attentional modulation in visual cortex, including V1 and extra-striate cortex (hV4 and hMT+), from the amblyopic eye was degraded in adults with strabismic amblyopia. This degraded attentional modulation in V1 was also correlated with the magnitude of interocular suppression and the depth of amblyopia, suggesting that interocular suppression may play a role of attention deficits in amblyopia. Supporting this, in a previous study (Wong-Kee-You et al., 2020), we found that feature counting under dichoptic viewing was impaired in the amblyopic eye of people with amblyopia with greater impairment in strabismic amblyopes than in anisometropic amblyopes. Chow et al. (2018) reported that attention was biased to the non-amblyopic fellow eye of amblyopia with dichoptic multiple-object tracking tasks. This bias was only found in strabismic amblyopes, but not in anisometropic amblyopes. These studies imply that in the natural visual environment, which is binocular and elicits interocular suppression, more severe deficits in feature counting in amblyopia may be revealed, compared to that under monocular viewing (Sharma et al., 2000). This speculation is based on previous studies that interocular suppression is stronger in strabismic amblyopes than in anisometropic amblyopes (Holopigian et al., 1988; Harrad and Hess, 1992; Agrawal et al., 2006; Narasimhan et al., 2012), although not all studies have found this (Li R. W. et al., 2011).

In the current study, we hypothesized that feature counting performance is further affected under binocular viewing when shifting attention between the eyes in strabismic amblyopia, as compared to the performance under monocular viewing reported in the Sharma et al. (2000) study. To test our hypothesis, we used a variant of the Sharma et al. (2000) paradigm that was modified for our binocular approach. We replicated the experiment in the Sharma et al. (2000) study and compared the counting performance between monocular viewing condition when maintaining attention in the same eye and binocular viewing condition when shifting attention between the eyes. We expected to reveal further deficits in feature counting under binocular viewing condition in strabismic amblyopia, given the experimental environment of interocular suppression from our stimulus setting. In addition to include participants with strabismic amblyopia, we also included participants with anisometropic amblyopia in the current study. Given the different findings between anisometropic and strabismic amblyopia from previous studies (Levi and Klein, 1982a,b; Thiel and Sireteanu, 2009; Hou et al., 2014; Chow et al., 2018; Wong-Kee-You et al., 2020), we expected to reveal different patterns of feature counting deficits between these subgroups as well.

MATERIALS AND METHODS

Participants

A total of 21 adults between 21 and 65 years old (mean ± SD, 43 ± 14) of both sexes (8 males) were recruited for this study from the San Francisco Bay Area via research advertisement.

Among them, 13 participants had unilateral amblyopia with visual acuity (VA) equal or worse than 20/25 (0.1 logMAR) in the amblyopic eye, and VA equal or better than 20/20 (0 logMAR) in the fellow eye, measured with Bailey-Lovie LogMAR chart. Normal vision participants (also referred to as "Normal"; $n = 8$) had 20/20 or better VA in each eye. There was no significant difference ($p = 0.89$) in age between normal (mean ± SD, 43 ± 16) and amblyopic participants (mean ± SD, 44 ± 13). All participants were refracted under noncycloplegic conditions by one of the authors (CH), a pediatric ophthalmologist, before the experiments. Participants with amblyopia were classified into two subgroups. Anisometropic amblyopia (referred to as "Aniso"; $n = 6$) was defined as unequal refractive error between the two eyes of at least 1 diopter in any meridian and with no constant ocular deviation or history of strabismus surgery. Strabismic amblyopia (referred to as "Strab"; $n = 7$) was defined as a constant ocular deviation or a history of prior strabismus surgery with or without anisometropia. All strabismic participants were non-alternating strabismus. There was no significant difference ($p = 0.20$) in logMAR VA in the amblyopic eye between the anisometropic (mean ± SD, 0.48 ± 0.16) and the strabismic (mean ± SD, 0.61 ± 0.18) groups. Stereoacuity was measured with the Random-dot stereo butterfly (Stereo Optical CO., INC). Normals had stereoacuity of at least 40 arcsec. The dominant and non-dominant eye in Normals was determined using the hole-in-card test. The demographic information of the amblyopic participants is provided in **Table 1**. Anisometropic participants had measurable stereoacuity while most strabismic participants had non-measurable stereoacuity, as seen in **Table 1**. Participants who had congenital cataract, eccentric fixation (measured by a direct ophthalmoscope) and nystagmus or latent nystagmus (nystagmus that appears when covering one eye) were excluded from the study. The research protocol conformed to the tenets of the Declaration of Helsinki and was approved by the Institutional Review Board of The Smith-Kettlewell Eye Research Institute. Written informed consent was obtained before the start of the experiments.

Stimuli and Experimental Design

We modified the Sharma et al. (2000) paradigm that was originally used for a monocular test for our binocular approach. The reason we used a variant of Sharma et al. (2000) paradigm was because this paradigm used highly visible Gabor patches and have ruled out low-level cortical feature deficits in amblyopia, such as feature visibility, crowding, positional jitter, abnormal temporal integration, and spatial scale shifts (Levi et al., 1994). We modified the Sharma et al. (2000) paradigm, in which we used the same display of Gabor patches that could be used for both monocular test (Experiment 1) and binocular test (Experiment 2).

Experiment 1

In this experiment, we repeated the experiment 1 in the Sharma et al. (2000) study. The stimuli (Gabor patches) were tested under monocular viewing condition with attention maintained in the same eye within a block of trials, while the untested eye remained open and viewed blank gray screen. There were 6 normal-vision observers, 5 anisometropic and 5 strabismic amblyopes participated this experiment.

In the attended eye, a random array of Gabor patches was presented for 200 ms in the central visual field (5.6° square frame) surrounded by noise in the periphery (21° x 18° in the visual field), followed by a 200 ms noise mask. A 100% valid spatial cue (5.6° black square) displayed for 500 ms preceded the stimuli to the tested eye. This spatial cue was critical in Experiment 2 to guide attention to the tested eye when the stimuli were randomly presented to the left or to the right eye. Thus, the cue in Experiment 1 was to keep the same stimulus parameters as in Experiment 2. The stimuli and the temporal sequence of a given trial are illustrated in **Figure 1**. Participants

TABLE 1 | Clinical details of the participants with amblyopia.

				Visual acuity (logMAR)					
Participant number	**Diagnosis**	**Age**	**Gender**	**Fellow eye**	**Amblyopic eye**	**Stereoacuity**	**Deviation**	**History**	**Experiment**
1	A	22	M	−0.097	0.341	200′	Ortho	Patching Done	1
2	A	52	F	0.04	0.518	200″	Ortho	Patching Done	1 and 2
3	A	51	F	0	0.739	200″	Ortho	Patching done	1 and 2
4	A	49	F	0	0.301	70″	Ortho	Patching done	1 and 2
5	A	50	F	−0.2	0.498	800′	Ortho	Patching done	1 and 2
6	A	21	M	0	0.498	140″	Ortho	No patching	1 and 2
7	S and A	59	M	−0.04	0.836	n/a	XT 14, L/R 14, DVD	Surgery and patching	1 and 2
8	S	38	M	−0.097	0.341	n/a	XT 12, R/L 4	Patching done	1
9	S and A	34	F	0	0.518	n/a	XT 8	Surgery and patching	1 and 2
10	S and A	62	M	0	0.756	n/a	XT 4, R/L 20, DVD	Patching done	1 and 2
11	S and A	65	F	−0.02	0.518	2000″	XT 8	Surgery and patching	1 and 2
12	S and A	36	F	−0.097	0.538	n/a	ET 4	Surgery and patching	1
13	S and A	46	F	0	0.756	n/a	ET 14	Patching done	1 and 2

A, anisometropic amblyopia; S, strabismic amblyopia; S and A, mixed strabismus and anisometropia. Deviation at near with correction is shown in prism diopters. DVD, disassociated vertical deviation; XT, exotropia. ET, esotropia; L/R, left-eye hypertropia; R/L, right-eye hypertropia. "n/a" indicates that stereoacuity was not measurable with Random-dot stereo butterfly (Stereo Optical CO., INC).

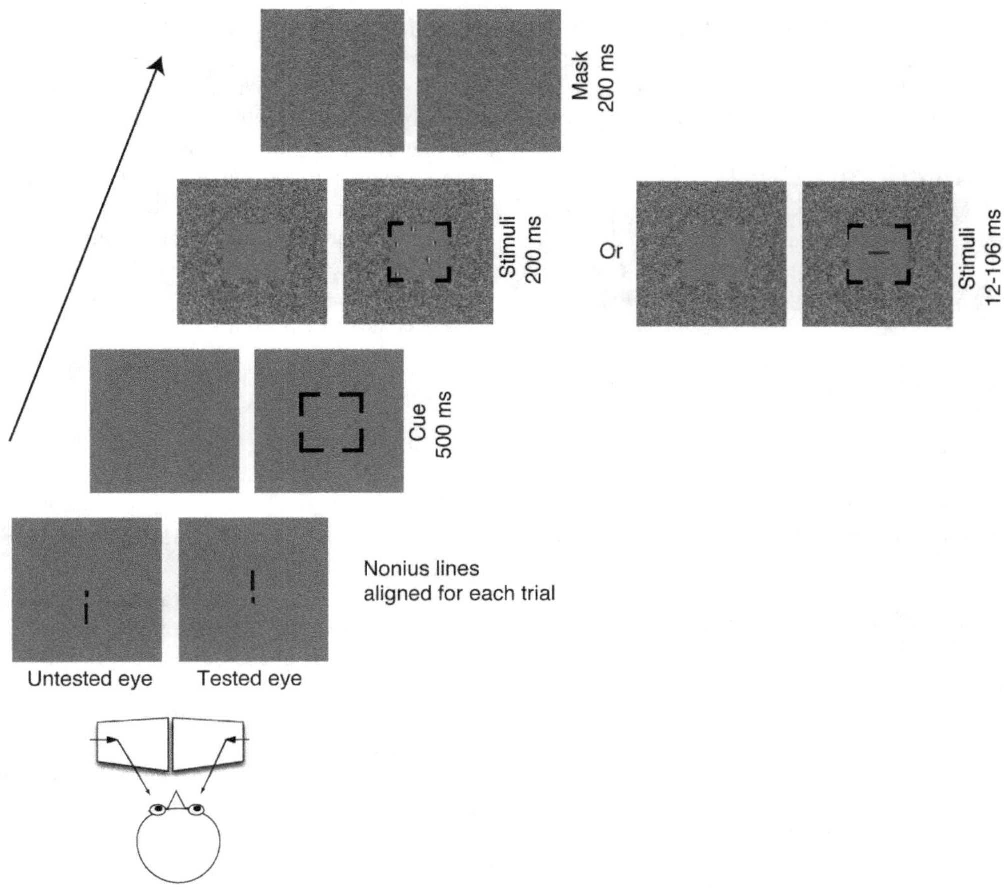

FIGURE 1 | Illustration of the stimuli and the temporal sequence of a given trial viewing through a mirror stereoscope. In Experiment 1, the targets (Gabors) were presented to the same eye within a block. In Experiment 2, the targets (Gabors) were randomly presented to the left eye or to the right eye within a block. The task for Experiments 1, 2 was to count the number of Gabors. In Experiment 3, the target (a rectangle in horizontal or vertical orientation) was randomly presented to the left eye or to the right eye within a block with a wide range of display durations between 12 and 106 ms. The task for Experiment 3 was to report the orientation of the rectangle.

were required to report the total number of Gabors (3-9) by pressing a button on the keyboard. In order to shorten the duration of the experiment, we skipped 4 Gabor patches in all experiments (including Experiments 1, 2). The spatial frequency of the presented Gabors was low (2 c/deg), as done in the Sharma et al. (2000) study, to compromise the poor visual acuity in the amblyopic eye of amblyopes. The contrast of Gabors was ≥ 25% for both eyes, but the contrast for the amblyopic eye was adjusted (matched) for equal visibility between the eyes (see below for details).

Experiment 2

In this experiment, the stimuli (Gabor patches) were tested under a "binocular" viewing condition requiring attentional shifts between the eyes within a block. The targets were always viewed by the tested eye, while the blank screen was viewed by the untested eye. Here we used the term "binocular" as a comparison to the monocular test from a previous study (Sharma et al., 2000). Eight normal observers, 6 anisometropic and 7 strabismic amblyopes participated in this experiment. Among the participants in Experiments 2, 6 normal observers, 5 anisometropic and 5 strabismic amblyopes also participated in Experiment 1, which are marked in **Table 1**.

A random array of highly visible Gabor patches was randomly presented to the left eye or to the right eye with an equal probability within a block. A 100% valid spatial cue (5.6° black square) was displayed for 500 ms preceded the stimuli to guide participants' attention to their tested eye. The task and stimulus parameters were the same as in Experiment 1.

Experiment 3

In this experiment, the stimulus sequence and spatial cue were presented in the same manner as in Experiment 2, but the target was a single rectangle, instead of Gabor patches. Two normal observers, 2 anisometropic and 3 strabismic amblyopes, who also participated in Experiment 2, participated in this experiment.

Using a psychophysical procedure of constant stimuli, a single stimulus (a horizontal or a vertical rectangle ranging in size from

0.23° x 0.94° to 1.64° x 5.16°) was randomly presented to one of two eyes at 35% contrast for 12, 35, 60, 82 and 106 ms. The size of the rectangle was adjusted so that its orientation was correctly identified for more than 75% of the trials where the rectangle was presented for 60 ms monocularly to the amblyopic eye.

Display and Procedure

Two Sony Trinitron Multiscan G400 CRT monitors, each with a frame rate of 85 Hz, were used to present the stimuli at a viewing distance of 85 cm. The stimuli were programmed in MATLAB (Mathworks, Natick, MA) with the Psychophysics Toolbox.

All participants were tested under their best-corrected vision. A practice block for each experiment was conducted to make sure the participant understood the task. Before the start of the trial, participants were required to adjust the mirror stereoscope to align nonius lines presented at the center of each screen. Participants repeated three blocks of trials and each block included 90 to 120 trials. The trials were self-initiated and the participants were required to respond as accurately as possible with no time limit and no feedback given.

Contrast Match in the Two Eyes

All amblyopic participants adjusted the contrast in the two eyes for equal perceptual visibilities before the experiments. Through a mirror stereoscope, two horizontal sinusoidal gratings (3 c/deg, 2.5°) were separately presented with one in the upper visual field of the left eye and another in the lower visual field of the right eye. The participants were unaware of which eye saw which grating. The contrast in the fellow eye was fixed at 25%, while the contrast in the amblyopic eye was adjusted to match the perceptual visibility of the fellow eye. This procedure was repeated 3 times, and the average of all 3 contrast adjustments was defined as the balanced contrast for the amblyopic eye in Experiments 1, 2.

Modeling

A Weibull cumulative distribution function with additional scaling coefficient and constant offset (equation 1) was used to fit the data as shown in **Figures 2, 3**. Fitting of these functions was done in KaleidaGraph to extract the scale (η) and shape (β) parameters.

$$y = \left\{1 - \exp\left[\left(\frac{-x}{\eta}\right)^{\beta}\right]\right\} \Delta_N + N_0 \qquad (1)$$

where η is a semi-saturation constant, β represents the slope of Weibull function, Δ_N is the amplitude scaling, and N_0 is the constant offset. The coefficient of determination (R^2) was used to assess goodness of fit of the model.

Statistical Analysis

The primary analyses were conducted using a mixture of between- and within-subjects design ANOVA (**Figures 2, 3**) and a within-subjects design ANOVA (**Figure 4**). ANOVA was conducted in R. The Bonferroni correction was used to control the familywise error rate for repeated-measures ANOVA in each eye of the participants, in which the significance level was at 0.05/2 = 0.025. Significant differences in age between amblyopes and controls and visual acuity (logMAR) in the amblyopic eye between anisometropic and strabismic amblyopes were identified with the two-tailed heteroscedastic t tests. The significance of Weibull fit parameters between groups (**Figures 2B, 3B**) and significant differences in the contrast balance between anisometropic and strabismic amblyopes (**Figure 5A**) were identified with the one-tailed, Mann-Whitney Test for two independent sample. Correlation coefficient and its significance were calculated with Spearman's rho with two-tails (**Figure 5**). Mann-Whitney Test and Spearman's rho were conducted using the Real Statistics Resource Pack software (Copyright: 2013 – 2020, Charles Zaiontz)[1].

RESULTS

Experiment 1

Visual Features Were Presented to the Same Eye Within a Block

In this experiment, our goal was to replicate the experiment 1 in the Sharma et al. (2000) study where Gabor patches were presented only to one eye within a block. For simplicity, we refer to the amblyopic eye as "AE," the fellow eye as "FE," the dominant eye of Normals as "dom" and the non-dominant eye of Normals as "nondom" in the figures. Our data showed that the amblyopic eye of both the anisometropic and the strabismic group underestimated the number of Gabors, which reproduced the findings in the Sharma et al. (2000) study for strabismic amblyopes.

Figure 2 plots the counting performances for 3 groups (normal, anisometropic and strabismic groups). As seen in **Figures 2A,C** (left panels), all 3 groups, when using their dominant/fellow eye, were accurately able to estimate the number of Gabors until a set-size of 7, with errors emerging at set-sizes of 8 and 9 Gabors. In contrast, when using their amblyopic eye, the anisometropic and strabismic groups were only able to accurately estimate the number of Gabors until a set-size of 5, whereas accurate estimation was maintained in the normal group at a set-size of 7 when using their non-dominant eye. Since the enumeration of the small and the large set-sizes of Gabors depends on different neural mechanisms, we separated the participants' performances into two Gabor groups. The Small Gabor Size group included trials with Gabor set-sizes of 3, 5 and 6, and the Large Gabor Size group included set-sizes of 7, 8 and 9. We expected to reveal counting deficits in amblyopia with the Large Gabor Size group, because their enumeration engages more attentional efforts than the Small Gabor Size group. An initial 4-factorial ANOVA (Group, Eye, Gabor Size Group and Gabor Set-size) revealed significant interactions among Group, Eye and Gabor Size Group ($F_{(2,12)} = 4.83$, $p = 0.029$). We therefore conducted sequential 1-factorial ANOVAs between groups for Large Gabor Size Group and Small Gabor Size Group to compare the performance of the amblyopic groups and the normal-vision group in each eye under higher levels of attention and lower

[1] www.real-statistics.com

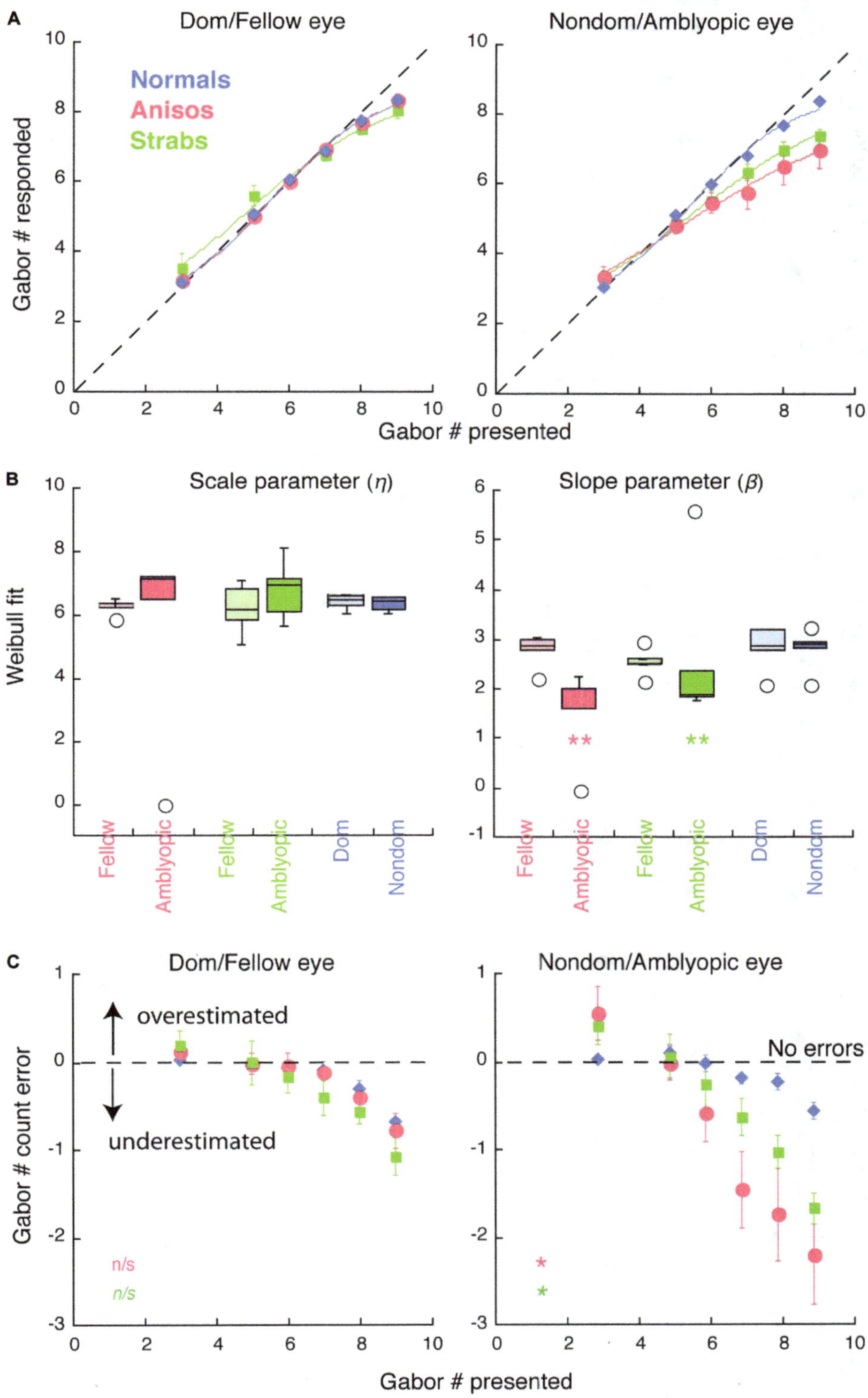

FIGURE 2 | Counting performance in anisometropic and strabismic amblyopes and normal-vision observers when visual features were presented to the same eye within a block in Experiment 1. **(A)** Group mean of counting performance, in which the subjective estimates of the number are plotted as a function of the number of Gabor patches present. Colors denote the group. Error bars denote SEM. The dashed lines indicate 1:1 ratio between reported and displayed number of Gabors, representing correct estimates. Data below the dashed line indicate underestimates of the number of Gabors. Solid curves are the average model fits of Weibull function. **(B)** Comparison of the model fit results from individual participants with scale (η) and slope (β) parameters. **(C)** Group mean of counting errors from **(A)**. *, and ** denotes $p < 0.025$ (significance level by Bonferroni correction) and $p < 0.01$, respectively.

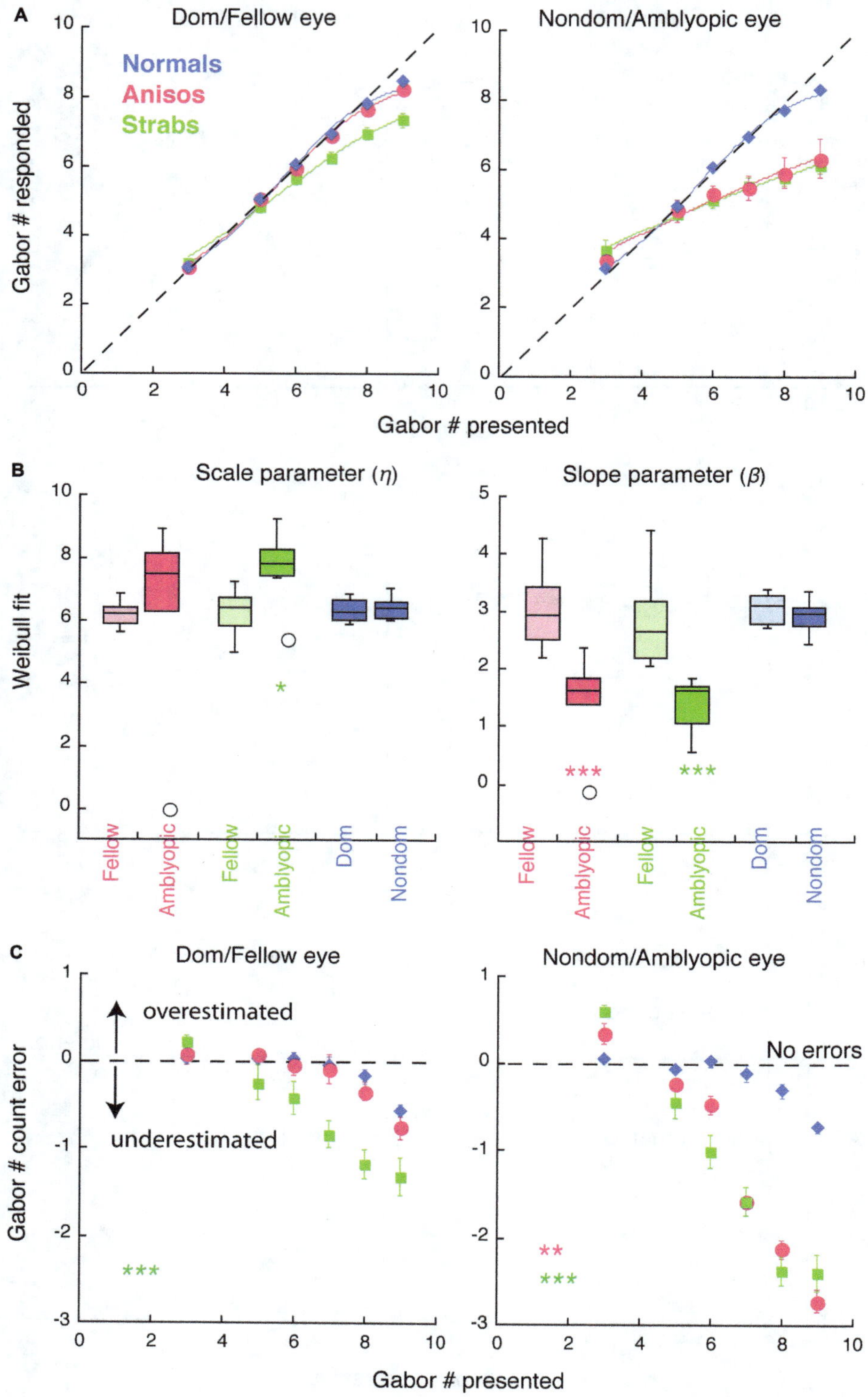

FIGURE 3 | Counting performance in anisometropic and strabismic amblyopes and normal-vision observers when visual features were randomly presented to the left or to the right eye within a block in Experiment 2. **(A)** Group mean of counting performance. Colors denote the group. Error bars denote SEM. The dashed lines indicate 1:1 ratio between reported and displayed number of Gabors, representing correct estimates. Data below the dashed line indicate underestimates of the number of Gabors. Solid curves are the model fits of Weibull function. **(B)** Comparison of model fit results from individual participants with scale (η) and slope (β) parameters. **(C)** Group mean of counting errors from **(A)**. *, **, and *** denote $p < 0.025$ (significance level by Bonferroni correction), $p < 0.01$ and $p < 0.001$, respectively.

levels of attention, respectively. For the Large Gabor Size trials, the results of the ANOVA revealed a significant difference only in the amblyopic eye of anisometropic amblyopes ($F_{(1,9)} = 10.23$, $p = 0.011$) and strabismic amblyopes ($F_{(1,9)} = 10.23$, $p = 0.014$), which underestimated the number of Gabors and made more errors (**Figure 2C**) as compared to the non-dominant eye of normal group. For the Small Gabor Size group trials, the results of the ANOVA revealed no significant difference between the eyes of amblyopes and the eyes of normal-vision observers ($p > 0.05$).

Furthermore, we quantified the counting performance by fitting the data with a variant of the Weibull cumulative distribution-function (see details in Methods). The model fits of the group mean for each eye and each group are shown with the solid curves in **Figure 2A**. The distribution of the data fits of individual participants are shown in **Figure 2B**. The goodness of fit (R^2) across all participants and both eyes was 0.9956 ± 0.0C77 (mean ± SD). In the left panel of **Figure 2B**, the scale parameter eta (η), which represents a semi-saturation constant, did not reveal significant difference between the eyes of both the amblyopic subgroups and the Normal group. However, the slope parameter beta (β) revealed a shallower slope in the AE of the anisometropic group ($p = 0.0019$) and the strabismic group ($p = 0.0012$) compared to the non-dominant eye of the normal group, indicating that performance in the amblyopic groups was impaired when using the amblyopic eye, specifically. Both amblyopic groups underestimated the number of visual features, as shown in **Figure 2C**. Notably, the fellow eye of the strabismic group achieved nearly perfect performance, as compared to the dominant eye of normal group ($F_{(1,9)} = 5.08$, $p = 0.051$). The results of the strabismic group are consistent with the findings in the Sharma et al. (2000) study. The amblyopic eye performance of the anisometropic group were similar to that of the strabismic group (FE: $F_{(1,8)} = 2.57$, $p = 0.148$; AE: $F_{(1,8)} = 2.45$, $p = 0.156$), which is the first report that the amblyopic eye of anisometropic amblyopes also undercounts visual features. These data analyses revealed that the amblyopic eye of both anisometropic and strabismic amblyopes underestimated features.

Experiment 2

Visual Features Were Randomly Presented to the Left or to the Right Eye Within a Block

In this experiment, we expected to reveal further deficits in feature counting when shifting attention between the eyes in strabismic amblyopia, as compared to the deficits when visual features were only presented to one eye within a block in Experiment 1. We particularly anticipated that these further deficits would be observed in our strabismic amblyopia group, given that the stimulus design of the current experiment was binocular, which induces greater levels of interocular suppression.

Both Eyes of Strabismic Amblyopes Undercounted Features When Shifting Attention Between the Eyes

Figure 3 plots the counting performance of the 3 groups. As seen in **Figures 3A,C** (green symbols), the strabismic group, when using their fellow (left panels) and amblyopic (right panels) eye, performed worse in comparison to normal-vision observers and started to make errors at the set-size of 5 Gabors. In contrast, when visual features were only presented to one eye within a block in Experiment 1, only the amblyopic eye of the strabismic group performed worse, with impairments starting at the set-size of 6 Gabors (**Figures 2A,C**). An initial 4-factorial ANOVA (Group, Eye, Gabor Size Group and Gabor Set-Size) revealed significant interactions among Group, Eye and Gabor Size Group ($F_{(10,17)} = 9.03$, $p = 0.002$). Thus, we further conducted sequential 1-factorial ANOVAs between groups for the Large Gabor Size trials and the Small Gabor Size trials, to compare performance between the amblyopic groups and the normal-vision group, across each eye. For the Large Gabor Size trials, the results of the ANOVA revealed significant differences in the amblyopic eye of both anisometropic ($F_{(1,12)} = 20.43$, $p = 0.001$) and strabismic ($F_{(1,13)} = 72.19$, $p < 0.001$) amblyopes, in which the amblyopic eye underestimated the number of Gabors and made more errors (**Figure 3C**) compared to the non-dominant eye of normal observers. Surprisingly, the fellow eye of strabismic amblyopes also underestimated number of Gabors compared to the dominant eye of normal observers ($F_{(1,13)} = 28.31$, $p < 0.001$, **Figure 3C** left panel), while no significant difference between the fellow eye of anisometropic amblyopes and the dominant eye of normal-vision observers ($F_{(1,12)} = 1.12$, $p = 0.311$) was found. For the Small Gabor Size group trials, the results of the ANOVA revealed no significant difference between the eyes of amblyopes and the eyes of normal-vision observers ($p > 0.05$).

As done in the Experiment 1, we also quantified the participants' performance by fitting their data with a Weibull function (**Figures 3A,B**). The goodness of fit (R^2) across all participants and two eyes was 0.9787 ± 0.0834 (mean ± SD). The slope parameter beta (β) revealed shallower slope for the amblyopic eye of the anisometropic group ($p < 0.001$) and the strabismic group ($p < 0.001$), compared to the non-dominant eye of normal group. Impaired performance in the amblyopic eye of both amblyopic groups, were primarily due to underestimations of the visual features, as shown in **Figure 3C**. The scale parameter eta (η) revealed a significant difference between the amblyopic eye of the strabismic group and the non-dominant eye of normal group ($p = 0.0103$).

Comparison of Feature Counting Between Monocular and Binocular Viewing Condition

We wanted to look at the performance across monocular and binocular viewing. Since 10 amblyopes participated in both Experiments 1, 2, we were able to compare counting performance between monocular and binocular viewing conditions within subjects.

Figure 4 plots the comparison of counting errors in group mean between monocular and binocular viewing condition in each eye of the normal, anisometropic and strabismic groups. As seen in **Figure 4B** and C (red and green symbols), both the amblyopic eye of the anisometropic and the strabismic groups undercounted the number of Gabors under binocular viewing (filled symbols) starting at the set-size of 5 Gabors, while under monocular viewing (open symbols), both groups undercounted from the set-size of 6 Gabors. This difference in

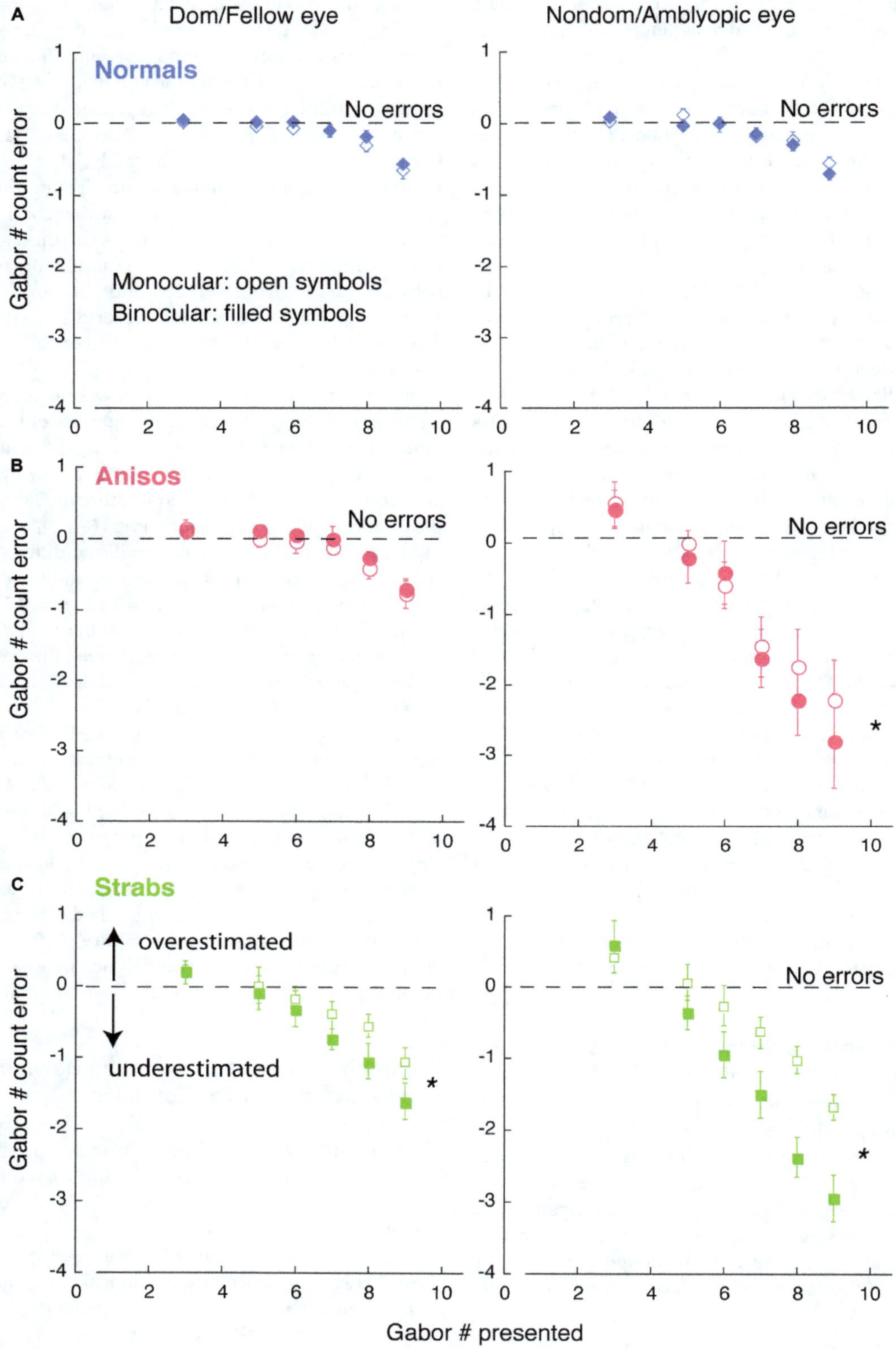

FIGURE 4 | Comparison of counting errors between monocular and binocular viewing in each eye of **(A)** Normals, **(B)** Anisos, and **(C)** Strabs. Left column: Dom/Fellow eye; Right column: Nondom/Amblyopic eye. Open symbols: monocular viewing; Filled symbols: binocular viewing. The horizontal dashed lines indicate no counting errors. Data below the dashed lines indicate underestimates of the number of Gabors; and data above the dashed lines indicate overestimates of the number of Gabors. * denotes $p < 0.025$ (Bonferroni correction).

impairment across binocular and monocular viewing, suggests that feature counting is further affected when attentional shifts between the eyes is required, such as under conditions of interocular suppression. In addition, the fellow eye of the strabismic group also undercounted the number of Gabors, from a set-size of 6 Gabors under binocular viewing and a set-size of 7 Gabors under monocular viewing. These findings in the strabismic group suggest that with the natural viewing that is binocular, strabismic amblyopes encounters attention deficits, either with the amblyopic eye viewing or the fellow eye viewing. By contrast, the fellow eye of the anisometropic group estimated the number of Gabors similarly to the normal group. Moreover, the amblyopic eye of both the anisometropic and strabismic groups always overestimated when the number of Gabors to be enumerated was small (Gabor set-size = 3), as was reported in strabismic amblyopes in Sharma et al. (2000) study.

The observations described above were also confirmed with statistical analysis. An initial 5-factorial ANOVA (Group, Eye, Viewing condition, Gabor Size and Gabor Set-Size) revealed significant interactions among Eye, Viewing condition and Gabor Size ($F_{(1,13)} = 4.78$, $p = 0.048$). We further conducted 1-factorial ANOVAs for Viewing Condition with the Large Gabor Size group trials and Small Gabor Size group trials, to compare the performances between viewing conditions in each eye of the amblyopic groups. For the Large Gabor Size trials, the results of the ANOVA revealed a significant difference between the monocular and binocular viewing conditions in the amblyopic eye of both anisometropic amblyopes ($F_{(1,4)} = 52.10$, $p = 0.002$) and strabismic amblyopes ($F_{(1,4)} = 17.72$, $p = 0.014$), as seen in **Figures 4B,C**. These findings indicate that under binocular viewing condition, anisometropic and strabismic amblyopes exhibit greater impairments and underestimate visual features to a greater extent, compared to monocular viewing conditions. The ANOVA also revealed a significant difference between the monocular and binocular viewing conditions in the fellow eye of strabismic amblyopes ($F_{(1,4)} = 21.12$, $p = 0.010$), but no significant difference in the fellow eye of anisometropic amblyopes ($F_{(1,4)} = 0.29$, $p = 0.620$) was found. Both eyes of normal group had no significant difference between viewing conditions ($p > 0.05$). For the Small Gabor Size group trials, the results of the ANOVA revealed no significant difference between viewing conditions in each eye of the 3 groups ($p > 0.05$).

Correlation Between Feature Counting Performance and Interocular Suppression

We have showed that the amblyopic eye of both anisometropic and strabismic amblyopes further undercounted the number of Gabors when shifting attention between the eyes, as compared to when maintaining attention in the same eye, suggesting that redirecting attention between the eyes is impaired in amblyopia under experimental environment of interocular suppression. Previous studies used contrast difference between the two eyes (i.e., contrast balance) to represent interocular suppression (Li et al., 2013; Cοi et al., 2013). Since we matched contrast in the amblyopic eye to obtain an equal perceptual visibility to the fellow eye in both Exp 1 and 2, we used contrast balance to index the magnitude of interocular suppression for our amblyopic participants. **Figure 5A** depicts the comparison of the degree of interocular suppression between anisometropic and strabismic groups. Stronger interocular suppression was found in the strabismic amblyopes compared to the anisometropic amblyopes (p = 0.011). To determine whether there is relationship between counting performance and interocular suppression, in **Figure 5B** we plotted the participants' feature counting errors from both Experiments 1, 2 at the set-size of 9 Gabors when using the amblyopic eye as a function of contrast balance. As seen in **Figure 5B**, there was no correlation between counting performance and interocular suppression in both Experiment 1 ($rho = 0.36$, $p = 0.31$) and 2 ($rho = -0.16$, $p = 0.59$).

Experiment 3

A Single Task Was Randomly Presented to the Left or to the Right Eye Within a Block

Our Experiment 2 has demonstrated further counting deficits when shifting attention between the eyes in amblyopia, as compared to Experiment 1 when maintaining attention in the same eye (**Figure 4**). This was particularly evident for strabismic amblyopes, who exhibited deficits in both eyes. We also showed that interocular suppression (i.e., contrast balance) was stronger in the strabismic group than in the anisometropic group (**Figure 5A**). These results suggest that interocular suppression may play a role in these additional deficits. On the other hand, it is also possible that the greater deficits found for binocular viewing (Experiment 2), especially in strabismic amblyopes, could be due to deviation of the eyes, which would require longer stimulus display durations to deal with the eye misalignment. However, our previous feature counting study with a dichoptic viewing (Wong-Kee-You et al., 2020) found that increasing the display duration from 200 ms to 350 ms did not improve counting performance in both anisometropic and strabismic amblyopes. Therefore, Experiment 3 was conducted to address two questions: 1) whether deficits in amblyopia would still be observed under the condition, where a simple target alternates between the eyes but little to no attention is required; 2) whether strabismic amblyopes need longer display durations to perform this simple task compared to normal-vision observers. If strabismic amblyopes can perform a simple eye-alternating task that requires little to no attention as accurately as normal-vision observers at various display durations, then it is unlikely that the deficits in feature counting we observed in Experiments 1, 2 are a result of display durations being too fast. Instead, it would indicate that the deficits in feature counting are a result of impairments in attention and high-level cortical function.

Figure 6 plots the proportion correct of single target orientation discrimination as a function of the target display duration for 2 normal-viewing observer, 2 anisometropic and 3 strabismic participants who also participated in Experiment 2. These amblyopic participants exhibited counting deficits, which were marked in **Figure 5B** (i.e., anisometropic amblyopes were marked as triangles; strabismic amblyopes were marked as diamonds). The data from all 7 participants showed about 75% correct for the single target orientation discrimination at the

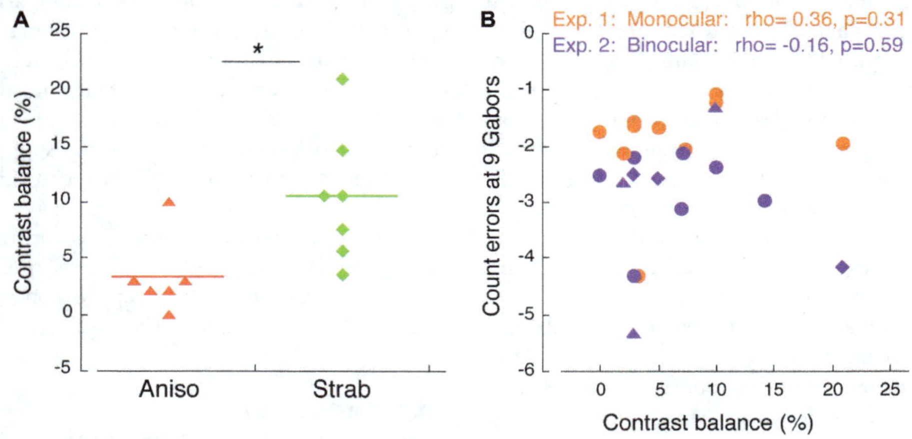

FIGURE 5 | Correlation of counting performance and contrast balance. **(A)** Contrast balance between anisometropic and strabismic amblyopes. * denotes $p < 0.05$. **(B)** Correlation of counting error at 9 Gabors and contrast balance in Experiment 1 (orange) and Experiment 2 (purple). Triangles indicate anisometropic amblyopes and diamonds indicate strabismic amblyopes, who also participated in Experiment 3.

shortest duration of 12 ms, and nearly 100% correct when the display was over 40 ms for both eyes. Notably, there were no differences between the two eyes in most display durations for all participants, as seen in **Figure 6**. Importantly, the strabismic group did not need longer display durations of the single target to perform this simple orientation discrimination task as accurately as the normal-vision observers. Thus, this experiment ruled out that the underestimates of multiple numbers of Gabors found in Experiments 1, 2 in strabismic amblyopes are due to the deviation of the eyes. Instead, the deficits are likely due to being unable to count multiple features accurately when the number of features is larger than 6.

DISCUSSION

Strabismic amblyopes have previously been found to undercount visual features when using their amblyopic eye under monocular viewing condition (Sharma et al., 2000). In the current study, we show that under binocular viewing condition where attentional shifts between the eyes are required, strabismic amblyopes further undercount when using their amblyopic eye. Notably, undercounting was found not only in the amblyopic eye, but also in the non-amblyopic fellow eye of strabismic amblyopes. Anisometropic amblyopes similarly undercounted visual features when using their amblyopic eye. However, when using their fellow eye, anisometropic amblyopes counted features as accurately as the normal-vision observers, whether attention was maintained on the same eye or shifted between the eyes.

High-Level Cortical Dysfunctions and Attention Deficits in Amblyopia

During feature counting, small or large numbers of visual features are believed to recruit different neural mechanisms (Pylyshyn et al., 1994; Trick and Pylyshyn, 1994). Normal-vision observers can achieve error-free performance when counting up to 4 briefly presented visual features (Atkinson et al., 1976). This fast and error-free counting is thought to be 'pre-attentive'. In contrast, the counting of briefly presented visual features at set-sizes above 5 requires spatial attention and the engagement of high-level cortical functions (Knudsen, 2007). In the current study, we used a variant of the Sharma et al. (2000) paradigm, which was originally used for monocular testing. The Sharma et al. (2000) paradigm had been tested for ruling out low-level cortical features, such as feature visibility, crowding, positional jitter, abnormal temporal integration, and spatial scale shifts in amblyopia (Levi et al., 1994). Therefore, in the current study the testing with a modified paradigm is believed to reflect high-level cortical functions, as claimed in Sharma et al. (2000) study. Our study found that both the amblyopic and fellow eyes of amblyopes, including both anisometropic and strabismic types of amblyopia, could achieve nearly accurate performance when counting from the Small Gabor Size group (**Figures 2–4**). This finding suggests that 'pre-attentive' processes, or the process with little attention are spared in the amblyopic brain. However, in both types of amblyopia, the amblyopic eye was unable to accurately count features when the set-sizes were in the Large Gabor Size group (i.e., large Gabor set-size of 7, 8 and 9), suggesting that attention processes are impaired in amblyopia, reflecting dysfunction of high-level cortices in the amblyopic brain.

Relation of Selective Visual Attention and Interocular Suppression

When counting large set-sizes of Gabors (i.e., Gabor 7, 8, and 9) with shifting attention between the eyes (Experiment 2), additional counting deficits in amblyopia were found (**Figure 4**), as compared to those with maintaining attention in the same eye (Experiment 1). This is particularly evident for strabismic amblyopes, who exhibited deficits in both eyes. This finding suggests that the ability to quickly redirect attention between the eyes is further impaired in amblyopia, especially under the

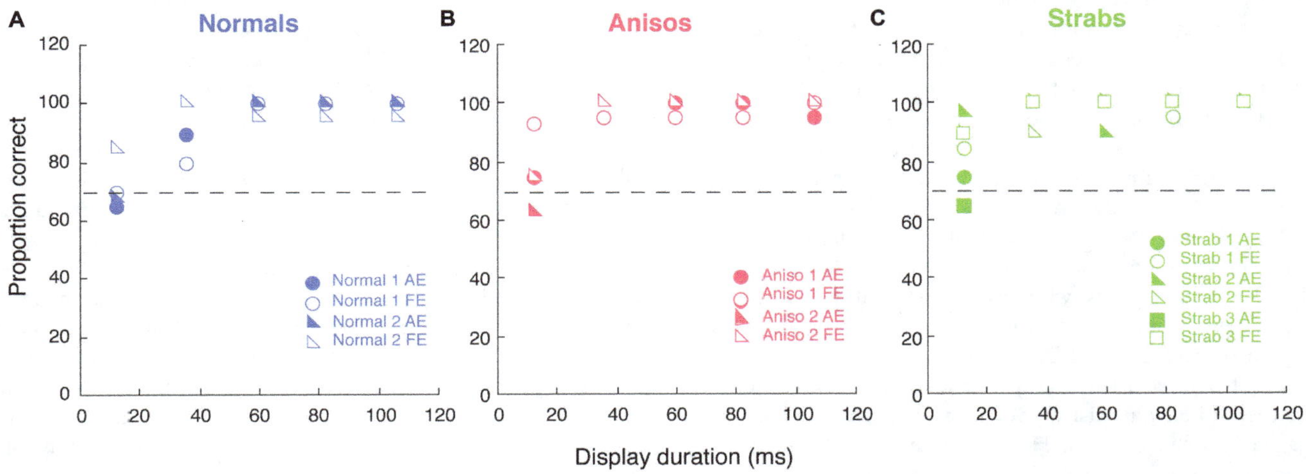

FIGURE 6 | Proportion correct of a single target orientation discrimination as a function of the target display duration for 2 Normals **(A)**, 2 Anisos **(B)**, and 3 Strabs **(C)**, who also participated in Experiment 2. Open symbols, dom/fellow eye; filled symbols, nondom/amblyopic eye. Horizontal dashed lines indicate 75% correct.

experimental environment of interocular suppression provided by our stimulus design with a binocular approach. People with strabismic amblyopia or anisometropic amblyopia usually suppress the visual percept from the deviating eye (strabismus) or from the higher refractive eye (anisometropia) to overcome diplopia (double vision) or visual blur. This long-term and chronic interocular suppression is believed to play an important role in amblyopic mechanisms (Jampolsky, 1955; Sireteanu, 1982; Holopigian et al., 1988). It has been reported that interocular suppression is stronger in strabismic amblyopia than in anisometropic amblyopia (Holopigian et al., 1988; Harrad and Hess, 1992; Agrawal et al., 2006; Narasimhan et al., 2012). We found this is also true in our amblyopic participants (**Figure 5A**). An fMRI study (Farivar et al., 2011) reported that the hemodynamic response function in response to amblyopic eye stimulation depended on whether the dominant fellow eye was open. When the fellow eye was open to a static pattern (not stimulated), the responses in the early visual cortex to amblyopic eye stimulation were reduced (suppressed) as compared to the responses when the fellow eye was patched and closed. This study demonstrated that interocular suppression exists once the fellow eye was open; no matter whether the fellow eye was stimulated or not. Consistent with this fMRI study, our findings revealed additional feature counting deficits in the amblyopic eye when redirecting attention randomly between the eyes, while the fellow eye was viewing a blank screen. Our results imply that there might be a relation between redirecting attention between the eyes and interocular suppression in the amblyopic brain. Such inability to redirect attention is unlikely related to poor visual acuity, because this defect was also found in the non-amblyopic fellow eye of strabismic amblyopes. Rather, it is likely related to selective attention deficits, particularly under interocular suppression. However, we did not find significant correlation between feature counting performance and interocular suppression (**Figure 5B**) in the current study. This might be due to our small sample size, or the measurement of interocular suppression that might not truly represent the magnitude of interocular suppression, because a certain number of strabismic amblyopes have a normal contrast sensitivity in their amblyopic eye (McKee et al., 2003). Thus, a future study with a better stimulus design is needed to reveal the correlation between feature counting performance and interocular suppression.

On the other hand, it also possible that shifting attention randomly between the eyes (Experiment 2) increased perceptual uncertainty between the eyes, as compared to the condition when attention was maintained in the same eye (Experiment 1). For example, individuals with amblyopia experience difficulty with spatial localiation tasks (e.g., Vernier tasks), and this is more evident in strabismic amblyopes than in anisometropic amblyopes (Levi and Klein, 1982a). When shifting attention between the eyes, this perceptual uncertainty could be more apparent for strabismic amblyopes under interocular suppression, as compared to that for anisometropic amblyopes. A previous study reported that perceptual uncertainty is a property of the cognitive system (Perea and Carreiras, 2012). It is not surprising to see more visual uncertainty in amblyopes than in normal-vision observers, as we have mentioned above regarding dysfunction of high-level cortices in the amblyopic brain. However, in our study, we were unable to know how much of perceptual uncertainty was created and how the interaction between interocular suppression and perceptual uncertainty was. Future studies are needed with well-designed experiments to manipulate and quantify the factors of interocular suppression and perceptual uncertainty in amblyopia.

Different Pattern of Visual Deficits in Anisometropic and Strabismic Amblyopia

Our results showed that different feature counting deficits are associated with anisometropic versus strabismic amblyopia. When shifting attention between the eyes, the fellow eye of anisometropic amblyopes, like normal-vision observers, counted Gabors accurately up to 7 and started to make errors at 8. In contrast, the fellow eye of strabismic amblyopes was able to count features accurately at 3 Gabors, but started to make errors at 5 Gabors. Since we skipped 4 Gabors to reduce the exam duration, we were unable to show the performance at 4 Gabors. These findings are consistent with our previous dichoptic feature counting study (Wong-Kee-You et al., 2020). Wong-Kee-You et al. (2020) reported that when different numbers of Gabors were simultaneously presented to the left and the right eyes, participants with strabismic amblyopia exhibited greater deficits in feature counting in comparison to those with anisometropic amblyopia. The greater deficits in feature counting from strabismic amblyopes might have also confounded with their binocular disruption, since the tasks in that study engaged binocular fusion. However, the current study, which presented visual features in the same eye, still exhibited greater deficits in feature counting in strabismic amblyopes than in anisometropic amblyopes. The current study further confirmed a different pattern of visual deficits in anisometropic and strabismic amblyopia. The findings in the current study are also consistent with our previous electrophysiological studies that the fellow eye of strabismic amblyopes showed abnormal SSVEP responses to illusory contours (Hou et al., 2014), motion coherence (Hou et al., 2008) and selective attention (Hou et al., 2016), while the fellow eye of anisometropic amblyopes had normal SSVEP responses to illusory contours (Hou et al., 2014). The fellow eye deficits in strabismic amblyopes have also been reported in behavioral studies with position tasks (Vernier) (Levi and Klein, 1982a) and global motion-discrimination tasks (Giaschi et al., 1992; Simmers et al., 2003; Ho et al., 2005). These fellow eye deficits reported in previous studies commonly use tasks that primarily represent function of extra-striate or higher level cortices, and are more commonly found in strabismic amblyopia than anisometropic amblyopia (Hess and Demanins, 1998). The results, as we found in the current study, with different patterns of feature counting deficits in anisometropic and strabismic amblyopia strongly support the view that different patterns of visual deficits are associated with amblyopia of different etiologies.

In summary, in this study we demonstrated that the amblyopic eye of both anisometropic and strabismic amblyopes were unable to count multiple visual features greater than 6 accurately, supporting the view of attention deficits and dysfunction in high-level cortex of the amblyopic brain. More importantly, we found that the performance of feature counting was further affected when shifting attention between the eyes in amblyopes, as compared to when maintaining attention in the same eye. Our findings suggest that the ability to quickly redirect attention, particularly under interocular suppression, is impaired in amblyopia. We also found different patterns of feature counting deficits in anisometropic and strabismic amblyopia, supporting the view that different patterns of visual deficits are associated with amblyopia of different etiologies.

AUTHOR CONTRIBUTIONS

CH designed research, performed research, and wrote the first draft of the manuscript. GA analyzed data and edited the manuscript. Both authors contributed to the article and approved the submitted version.

ACKNOWLEDGMENTS

The authors thank Xie Jie Lai for programming the early version of the stimuli and part of data collection. The authors also thank Spero C. Nicholas for programming the stimuli, Margaret Q. McGovern for assistance in recruiting the participants, and Audrey Wong-Kee-You for help with manuscript revision.

REFERENCES

Agrawal, R., Conner, I. P., Odom, J. V., Schwartz, T. L., and Mendola, J. D. (2006). Relating binocular and monocular vision in strabismic and anisometropic amblyopia. *Arch. Ophthalmol.* 124, 844–850. doi: 10.1001/archopht.124.6.844

Anobile, G., Cicchini, G. M., and Burr, D. C. (2012). Linear mapping of numbers onto space requires attention. *Cognition* 122, 454–459. doi: 10.1016/j.cognition.2011.11.006

Atkinson, J., Campbell, F. W., and Francis, M. R. (1976). The magic number 4 +/- 0: a new look at visual numerosity judgements. *Perception* 5, 327–334. doi: 10.1068/p050327

Balakrishnan, J. D., and Ashby, F. G. (1992). Subitizing: magical numbers or mere superstition? *Psychol. Res.* 54, 80–90. doi: 10.1007/BF00937136

Bressler, S. L., Tang, W., Sylvester, C. M., Shulman, G. L., and Corbetta, M. (2008). Top-down control of human visual cortex by frontal and parietal cortex in anticipatory visual spatial attention. *J. Neurosci.* 28, 10056–10061. doi: 10.1523/JNEUROSCI.1776-08.2008

Chandna, A., Pennefather, P. M., Kovacs, I., and Norcia, A. M. (2001). Contour integration deficits in anisometropic amblyopia. *Invest. Ophthalmol. Vis. Sci.* 42, 875–878.

Chow, A., Giaschi, D., and Thompson, B. (2018). Dichoptic attentive motion tracking is biased toward the nonamblyopic eye in strabismic amblyopia. *Invest. Ophthalmol. Vis. Sci.* 59, 4572–4580. doi: 10.1167/iovs.18-25236

Egeth, H., Leonard, C. J., and Palomares, M. (2008). The role of attention in subitizing: is the magical number 1? *Vis. Cognit.* 16, 463–473. doi: 10.1080/13506280801937939

Farivar, R., Thompson, B., Mansouri, B., and Hess, R. F. (2011). Interocular suppression in strabismic amblyopia results in an attenuated and delayed hemodynamic response function in early visual cortex. *J. Vis.* 11, 1–12. doi: 10.1167/11.14.16

Farzin, F., and Norcia, A. M. (2011). Impaired visual decision-making in individuals with amblyopia. *J Vis.* 11, 1–15. doi: 10.1167/11.14.6

Giaschi, D. E., Regan, D., Kraft, S. P., and Hong, X. H. (1992). Defective processing of motion-defined form in the fellow eye of patients with unilateral amblyopia. *Invest. Ophthalmol. Vis. Sci.* 33, 2483–2489.

Harrad, R. A., and Hess, R. F. (1992). Binocular integration of contrast information in amblyopia. *Vision Res.* 32, 2135–2150. doi: 10.1016/0042-6989(92)90075-t

Hess, R. F., and Demanins, R. (1998). Contour integration in anisometropic amblyopia. *Vision Res.* 38, 889–894. doi: 10.1016/s0042-6989(97)00233-2

Hess, R. F., McIlhagga, W., and Field, D. J. (1997). Contour integration in strabismic amblyopia: the sufficiency of an explanation based on positional uncertainty. *Vision Res.* 37, 3145–3161. doi: 10.1016/s0042-6989(96)00281-7

Ho, C. S., and Giaschi, D. E. (2006). Deficient maximum motion displacement in amblyopia. *Vision Res.* 46, 4595–4603. doi: 10.1016/j.visres.2006.09.025

Ho, C. S., and Giaschi, D. E. (2007). Stereopsis-dependent deficits in maximum motion displacement in strabismic and anisometropic amblyopia. *Vision Res.* 47, 2778–2785. doi: 10.1016/j.visres.2007.07.008

Ho, C. S., and Giaschi, D. E. (2009). Low- and high-level motion perception deficits in anisometropic and strabismic amblyopia: evidence from fMRI. *Vision Res.* 49, 2891–2901. doi: 10.1016/j.visres.2009.07.012

Ho, C. S., Giaschi, D. E., Boden, C., Dougherty, R., Cline, R., and Lyons, C. (2005). Deficient motion perception in the fellow eye of amblyopic children. *Vision Res.* 45, 1615–1627. doi: 10.1016/j.visres.2004.12.009

Ho, C. S., Paul, P. S., Asirvatham, A., Cavanagh, P., Cline, R., and Giaschi, D. E. (2006). Abnormal spatial selection and tracking in children with amblyopia. *Vision Res.* 46, 3274–3283. doi: 10.1016/j.visres.2006.03.029

Holmes, J. M., and Clarke, M. P. (2006). Amblyopia [Research support, N.I.H., extramural research support, Non-U.S. Gov't review]. *Lancet* 367, 1343–1351. doi: 10.1016/S0140-6736(06)68581-4

Holopigian, K., Blake, R., and Greenwald, M. J. (1988). Clinical suppression and amblyopia. *Invest. Ophthalmol. Vis. Sci.* 29, 444–451.

Hou, C., Kim, Y.-J., Lai, X. J., and Verghese, P. (2016). Degraded attentional modulation of cortical neural populations in strabismic amblyopia. *J. Vis.* 16:16. doi: 10.1167/16.3.16

Hou, C., Pettet, M. W., and Norcia, A. M. (2008). Abnormalities of coherent motion processing in strabismic amblyopia: visual-evoked potential measurements. *J. Vis.* 8, 2.1–12.

Hou, C., Pettet, M. W., and Norcia, A. M. (2014). Acuity-independent effects of visual deprivation on human visual cortex. *Proc. Natl. Acad. Sci. U.S.A.* 111, E3120–E3128. doi: 10.1073/pnas.1404361111

Jampolsky, A. (1955). Characteristics of suppression in strabismus. *AMA Arch. Ophthalmol.* 54, 683–696. doi: 10.1001/archopht.1955.00930020689010

Kiorpes, L., Kiper, D. C., O'Keefe, L. P., Cavanaugh, J. R., and Movshon, J. A. (1998). Neuronal correlates of amblyopia in the visual cortex of macaque monkeys with experimental strabismus and anisometropia. *J. Neurosci.* 18, 6411–6424. doi: 10.1523/jneurosci.18-16-06411.1998

Knudsen, E. I. (2007). Fundamental components of attention. *Annu. Rev. Neurosci.* 30, 57–78. doi: 10.1146/annurev.neuro.30.051606.094256

Kovacs, I., Polat, U., Pennefather, P. M., Chandna, A., and Norcia, A. M. (2000). A new test of contour integration deficits in patients with a history of disrupted binocular experience during visual development. *Vision Res.* 40, 1775–1783. doi: 10.1016/s0042-6989(00)00008-0

Kozma, P., and Kiorpes, L. (2003). Contour integration in amblyopic monkeys. *Vis. Neurosci.* 20, 577–588. doi: 10.1017/s0952523803205113

Levi, D. M., and Klein, S. (1982a). Differences in vernier discrimination for grating between strabismic and anisometropic amblyopes. *Invest. Ophthalmol. Vis. Sci.* 23, 398–407.

Levi, D. M., and Klein, S. (1982b). Hyperacuity and amblyopia. *Nature* 298, 268–270. doi: 10.1038/298268a0

Levi, D. M., and Klein, S. A. (1985). Vernier acuity, crowding and amblyopia. *Vision Res.* 25, 979–991. doi: 10.1016/0042-6989(85)90208-1

Levi, D. M., and Klein, S. A. (1986). Sampling in spatial vision. *Nature* 320, 360–362. doi: 10.1038/320360a0

Levi, D. M., Waugh, S. J., and Beard, B. L. (1994). Spatial scale shifts in amblyopia. *Vision Res.* 34, 3315–3333. doi: 10.1016/0042-6989(94)90067-1

Li, J., Thompson, B., Deng, D., Chan, L. Y., Yu, M., and Hess, R. F. (2013). Dichoptic training enables the adult amblyopic brain to learn. *Curr. Biol.* 23, R308–R309. doi: 10.1016/j.cub.2013.01.059

Li, J., Thompson, B., Lam, C. S. Y., Deng, D., Chan, L. Y. L., Maehara, G., et al. (2011). The role of suppression in amblyopia. [Comparative study]. *Invest. Opthalmol. Vis. Sci.* 52, 4169–4176. doi: 10.1167/iovs.11-7233

Li, R. W., Ngo, C., Nguyen, J., and Levi, D. M. (2011). Video-game play induces plasticity in the visual system of adults with amblyopia. *PLoS Biol.* 9:e1001135. doi: 10.1371/journal.pbio.1001135

McKee, S. P., Levi, D. M., and Movshon, J. A. (2003). The pattern of visual deficits in amblyopia. *J. Vis.* 3, 380–405.

Narasimhan, S., Harrison, E. R., and Giaschi, D. E. (2012). Quantitative measurement of interocular suppression in children with amblyopia. *Vision Res.* 66, 1–10. doi: 10.1016/j.visres.2012.06.007

Nieder, A., and Dehaene, S. (2009). Representation of number in the brain. *Annu. Rev. Neurosci.* 32, 185–208. doi: 10.1146/annurev.neuro.051508.135550

Nieder, A., Diester, I., and Tudusciuc, O. (2006). Temporal and spatial enumeration processes in the primate parietal cortex. *Science* 313, 1431–1435. doi: 10.1126/science.1130308

Ooi, T. L., Su, Y. R., Natale, D. M., and He, Z. J. (2013). A push-pull treatment for strengthening the 'lazy eye' in amblyopia. *Curr. Biol.* 23, R309–R310. doi: 10.1016/j.cub.2013.03.004

Perea, M., and Carreiras, M. (2012). Perceptual uncertainty is a property of the cognitive system. *Behav. Brain Sci.* 35, 298–299. doi: 10.1017/S0140525X12000118

Popple, A. V., and Levi, D. M. (2000). Amblyopes see true alignment where normal observers see illusory tilt. *Proc. Natl. Acad. Sci. U.S.A.* 97, 11667–11672. doi: 10.1073/pnas.97.21.11667

Popple, A. V., and Levi, D. M. (2008). The attentional blink in amblyopia. *J. Vis.* 8, 12.11–19.

Pylyshyn, Z. (1994). Some primitive mechanisms of spatial attention. *Cognition* 50, 363–384. doi: 10.1016/0010-0277(94)90036-1

Pylyshyn, Z., Burkell, J., Fisher, B., Sears, C., Schmidt, W., and Trick, L. (1994). Multiple parallel access in visual attention. *Can. J. Exp. Psychol.* 48, 260–283. doi: 10.1037/1196-1961.48.2.260

Sathian, K., Simon, T. J., Peterson, S., Patel, G. A., Hoffman, J. M., and Grafton, S. T. (1999). Neural evidence linking visual object enumeration and attention. *J. Cogn. Neurosci.* 11, 36–51. doi: 10.1162/089892999563238

Secen, J., Culham, J., Ho, C., and Giaschi, D. (2011). Neural correlates of the multiple-object tracking deficit in amblyopia. *Vision Res.* 51, 2517–2527. doi: 10.1016/j.visres.2011.10.011

Sharma, V., Levi, D. M., and Klein, S. A. (2000). Undercounting features and missing features: evidence for a high-level deficit in strabismic amblyopia. *Nat. Neurosci.* 3, 496–501. doi: 10.1038/74872

Simmers, A. J., Ledgeway, T., Hess, R. F., and McGraw, P. V. (2003). Deficits to global motion processing in human amblyopia. *Vision Res.* 43, 729–738. doi: 10.1016/s0042-6989(02)00684-3

Sireteanu, R. (1982). Human amblyopia: consequence of chronic interocular suppression. *Hum. Neurobiol.* 1, 31–33.

Smith, E. L. III, Chino, Y. M., Ni, J., Cheng, H., Crawford, M. L., and Harwerth, R. S. (1997). Residual binocular interactions in the striate cortex of monkeys reared with abnormal binocular vision. *J. Neurophysiol.* 78, 1353–1362. doi: 10.1152/jn.1997.78.3.1353

Thiel, A., and Sireteanu, R. (2009). Strabismic amblyopes show a bilateral rightward bias in a line bisection task: evidence for a visual attention deficit [Research support, Non-U.S. Gov't]. *Vision Res.* 49, 287–294. doi: 10.1016/j.visres.2008.08.005

Trick, L. M., and Pylyshyn, Z. W. (1994). Why are small and large numbers enumerated differently? A limited-capacity preattentive stage in vision. *Psychol. Rev.* 101, 80–102. doi: 10.1037/0033-295x.101.1.80

Tripathy, S. P., and Levi, D. M. (2008). On the effective number of tracked trajectories in amblyopic human vision. *J. Vis.* 8, 8.1–22.

Tsirlin, I., Colpa, L., Goltz, H. C., and Wong, A. M. F. (2018). Visual search deficits in amblyopia. *J. Vis.* 18:17. doi: 10.1167/18.4.17

Wong-Kee-You, A. M. B., Wei, H., and Hou, C. (2020). Feature counting under dichoptic viewing in anisometropic and strabismic amblyopia. *Transl. Vis. Sci. Technol.* 9:13. doi: 10.1167/tvst.9.6.13

12

Investigation of the Relationship Between Subjective Symptoms of Visual Fatigue and Visual Functions

*Fuhao Zheng, Fang Hou, Ruru Chen, Jianhui Mei, Pingping Huang, Bingzhen Chen and Yuwen Wang**

Eye Hospital, Wenzhou Medical University, Wenzhou, China

Correspondence:
Yuwen Wang
wyw-0721@163.com

Purpose: To investigate whether the severity of symptoms of visual fatigue might be associated with clinical visual measures and basic visual functions, such as accommodation, vergence, and contrast sensitivity.

Methods: In this study, 104 students were recruited (25 males, 79 females, Age 23.4 $\pm$ 2.5) for this study. Those with high myopia, strabismus, anisometropia, eye disease or history of ophthalmological surgery were excluded. The included subjects completed a questionnaire that assesses the severity of visual fatigue. Then, binocular accommodative facility, vergence facility and contrast sensitivity using a quick contrast sensitivity function approach were measured in a random sequence. Next, the correlations between each symptom of visual fatigue in the questionnaire and accommodative facility, vergence facility and contrast sensitivity were examined.

Results: Factor analysis indicated that visual fatigue, as captured by the scores of a subset of the questionnaire items, could be strongly related to binocular accommodative facility and binocular contrast sensitivity, but not to vergence facility. We also found that binocular accommodative facility and contrast sensitivity at high spatial frequencies are related.

Conclusion: Our findings suggest that visual fatigue is related to the ability of human observers to encode visual details through their binocular vision.

Keywords: visual fatigue, contrast sensitivity, subjective symptoms, vergence facility, binocular accommodative facility, factor analysis, binocular vision

INTRODUCTION

Visual fatigue refers to a group of somatic or perceptive symptoms that usually occur following using a computer, reading, or other performing near visual activities (Bhanderi et al., 2008). The prevalence of visual fatigue is 12.4-32.2% in children below 18 years (Ip et al., 2006; Sterner et al., 2006; Tiwari et al., 2011; Tiwari, 2013) and 46–71% in university students around the world (Bhanderi et al., 2008; Han et al., 2013; Hashemi et al., 2019). Moreover, the prevalence of visual fatigue has been increasing (Sheppard and Wolffsohn, 2018).

Common symptoms of visual fatigue are blurred vision, diplopia, and illusory movement or flicker of words at a near viewing distance. These characteristics are related to near vision and binocular anomalies (Chen, 1986; Sheedy et al., 2003; Blehm et al., 2005; García-Muñoz et al., 2014).

A questionnaire has been used as a quick method to assess the severity of symptoms and distinguish patients with symptoms from those who have normal vision (García-Muñoz et al., 2014).

Visual acuity is measured to evaluate the severity of visual fatigue. For instance, the larger the visual extent required to resolve a spatial pattern, the more severe the visual fatigue (Leroy, 2016) However, measurement of visual acuity might not be ideal. For example, blurred vision is a cardinal symptom of visual fatigue. Patients who suffer from visual fatigue often complain about blurred vision. However, studies show that their visual acuity is normal (Vilela et al., 2015). A 10-year follow-up study about visual fatigue reveals no relationship among visual fatigue and age, sex, seniority of work, visual acuity, and refractory disorders (Larese et al., 2019). In addition, a visual acuity test only utilizes optotypes with high degrees of contrast. Therefore, it might not reflect the visual performance in the real world (Marmor, 1986) where visual targets could appear at a relatively lower contrast, such as high spatial frequency content. High spatial frequency information can appear at a relatively lower contrast because the contrast sensitivity for higher spatial frequency content is much lower in humans. For this reason, measurement of contrast sensitivity across spatial frequency might better capture the ability of human observers to detect and encode the details (Arden, 1978; Marmor, 1986). In addition, studies show that contrast sensitivity, but not visual acuity, is impaired in patients who have visual disorders such as high myopia, asthenopia, foggy vision, and ocular hypertension (Quant, 1992; Järvinen and Hyvärinen, 1997; Gandolfi et al., 2005). These findings suggest that contrast sensitivity, rather than visual acuity, might be a more appropriate measure to diagnose a wide range of visual disorders.

Additionally, visual fatigue can occur to demands on early visual functions such as focusing and converging the eyes at a near object (Wilkins, 1995; Scheiman and Wick, 2014). Thus, accommodative and binocular dysfunctions might play a pivotal role in causing visual fatigue (Rosenfield, 2011; Sheppard and Wolffsohn, 2018; Golebiowski et al., 2020). Accommodation function is measured by accommodative amplitude and accommodative facility. Vergence function is measured by phoria, fusional range reserves, and vergence facility (Scheiman and Wick, 2014). Importantly, facility of accommodation and binocular vision can be more informative than the amplitude of accommodation and vergence (Liu et al., 1979; Hennessey et al., 1984; Scheiman and Wick, 2014) for clinical assessment. For instance, vergence facility and accommodative facility are central indexes of binocular vision (Buzzelli, 1991; Grisham et al., 2007; Palomo-Alvarez and Puell, 2008; Dusek et al., 2010; Quaid and Simpson, 2013; Scheiman and Wick, 2014). Many patients suffering from visual fatigue experience a decline in vergence or accommodative facility (Hennessey et al., 1984; Levine et al., 1985; Momeni-Moghaddam et al., 2014). Moreover, patients, whose amplitudes of accommodation and vergence are normal, have been shown to have severe visual symptoms if their accommodative and vergence facility are abnormal (Gall and Wick, 2003).

In this study, we investigated relationships between subjective symptoms (i.e., each item score of the questionnaire) and results from visual measurements, such as contrast sensitivity and accommodative and vergence facility. Contrast sensitivity, accommodation, vergence were measured using a qCSF method and lenses and prism flippers in 104 college students, respectively.

MATERIALS AND METHODS

Participants

This study followed the tenets of the Declaration of Helsinki and was approved by the Hospital Committee of Wenzhou Medical University for the Protection of Human Subjects. For this study, 104 college students, 25 males and 79 females, ranged from 18 to 30 years ($M = 23.4$, $SD = 2.5$), were recruited from Wenzhou Medical University. Those with eye disease, ocular surgery, history of amblyopic or strabismus had been excluded. Their refractive error was between +1.00 Diopter (D) and −6.00 Diopter (D), astigmatism was less than 1.25 D. Their visual acuity was above or corrected to 20/20 with a normal monocular accommodative amplitude. All subjects were naïve to the purpose of the study.

Questionnaire

A questionnaire of visual discomfort (Yang and James, 2011) was used to evaluate subjective symptoms of visual fatigue (see **Appendix Table 1**). In this paper, we define subjective symptom as each item in the questionnaire. Before their clinical examination, all subjects were asked to finish the questionnaire. Scores of the questionnaire for each symptom ranged from 0 (none) to 4 (extremely so). Visual fatigue was defined as the presence of one or more visual symptoms (subjective symptoms #2,3,6,7,9,10,13) (Han et al., 2013). In our study, there were about 53 of 104 (50.96%) participants who had more than one subjective symptom (score of symptoms is no less than two, which is the mean of the empirical distribution of the scores from all our participants) in the questionnaire, so they were categorized as having visual fatigue.

Procedure

First, all subjects were asked to finish the questionnaire. Then accommodative facility and vergence facility were examined in a brightly lit room. Binocular contrast sensitivity was measured in a dark room on another day. All subjects performed the tests with best-corrected glasses. Some subject had good visual acuity without glasses, but some were corrected to 20/20. They had to wear their best-corrected glasses if they had ametropia.

Accommodative Facility test

Binocular accommodative facility was measured using a flipper lens. A card had 6/9 (20/30) sized of letters. The card was positioned at a viewing distance of 40 cm. The participants were asked to report if the letters were clear while they were viewed with alternating +2.00 D and −2.00 D lenses. As an index of binocular accommodative facility, the number of cycles per minute (cpm) was measured. It denotes the ability of the observers to clear the plus lens followed by the minus lens. Any difficulties in responding between +2.00 D and −2.00 D was

TABLE 1 | Factor analysis for 15 items in the questionnaire after Varimax with Kaiser Normalization.

	Factor 1 Disorientation and difficulty in focusing	Factor 2 Discomfort after near work	Factor 3 Unclear mind	Factor 4 Physical discomfort
Q1		0.777		
Q2		0.582		
Q3				0.699
Q4	0.600			
Q5	0.781			
Q6	0.526	0.600		
Q7	0.722			
Q8			0.791	
Q9	0.692			
Q10	0.586	0.503		
Q11				0.692
Q12			0.880	
Q13		0.647		
Q14			0.619	
Q15				0.659

The values are factor loading scores that have been standardized.

noted (Chen et al., 2021). F(+) means that the subjects had more difficulty in +2.00 D, whereas F(−) means that they experienced more difficulty in −2.00 D.

Vergence Facility test

Vergence facility was evaluated at a viewing distance of 40 cm with a flipper prism. The power for the flippers was chosen as $3^{\triangle}$BI/$12^{\triangle}$BO. A vertical column of small letter "E" at a 20/30 [6/9] size was presented as an accommodative target. The subjects observed the fixation target while their vision underwent best-correction. They reported when there was a clear and one visual target. We changed the flipper prism from BI to BO and from BO to BI, which makes up one cycle. Vergence facility was measured as cycles per minute, which is the number of cycles that each observer reported as clear and single visual percept for 1 min. In other words, this test measured the ability of the participants to form a fusion through BI and BO prisms. We noted if there were difficulty in the fusion through the BI and BO prisms during testing (Momeni-Moghaddam et al., 2014).

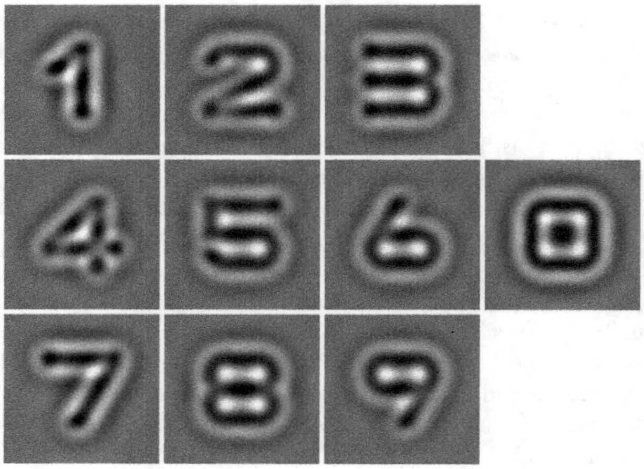

FIGURE 1 | Ten Band-pass filtered digits were used as stimuli in the qCSF method.

Quick CSF test

We measured binocular contrast sensitivity using a qCSF method, which was written in MATLAB (MathWorks, Natick, MA) with PsychToolBox extensions (Kleiner et al., 2007). Stimuli (Zheng et al., 2018) were displayed on a gamma-corrected screen (KD-55 × 9300E, SONY, Tokyo, Japan). The display had a spatial resolution of 1920 × 1080 pixels and a refresh rate of 60 Hz. Each pixel subtended 0.908° at a viewing distance of 4 m. Observers viewed the display binocularly with their best corrections in a dark room.

In the CSF test, the participants were asked to perform a 10-digit identification task. Ten digits stimuli (0∼9, see **Figure 1**) were filtered using a raised cosine filter (Chung et al., 2002; Hou et al., 2016). The quick CSF changes the stimulus parameters based on the most recent response of the observer. In other words, a quick CSF algorithm automatically selects the most optimal contrast and spatial frequency of the stimulus for each subsequent trial (Lesmes et al., 2010). The responses of the observer revised posterior probability of the stimulus parameters.

Before starting the experiment, the observers spent 5 min adapting to the dark in the testing room. Besides the stimulus with the optimal contrast and spatial frequency (selected from the Bayesian posterior probability), two stimuli at higher contrasts were displayed during each trial. The presentation of these two additional stimuli enhanced the subject's task performance. The three digits were randomly sampled from the 10 digits stimuli with replacement. Their positions were aligned in a single row; the distance between the neighboring digits was 1.1 times of the letter size. These three digits were displayed at the same spatial frequency but not in contrast.

Observers verbally identified the numbers. The experimenter recorded the response with the computer. When uncertain, observers reported by saying "I don't know," which was categorized as incorrect. There was no feedback to the response. A new trial began 500 ms after the subjects verbally identified the numbers (Hou et al., 2016).

Data Analysis

The number of cpm of binocular accommodative facility and vergence facility was analyzed. There were 21 subjects who experienced difficulty during the accommodative facility test for +2.00D, and 7 subjects for −2.00D, two of whom had double vision in −2.00D. For vergence facility, there were 16 subjects who experienced difficulty in achieving fusion in $12^{\triangle}$BO and 3 subjects in $3^{\triangle}$BI. Since the number of subjects of infacility was too small to yield a reliable statistical result, we did not do further analysis.

We used a qCSF method, which is a parametric procedure, to estimate the entire CSF curve. After estimating a CSF, we computed the area under a curve. We used the areal measure as an index to describe contrast sensitivity as a function of spatial frequency. We computed four variations of the areal measure. These were an area under low frequency (1.5–3 cpd) of the CSF curve (Low CSF), the area under middle frequency (3–12 cpd) of the CSF curve (Mid CSF), the area under high spatial frequency (12–18 cpd) of the CSF curve (High CSF), and the area under the log CSF curve (AULCSF), which is a summary metric of the CSF function (Applegate et al., 1998; Oshika et al., 2006; Yan et al., 2010). They have been reported that the area under log CSF curve is correlated with optical aberration of the human eye and has been used as an image quality indicator (Barten, 1999). The area in different spatial frequency ranges may be a powerful metric to represent different aspects of visual performance. Moreover, a cutoff spatial frequency (Cut-off SF) was calculated; it is a spatial frequency at which the contrast threshold of CSF is 0.50 and characterizes the high frequency resolution of the visual system (Regan and Beverley, 1983; Kwon and Legge, 2011; Zhang et al., 2015). The illustration of these areal measures and Cut-off SF is shown in **Figure 2**.

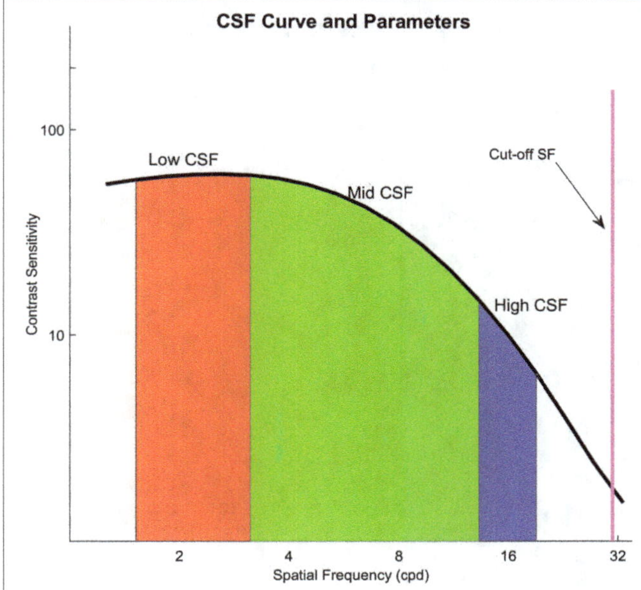

FIGURE 2 | The black curve in the figure is the contrast sensitivity curve; the red area means an area under low frequency (1.5–3 cpd) of the CSF curve (Low CSF); the green area means the area under middle frequency (3–12 cpd) of the CSF curve (Mid CSF); the blue area means the area under high spatial frequency (12–18 cpd) of the CSF curve (High CSF); the purple line shows Cut-off SF.

A Shapiro-Wilk test was used to evaluate whether the data were normally distributed. The score of each item in the questionnaire, data of Low CSF and Cut-off SF had non-normal distributions. On the other hand, datasets of binocular accommodative facility, vergence facility, Mid CSF, High CSF had normal distributions. We compared binocular accommodative facility, vergence facility and contrast sensitivity between participants with or without visual fatigue. For normally distributed datasets, we used methods such as two independent sample *t*-test or a Pearson correlation test. Otherwise, we used a Mann-Whitney *U* test or a Spearman correlation test.

To map out the association between different subjective symptoms, we performed factor analysis using 15 items of the questionnaire. All the scores from the questionnaire were first standardized before factor analysis. To confirm whether factor analysis was appropriate for our datasets, we performed the Kaiser-Meyer-Olkin (KMO) test, which revealed 0.817; this is much higher than the necessary 0.7 which warrants factor analysis. Moreover, we performed Bartlett's Test of Sphericity to see if the scores of the 15 items were unrelated to each other. It revealed $p < 0.05$, indicating that our datasets were related to each other. Hence, Bartlett's Test also indicated that factor analysis was necessary.

Factor analysis enabled us to find latent factors (exogenous variables) that influenced the scores of the items in the questionnaire (endogenous variables). Next, we also examined the relationship between the latent factors and clinical measurements of visual functions, such as Cut-off SF, binocular accommodative facility, and vergence facility. Varimax with Kaiser Normalization was the rotation method to find rotated component. To make matrix clearer, we suppressed small coefficients when their absolute values were below 0.50. Then, multiple linear regression was used among variates with significant correlation.

The statistical analyses were performed using the software package SPSS (Windows version 22.0; IBM-SPSS). As for statistical significance, an alpha of 0.05 was established to reject the null hypothesis. When necessary, Bonferroni correction was applied.

RESULTS

In our study, scores of the subjective symptoms in the questionnaire, visual acuity, Low CSF, Cut-off SF were not normally distributed, and binocular accommodative facility, vergence facility, Mid CSF, High CSF, and AULCSF were

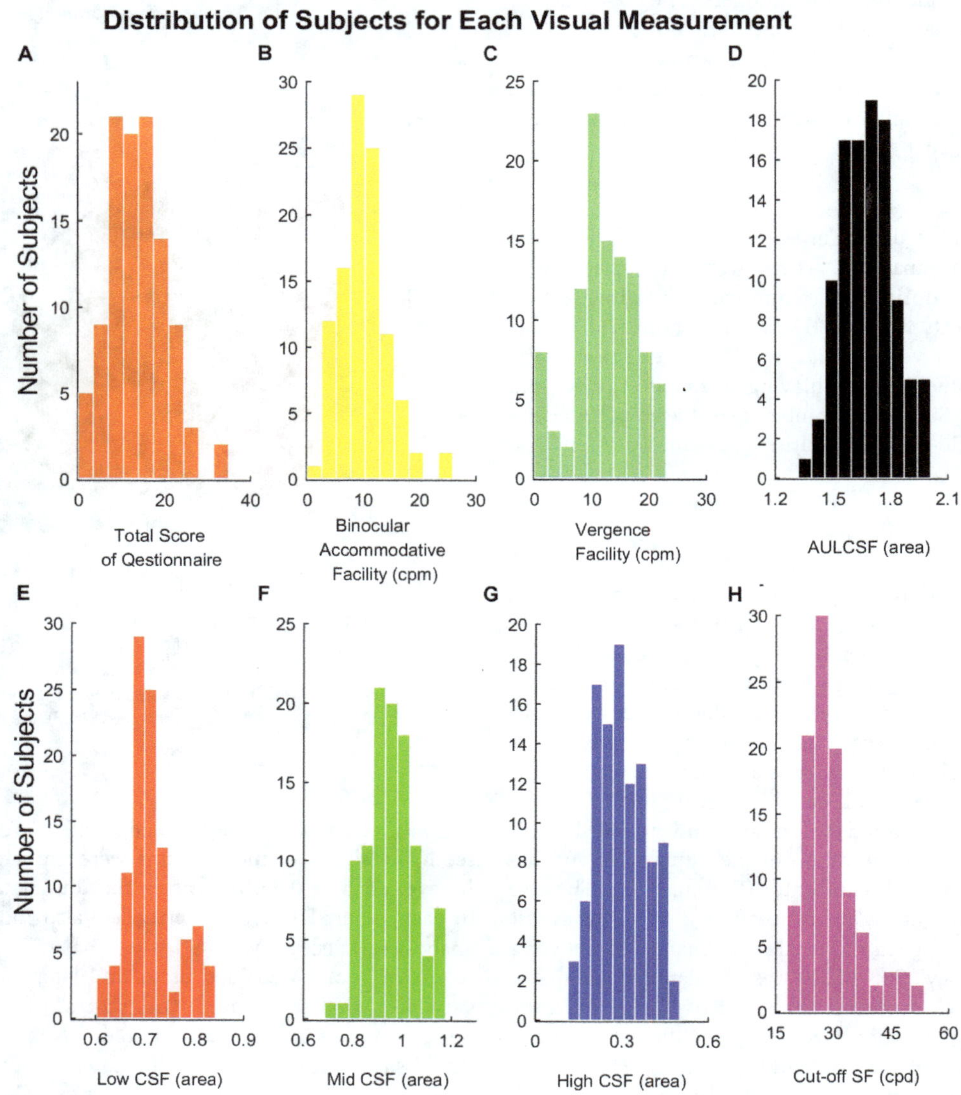

FIGURE 3 | (A) Histograms of total score of the questionnaire. **(B)** Binocular accommodative facility. **(C)** Vergence facility. **(D)** AULCSF. **(E)** Low CSF. **(F)** Mid CSF. **(G)** High CSF. **(H)** Cut-off SF.

normally distributed (shown in **Figure 3**). Total points of the questionnaire in 104 participants ranged from 0 to 16 out of 28 (median = 6, Q1 = 4, Q3 = 8.125). Median of visual acuity (log MAR) was 0.00, the first quartile was −0.08 and the third quartile was 0.00. Parameters of CSF (Low CSF: median = 0.70, Q1 = 0.68, Q3 = 0.73); Mid CSF: M = 0.95, SD = 0.09; High CSF: M = 0.29, SD = 0.09; AULCSF: M = 1.68, SD = 0.14; Cut-off SF: median = 28.30, Q1 = 24.78, Q3 = 31.10), binocular accommodative facility (M = 10.29, SD = 4.31) and vergence facility (M = 12.25, SD = 5.50) were detected from participants, respectively.

Those with more than one subjective symptom of visual symptoms were categorized as symptomatic of visual fatigue (see Methods). There were significant differences between asymptomatic (N = 51) and symptomatic (N = 53) participants in binocular accommodative facility [$t(102)$ = 2.508, P = 0.013], vergence facility [$t(102)$ = 2.944, P = 0.004], Cut-off SF (Z = −2.270, P = 0.023), shown in **Figure 4**. There was no significant difference in AULCSF, Low CSF, Mid CSF, and High CSF.

Factor Analysis

The scores of the 15 items in the questionnaire showed inter-correlation amongst clusters of items (shown by the Bartlett's test). For this reason, we performed factor analysis. We found that we could reduce our entire dataset based on four factors (shown in **Table 1**) because there were four factors which had eigenvalues larger than 1. These four factors are disorientation and difficulty in focusing, discomfort after near work, unclear mind and physical discomfort.

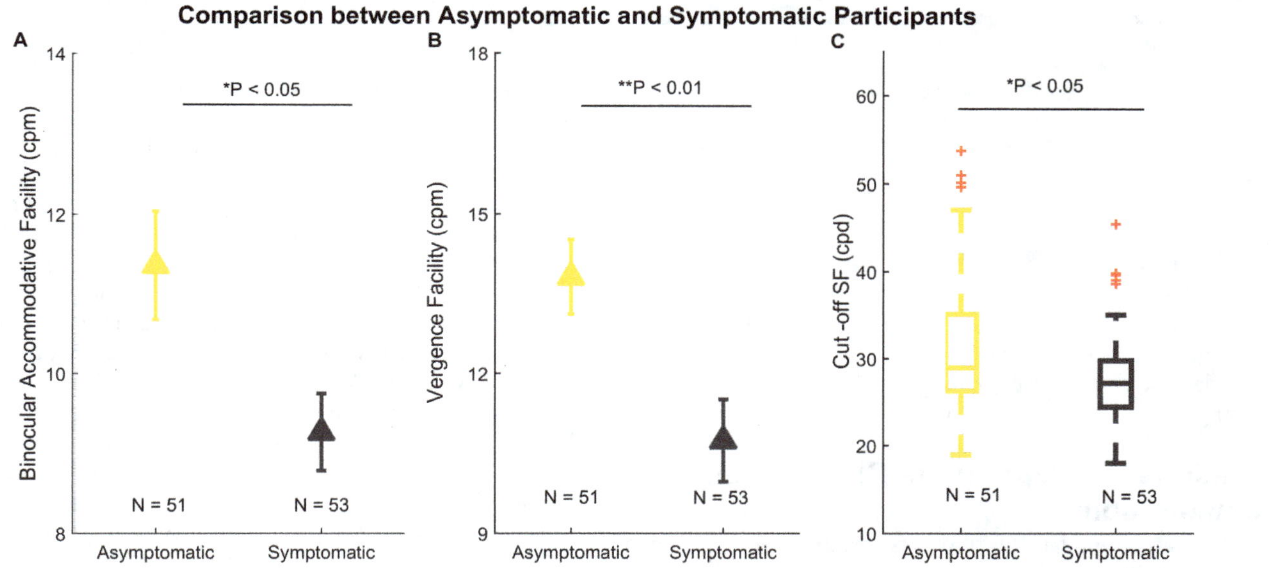

FIGURE 4 | Comparison between asymptomatic ($N = 51$) and symptomatic participants ($N = 53$). **(A)** Binocular accommodative facility. **(B)** Vergence facility. **(C)** A boxplot of Cut-off SF. In panels **(A)** and **(B)**, the error bars denote standard errors. In panel **(C)**, the line within each box is the median. The box spans the interquartile range (Q1 and Q3). The whiskers represent 1.5 × interquartile above the upper quartile (Q3) and below the lower quartile (Q1). The red crosses outside the whiskers are outliers. $^*p < 0.05$; $^{**}p < 0.01$.

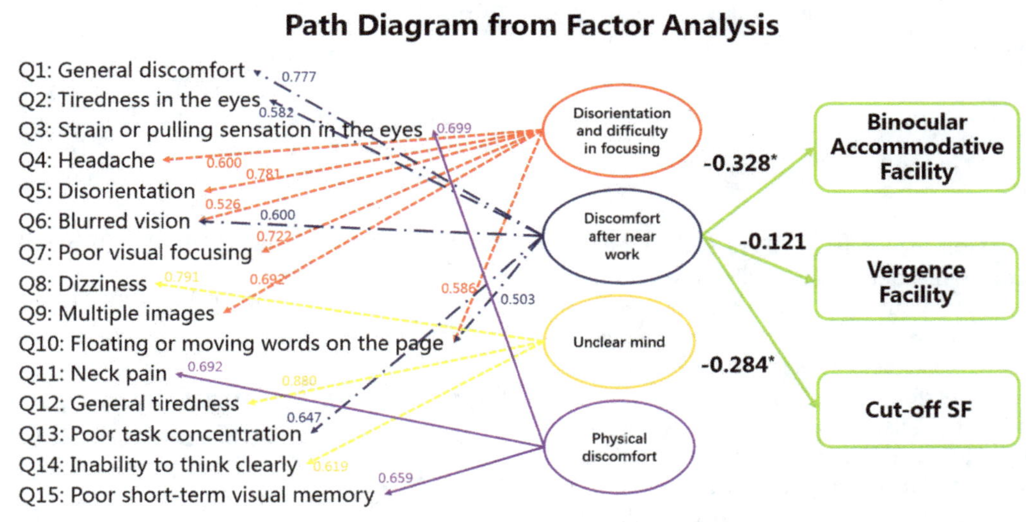

FIGURE 5 | Statistical analysis among subjective symptoms and visual functions (binocular accommodative facility, vergence facility and Cut-off SF). The values between the score of each item in the questionnaire and the latent factors indicate the standardized factor loading scores from the factor analysis. Factor #2 is the focus here because it seems to be strictly concerned with visual fatigue. The values between the latent factor "discomfort after near work" and the visual measures were obtained from bivariate correlation. $^*p < 0.05$.

We believe that factor #2 (discomfort after near work) is most representative of visual fatigue because factor #1 (disorientation and difficulty in focusing) is associated with both physical and visual discomfort, whereas factor #2 is strictly associated with visual discomfort. For this reason, we performed bivariate correlation between the factor "discomfort after near work" and results from clinical visual measurements but not between the other factors and the visual measurements. The results are shown in **Figure 5**, which indicates that the factor "discomfort after near work" is strongly associated with binocular accommodative facility (Spearman's $r = -0.328$, $p < 0.001$) and Cut-off SF (Spearman's $r = -0.284$, $P = 0.0018$), but not with vergence facility (Spearman's $r = -0.121$, $P = 0.111$).

In addition, multiple linear regression between the factor 'discomfort after near work' (Y) and binocular accommodative facility (X_1) and Cut-off SF (X_2) was $Y = -0.215^*X_1 - 0.278^*X_2$

TABLE 2 | Correlation coefficients (r) between binocular accommodative facility (BAF)/vergence facility (VF) and contrast sensitivity (Low CSF, Mid CSF, High SF) in 104 participants.

	Contrast sensitivity		
	Low CSF	**Mid CSF**	**High CSF**
BAF	0.198	0.180	0.267*
VF	−0.271*	−0.213	−0.026

$P < 0.05/6$ due to Bonferroni correction.

($F = 9.196$, $P < 0.001$). The values between the latent factor "discomfort after near work" and the visual measures indicate binocular accommodative facility and Cut-off SF are sensitive measurements that may also inform about visual fatigue.

Relationships Among the Clinical Visual Measurements

Binocular accommodative facility was correlated positively with vergence facility (Pearson's $r = 0.249$, $P = 0.011$).

Correlation coefficients between binocular accommodative facility/vergence facility and contrast sensitivity are listed in **Table 2**. Binocular accommodative facility was moderately correlated with High CSF (Pearson's $r = 0.267$, $P = 0.006$), but not so with Low CSF (Spearman's $r = 0.198$, $P = 0.044$) and Mid CSF (Pearson's $r = 0.180$, $P = 0.068$). Vergence facility was moderately correlated with Low CSF (Spearman's $r = -0.271$, $P = 0.005$), but not with Mid CSF (Pearson's $r = -0.213$, $P = 0.028$) and High CSF (Pearson's $r = -0.026$, $P = 0.793$).

DISCUSSION

In our study, we investigated whether there is an association between the scores of the questionnaire about visual fatigue and results from clinical visual measurements. We performed factor analysis to find associations between the exogenous latent factors (ex. visual fatigue) and endogenous scores of the questionnaire. Then we performed a bivariate correlation analysis between the latent factor "discomfort after near work," which represents visual fatigue, and the results from clinical visual measurements for binocular accommodative facility, vergence facility and contrast sensitivity. Lastly, we assessed whether there is an association between the measures from the clinical visual measurements themselves.

Relationship Between Visual Fatigue and Visual Clinical Measurements Based on Factor Analysis

Factor analysis showed that visual fatigue, which is represented by the factor "discomfort after near work," is strongly correlated with the results of binocular accommodative facility and Cut-off SF but not with vergence facility (see **Figure 5**). This finding is unexpected because both binocular accommodative facility and vergence facility are related to binocular vision. However, as our results from the subsequent section indicate, results between vergence facility and High CSF are not correlated, whereas those between binocular accommodative facility and High CSF are correlated. These findings indicate that binocular accommodative facility captures not only binocular visual function but also the ability of observers to encode visual details (i.e., high spatial frequency content). Hence, our results from factor analysis indicate that visual fatigue is strongly correlated with the ability of the adult observers to encode visual details at the binocular (cut-off SF, binocular accommodative facility) level.

Moreover, the subsequent section (section #2) of our study indicates that binocular accommodative facility is correlated with vergence facility. This finding indicates that binocular accommodative facility, rather than vergence facility, might be a more sensitive index. A high incidence rate of binocular vision dysfunction in Chinese young adults has been reported (Ma et al., 2019). For this reason, it is critical to come up with a sensitive quantitative measurement to evaluate visual fatigue caused by binocular dysfunction.

In our study, all participants had 20/20 or corrected to 20/20 in their visual acuity, but there were some individuals who reported blurred vision. This observation seems to be in line with results from some studies which indicate that the experience of mild symptoms of asthenopia and foggy vision can decrease contrast sensitivity even if the visual acuity remains intact (Quant, 1992; Järvinen and Hyvärinen, 1997). Since high spatial frequency information can appear at a relatively lower contrast, the contrast sensitivity for higher spatial frequency content is much lower in humans. For this reason, a measurement of contrast sensitivity, Cut-off SF, which reveals the best resolution of visual performance, might better capture the ability of human observers to detect and encode the details (Arden, 1978; Marmor, 1986) than the measurement of visual acuity.

These results indicate that symptoms originating from accommodative and binocular dysfunction primarily impact the feeling of eyes and visual performance. Cut-off SF and binocular accommodative facility seem to be robust predictors of visual fatigue.

Correlations Among Accommodative Facility, Vergence Facility, and Contrast Sensitivity

Our results show that there are moderate correlations between accommodation/vergence and contrast sensitivity. We found that binocular accommodative facility is positively correlated with High CSF (shown in **Table 2**). Our results are consistent with those from previous studies. To illustrate, Muck (Mucke et al., 2010) reported that dynamic accommodation is related with contrast sensitivity at high spatial frequency. The faster the dynamic response, the more reduced the contrast sensitivity for high but not low spatial frequency (Mucke et al., 2010). To perform well in an accommodative facility test, individuals should have a good contrast sensitivity for high spatial frequency.

We found a strong negative correlation ($p < 0.01$) between vergence facility and Low CSF. This indicates that when Low CSF is lower, vergence facility is better. Vergence causes a rapid shift of the retina image, which causes one to neglect high spatial frequency information (Campbell and Wurtz, 1978; Burr and Ross, 1982). Suppression of low spatial frequency content takes place during convergence eye movement (i.e., vergence dynamics) (Mucke et al., 2013). This recent study agrees to what we report here, namely no correlation between vergence facility and High CSF, and the negative correlation between vergence facility and Low CSF (shown in **Table 2**).

Moreover, according to our results, symptomatic participants had worse binocular accommodative facility and vergence facility than asymptomatic ones. There are many studies that show similar findings to our results. For example, Hennessey et al. (1984); Levine et al. (1985) and Momeni-Moghaddam et al. (2014) found that accommodative facility and vergence facility are primary functions for accommodation and vergence. They also found that these two functions have a strong relationship with symptoms of visual fatigue (Garcia-Munoz et al., 2014). In addition, accommodative facility and vergence facility are important for reading (Dusek et al., 2011; CITT-ART Investigator Group et al., 2015). Compared to static accommodative amplitude and fusional range, dynamic function, such as facility, could be more pertinent to reading performance (Buzzelli, 1991; Grisham et al., 2007; Palomo-Alvarez and Puell, 2008; Dusek et al., 2010; Quaid and Simpson, 2013).

Moreover, our study uses the qCSF method (Lesmes et al., 2010), which is quick and reliable (Hou et al., 2010; Lesmes, 2010; Hou et al., 2016). In this study, we show that the correlation between clinical characteristics and areal measure from CSF can be used to explain the relationship between binocular dysfunction and visual performance (contrast sensitivity). This approach can be used not just for assessing visual fatigue but also other visual disorders.

In summary, visual fatigue disrupts the binocular ability of adult observers to encode fine details from their visual environment. Binocular accommodative facility and Cut-off SF were sensitive indexes to detect the influence of visual fatigue.

AUTHOR CONTRIBUTIONS

FZ, FH, and WYW contributed to conception and design of the study and performed the statistical analysis. FZ, JM, PH, and BC organized the database. FZ wrote the first draft of the manuscript. All authors contributed to manuscript revision, read, and approved the submitted version.

ACKNOWLEDGMENTS

We thank Chunwen Tao and Weiwei Lu for their help in data collection in this study. We thank Seung Hyun (Sam) Min (www.ses21.com) for editing the manuscript.

REFERENCES

Applegate, R. A., Howland, H. C., Sharp, R. P., Cottingham, A. J., and Yee, R. W. (1998). Corneal aberrations and visual performance after radial keratotomy. *J. Refract. Surg.* 14, 397–407. doi: 10.3928/1081-597x-19980701-05

Arden, G. B. (1978). The importance of measuring contrast sensitivity in cases of visual disturbance. *Br. J. Ophthalmol.* 62, 198–209. doi: 10.1136/bjo.62.4.198

Barten, P. G. J. (1999). *Contrast Sensitivity of the Human Eye and Its Effects on Image Quality*. USA: SPIE.

Bhanderi, D. J., Choudhary, S., and Doshi, V. G. (2008). A community-based study of asthenopia in computer operators. *Indian J. Ophthalmol.* 56, 51–55. doi: 10.4103/0301-4738.37596

Blehm, C., Vishnu, S., Khattak, A., Mitra, S., and Yee, R. W. (2005). Computer vision syndrome: a review. *Surv. Ophthalmol.* 50, 253–262.

Burr, D. C., and Ross, J. (1982). Contrast sensitivity at high velocities. *Vision Res.* 22, 479–484. doi: 10.1016/0042-6989(82)90196-1

Buzzelli, A. R. (1991). Stereopsis, accommodative and vergence facility: do they relate to dyslexia? *Optom. Vis. Sci.* 68, 842–846. doi: 10.1097/00006324-199111000-00002

Campbell, F. W., and Wurtz, R. H. (1978). Saccadic omission: why we do not see a grey-out during a saccadic eye movement. *Vision Res.* 18, 1297–1303. doi: 10.1016/0042-6989(78)90219-5

Chen, A. M., Roberts, T. L., Cotter, S. A., Kulp, M. T., Sinnott, L. T., Borsting, E. J., et al. (2021). Effectiveness of vergence/accommodative therapy for accommodative dysfunction in children with convergence insufficiency. *Ophthalmic. Physiol. Opt.* 41, 21–32.

Chen, M. K. (1986). The epidemiology of self-perceived fatigue among adults. *Prev. Med.* 15, 74–81. doi: 10.1016/0091-7435(86)90037-x

Chung, S. T. L., Legge, G. E., and Tjan, B. S. (2002). Spatial-frequency characteristics of letter identification in central and peripheral vision. *Vision Res.* 42, 2137–2152. doi: 10.1016/s0042-6989(02)00092-5

CITT-ART Investigator Group, M., Mitchell, G. L., Cotter, S. A., Kulp, M., Chase, C., et al. (2015). Convergence Insufficiency Treatment Trial - Attention and Reading Trial (CITT-ART): design and Methods. *Vis. Dev. Rehabil.* 1, 214–228. doi: 10.31707/vdr2015.1.3.p214

Dusek, W. A., Pierscionek, B. K., and McClelland, J. F. (2011). An evaluation of clinical treatment of convergence insufficiency for children with reading difficulties. *BMC Ophthalmol.* 11:21. doi: 10.1186/1471-2415-11-21

Dusek, W., Pierscionek, B. K., and McClelland, J. F. (2010). A survey of visual function in an Austrian population of school-age children with reading and writing difficulties. *BMC Ophthalmol.* 10:16. doi: 10.1186/1471-2415-10-16

Gall, R., and Wick, B. (2003). The symptomatic patient with normal phorias at distance and near: what tests detect a binocular vision problem? *Optometry* 74, 309–322.

Gandolfi, S. A., Cimino, L., Sangermani, C., Ungaro, N., Mora, P., and Tardini, M. G. (2005). Improvement of spatial contrast sensitivity threshold after surgical reduction of intraocular pressure in unilateral high-tension glaucoma. *Invest Ophthalmol. Vis. Sci.* 46, 197–201. doi: 10.1167/iovs.04-0199

García-Muñoz, Á, Carbonell-Bonete, S., and Cacho-Martínez, P. (2014). Symptomatology associated with accommodative and binocular vision anomalies. *J. Optom.* 7, 178–192. doi: 10.1016/j.optom.2014.06.005

Garcia-Munoz, A., Carbonell-Bonete, S., and Cacho-Martinez, P. (2014). Symptomatology associated with accommodative and binocular vision anomalies. *J. Optom.* 7, 178–192. doi: 10.1016/j.optom.2014.06.005

Golebiowski, B., Long, J., Harrison, K., Lee, A., Chidi-Egboka, N., and Asper, L. (2020). Smartphone Use and Effects on Tear Film, Blinking and Binocular Vision. *Curr. Eye Res.* 45, 428–434. doi: 10.1080/02713683.2019.1663542

Grisham, D., Powers, M., and Riles, P. (2007). Visual skills of poor readers in high school. *Optometry* 78, 542–549. doi: 10.1016/j.optm.2007.02.017

Han, C. C., Liu, R., Liu, R. R., Zhu, Z. H., Yu, R. B., and Ma, L. (2013). Prevalence of asthenopia and its risk factors in Chinese college students. *Int. J. Ophthalmol.* 6, 718–722.

Hashemi, H., Saatchi, M., Yekta, A., Ali, B., Ostadimoghaddam, H., Nabovati, P., et al. (2019). High Prevalence of Asthenopia among a Population of University Students. *J Ophthalmic Vis. Res.* 14, 474–482.

Hennessey, D., Iosue, R. A., and Rouse, M. W. (1984). Relation of symptoms to accommodative infacility of school-aged children. *Am. J. Optom. Physiol. Opt.* 61, 177–183. doi: 10.1097/00006324-198403000-00005

Hou, F., Huang, C. B., Lesmes, L., Feng, L. X., Tao, L., Zhou, Y. F., et al. (2010). qCSF in clinical application: efficient characterization and classification of contrast sensitivity functions in amblyopia. *Invest Ophthalmol. Vis. Sci.* 51, 5365–5377. doi: 10.1167/iovs.10-5468

Hou, F., Lesmes, L. A., Kim, W., Gu, H., Pitt, M. A., Myung, J. I., et al. (2016). Evaluating the performance of the quick CSF method in detecting contrast sensitivity function changes. *J. Vis.* 16:18. doi: 10.1167/16.6.18

Ip, J. M., Robaei, D., Rochtchina, E., and Mitchell, P. (2006). Prevalence of eye disorders in young children with eyestrain complaints. *Am. J. Ophthalmol.* 142, 495–497. doi: 10.1016/j.ajo.2006.03.047

Järvinen, P., and Hyvärinen, L. (1997). Contrast sensitivity measurement in evaluations of visual symptoms caused by exposure to triethylamine. *Occup. Environ. Med.* 54, 483–486. doi: 10.1136/oem.54.7.483

Kleiner, M. B., Brainard, D. H., Pelli, D. G., Ingling, A., and Broussard, C. (2007). What's new in Psychtoolbox-3? *Perception* 36, 301–307.

Kwon, M., and Legge, G. E. (2011). Spatial-frequency cutoff requirements for pattern recognition in central and peripheral vision. *Vision Res.* 51, 1995–2007. doi: 10.1016/j.visres.2011.06.020

Larese, F. F., Drusian, A., Ronchese, F., and Negro, C. (2019). Video Display Operator Complaints: a 10-Year Follow-Up of Visual Fatigue and Refractive Disorders. *Int. J. Environ. Res. Public Health* 16:2501. doi: 10.3390/ijerph16142501

Leroy, L. (2016). *Eyestrain Reduction in Stereoscopy.* United States: Wiley.

Lesmes, L. A. (2010). Bayesian adaptive estimation of the contrast sensitivity function: The quick CSF method. *J. Vis.* 10, 1–21. doi: 10.1167/10.3.17

Lesmes, L. A., Lu, Z. L., Baek, J., and Albright, T. D. (2010). Bayesian adaptive estimation of the contrast sensitivity function: the quick CSF method. *J. Vis.* 10, 17, 11–21.

Levine, S., Ciuffreda, K. J., Selenow, A., and Flax, N. (1985). Clinical assessment of accommodative facility in symptomatic and asymptomatic individuals. *J. Am. Optom. Assoc.* 56, 286–290.

Liu, J. S., Lee, M., Jang, J., Ciuffreda, K. J., Wong, J. H., Grisham, D., et al. (1979). Objective assessment of accommodation orthoptics. I. Dynamic insufficiency. *Am. J. Optom. Physiol. Opt.* 56, 285–294. doi: 10.1097/00006324-197905000-00002

Ma, M. M., Yeo, A. C. H., Scheiman, M., and Chen, X. (2019). Vergence and Accommodative Dysfunctions in Emmetropic and Myopic Chinese Young Adults. *J. Ophthalmol.* 2019:5904903.

Marmor, M. F. (1986). Contrast sensitivity versus visual acuity in retinal disease. *Br. J. Ophthalmol.* 70, 553–559. doi: 10.1136/bjo.70.7.553

Momeni-Moghaddam, H., Goss, D. A., and Dehvari, A. (2014). Vergence facility with stereoscopic and nonstereoscopic targets. *Optom. Vis. Sci.* 91, 522–527. doi: 10.1097/opx.0000000000000227

Mucke, S., Manahilov, V., Strang, N. C., Seidel, D., Gray, L. S., and Shahani, U. (2010). Investigating the mechanisms that may underlie the reduction in contrast sensitivity during dynamic accommodation. *J. Vis.* 10:5. doi: 10.1167/10.5.5

Mucke, S., Strang, N. C., Aydin, S., Mallen, E. A., Seidel, D., and Manahilov, V. (2013). Spatial frequency selectivity of visual suppression during convergence eye movements. *Vision Res.* 89, 96–101. doi: 10.1016/j.visres.2013.07.008

Oshika, T., Okamoto, C., Samejima, T., Tokunaga, T., and Miyata, K. (2006). Contrast Sensitivity Function and Ocular Higher-Order Wavefront Aberrations in Normal Human Eyes. *Ophthalmology* 113, 1807–1812. doi: 10.1016/j.ophtha.2006.03.061

Palomo-Alvarez, C., and Puell, M. C. (2008). Accommodative function in school children with reading difficulties. *Graefes Arch. Clin. Exp. Ophthalmol.* 246, 1769–1774. doi: 10.1007/s00417-008-0921-5

Quaid, P., and Simpson, T. (2013). Association between reading speed, cycloplegic refractive error, and oculomotor function in reading disabled children versus controls. *Graefes Arch. Clin. Exp. Ophthalmol.* 251, 169–187. doi: 10.1007/s00417-012-2135-0

Quant, J. R. (1992). The effect of sleep deprivation and sustained military operations on near visual performance. *Aviat Space Environ. Med.* 63, 172–176.

Regan, D., and Beverley, K. I. (1983). Visual fields described by contrast sensitivity, by acuity, and by relative sensitivity to different orientations. *Invest. Ophthalmol. Vis. Sci.* 24, 754–759.

Rosenfield, M. (2011). Computer vision syndrome: a review of ocular causes and potential treatments. *Ophthalmic Physiol. Opt.* 31, 502–515. doi: 10.1111/j.1475-1313.2011.00834.x

Scheiman, M., and Wick, B. (2014). *Clinical Management of Binocular Vision-Heterophoric, Accommodative, and Eye Movement Disorders.* Philadelphia, PA: Lippincott, Williams & Wilkins.

Sheedy, J. E., Hayes, J. N., and Engle, J. (2003). Is all asthenopia the same? *Optom. Vis. Sci.* 80, 732–739. doi: 10.1097/00006324-200311000-00008

Sheppard, A. L., and Wolffsohn, J. S. (2018). Digital eye strain: prevalence, measurement and amelioration. *BMJ Open Ophthalmol.* 3:e000146. doi: 10.1136/bmjophth-2018-000146

Sterner, B., Gellerstedt, M., and Sjostrom, A. (2006). Accommodation and the relationship to subjective symptoms with near work for young school children. *Ophthalmic Physiol. Opt.* 26, 148–155. doi: 10.1111/j.1475-1313.2006.00364.x

Tiwari, R. R. (2013). Eyestrain in working children of footwear making units of Agra, India. *Indian Pediatr.* 50, 411–413. doi: 10.1007/s13312-013-0117-x

Tiwari, R. R., Saha, A., and Parikh, J. R. (2011). Asthenopia (eyestrain) in working children of gem-polishing industries. *Toxicol. Ind. Health* 27, 243–247. doi: 10.1177/0748233710386407

Vilela, M. A., Pellanda, L. C., Fassa, A. G., and Castagno, V. D. (2015). Prevalence of asthenopia in children: a systematic review with meta-analysis. *J. Pediatr.* 91, 320–325. doi: 10.1016/j.jped.2014.10.008

Wilkins, A. (1995). *Visual Stress.* Oxford: Oxford University Press.

Yan, F. F., Hou, F., Lu, Z. L., Hu, X., and Huang, C. B. (2010). qCSF in Clinical Application: efficient Characterization and Classification of Contrast Sensitivity Functions in Amblyopia. *Invest Ophthalmol. Vis. Sci.* 7, 5365–5377.

Yang, S., and James, S. E. (2011). *Effects of Vergence and Accommodative Responses on Viewer's Comfort in Viewing 3D Stimuli.* United States: Pacific University College of Optometry.

Zhang, X., An, X., Liu, H., Peng, J., Cai, S., Wang, W., et al. (2015). The Topographical Arrangement of Cutoff Spatial Frequencies across Lower and Upper Visual Fields in Mouse V1. *Entific Rep.* 5:7734.

Zheng, H., Wang, C., Cui, R., He, X., Shen, M., Lesmes, L. A., et al. (2018). Measuring the Contrast Sensitivity Function Using the qCSF Method With 10 Digits. *Transl. Vis Sci. Technol.* 7:9. doi: 10.1167/tvst.7.6.9

13

Time Course of Perceived Visual Distortion and Axial Length Growth in Myopic Children Undergoing Orthokeratology

Guihua Liu[1], Yiyuan Wu[1], Hua Bi[2], Biying Wang[1], Tianpu Gu[1], Bei Du[1], Jianliang Tong[3], Bin Zhang[2†] and Ruihua Wei[1*†]*

[1] *Tianjin Key Laboratory of Retinal Functions and Diseases, Tianjin Branch of National Clinical Research Center for Ocular Disease, Eye Institute and School of Optometry, Tianjin Medical University Eye Hospital, Tianjin, China,* [2] *College of Optometry, Nova Southeastern University, Davie, FL, United States,* [3] *Doctor's Exchange of Georgia PC, Lawrenceville, GA, United States*

***Correspondence:**
Bin Zhang
bz52@nova.edu
Ruihua Wei
rwei@tmu.edu.cn

† These authors have contributed equally to this work

Purpose: To establish the time course of the subjective visual function changes during the first month of orthokeratology treatment in myopic children, and to investigate how the time course variations are associated with the objective optical quality changes and the axial length growth (ALG) after 1 year of treatment.

Methods: A total of 58 myopic children aged from 8 to 16 years participated in this self-controlled prospective study. All subjects were fitted with designed spherical four-zone orthokeratology lenses. Subjective visual function was evaluated with orientation discrimination threshold (ODT), and objective optical quality was quantified with the high-order aberration root-mean-square (HOA-RMS) and the changing speed of HOA. The measurements were done before the lens fitting and 1 day, 1-, 2-, and 4-weeks after lens wear. Axial length was obtained at baseline and 1-year follow-up, and ALG was defined as the difference. One-way ANOVA was conducted to compare the difference for statistical analysis.

Results: After lens fitting, the ODT time courses peaked on day 1 in 28 children, 1 week in 15 children, 2 weeks in 11 children, and 4 weeks in 4 children. In contrast, the HOA-RMS steadily rose during the first month, and the changing speed of HOA was only transiently elevated on day 1 after the initial lens wear. The ALG was 0.12 ± 0.20 mm in subjects whose ODT peaked at day 1, 0.08 ± 0.09 mm in subjects whose ODT peaked on 1-week, and 0.12 ± 0.15 mm in subjects whose ODT peaked on 2-week or later. There was no difference in axial growth among the subjects whose ODT peaked at different days ($P = 0.734$).

Conclusion: While half ODT time course resembled the changing speed of HOA with a transient elevation on day 1, about a quarter of the ODT time course resemble the steadily rising of HOA-RMS, and the rest was located in the middle. The ALGs in children with different types of ODT time courses were similar.

Keywords: orientation discrimination threshold, high-order aberration, visual distortion, axial length, orthokeratology

INTRODUCTION

The prevalence of myopia has dramatically elevated over the past several decades, especially in East Asian countries and regions (Pan et al., 2015; Holden et al., 2016), where up to 90% of teenagers and young adults in China and 96.5% of 19-year-old men in Seoul are myopic (Dolgin, 2015). It is also one of the World Health Organization's immediate concerns (Fricke et al., 2012). Among optical methods developed to retard myopia progress, orthokeratology is one of the most often applied devices in clinics. It is a rigid contact lens with a reverse geometry on its back surface. It alters the shape of the front corneal surface through overnight wearing (Nichols et al., 2000). During the daytime, the cornea's flattened central portion reduces refractive errors and improves visual acuity (Swarbrick, 2006). The steepened mid-peripheral cornea can induce a myopic defocus shift on the retina, which may be the underlying mechanism for axial growth retardation. Orthokeratology lens can reduce 32–63% per year in subjects of different ethnicities (Charm and Cho, 2013; Li et al., 2017; Santodomingo-Rubido et al., 2017).

With an altered front optical surface, the OK lens also leads to increased optical aberrations and straying light in the patients undergoing such treatment (Hiraoka et al., 2007; Liu et al., 2017). Higher-order aberrations sharply increased 7 days after lens wearing and remained high when measured 1-year treatment (Stillitano et al., 2008; Santolaria Sanz et al., 2015; Santolaria-Sanz et al., 2016; Xia et al., 2020). However, patients' visual performances wearing orthokeratology lenses were surprisingly good. In adult patients aged 18–43, the perceived visual distortion was measured by reporting if the briefly turn-on LED lights were visible in the peripheral visual field. It transiently increased 1 day after lens fitting and returned to baseline level 1 week after lens wearing (Santolaria Sanz et al., 2015; Santolaria-Sanz et al., 2016). In children aged between 8 and 14, the threshold to detect shape distortion was not significantly different from the baseline level at 1 week and 1 month after the lens wear (Xia et al., 2020). Rapid neural adaptation was proposed to explain the disparity between subjective visual function and optical quality.

However, several vital questions remained unclear. Firstly, the adult study reported the average trend of light distortion perceived and did not disclose the variance among individuals' time courses. Since it is unlikely that everyone returned to baseline level at 1 week, it would be more informative by revealing the time course variations. Secondly, the children's study had the first follow-up visit scheduled 1 week after the initial lens wear. It is not clear if the transient elevation in light distortion reported in adults also exists in children or only in a part of the children. More importantly, neither study provided the axial growth data. The children's research stopped at 1 month. Although the adult study had a 1-year follow-up, the author did not report the axial length growth probably because axial length in adults was insignificant. It is unclear if the variations in light distortion time course are associated with differential axial length growth.

In the present study, we aimed to track the changes in visual distortion with the orientation discrimination threshold (ODT) method during the first month of lens-wear and measure the axial length growth over a year. Moreover, we attempted to clarify if the variations in light distortion time course are associated with axial length growth.

MATERIALS AND METHODS

Subjects

This self-controlled prospective study was conducted at the Tianjin Medical University Eye Hospital (Tianjin, China) between September 2019 and November 2020. The inclusion criteria were: aged between 8 and 16 years; myopia greater than −0.75 D and less than −5.00 D; with-the-rule astigmatism less than −1.5 D; best-corrected monocular optical acuity better than 20/20; no strabismus or ocular surface disease; no history of surgery or contact lens wear. This study protocol adhered to the Declaration of Helsinki's tenets and was approved by the Ethics Committee of Tianjin Medical University Eye Hospital. After being informed of the potential risks related to this study, all subjects and their guardians signed informed consent forms before any procedures were performed. Only right eye data were taken into analysis to avoid the interference caused by the interocular correlation.

Measurements

Uncorrected visual acuity, subjective refraction, high-order aberration, and orientation discrimination threshold (ODT) tests were measured before the lens fitting and 1 day, 7 days, 14 days, and 1 month after lens dispatch. Axial length was measured at baseline and 1-year follow-up.

Orthokeratology

Subjects were fitted with spherical four-zone orthokeratology lenses (Euclid Systems Corporation, Herndon, United States) composed of oprifocon A (Boston EQUALENS II) with an oxygen permeability (DK) of 85×10^{-11} ($cm^{2/}s$) (mL O_2/mL mmHg). Total lens diameter ranged from 10.6 to 10.8 mm, the back optic zone diameter (BOZD) was 6.0 mm, and the reverse curve (RC) width was between 0.6 and 0.8 mm. The lens fitting procedures strictly followed the guidelines provided by the lens manufacturer. In brief, lenses were first selected based on the measurements of a subject's horizontal visible iris diameter (Lenstar LS900; Haag-Streit AG, Bern, Switzerland), the flat-*K* value of the 3 mm zone, and corneal eccentricity value (Medmont E300; Medmont International Pty., Ltd., Nunawading, VIC, Australia). Fitting quality was evaluated by fluorescence staining 1 h after the lens dispatch. A good fitting was indicated by an optical zone coving the pupil, no apparent decentration of the lens, lens movement less than 1 mm with blinks, and a bulls-eye pattern with fluorescence staining. After lens delivery, subjects were required to wear the lens for more than 8 h per night and at least 6 days per week.

High-Order Aberration

Corneal topography was obtained with Pentacam (OCULUS Optikgeräte GmbH, Wetzlar, Germany) (Pinero et al., 2009; Greenstein et al., 2012; Rudolph et al., 2012; Gyldenkerne et al., 2015). The system's internal software

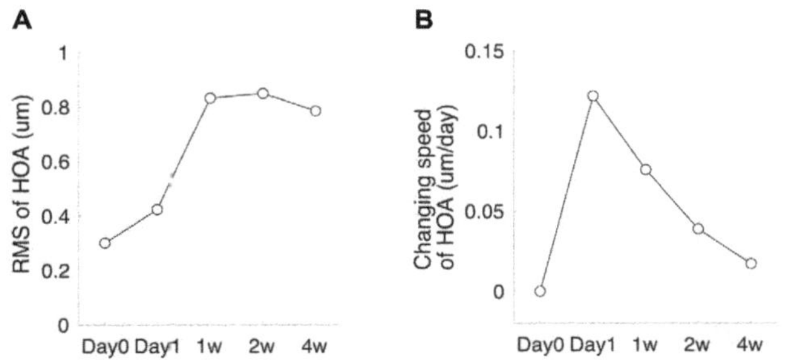

FIGURE 1 | High-order aberration (HOA) measurement schedule. **(A)** A subject's HOA-FMS. **(B)** The subject's changing speed of HOA at each follow-up visit.

automatically decomposed the corneal elevation data into Zernike polynomials up to the 10th order (Pinero et al., 2009). The root-mean-square (RMS) of total higher-order aberrations (HOA, 3rd–6th orders) aberrations were extracted from the central corneal zones with a diameter of 6 mm. During the measurement, the Pentacam uses a blue Light Emitting Diode (LED) slit beam to illuminate a cornea and anterior chamber. The subject was instructed to fixate on a target in the center of the slit beam. Three scans were taken per eye. Each scan was automatically assigned a quality score by the system, and only the scan with an acceptable score was taken into analysis. Low-quality scans were deleted, and the measurements were repeated. The changing speed of HOA-RMS was calculated as the difference between the two follow-up visits divided by the number of days between the two visits (**Figure 1**).

Orientation Discrimination Threshold Test

Orientation discrimination threshold test stimuli were presented on a 24.1-inch (48 cm × 26 cm) screen (AOC22732, 1920 × 1080 pixels, 60 Hz) at a viewing distance of 1 m. Each pixel subtended a visual angle of 0.66 arcmins horizontally and vertically. All patients were tested monocularly as the non-tested eye occluded with an opaque patch. The tested eye's distance refractive error was corrected if the visual acuity was less than 20/20. Before each trial, a subject fixated at the center of a 4-degree-diameter ring, within which test stimuli were presented. Following a button press, the ring disappeared and, after a 1 s delay, the first stimulus pattern was presented for 50 ms, followed by a 200 ms blank interval. The fixation ring then reappeared for 50 ms; the second stimulus pattern was presented 1 s later for 50 ms and was followed by a 200 ms blank interval. The duration of each pattern was set at 50 ms to minimize the effect of scanning eye movements (Fu et al., 2017; Chen et al., 2018). All ODT tests were performed with full optical correction to remove the lower order aberrations, including defocus and astigmatism.

One stimulus pattern presented at each trial consisted of four bright parallel lines, each of which was two pixels (1.3 arcmin) wide and 0.4° in length, presented vertically on a dark background. Each line was randomly located inside the preceding fixation ring, and the distance between two adjacent lines was at least 0.5° to prevent overlap. The other stimulus pattern had the same arrangement except that the orientations of the four lines were randomly deviated from the vertical direction according to a standard deviation (SD). At each trial, the subject had to decide which pattern contained the parallel vertical lines. The order of the parallel and non-parallel line patterns varied randomly from trial to trial (**Figure 2**).

The test was programmed in MATLAB (MathWorks, Natick, MA, United States) and Psychophysics Toolbox version 3 (Brainard, 1997). A Bayesian adaptive two-alternative forced-choice task based on the ZEST algorithm was used (King-Smith et al., 1994). From trial to trial, the program adjusted the non-parallel lines' SD based on the subject's previous responses. A Weibull function with a slope of 3.5 was used as the likelihood function in the ZEST algorithm. The initial angular SD was set at 8° according to values from a previous study. After each trial, the probability density function (PDF) of the experimentally determined angular SD was updated by multiplying the likelihood function with the prior PDF until the confidence interval for the PDF was less than 0.3 log units or a total of 30 trials were finished. The output SD, which was equal

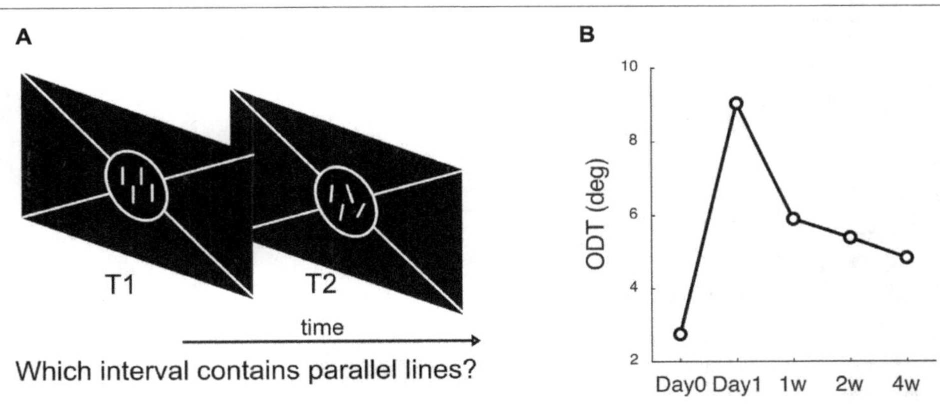

FIGURE 2 | Methods to measure ODT. **(A)** The subject's task was to answer which interval contains the parallel lines, 1st or 2nd. **(B)** A subject's ODT measured at each follow-up visit.

to the final PDF's mean, was defined as the ODT. Testing of each eye required about 2 min to finish.

Each subject's ODT was measured three times at each visit, and the average value was taken into analysis. The test-retest reproducibility was quantified with the intraclass correlation coefficient (ICC), and a value greater than 0.75 indicated good reliability (Chen et al., 2018).

Axial Length

Axial length was measured with a non-contact biometer (Lenstar LS-900; Haag-Streit AG, Bern, Switzerland). Subjects were asked to keep both eyes open and fixate on the target. Between measurements, subjects blinked multiple times to ensure an intact tear film to minimize potential measurement errors. Five measurements were taken for each axial length measurement, and only the repeats with intra-session differences less than 0.02 mm were averaged and recorded.

Statistical Analysis

The means and standard deviations of ODT, HOA-RMS, HOA changing speed, axial length growth were computed for descriptive purposes. One-way ANOVA was used to compare if the differences among groups were significant. All statistical analyses were performed using R software (version 3.2.2)[1]. A p-value < 0.05 value was defined as statistically significant.

RESULTS

Among a total of 65 subjects who were enrolled initially, 58 completed all follow-up examinations [30 males and 28 females, mean age 12.10 ± 2.01 years (range: 8 –16 years)]. All participants were first categorized according to the time at which ODT peaked. In 28 children, ODT reached the peak 1 day of OK lens wear and declined afterward. Fifteen children had ODT reaching the peak at 1 week and decreased thereafter. In 11 and 4 children, the ODT reached the peak at 2 weeks and 4 weeks after the initial lens wearing, respectively (top tows, **Figure 3**). However, regardless of the peaking time of ODT, HOA-RMS increased steadily during the first month after lens wear (middle row, **Figure 3**). The changing speed of HOA was transiently elevated

[1]http://www.R-project.org/

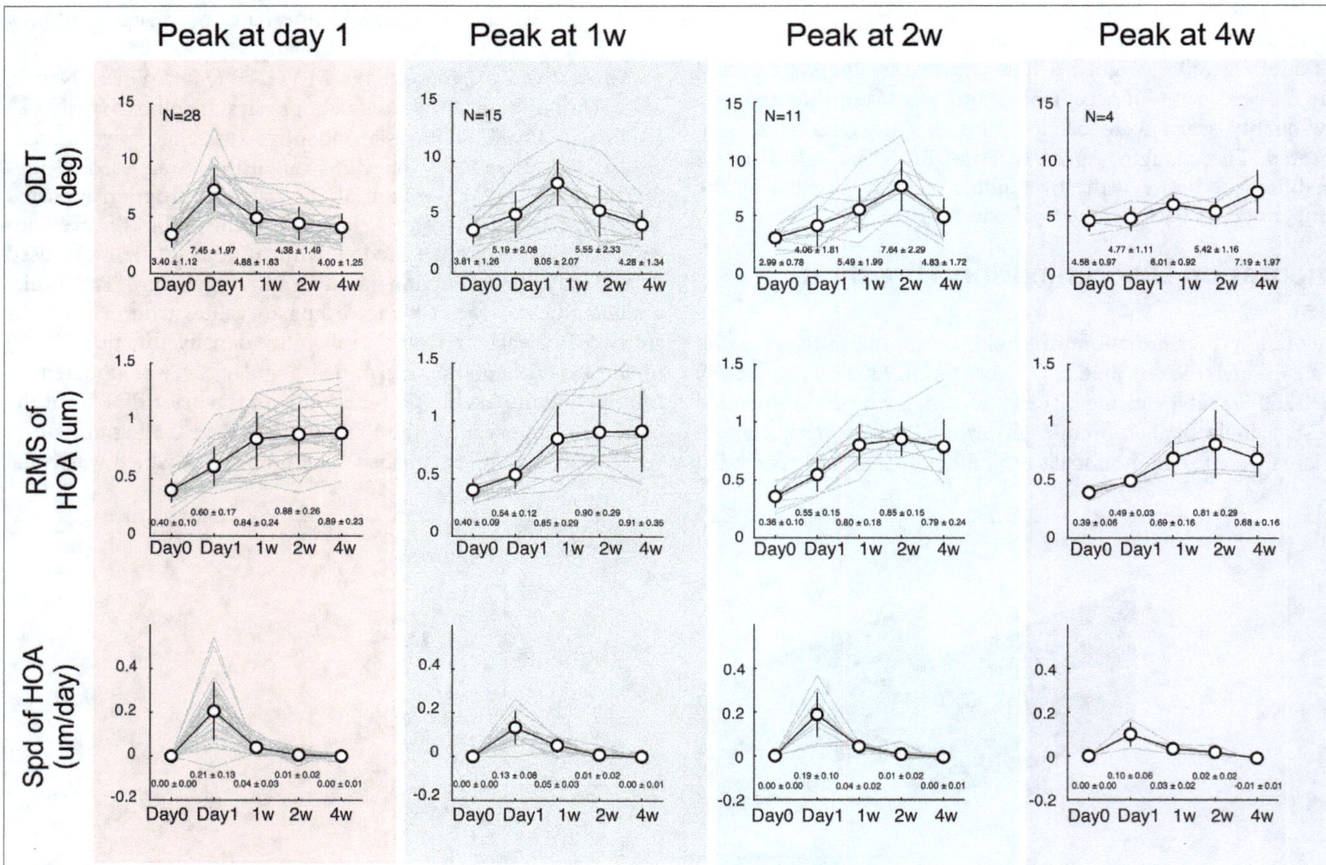

FIGURE 3 | Time courses separated according to the ODT peaking time. Top row: discrimination threshold (ODT), Middle row: Residua Mean Square (RMS) of high-order aberrations (HOA), Bottom row: changing speeding of HOA. The left column shows subjects whose ODT peaked at day 1 (red shade); the middle column shows subjects whose ODT peaked at 1 week (gray shade), and the right two columns show subjects whose ODT peaked at 2 weeks (blue shade) or 4 weeks (purple shade), respectively.

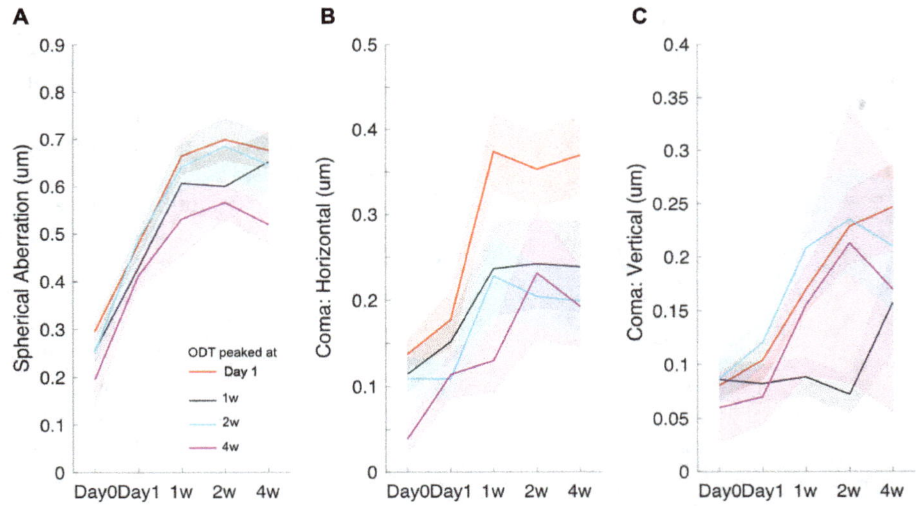

FIGURE 4 | Time courses of spherical aberration **(A)**, horizontal coma **(B)**, and vertical coma **(C)**. Redline: subjects whose ODT peaked at day 1, black line: subjects whose ODT peaked at 1 week, blue line: subjects whose ODT peaked at 2 weeks, and purple line: subjects whose ODT peaked at 4 weeks. The shaded area indicates mean ± one standard error.

on the first day after the lens wear and immediately declined afterward (bottom row, **Figure 3**).

The time course for spherical aberration (**Figure 4A**), coma horizontal (**Figure 4B**), and coma vertical (**Figure 4C**) did not appear to match the ODT time course. Spherical aberration significantly increased in all subjects and reached the peak mostly around 2 weeks (one-way ANOVA, $p < 0.001$ in all four groups). Horizontal coma component significantly increased in the subjects whose ODT peaked at day 1 (one-way ANOVA, $p < 0.001$). However, the peak value of horizontal coma was reached at 1 week and remained high afterward. Horizontal coma in other groups showed increased trend, but not reaching significant level [one-way ANOVA, $p = 0.15$ for subjects whose ODT peaked at 1 week (black), $p = 0.06$ for subjects whose ODT peaked at 2 weeks (blue), and $p = 0.08$ for subjects whose ODT peaked at 4 weeks (purple)]. Similar patterns were found in vertical coma component.

To explore the effect of age on the ODT time course, subjects were separated into three age groups (8–11 years, 12–14 years, and 15–16 years), and the mean ODT time courses were computed (**Figure 5**). Subjects in the youngest group and oldest group both reached the peak on day 1.

In each subject, we normalized the HOA-RMS and the changing speed of HOA to its peak value, respectively. Normalization did not change the shape of the time courses, and there was no significant correlation between the two normalized indexes ($r = -0.24$, $p = 0.09$) population-wise. Therefore, the ODT time course could be decomposed as a linear combination of the time courses of the normalized HOA-RMS and the changing speed of HOA (**Figure 6A**). The subjects whose ODT peaked at 2-week or later had greater coefficient values in HOA-RMS and small coefficient values in HOA changing speed (Blue dots, **Figure 6B**). Those subjects' ODT time courses had a high resemblance to the HOA-RMS time course and were less parallel to the HOA changing speed time course. In other words, they may have weak adaptation to HOA-RMS and strong adaptation to HOA changing speed. The subjects whose ODT time course peaked at day 1 had a small coefficient on HOA-RMS and a large coefficient value on HOA changing speed. Their ODT time courses had less resemblance to the HOA-RMS time course and were more parallel to the HOA-changing speed's time course. In other words, they may have a strong adaptation to HOA-RMS and a weak adaptation to the HOA changing speed (Red dots, **Figure 6**). The subjects with ODT peaked at 1 week were located in the middle and had similar coefficient values to either HOA-RMS or HOA changing speed (Black dots, **Figure 6**).

The axial length growth was significantly correlated with baseline age ($r = -0.61$, $P < 0.001$). However, there was no difference in axial growth among the subjects whose ODT peaked at different days (one-way ANOVA, $P = 0.73$). There was also no difference in age among the subjects who showed ODT peak at different days (One-way ANOVA, $P = 0.44$) (**Figure 7**).

DISCUSSION

The most critical finding in the present study is ODT time courses' variations. Instead of uniformly peaking 1 week after the initial lens-wear, about half of the subjects experienced a transient increase in ODT, a quarter reached the peak at 1 week, and a quarter peaked relatively late at 2 weeks or later. In contrast, the time course of HOA-RMS and HOA changing speed were quite similar across different subjects. HOA changing speed only had a transient increment on day 1, and the HOA-RMS time course steadily rose during the first month. We proposed that the ODT time course could be interpreted as a combination of the time courses of HOA changing speed and HOA-RMS, and neural adaptation plays an important role underlying the

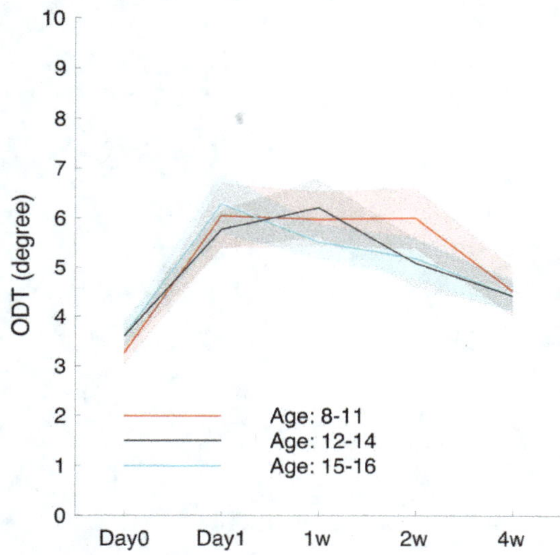

FIGURE 5 | The averaged ODT time course for subjects grouped by age.

variance in the ODT time course. The other essential finding was that ODT time courses' variations were not associated with axial length growth and age.

Orientation Discrimination Threshold Peaking After 1 Week

One key difference between the present study and previous studies was that half of the subjects had ODT peaking at 1 week or later. Previous studies done in both adults and children reported no changes in visual performance 1 week after the initial lens-wear (Santolaria Sanz et al., 2015; Santolaria-Sanz et al., 2016; Xia et al., 2020). This study captured the ODT peaking both before and after 1 week of lens wear. The difference could partially be attributed to the different methods used to evaluate subjective visual distortion. The human visual system may utilize two mechanisms to minimize distortion perception. When the information sent from a retina region is distorted or missing, the central visual system can take the information from surrounding regions into processing to "fill in" or complete the visual scene (Ramachandran and Gregory, 1991; De Weerd et al., 1995). Moreover, due to the relatively long stimulus presentation duration, subjects may not maintain steady fixation throughout the examination (Tarita-Nistor et al., 2012, 2017). Unstable fixation may "average" all distorted or missing lines over time. The spatial and temporal redundancy embedded in the methods used by previous studies facilitates the process of "filling-in" and "averaging." In the children's study, the visual stimulus used was a radial pattern covering 360°, making the filling-in easier (Xia et al., 2020). The visual stimulus used in the adult study was not static. Instead, it moved from the periphery toward the center along the pre-defined semi-meridians, which increased the possibility of unstable fixation. The stimulus presentation duration was 250–750 ms in the adult studies (Santolaria Sanz et al., 2015; Santolaria-Sanz et al., 2016) and 500 ms in the children study (Xia et al., 2020). That long fixation time allows for unstable eye fixation and eye movements. Such two processes can mask the early and subtle functional changes until the function's loss becomes sufficient to exceed the threshold. For the ODT test used in this present study, a short and randomly distributed set

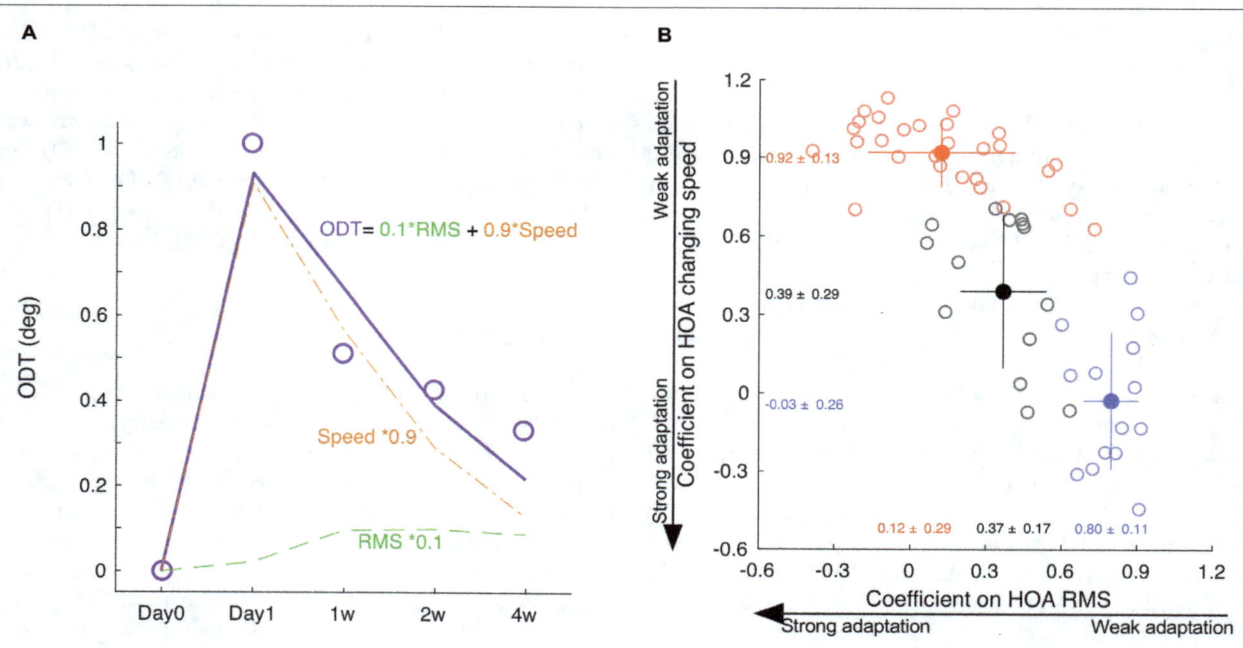

FIGURE 6 | The decomposition of ODT time course. **(A)** The ODT time course is decomposed as a linear combination of the time courses of HOA-RMS and HOA changing speed. **(B)** The distribution of coefficients of subjects peaked at day 1 (red), day 7 (black), and at or after day 14 (blue). SPD, speed. * means multiplication.

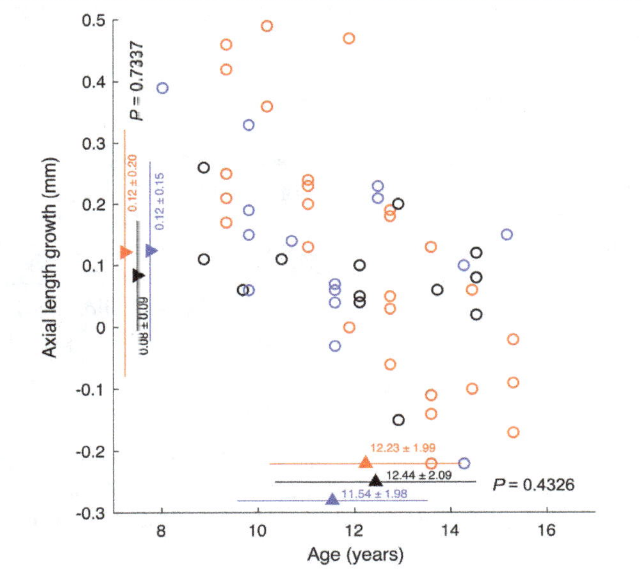

FIGURE 7 | The correlation between axial length growth and age. Circles indicating subjects whose ODT peaked at day 1 (red), 1 week (black), and 2 weeks or later (blue).

of line segments was used to minimize the "fill in" phenomenon (Williams et al., 1984). The present study's stimulus duration was only 50 ms, too short to trigger saccadic eye movements. Such a design minimizes the possibility of "average."

Variations in Orientation Discrimination Threshold Time Course and Adaptation

When the environment changes, the visual system's adaptation is a mechanism to achieve satisfactory performance (Clifford et al., 2007). Adaptation has been displayed in light (Matesanz et al., 2011; Takemura et al., 2020), color (Eisner and Enoch, 1982; Neitz et al., 2002; Delahunt et al., 2004; Belmore and Shevell, 2008, 2011), contrast (Kwon et al., 2009; Bao and Engel, 2012; Bao et al., 2013), distortion and blur (Adams et al., 2001; Yehezkel et al., 2010; Habtegiorgis et al., 2017, 2018). The significantly increased high order aberrations reported in this study were consistent with previous studies on orthokeratology lens (Santolaria Sanz et al., 2015; Santolaria-Sanz et al., 2016; Xia et al., 2020). Here, we propose that neural adaptation may have played an essential role in the emergence of different types of time courses of ODT. HOA's changing speed was only significantly elevated on day 1, while the HOA-RMS steadily rose during the first month following lens-wear. The subjects whose ODT peaked at day 1 did not adapt well to the transient elevation in the changing speed of HOA and adapted well to the steadily rising HOA-RMS. This may explain the large coefficient in changing speed of HOA and the small coefficient in HOA-RMS. On the other extreme, the subjects whose ODT peaked at 2 weeks or later adapted well to the transient elevation in HOA changing speed but were slow at adapting to the steadily rising HOA-RMS. This may explain the small coefficient in changing speed of HOA and the large coefficient in HOA-RMS. With only four subjects peaking at 4-week, the steadily rising HOA-RMS adaptation was mostly completed by the end of the first month. This was consistent with a previous study showing that the lack of adaptation to image distortion is the cause of long-term visual discomfort for some novices with progressive extra glasses (Meister and Fisher, 2008). The 15 subjects whose ODT peaked at 1 week were mixed cases in the middle, with relatively balanced adaptation to either the transient elevation of HOA changing speed and steadily rising HOA-RMS.

No Correlation Between Orientation Discrimination Threshold Time Course and Axial Length Growth

The second vital finding from this present study was that axial length growth was not different in the three different categories of subjects. This indicates that whether a subject can adapt to the HOA-RMS or HOA change is not influential in determining the axial growth. This result was consistent with the findings that an intact retina-brain link was not required for axial growth. In chicks with optic nerve sectioned, optically occluded eyes demonstrated longer axial growth than those of non-occluded eyes (Troilo et al., 1987). Compensation to hyperopic defocus was found in chicks with either or both optic nerve section (ONS) and ciliary nerve section (CNS; Miles and Wallman, 1990; Diether and Schaeffel, 1997; Wildsoet, 2003). The myopia progression depends on retina local cues (Wallman et al., 1987). Such a mechanism was also confirmed in primates (Smith et al., 2009; Read et al., 2010).

In this study, the subjects who peaked at different days had no age difference. This is in contrast to the findings in other previous studies. For example, Li reported that younger children might have an easier or faster adaptation to the lenses, which could compensate for the optical disturbance induced by lenslets while looking through the lenses' peripheral parts. Better adaptation of blur and acceptance of the lenses were also found in younger children wearing Defocus Incorporated Multiple Segments (DIMS; Lu et al., 2020). Adults were more sensitive to the visual symptoms by reporting headaches and dizziness after wearing DIMS. Furthermore, in contrast to 85% of the children who were willing to wear DIMS lenses, the acceptance rate in adults was only 60% due to unbearable discomfort. Chang and Cheng (2020) reported decreased contrast sensitivity resulting from optical and neural components of visual processing and revealed a greater extent in adults than children after wearing orthokeratology for 28 days.

Limitations of Our Study

This present study has several limitations. First, we only measured cornea HOA, but the whole-eye HOA. With orthokeratology lens alters the front surface of the cornea, the difference between these two types of HOA should be slight. Second, both HOA measurement and ODT test were done in monocular conditions, which is different from the daily use of binocular vision (Brito et al., 2015; Santolaria Sanz et al., 2015). Third, the association between ODT values and the subjects' visual distortions, such as ghosts, haloes, and starbursts, is unclear. Fourth, we did not evaluate other factors contributing to visual distortion, such as contrast sensitivity changes (Santolaria Sanz et al., 2015; Santolaria-Sanz et al., 2016) and pupil size (Chen et al., 2012).

Clinical Significance

The time course revealed from this present study provided guidance on expecting visual discomforts reported by children who received orthokeratology. Half of the complaints would be anticipated at day 1, and the majority of the visual discomforts should be reported within the first week. Any visual discomforts reported beyond 2 weeks deserve more attention from the clinicians. Recently, it has been reported that persons with different personalities may have different sensitivity to image quality (Woods-2010). People who lack confidence tend to hesitate at reporting blurred images and choose to endure them while waiting for more substantial evidence to emerge. Therefore, a questionnaire on personality would help predict the subjective complaints from the children undergoing orthokeratology. Meanwhile, the clinician should have confidence in the outcome of orthokeratology. Even a patient who has late visual discomfort can achieve good axial growth retardation.

CONCLUSION

In children who underwent orthokeratology treatment, their ODT significantly increased during the first month after the initial lens wear. While 25% of the children, the ODT time course resembles the HOA-RMS, which showed a steady increase, about half ODT time course resemble the changing speed of HOA, which was most significant during the first day. Children with different types of ODT time courses showed similar axial growth.

AUTHOR CONTRIBUTIONS

BZ, RW, and GL conceived the experiments. HB, GL, and JT determined the experimental methods. YW, TG, and BD performed the experiments. BZ and GL analyzed and interpreted the data. BW and GL wrote the manuscript. BZ and RW modified the manuscript. All authors contributed to manuscript revision, read, and approved the submitted version.

REFERENCES

Adams, W. J., Banks, M. S., and van Ee, R. (2001). Adaptation to three-dimensional distortions in human vision. *Nat. Neurosci.* 4, 1063–1064. doi: 10.1038/nn729

Bao, M., and Engel, S. A. (2012). Distinct mechanism for long-term contrast adaptation. *Proc. Natl. Acad. Sci. U.S.A.* 109, 5898–5903. doi: 10.1073/pnas.1113503109

Bao, M., Fast, E., Mesik, J., and Engel, S. (2013). Distinct mechanisms control contrast adaptation over different timescales. *J. Vis.* 13:14. doi: 10.1167/13.10.14

Belmore, S. C., and Shevell, S. K. (2008). Very-long-term chromatic adaptation: test of gain theory and a new method. *Vis. Neurosci.* 25, 411–414. doi: 10.1017/S0952523808080450

Belmore, S. C., and Shevell, S. K. (2011). Very-long-term and short-term chromatic adaptation: are their influences cumulative? *Vis. Res.* 51, 362–366. doi: 10.1016/j.visres.2010.11.011

Brainard, D. H. (1997). The psychophysics toolbox. *Spat. Vis.* 10, 433–436.

Brito, P., Salgado-Borges, J., Neves, H., Gonzalez-Meijome, J., and Monteiro, M. (2015). Light-distortion analysis as a possible indicator of visual quality after refractive lens exchange with diffractive multifocal intraocular lenses. *J. Cataract Refract. Surg.* 41, 613–622. doi: 10.1016/j.jcrs.2014.07.033

Chang, C. F., and Cheng, H. C. (2020). Effect of orthokeratology lens on contrast sensitivity function and high-order aberrations in children and adults. *Eye Contact Lens* 46, 375–380. doi: 10.1097/ICL.0000000000000667

Charm, J., and Cho, P. (2013). High myopia-partial reduction ortho-k: a 2-year randomized study. *Optom. Vis. Sci.* 90, 530–539. doi: 10.1097/OPX.0b013e318293657d

Chen, T., Su, B., Chen, Z., Tong, J., Bedell, H., Song, Z., et al. (2018). The associations among metamorphopsia, orientation discrimination threshold, and retinal layer thickness in patients with idiopathic epiretinal membrane. *Curr. Eye Res.* 43, 1151–1159. doi: 10.1080/02713683.2018.1481515

Chen, Z., Niu, L., Xue, F., Qu, X., Zhou, Z., Zhou, X., et al. (2012). Impact of pupil diameter on axial growth in orthokeratology. *Optom. Vis. Sci.* 89, 1636–1640. doi: 10.1097/OPX.0b013e31826c1831

Clifford, C. W., Webster, M. A., Stanley, G. B., Stocker, A. A., Kohn, A., Sharpee, T. O., et al. (2007). Visual adaptation: neural, psychological and computational aspects. *Vis. Res.* 47, 3125–3131. doi: 10.1016/j.visres.2007.08.023

De Weerd, P., Gattass, R., Desimone, R., and Ungerleider, L. G. (1995). Responses of cells in monkey visual cortex during perceptual filling-in of an artificial scotoma. *Nature* 377, 731–734. doi: 10.1038/377731a0

Delahunt, P. B., Webster, M. A., Ma, L., and Werner, J. S. (2004). Long-term renormalization of chromatic mechanisms following cataract surgery. *Vis. Neurosci.* 21, 301–307. doi: 10.1017/s0952523804213025

Diether, S., and Schaeffel, F. (1997). Local changes in eye growth induced by imposed local refractive error despite active accommodation. *Vis. Res.* 37, 659–668. doi: 10.1016/s0042-6989(96)00224-6

Dolgin, E. (2015). The myopia boom. *Nature* 519, 276–278. doi: 10.1038/519276a

Eisner, A., and Enoch, J. M. (1982). Some effects of 1 week's monocular exposure to long-wavelength stimuli. *Percept. Psychophys.* 31, 169–174. doi: 10.3758/bf03206217

Fricke, T. R., Holden, B. A., Wilson, D. A., Schlenther, G., Naidoo, K. S., Resnikoff, S., et al. (2012). Global cost of correcting vision impairment from uncorrected refractive error. *Bull. World Health Organ.* 90, 728–738. doi: 10.2471/BLT.12.104034

Fu, H., Zhang, B., Tong, J., Bedell, H., Zhang, H., Yang, Y., et al. (2017). Relationships of orientation discrimination threshold and visual acuity with macular lesions in age-related macular degeneration. *PLoS One* 12:e0185070. doi: 10.1371/journal.pone.0185070

Greenstein, S. A., Fry, K. L., Hersh, M. J., and Hersh, P. S. (2012). Higher-order aberrations after corneal collagen crosslinking for keratoconus and corneal ectasia. *J. Cataract. Refract. Surg.* 38, 292–302. doi: 10.1016/j.jcrs.2011.08.041

Gyldenkerne, A., Ivarsen, A., and Hjortdal, J. O. (2015). Comparison of corneal shape changes and aberrations induced By FS-LASIK and SMILE for myopia. *J. Refract. Surg.* 31, 223–229. doi: 10.3928/1081597X-20150303-01

Habtegiorgis, S. W., Rifai, K., Lappe, M., and Wahl, S. (2017). Adaptation to skew distortions of natural scenes and retinal specificity of its aftereffects. *Front. Psychol.* 8:1158. doi: 10.3389/fpsyg.2017.01158

Habtegiorgis, S. W., Rifai, K., Lappe, M., and Wahl, S. (2018). Experience-dependent long-term facilitation of skew adaptation. *J. Vis.* 18:7. doi: 10.1167/18.9.7

Hiraoka, T., Okamoto, C., Ishii, Y., Kakita, T., and Oshika, T. (2007). Contrast sensitivity function and ocular higher-order aberrations following overnight orthokeratology. *Invest. Ophthalmol. Vis. Sci.* 48, 550–556. doi: 10.1167/iovs.06-0914

Holden, B. A., Fricke, T. R., Wilson, D. A., Jong, M., Naidoo, K. S., Sankaridurg, P., et al. (2016). Global prevalence of myopia and high myopia and temporal trends from 2000 through 2050. *Ophthalmology* 123, 1036–1042. doi: 10.1016/j.ophtha.2016.01.006

King-Smith, P. E., Grigsby, S. S., Vingrys, A. J., Benes, S. C., and Supowit, A. (1994). Efficient and unbiased modifications of the QUEST threshold method: theory, simulations, experimental evaluation and practical implementation. *Vis. Res.* 34, 885–912. doi: 10.1016/0042-6989(94)90039-6

Kwon, M., Legge, G. E., Fang, F., Cheong, A. M., and He, S. (2009). Adaptive changes in visual cortex following prolonged contrast reduction. *J. Vis.* 9, 20.1–16. doi: 10.1167/9.2.20

Li, X., Friedman, I. B., Medow, N. B., and Zhang, C. (2017). Update on orthokeratology in managing progressive myopia in children: efficacy, mechanisms, and concerns. *J. Pediatr. Ophthalmol. Strabismus* 54, 142–148. doi: 10.3928/01913913-20170106-01

Liu, G., Chen, Z., Xue, F., Li, J., Tian, M., Zhou, X., et al. (2017). Effects of myopic orthokeratology on visual performance and optical quality. *Eye Contact Lens* 44, 316–321. doi: 10.1097/ICL.0000000000000372

Lu, Y., Lin, Z., Wen, L., Gao, W., Pan, L., Li, X., et al. (2020). The adaptation and acceptance of defocus incorporated multiple segment lens for chinese children. *Am. J. Ophthalmol.* 211, 207–216. doi: 10.1016/j.ajo.2019.12.002

Matesanz, B. M., Issolio, L., Arranz, I., de la Rosa, C., Menendez, J. A., Mar, S., et al. (2011). Temporal retinal sensitivity in mesopic adaptation. *Ophthalmic Physiol. Opt.* 31, 615–624. doi: 10.1111/j.1475-1313.2011.00859.x

Meister, D. J., and Fisher, S. W. (2008).). Progress in the spectacle correction of presbyopia. Part 1: design and development of progressive lenses. *Clin. Exp. Optom.* 91, 240–250. doi: 10.1111/j.1444-0938.2007.00245.x

Miles, F. A., and Wallman, J. (1990). Local ocular compensation for imposed local refractive error. *Vis. Res.* 30, 339–349. doi: 10.1016/0042-6989(90)90076-w

Neitz, J., Carroll, J., Yamauchi, Y., Neitz, M., and Williams, D. R. (2002). Color perception is mediated by a plastic neural mechanism that is adjustable in adults. *Neuron* 35, 783–792. doi: 10.1016/s0896-6273(02)00818-8

Nichols, J. J., Marsich, M. M., Nguyen, M., Barr, J. T., and Bullimore, M. A. (2000). Overnight orthokeratology. *Optom. Vis. Sci.* 77, 252–259.

Pan, C. W., Dirani, M., Cheng, C. Y., Wong, T. Y., and Saw, S. M. (2015). The age-specific prevalence of myopia in Asia: a meta-analysis. *Optom. Vis. Sci.* 92, 258–266. doi: 10.1097/OPX.0000000000000516

Pinero, D. P., Alio, J. L., Aleson, A., Escaf, M., and Miranda, M. (2009). Pentacam posterior and anterior corneal aberrations in normal and keratoconic eyes. *Clin. Exp. Optom.* 92, 297–303. doi: 10.1111/j.1444-0938.2009.00357.x

Ramachandran, V. S., and Gregory, R. L. (1991). Perceptual filling in of artificially induced scotomas in human vision. *Nature* 350, 699–702. doi: 10.1038/350699a0

Read, S. A., Collins, M. J., and Sander, B. P. (2010). Human optical axial length and defocus. *Invest. Ophthalmol. Vis. Sci.* 51, 6262–6269. doi: 10.1167/iovs.10-5457

Rudolph, M., Laaser, K., Bachmann, B. O., Cursiefen, C., Epstein, D., and Kruse, F. E. (2012). Corneal higher-order aberrations after Descemet's membrane endothelial keratoplasty. *Ophthalmology* 119, 528–535. doi: 10.1016/j.ophtha.2011.08.034

Santodomingo-Rubido, J., Villa-Collar, C., Gilmartin, B., Gutierrez-Ortega, R., and Sugimoto, K. (2017). Long-term efficacy of orthokeratology contact lens wear in controlling the progression of childhood myopia. *Curr. Eye Res.* 42, 713–720. doi: 10.1080/02713683.2016.1221979

Santolaria Sanz, E., Cervino, A., Queiros, A., Villa-Collar, C., Lopes-Ferreira, D., and Gonzalez-Meijome, J. M. (2015). Short-term changes in light distortion in orthokeratology subjects. *Biomed. Res. Int.* 2015:278425. doi: 10.1155/2015/278425

Santolaria-Sanz, E., Cervino, A., and Gonzalez-Meijome, J. M. (2016). Corneal aberrations, contrast sensitivity, and light distortion in orthokeratology patients: 1-year results. *J. Ophthalmol.* 2016:8453462. doi: 10.1155/2016/8453462

Smith, E. L. III, Huang, J., Hung, L. F., Blasdel, T. L., Humbird, T. L., and Bockhorst, K. H. (2009). Hemiretinal form deprivation: evidence for local control of eye growth and refractive development in infant monkeys. *Invest. Ophthalmol. Vis. Sci.* 50, 5057–5069. doi: 10.1167/iovs.08-3232

Stillitano, I., Schor, P., Lipener, C., and Hofling-Lima, A. L. (2008). Long-term follow-up of orthokeratology corneal reshaping using wavefront aberrometry and contrast sensitivity. *Eye Contact Lens* 34, 140–145. doi: 10.1097/ICL.0b013e318145ab5d

Swarbrick, H. A. (2006). Orthokeratology review and update. *Clin. Exp. Optom.* 89, 124–143. doi: 10.1111/j.1444-0938.2006.00044.x

Takemura, Y., Ito, M., Shimizu, Y., Okano, K., and Okano, T. (2020). Adaptive light: a lighting control method aligned with dark adaptation of human vision. *Sci. Rep.* 10:11204. doi: 10.1038/s41598-020-68119-7

Tarita-Nistor, L., Brent, M. H., Steinbach, M. J., and Gonzalez, E. G. (2012). Fixation patterns in maculopathy: from binocular to monocular viewing. *Optom. Vis. Sci.* 89, 277–287. doi: 10.1097/OPX.0b013e318244e8b1

Tarita-Nistor, L., Gill, I., Gonzalez, E. G., and Steinbach, M. J. (2017). Fixation stability recording: how long for eyes with central vision loss? *Optom. Vis. Sci.* 94, 311–316. doi: 10.1097/OPX.0000000000001033

Troilo, D., Gottlieb, M. D., and Wallman, J. (1987). Visual deprivation causes myopia in chicks with optic nerve section. *Curr. Eye Res.* 6, 993–999. doi: 10.3109/02713688709034870

Wallman, J., Gottlieb, M. D., Rajaram, V., and Fugate-Wentzek, L. A. (1987). Local retinal regions control local eye growth and myopia. *Science* 237, 73–77. doi: 10.1126/science.3603011

Wildsoet, C. (2003). Neural pathways subserving negative lens-induced emmetropization in chicks–insights from selective lesions of the optic nerve and ciliary nerve. *Curr. Eye Res.* 27, 371–385. doi: 10.1076/ceyr.27.6.371.18188

Williams, R. A., Enoch, J. M., and Essock, E. A. (1984). The resistance of selected hyperacuity configurations to retinal image degradation. *Invest. Ophthalmol. Vis. Sci.* 25, 389–399.

Xia, R., Su, B., Bi, H., Tang, J., Lin, Z., Zhang, B., et al. (2020). Good visual performance despite reduced optical quality during the first month of orthokeratology lens wear. *Curr. Eye Res.* 45, 440–449. doi: 10.1080/02713683.2019.1668950

Yehezkel, O., Sagi, D., Sterkin, A., Belkin, M., and Polat, U. (2010). Learning to adapt: dynamics of readaptation to geometrical distortions. *Vis. Res.* 50, 1550–1558. doi: 10.1016/j.visres.2010.05.014

14

A New Dichoptic Training Strategy Leads to Better Cooperation between the Two Eyes in Amblyopia

Zitian Liu[1†], Zidong Chen[1†], Le Gao[1], Manli Liu[1], Yiru Huang[1], Lei Feng[1], Junpeng Yuan[1], Daming Deng[1], Chang-Bing Huang[2,3] and Minbin Yu[1]**

[1] State Key Laboratory of Ophthalmology, Guangdong Provincial Key Laboratory of Ophthalmology and Visual Science, Zhongshan Ophthalmic Center, Sun Yat-sen University, Guangzhou, Guangdong, China, [2] Key Laboratory of Behavioral Science, Institute of Psychology, Chinese Academy of Sciences (CAS), Beijing, China, [3] Department of Psychology, University of Chinese Academy of Sciences, Beijing, China

***Correspondence:**
Minbin Yu
yuminbin@mail.sysu.edu.cn
Chang-Bing Huang
huangcb@psych.ac.cn

† These authors have contributed

Recent clinical trials failed to endorse dichoptic training for amblyopia treatment. Here, we proposed an alternative training strategy that focused on reducing signal threshold contrast in the amblyopic eye under a constant and high noise contrast in the fellow eye (HNC), and compared it to a typical dichoptic strategy that aimed at increasing the tolerable noise contrast in the fellow eye (i.e., TNC strategy). We recruited 16 patients with amblyopia and divided them into two groups. Eight patients in Group 1 received the HNC training, while the other eight patients in Group 2 performed the TNC training first (Phase 1) and then crossed over to the HNC training (Phase 2). We measured contrast sensitivity functions (CSFs) separately in the amblyopic and fellow eyes when the untested eye viewed mean luminance (monocularly unmasked) or noise stimuli (dichoptically masked) before and after training at a particular frequency. The area under the log contrast sensitivity function (AULCSF) of masked and unmasked conditions, and dichoptic gain (the ratio of AULCSF of masked to unmasked condition) were calculated for each eye. We found that both dichoptic training paradigms substantially improved masked CSF, dichoptic gain, and visual acuity in the amblyopic eye. As opposed to the TNC paradigm, the HNC training produced stronger effects on masked CSFs, stereoacuity, dichoptic gain, and visual acuity in the amblyopic eye. Interestingly, the second-phase HNC training in Group 2 also induced further improvement in the masked contrast sensitivity and AULCSF in the amblyopic eye. We concluded that the HNC training strategy was more effective than the TNC training paradigm. Future design for dichoptic training should not only focus on increasing the tolerable noise contrast in the fellow eye but should also “nurture” the amblyopic eye under normal binocular viewing conditions and sustained interocular suppression.

Keywords: amblyopia, dichoptic training, dichoptic masking, contrast sensitivity functions, interocular suppression

INTRODUCTION

Amblyopia, a neurodevelopmental vision disorder caused by abnormal visual experience during early childhood, affects about 2–5% of the population (Kiorpes et al., 1998; Holmes and Clarke, 2006). Amblyopia leads to both monocular deficits in the amblyopic eye, e.g., impaired visual acuity (Levi, 2006), reduced contrast sensitivity (Hess and Howell, 1977; McKee et al., 2003), unsteady monocular fixation (Subramanian et al., 2013), and abnormal binocular vision, e.g., interrupted binocular summation (Huang et al., 2009) and binocular rivalry (Lunghi et al., 2016), asymmetric dichoptic masking (Shooner et al., 2017; Zhou et al., 2018) and interocular suppression (Li J. et al., 2011), and reduced stereoacuity (Levi et al., 2015).

Focusing on improving monocular deficits in the amblyopic eye, patching or penalizing the fellow eye is still the clinical norm in amblyopia treatment (Holmes et al., 2006; Tailor et al., 2016). It is effective at improving visual acuity in the amblyopic eye during early childhood, with efficacy dropped sharply after the age of 7 years (Holmes and Levi, 2018). On the other hand, contrast sensitivity at high frequency, stereoacuity, binocular combination/summation were found to be still deficient in clinically "treated" amblyopia (Zhao et al., 2017), demonstrating the limits of monocular patching and penalization. In the past decades, monocular perceptual learning (PL) of different tasks, e.g., contrast detection with (Polat et al., 2004, 2009; Campana et al., 2014) and without flankers (Zhou et al., 2006; Huang et al., 2008; Hou et al., 2011; Jia et al., 2018), Vernier offset judgment (Levi et al., 1997) and position discrimination (Li R.W. et al., 2005, 2008), was also proposed to recover visual acuity in the amblyopic eye and showed promising results (Levi and Li, 2009; Astle et al., 2011). However, it has been found that monocular training cannot fully normalize binocular vision (Jia et al., 2018). In addition, the improvement of monocular and binocular functions following monocular PL did not correlate with each other, indicating (at least) partially different mechanisms underlying monocular and binocular deficits (Jia et al., 2018). The development of binocular treatment for amblyopia is thus necessary to recover deficient binocular vision in amblyopia.

Emphasizing on the binocular deficits in amblyopia and normalization of interocular balance between the two eyes, several dichoptic training paradigms had been developed to reduce disproportional interocular suppression (Hess et al., 2010; Knox et al., 2012; Li J. et al., 2013b; Ooi et al., 2013; Li J. et al., 2015; Kelly et al., 2018). Using relatively limited number of patients, early well-controlled laboratory-based studies mostly adopted playing video games, such as Tetris (Li J. et al., 2013b) and Dig Rush (Hess et al., 2010; Kelly et al., 2016, 2018), or watching films (Li S.L. et al., 2015; Bossi et al., 2017; Birch et al., 2019), and showed promising results in both children (Birch et al., 2015; Li S.L. et al., 2015; Bossi et al., 2017) and adults (Hess et al., 2010; Li J. et al., 2013b; Ooi et al., 2013; Li J. et al., 2015; Vedamurthy et al., 2015a,b) with amblyopia. However, recent clinical trials that recruited large diversified samples found only mild or modest treatment effect for both children (Holmes et al., 2016; Pediatric Eye Disease Investigator Group, et al., 2019) and adult amblyopia (Gao et al., 2018b), questioned the effectiveness and feasibility of binocular paradigm in recovering both binocular and monocular functions in clinical practice. One possibility is that, with the hope of achieving balanced contribution from the two eyes, typical application usually utilized presentation of low-contrast image, animated pictures, or video to the fellow eye and complimentary high-contrast contents to the amblyopic eye (Hess et al., 2010; Li J. et al., 2013b), which was inherently different from normal binocular viewing condition, in which the incoming stimuli in the amblyopic and fellow eyes are of similar images with the same contrast, and the fellow eye imposes strong and sustained suppression upon the amblyopic eye. Another possibility, e.g., failure to comply and engage continuously, was also proposed (Sloper, 2016), although gaming or film watching was thought to be more enjoyable in the original design.

Motivated by the well-recognized effectiveness of refractive adaptation in improving monocular visual acuity and reducing interocular suppression (Moseley et al., 2002; Cotter et al., 2006; Gao et al., 2018a; Wang et al., 2018), in which patients were prescribed only appropriate refractive correction, received roughly comparable physical inputs to both eyes, and maintained a high-energy stimulation in the fellow eye, we proposed a new binocular training paradigm that involves presenting high-contrast noise to the fellow eye and gradually decreasing image contrast in the amblyopic eye (or HNC, **Figure 1A**), aiming to actively "nurture" the amblyopic eye with strong inhibition from the fellow eye. Our HNC approach was related to the monocular contrast detection paradigm, which was found to be effective in improving contrast sensitivity and visual acuity in the amblyopic eye (Zhou et al., 2006; Huang et al., 2008), but prescribed strong and sustained interocular inhibition from the fellow to the amblyopic eye. The HNC paradigm was also related to the dichoptic TNC training paradigm (i.e., tolerable noise contrast; **Figure 1B**), which was believed to be effective in reducing interocular suppression (Liu and Zhang, 2018, 2019), but differed with it in two aspects: (1) We used contrast detection, a hallmark of spatial vision disorder in amblyopia (Kiorpes et al., 1999), instead of contrast discrimination task, an essentially veridical function in amblyopia (Hess and Bradley, 1980), and (2) We kept noise contrast in the fellow eye constant and adjusted the contrast of the grating in the amblyopic eye, posing a strong suppressive effect to the amblyopic eye and simulating a more typical binocular viewing condition (Li J. et al., 2013a).

By comparing the efficacy of the TNC and HNC strategies in amblyopic patients, we found that the HNC approach not only produced stronger monocular and binocular training effects than the TNC training did but also provided extra visual gains

Abbreviations: HNC, high noise contrast, referred to the new dichoptic training strategy with high-contrast noise in the fellow eye in this study; TNC, tolerable noise contrast, referred to the typical dichoptic training strategy aimed at increasing the tolerable noise contrast in the fellow eye; CSFs, contrast sensitivity functions; AULCSF, the area under the log contrast sensitivity function; FEU, fellow eye unmasked, CSF of the fellow eye with no mask but background luminance in the amblyopic eye; AEU, amblyopic eye unmasked, CSF of the amblyopic eye with no mask but background luminance in the fellow eye; FEM, fellow eye masked, CSF of the fellow eye with masks in the amblyopic eye; AEM, amblyopic eye masked, CSF of the amblyopic eye with masks in the fellow eye.

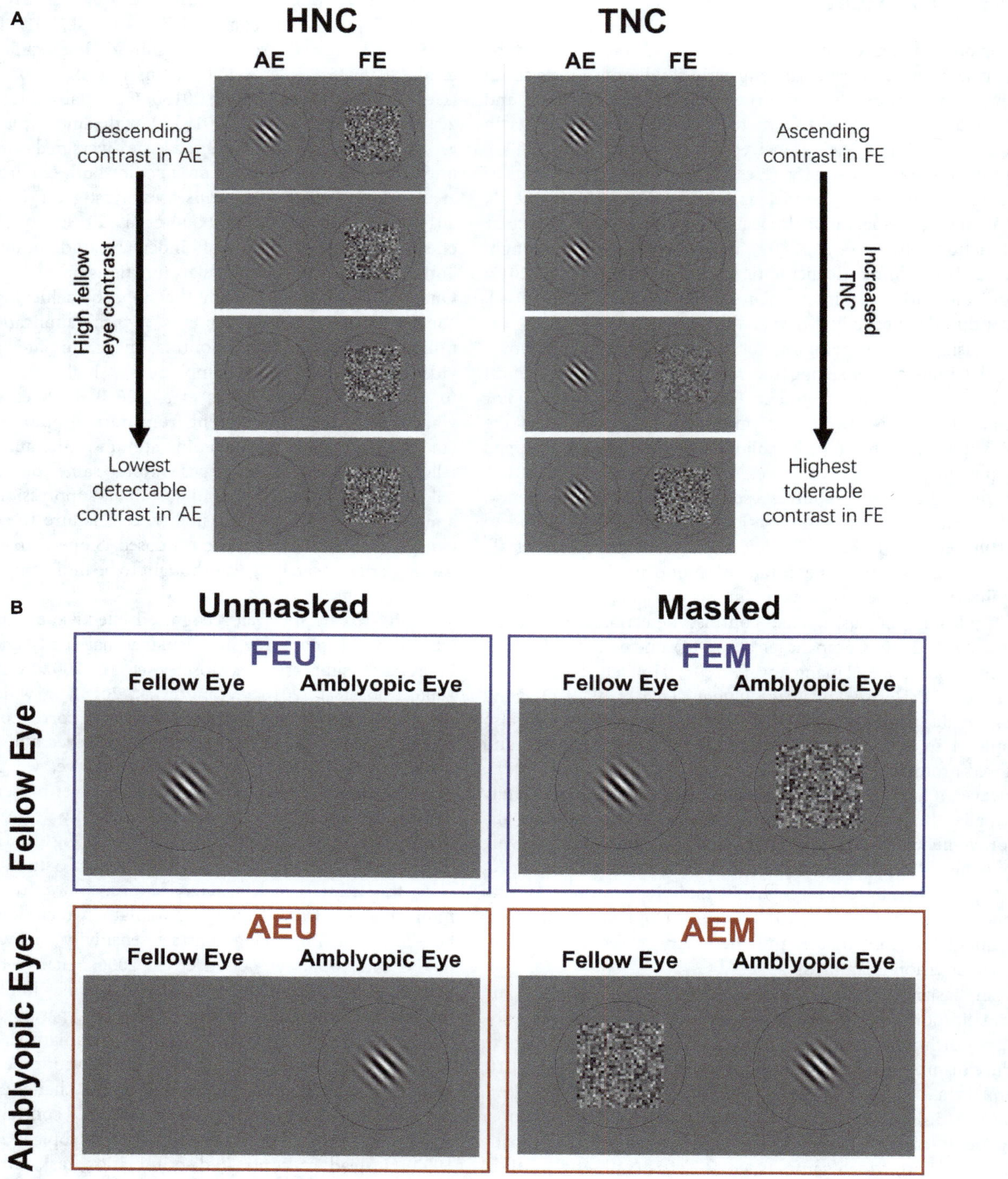

FIGURE 1 | (A) Two strategies of dichoptic training used in this study. Left: High noise contrast (HNC) protocol; Sinusoidal gratings were presented to one eye, while a mean background luminance (monocular unmasked condition) or a Gaussian white noise mask (dichoptic masked condition) was presented to the untested eye. From top to bottom: the contrast of gratings in an amblyopic eye (AE) was manipulated from high to low, while noise mask in a fellow eye (FE) was fixed at high contrast ($\sigma = 0.33$). With training, the contrast of grating was adjusted (usually decreased) to maintain stable performance. Right: tolerable noise contrast (TNC) protocol; grating contrast in AE was fixed while mask contrast in FE was manipulated from low to high to maintain stable performance. **(B)** Four conditions of CSFs were measured: unmasked fellow eye (FEU), unmasked amblyopic eye (AEU), masked fellow eye (FEM), and masked amblyopic eye (AEM).

in patients who have previously received the TNC training, demonstrating greater potential in recovering both monocular and binocular deficits in amblyopia.

MATERIALS AND METHODS

Participants

Sixteen amblyopic patients (13 anisometropic, 1 strabismic, and 2 combined) aged 12–32 years (mean ± S.D., 21.1 ± 6.4 years) participated in this study. Participants were recruited from Zhongshan Ophthalmic Center (Guangzhou, China), had no visual training experience, and were all naive to the purpose of the study. Clinical details of all participants are summarized in **Table 1**.

Inclusion criteria for amblyopic patients were as follows: Patients older than 12 years of age were diagnosed with amblyopia due to a history of anisometropia, strabismus, or both. Amblyopia was defined as an interocular difference in best-corrected visual acuity (BCVA) of 0.2 logMAR or greater (≥2 lines), with a logMAR acuity of at least 0.9 in the amblyopic eye and 0.1 in the fellow eye. Anisometropia was defined as an interocular spherical equivalent difference of 1.50 diopters or more, with or without microtropia. Patients with strabismus were initially diagnosed with esotropia, but were re-aligned with refractive correction and/or surgery to within four prism diopters of orthotropia at near and distance fixations for more than 1 year. Eligible patients had stable visual acuity (no improvement over the most recent three hospital visits) and had worn appropriate glasses for more than 8 weeks, if needed. Patients with combined mechanism had a history of acquired anisometropia and strabismus. Exclusion criteria were inability to cooperate with the eye examinations or psychophysical tests, presence of any coexisting ocular or systemic diseases, congenital infections/malformations, or developmental delay. Three patients were excluded due to the inability to perform the dichoptic training or unstable visual acuity.

Clinical Measurements

All participants underwent a set of ophthalmologic examinations, including cycloplegic objective and subjective refraction, cover tests at near and distance fixations, slit-lamp and funduscopic examinations. Full refractive correction was provided for all subsequent tests. Visual acuity was measured using a Chinese tumbling E logMAR chart (Mou, 2005; Xi et al., 2014; Jia et al., 2018). Stereopsis was measured using the Random Dot Stereo Acuity Test (Vision Assessment Corp., Elk Grove Village, IL). For patients who were unable to perceive depth at the 500 arcsec, we designated their stereoacuity as 800 arcsec (Liu and Zhang, 2019). All ophthalmologic examination procedures were conducted in the same clinic room under constant lighting conditions.

Design

The experiment consisted of three phases: pre-training measurement, training, and post-training measurement. In pre- and post-training measurements, visual acuity, different conditions of contrast sensitivity functions (CSFs) for amblyopic and fellow eyes, and stereoacuity were assessed for all patients. The scheme for different conditions of CSF measurement is presented in **Figure 1B**. We measured each eye's monocular unmasked CSF in which the untested eye viewed a background with mean luminance, and dichoptically masked CSF in which the untested eye viewed a high-energy noise mask. As a result, four conditions of CSFs were obtained for each patient: fellow eye unmasked (FEU), amblyopic eye unmasked (AEU), fellow eye masked (FEM), and amblyopic eye masked (AEM).

Contrast sensitivity, defined as the reciprocal of contrast threshold, was calculated from sinusoidal grating detection thresholds at spatial frequencies 0.5, 1, 2, 4, 8, and 16 cycles per degree (c/d) for each eye in the unmasked and masked conditions. Since the amblyopic eye is much weaker than the fellow eye and the magnitude of interocular inhibition varied significantly across patients (Chen et al., 2014; Zhou et al., 2018), we measured contrast sensitivity at the masked condition from low to high spatial frequency in sequence and terminated the measurement if contrast sensitivity was below 2.0 (i.e., contrast threshold > 50%) at a particular spatial frequency. As a result, masked CSF in the two eyes was measured with different number of frequencies.

In the training session, we applied and compared the TNC and HNC training strategies in 16 patients, who were randomly divided into two groups. Eight patients in Group 1 performed 8–10 sessions of dichoptic training following the HNC strategy. The other eight patients in Group 2 performed 8–10 sessions of dichoptic TNC training in the first training phase and then crossed over to the HNC training in the second training phase for another 8–10 sessions. Retention of training effects was evaluated in 5 out of 16 patients at 12 months post-training.

Apparatus and Stimuli

All stimuli were generated and controlled by a PC computer running Matlab (MathWorks, Natick, MA, United States) and Psychtoolbox (version 3.0) (Brainard, 1997; Pelli, 1997). Dichoptic stimuli were rendered on a 3D-ready gamma-corrected computer monitor (ASUS VG278HE; refresh rate: 144 Hz; resolution: 1,920 × 1,080 pixels; background luminance: 54 cd/m^2), with participants viewing through a pair of polarized glasses (NVIDIA 3D shutter glasses). The viewing distance was 114 cm, and a chin-forehead rest was used to secure the head position. All experiments were conducted in a dimly lit room (<5 lx).

The "signal" stimuli consisted of oriented (± 45° from vertical) sinusoidal gratings at six spatial frequencies (0.5, 1, 2, 4, 8, and 16 c/d) with random phase. Each grating consisted of eight cycles. The size of gratings was inversely proportional to the spatial frequency (i.e., 16°, 8°, 4°, 2°, 1°, and 0.5°), keeping the number of cycles the same across different spatial frequencies. Pixel intensities of the random "noise" stimuli were sampled from a Gaussian distribution (μ = 0, σ = 0.33). Noise stimuli in each trial were sampled independently. The size of the noise mask was the same as that of the signal grating (Chen et al., 2014).

TABLE 1 | Clinical details of all participants by group.

Group	Patient	Age, y/sex[a]	Eye[b]	Refractive error diopter	Visual acuity LogMAR[c]	Strabismus[d], prism diopter △	History[e]
1	P1	12/M	AE FE	+4.50/−1.00 × 165° +1.00	0.3 −0.04	None	Detected at 6 y, refractive correction from 6 y, patching for 4 y (2–4 hr/day)
	P2	32/F	AE FE	+5.75 +0.75/−0.50 × 90°	0.3 0	None	Detected at 6 y, refractive correction from 6 y, patching for 1 y (2 hr/day)
	P3	24/F	AE FE	+4.25/−0.50 × 45° −1.50/−0.75 × 90°	0.34 0	None	Detected at 12 y, refractive correction from 12 y, patching for 1 y (2 hr/day)
	P4	20/M	AE FE	−8.25/−1.75 × 170° −3.50/−0.75 × 10°	0.3 0	None	Detected at 6 y, refractive correction from 6 y, patching for 0.5 y (2 hr/day)
	P5	20/M	AE FE	+2.50/−1.50 × 10° −1.00/−0.75 × 175°	0.5 0	None	Detected at 6 y, refractive correction from 6 y, patching for 0.5 y (2 hr/day)
	P6	24/F	AE FE	−3.00 −3.00	0.32 0	ET 5△	Detected at 17 y, used to be ET 40△, refractive correction from 17 y, patching for 0.5y (2 hr/day), surgery at 20 y, ET 5△ now
	P7	16/F	AE FE	+7.75/−2.00 × 175° −3.75/−0.75 × 155°	0.86 0	None	Detected at 8 y, refractive correction from 8 y, patching for 2 y (2 hr/day)
	P8	16/F	AE FE	+3.00 −0.75	0.14 −0.08	None	Detected at 8 y, refractive correction from 8 y, patching for 2 y (2 hr/day)
2	P9	12/M	AE FE	+4.75/−1.50 × 160° +0.75/−0.50 × 175°	0.6 −0.04	None	Detected at 5 y, refractive correction from 5 y, patching for 3 y (2–4 hr/day)
	P10	26/F	AE FE	+9.25/−4.00 × 5° +7.50/−3.00 × 175°	0.2 0	ET40△ (Uncorrected) ET 5△ (Corrected)	Detected accommodative esotropia at 6 y, refractive correction from 6 y, patching for 1 y (2–4 hr/day)
	P11	26/F	AE FE	+2.75/−1.00 × 15° −2.50/−0.50 × 5°	0.34 0	None	Detected at 12 y, refractive correction from 12 y, no patching
	P12	13/M	AE FE	+4.25 +0.25/−0.50 × 180°	0.7 −0.06	None	Detected at 11 y, refractive correction from 11 y, patching for 2 y (4 hr/day)
	P13	14/F	AE FE	+6.00/−1.00 × 15° +1.50/−1.00 × 180°	0.5 0	ET 5△	Detected at 3 y, used to be ET 35△, refractive correction from 3 y, patching for 0.5 y (2 hr/day), surgery at 12 y, ET 5△ now
	P14	30/M	AE FE	+4.75/−1.50 × 180° −1.75/−1.25 × 5°	0.46 0	None	Detected at 12 y, refractive correction from 25 y, no patching
	P15	25/F	AE FE	+6.25/−1.75 × 135° +2.75	0.42 0	None	Detected at 12 y, refractive correction from 12 y, no patching
	P16	28/M	AE FE	+4.50/−1.50 × 180° −1.50	0.4 −0.1	None	Detected at 16 y, refractive correction from 16 y, no patching

[a]*M, male; F, female.* [b]*AE, amblyopic eye; FE, fellow eye.* [c]*LogMAR, the logarithm of the minimum angle of resolution.* [d]*△, prism diopter; ET, esotropia.* [e]*y, year; hr, hour.*

To minimize edge effects, a half-Gaussian ramp was added around the stimulus.

Procedure

Before the measurement of CSF and each training sessions, a 0.2° red fixation point and a circle, which was slightly larger than the size of grating, were presented to both eyes in the middle of the screen. Participants were asked to use a computer keyboard to adjust the position of the circles until the two eyes were able to fuse the stimulus. The generated coordinates that marked proper fusion were then used in the subsequent measurement and training.

In a typical trial, an oriented sinusoidal grating and a noise mask or mean luminance background were dichoptically presented for 200 ms to the tested and untested eye, respectively. The orientation was randomly set to be either +45° or −45° from the vertical, with equal probability. Participants were asked to indicate the orientation of the grating by using the "left" or "right" arrow key on the computer keyboard. The red fixation point will change to green for each correct response. The response also initiated the next trial after a 500-ms intertrial interval. Prior to the study, each participant had a chance to practice for 100 trials with high-contrast gratings (80%).

Contrast threshold at each spatial frequency was measured with an adaptive two-down one-up staircase procedure, converging to a performance level of 70.7% correct. Specifically, two consecutive correct responses decreased the grating contrast, and one error raised the grating contrast, and contrast changing from increase to decrease or vice versa was counted as one reversal. Step size of contrast change was 50% ($C_{n+1} = C_n{}^* \ 0.50$) before the first reversal and 10% ($C_{n+1} = C_n{}^* \ 0.90$) thereafter (Levitt, 1971). Contrast thresholds were calculated as the mean of the last four reversals of the staircase.

Training

In the dichoptic training phase, grating stimuli were only presented to the amblyopic eye, while the noise stimuli were presented to the fellow eye. Patients in Group 1 performed dichoptic training based on the HNC strategy, in which the amblyopic eye (AE) was trained with a contrast detection task under a high and fixed noise mask ($\sigma = 0.33$) in the fellow eye. An adaptive two-down one-up staircase controlled the contrast of the sinusoidal grating in the amblyopic eye upon subject's judgment and tracked performance of 70.7% correct. Training lasted 8–10 sessions.

Patients in Group 2 first performed dichoptic training based on the TNC strategy, in which the contrast of gratings in AE was fixed at 50% and the contrast energy of noise mask in FE was manipulated by an adaptive two-up one-down staircase that converged to a performance level of 70.7% correct. Specifically, two consecutive correct responses increased the noise level, and one error decreased the noise level, and noise level changing from increase to decrease or vice versa was counted as one reversal. The mean of the last four reversals of the staircase was taken as the maximally tolerable noise level. After the TNC training, patients in Group 2 went through the measurement of visual acuity, stereoacuity, and CSFs. They then received dichoptic HNC training, as described above.

In both Group 1 and Group 2, patients were trained at their individual cut-off spatial frequencies, as determined from the masked CSF measured in the amblyopic eye (average SF in Group 1: 4.00 ± 2.98 c/d; Group 2: 3.75 ± 1.98 c/d; $t_{14} = 0.245$, $P = 0.810$) and defined as the spatial frequency at which the contrast threshold under noise mask was 50% (or contrast sensitivity of 2.0).

Statistical Analysis and Model Fitting

Data are presented as mean ± SEM, unless otherwise specified. Learning curve (i.e., $\log_{10}$ contrast sensitivity as a function of log [training session]) was fitted with a linear function (Zhou et al., 2006; Huang et al., 2008):

$$\log_{10} CS(session) = CS_0 + \alpha \times \log_{10}(session),$$

where CS denotes contrast sensitivity at a particular session, CS_0 is the intercept, and α is the slope of the learning curve (learning rate, or unit improvement at the trained condition). When analyzing CSF in the amblyopic eye, only spatial frequencies with measurable contrast sensitivity (contrast threshold < 100%) in most patients were included (0.5–8 c/d for unmasked condition, 0.5–2 c/d for masked condition), while CSF across all spatial frequencies (0.5–16 c/d) was analyzed for the fellow eye.

The average CSF of each group measured before and after training was fitted by a parabolic function in log–log scale (Huang et al., 2008; Chen et al., 2016; Zhou et al., 2018). An overall contrast sensitivity metric, the area under the log contrast sensitivity function (AULCSF), was determined by calculating the definite integration of the best-fitted function from 0.5 c/d to the cut-off spatial frequency (Lesmes et al., 2010; Chen et al., 2016). To index the effect of dichoptic masking on CSF, or dichoptic gain (Shooner et al., 2017), we calculated the ratio of AULCSF of masked to unmasked CSF, varying from 0 (completely masked by the other untested eye) to 1 (no masking effect from the other eye).

For each patient, the magnitude of improvements (Zhou et al., 2006) for each measure (e.g., AULCSF, dichoptic gain magnitude, visual acuity, and stereoacuity) was defined as:

$$\textit{Improvement} = \frac{\text{Post\_training Measure} - \text{Pre\_training Measure}}{\text{Post\_training Measure}} \times 100\% \quad (1)$$

Data from pre-training and post-training measurements were compared using a two-tailed paired t-test. The magnitude of improvements for the two groups was compared using a two-tailed independent sample t-test.

To evaluate the retention effect of training, we calculated the retention coefficient (Zhou et al., 2006) of each measure (e.g., AULCSF, dichoptic gain, visual acuity, and stereoacuity) as:

$$\textit{Retention Coefficient} = \frac{\text{Retested Measure} - \text{Pre\_training Measure}}{\text{Post\_training Measure} - \text{Pre\_training Measure}} \times 100\% \quad (2)$$

RESULTS

Outcomes of HNC Protocol Training (Group 1)

Eight to ten sessions of contrast detection training in the amblyopic eye under constant and high-energy noise mask from the fellow eye led to significant improvement in contrast sensitivity at the trained spatial frequency (254.51 ± 64.08%; t_7 = 5.100, P = 0.001; calculated from pre- and post-training masked CSF measurement). The average learning curve (i.e., contrast sensitivity as a function of training sessions) is shown in **Figure 2A**. The HNC training improved contrast sensitivity with a slope of 1.55 log units per log training session (R^2 = 0.97, P < 0.01).

Training at one spatial frequency also facilitated contrast sensitivity at other untrained frequencies in the amblyopic eye, if tested under high masking from the fellow eye. Treating practice level (pre-/post- training) and spatial frequency (0.5, 1, and 2 c/d) as within-subject factors, a repeated-measure analysis of variance (ANOVA) showed that the AEM contrast sensitivity varied significantly with practice level [$F_{(1, 7)}$ = 31.411, P = 0.001, η^2 = 0.818], but not with spatial frequency [$F_{(2, 14)}$ = 0.429, P = 0.660, η^2 = 0.058] and interaction of the two factors [$F_{(2, 14)}$ = 0.013, P = 0.987, η^2 = 0.002], indicating a general contrast sensitivity improvement. CSF also showed significant change with practice level [$F_{(1, 7)}$ = 10.436, P = 0.014, η^2 = 0.599], spatial frequency [0.5–8 c/d, $F_{(4, 28)}$ = 155.321, P < 0.001, η^2 = 0.957], and interaction of the two factors [$F_{(4, 28)}$ = 3.005, P = 0.035, η^2 = 0.300] in the amblyopic eye, if tested with mean background in the fellow eye (AEU condition; **Figure 3A**). On the contrary, CSF in the fellow eye did not change significantly with practice, either at the FEU condition [$F_{(1, 7)}$ = 3.615, P = 0.099, η^2 = 0.341] or the FEM condition [$F_{(1, 7)}$ = 0.439, P = 0.529, η^2 = 0.059].

Averaged across patients, AULCSF improved about 266.21 ± 66.04% (t_7 = 7.066, P < 0.001) in the AEM condition and 13.32 ± 4.01% (t_7 = 3.370, P = 0.012) in the AEU condition. The AULCSF improvement showed significant difference between the two conditions (t_7 = 3.871, P = 0.006) but without correlation (r = 0.206, P = 0.624), which implied at least partially different mechanisms underlying the improvement of AEM and AEU contrast sensitivity. For the fellow eye, the AULCSF improvement in neither the FEM (t_7 = 1.303, P = 0.234) nor the FEU (t_7 = 2.092, P = 0.075) condition reached significance, indicating eye-specific learning.

To estimate the effects of HNC training on interocular interaction in amblyopia, we calculated and compared the magnitude of dichoptic gain before and after training. After HNC training, dichoptic gain improved in the amblyopic eye by 222.28 ± 56.71% (t_7 = 6.546, P < 0.001), but remained unchanged in the fellow eye (2.16 ± 3.48%, t_7 = 0.372, P = 0.721, **Figure 3B**). In other words, the masked CSF improved more than the unmasked CSF did in the amblyopic eye, demonstrating the increased strength of the amblyopic eye in counteracting the inhibition from the fellow eye.

After the HNC training, visual acuity in the amblyopic eye improved by 0.83 ± 0.14 lines (t_7 = 5.954, P = 0.001), while that of the fellow eye remained unchanged (t_7 = 0.798, P = 0.451). The HNC training also improved stereoacuity from 362.50″ ± 82.24″ to 272.00″ ± 88.84″ (t_7 = 2.695, P = 0.031). Interestingly, two out of three stereoblind patients (unable to identify geometric shapes at the largest disparity of 500 arcsecs) obtained measurable stereopsis after HNC training (to 500″ and 400″, respectively). The improvement of visual acuity in the amblyopic eye, dichoptic gain, and stereoacuity did not correlate with each other (all P > 0.10).

Outcomes of TNC Protocol Training (Group 2; Phase 1)

Patients in Group 2 first performed TNC training for 8–10 sessions (Phase 1), in which signal contrast in the amblyopic eye was fixed and noise in the fellow eye was progressively elevated (Liu and Zhang, 2018, 2019), and then underwent HNC training for an additional 8–10 sessions (Phase 2) to test if HNC training could bring extra benefits.

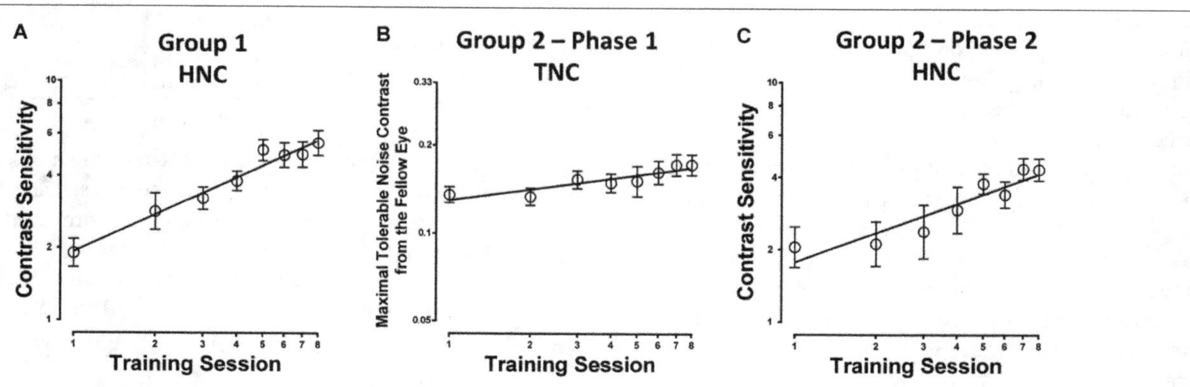

FIGURE 2 | Learning curves for the two different training protocols in amblyopic participants from **(A)** Group 1 with constant and high noise contrast in the fellow eye (HNC), **(B)** Group 2 (Phase 1) with progressively elevated noise contrast in the fellow eye (TNC); **(C)** Group 2 (Phase 2), HNC training.

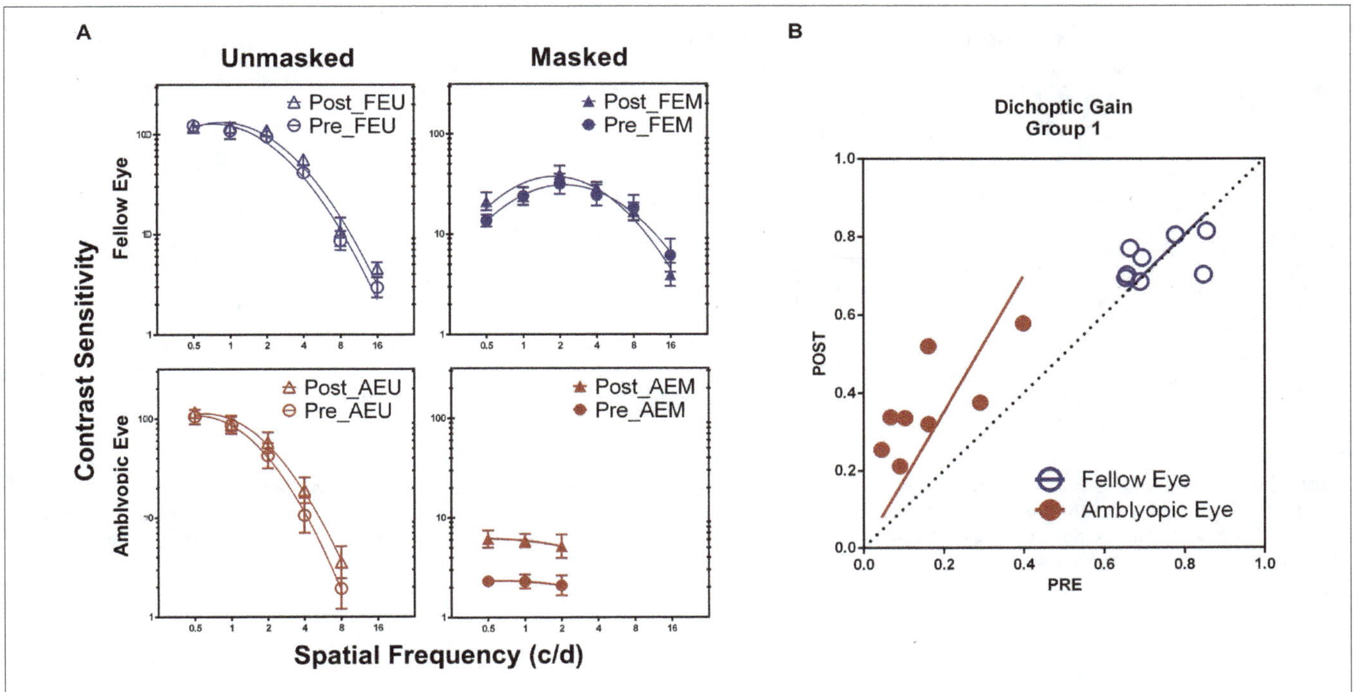

FIGURE 3 | (A) Pre- and post-training contrast sensitivity functions (CSFs) under different conditions in Group 1. **(B)** Dichoptic gains for the two eyes before HNC training (*x*-axis) are plotted against those after training (*y*-axis). The diagonal unity line represents unchanged dichoptic gain between pre- and post-training assessment.

The average learning curve (i.e., the maximal tolerable noise contrast in the fellow eye as a function of training sessions) for Phase 1 is shown in **Figure 2B**. TNC training increased maximal tolerable noise contrast in the fellow eye with a slope of 0.013 units per training session (R^2 = 0.83, P = 0.002). The maximal tolerable noise contrast significantly elevated by 48.9 ± 12.5% (t_7 = 7.408, P < 0.001; calculated from the measurement at the first and last training sessions).

After TNC training, AEM contrast sensitivity at the training spatial frequency was significantly improved by 60.30 ± 26.19% (t_7 = 4.364, P = 0.003; calculated from pre- and post-training masked CSF). Contrast sensitivity at other untrained frequencies in the amblyopic eye also elevated significantly, if tested under high masking from the fellow eye (AEM condition). ANOVA revealed that AEM contrast sensitivity varied significantly with practice level [$F_{(1,\ 7)}$ = 7.924, P = 0.026, η^2 = 0.531] and spatial frequency [$F_{(2,\ 14)}$ = 6.363, P = 0.011, η^2 = 0.476] but not with interaction of the two factors [$F_{(2,\ 14)}$ = 0.442, P = 0.651, η^2 = 0.059, **Figure 4A**]. On the other hand, CSF did not change significantly following training at all other conditions [AEU condition, $F_{(1,\ 7)}$ = 4.921, P = 0.062, η^2 = 0.413; FEU condition, $F_{(1,\ 7)}$ = 2.299, P = 0.173, η^2 = 0.247; FEM condition, $F_{(1,\ 7)}$ = 1.328, P = 0.287, η^2 = 0.159].

Averaged across patients, the AULCSF of the AEM condition significantly improved by 97.52 ± 26.82% (t_7 = 3.948, P = 0.006), whereas the AULCSFs of the other conditions showed no significant changes (AEU, 7.89 ± 4.08%, t_7 = 2.296, P = 0.055; FEU, 2.88 ± 1.76%, t_7 = 1.529, P = 0.170; FEM, 6.57 ± 3.13%, t_7 = 1.097, P = 0.309). For dichoptic gain, we also found significant change in the amblyopic eye (82.20 ± 23.03%; t_7 = 3.666, P = 0.008) instead of the fellow eye (3.66 ± 4.86%; t_7 = 0.643, P = 0.540, **Figure 4C**).

TNC training improved amblyopic visual acuity by 0.34 ± 0.13 lines (t_7 = 2.664, P = 0.032), while that of the fellow eye remained unchanged (t_7 = 1.001, P = 0.351). However, we found no significant changes in stereoacuity after TNC training (t_7 = 1.000, P = 0.351). No significant correlation was found among the three measures (all P > 0.10).

Additional Benefits of HNC Training in Patients With TNC Training History (Group 2; Phase 2)

After the second phase of HNC training, AEM contrast sensitivity got a further improvement of 179.84 ± 31.88% (t_7 = 10.076, P < 0.001; calculated from pre- and post-training masked CSF, **Figure 5**) at the training spatial frequency, with a slope of 1.22 log units per log training session (R^2 = 0.87, P = 0.001, **Figure 2C**).

A within-subject analysis of variance (ANOVA) showed that AEM contrast sensitivity varied significantly with practice level [$F_{(1,\ 7)}$ = 10.914, P = 0.016, η^2 = 0.609], but not with spatial frequency [$F_{(2,\ 14)}$ = 3.472, P = 0.065, η^2 = 0.332; **Figure 4B**]. Interaction between the two factors was also not significant [$F_{(2,\ 14)}$ = 0.681, P = 0.525, η^2 = 0.089]. In contrast, there was no significant changes in the AEU condition [$F_{(1,7)}$ = 0.816, P = 0.369, η^2 = 0.104], FEU condition [$F_{(1,\ 7)}$ = 0.291, P = 0.606,

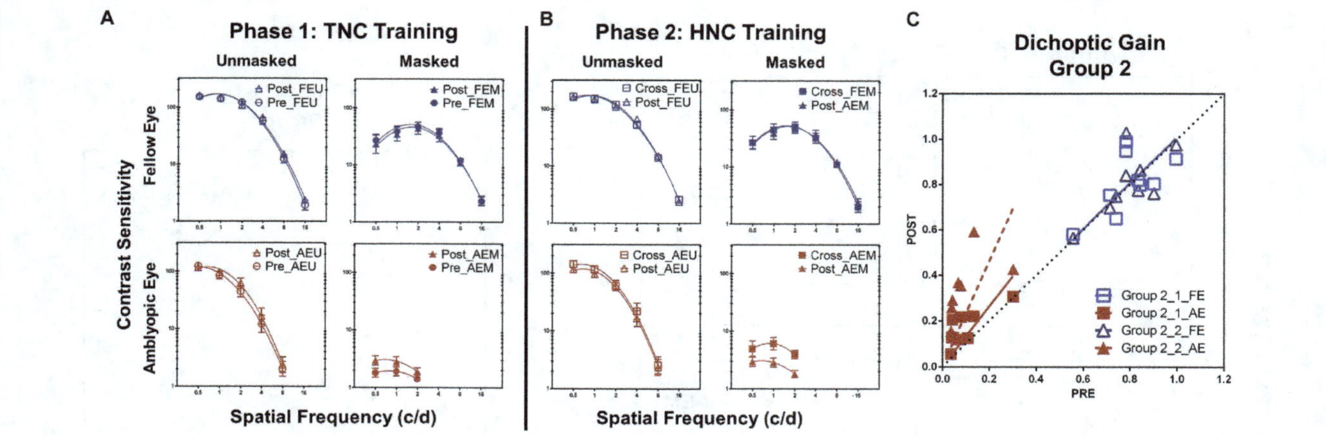

FIGURE 4 | (A) CSFs under different conditions in Group 2 before (Pre, circle) and after (Post, triangle) the TNC training (Phase 1). **(B)** CSFs under different conditions in Group 2 after the TNC training (Post, triangle) and after crossed over to the HNC training (Cross, square) (Phase 2). **(C)** Dichoptic gains for the two eyes in Group 2 before training (*x*-axis) is plotted against those after training (*y*-axis) for the two phases. The diagonal unity line represents unchanged dichoptic gain between pre- and post-training assessment.

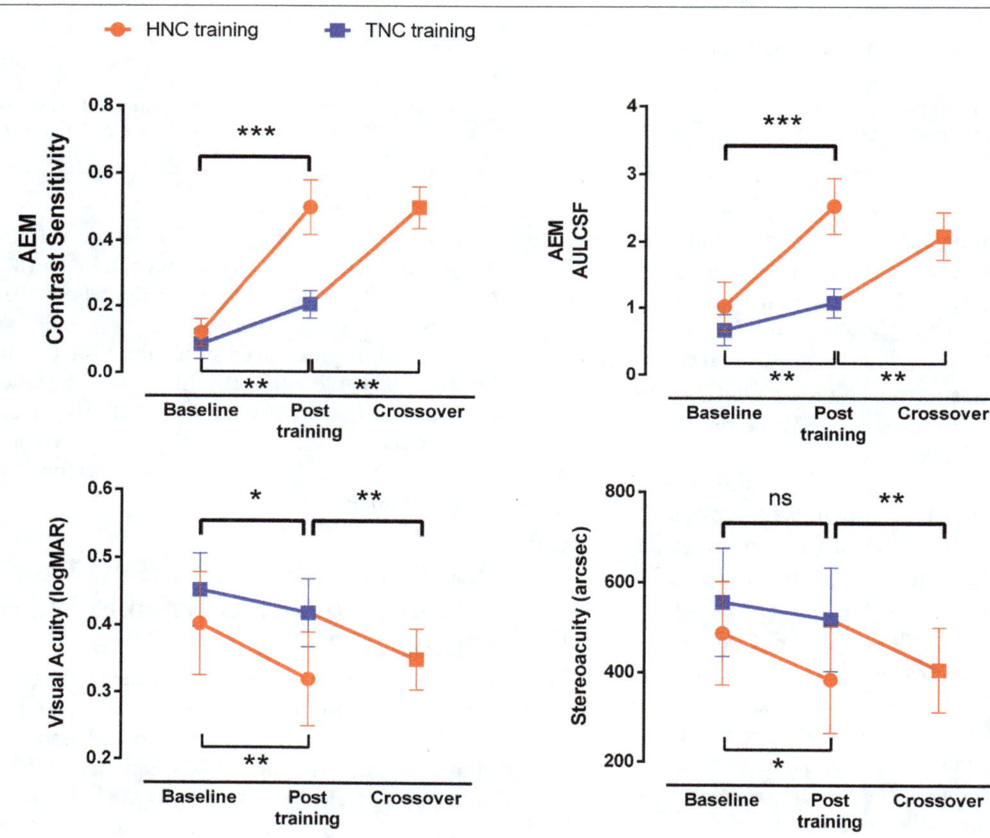

FIGURE 5 | Improvements in visual function after HNC vs. TNC training. Error bars represent SEM. $^{*}p < 0.05$; $^{**}p < 0.01$; $^{***}p < 0.001$.

$\eta^2 = 0.040$] and FEM condition [$F_{(1,\ 7)} = 0.078$, $P = 0.788$, $\eta^2 = 0.011$].

Patients in Group 2 gained additional improvement in AULCSF of AEM condition (113.99 ± 26.60%, $t_7 = 4.333$, $P = 0.003$, **Figure 5**), but not in the AEU condition (2.19 ± 3.05%, $t_7 = 2.070$, $P = 0.077$) and the fellow eye conditions (FEU: $t_7 = 0.887$, $P = 0.405$; FEM: $t_7 = 0.157$, $P = 0.880$). A further improvement was found in dichoptic gain in the amblyopic eye

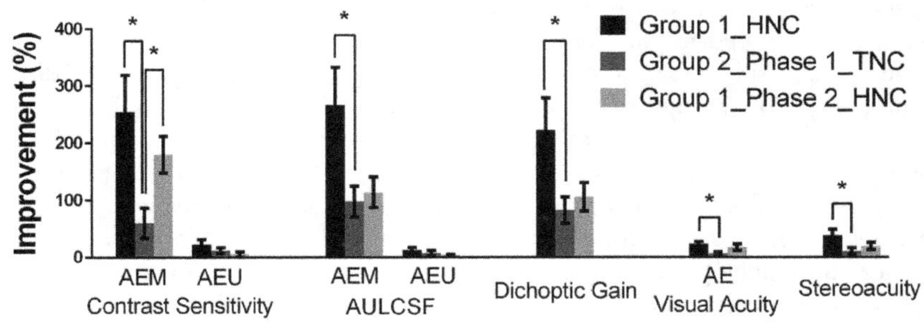

FIGURE 6 | Summary of training effects. Groups were represented by different colors: black (Group 1), dark gray (Group 2, Phase 1), and light gray (Group 2, Phase 2). Error bars represent SEM. $^*p < 0.05$.

(105.63 ± 25.25%, $t_7 = 3.987$, $P = 0.005$), instead of the fellow eye ($t_7 = 0.190$, $P = 0.855$, **Figure 4C**).

After HNC training in Phase 2, a significant further improvement in visual acuity of 0.69 ± 0.18 lines was observed in the amblyopic eye ($t_7 = 3.847$, $P = 0.006$, **Figure 5**), but not in the fellow eye ($t_7 = 0.357$, $P = 0.732$). There was also significant improvement in stereoacuity (from 418.75″ ± 81.25″ to 368.75″ ± 78.45″; $t_7 = 2.646$, $P = 0.033$, **Figure 5**). Similarly, there was no significant correlation among the acuity improvement in the amblyopic eye, the improvement in stereoacuity, and the improvement of dichoptic gain in the amblyopic eye (all $P > 0.10$).

Comparison of Training Strategies

By comparing the data from Group 1 and the first training phase of Group 2, we evaluated the efficacies of the two training strategies (HNC vs. TNC) on recovering monocular and binocular performance in amblyopia, e.g., the magnitudes of improvement, measured in terms of percent change of AULCSF at AEM, AEU, dichoptic gain, visual acuity, and stereoacuity (**Figure 6**).

For the amblyopic eye, we found that the HNC training produced significantly greater improvements in the AEM contrast sensitivity ($t_{14} = 2.841$, $P = 0.025$) at the training spatial frequency, AEM AULCSF ($t_{14} = 2.367$, $P = 0.033$) and dichoptic gain ($t_{14} = 2.289$, $P = 0.038$), indicating that the HNC strategy is more effective than the TNC strategy in promoting the amblyopic eye to counteract the masking effect from the fellow eye. On the contrary, no significant difference between the two strategies was found in the magnitude of improvements of AEU AULCSF ($t_{14} = 0.947$, $P = 0.359$) and AEU contrast sensitivity ($t_{14} = 0.118$, $P = 0.908$) at the training spatial frequency. Both training strategies produced no significant change in FEU and FEM CSFs in the fellow eye.

The HNC training strategy also produced significantly greater improvement in visual acuity in the amblyopic eye ($t_{14} = 2.670$, $P = 0.018$) and stereoacuity ($t_{14} = 2.998$, $P = 0.010$) than the TNC strategy did. Both training strategies produced no significant change in visual acuity of the fellow eye.

Retention

Retention of training effects was evaluated for five patients (two patients from Group 1, the other three from Group 2) 12 months after training. The AEM contrast sensitivity and AEM AULCSF were almost fully retained, with mean retention coefficients of 90.1 ± 49.3 and 106.90 ± 14.52% (mean ± SEM). The AEU contrast sensitivity at cut-off spatial frequency and AEU AULCSF were also retained, with mean retention coefficients of 79.4 ± 34.2 and 93.65 ± 16.78%, respectively. The dichoptic gain for the amblyopic eye was also well retained, with a mean retention coefficient of 106.14 ± 14.29%. The average retention coefficient of improvement on visual acuity and stereoacuity was 82.28 ± 23.70 and 110.0 ± 22.4%. Overall, the training effects of both dichoptic training paradigms were robust.

DISCUSSION

In the current study, we proposed a new binocular training paradigm (i.e., HNC) and compared the efficacy of HNC and TNC protocols in adults with amblyopia. Although both strategies triggered significant learning, the HNC strategy produced more improvements in dichoptically masked CSF, dichoptic gain, visual acuity, and stereoacuity in the amblyopic eye. Furthermore, patients who had been trained with TNC strategy gained additional benefits in monocular and binocular performances from extra phase of HNC training.

Unlike recent dichoptic training paradigms that usually penalized the fellow eye to construct an artificial environment of equal contribution from two eyes in performing particular tasks, e.g., playing a video game and/or watching a film (Hess et al., 2010; Knox et al., 2012; Li J. et al., 2013b, Li J. et al., 2015; Li S.L. et al., 2015; Birch et al., 2015; Vedamurthy et al., 2015a,b; Kelly et al., 2016, 2018; Bossi et al., 2017; Birch et al., 2019), refractive correction provided roughly comparable physical inputs to both eyes and maintained a high-energy stimulation in the fellow eye. In other words, refractive adaptation could be considered as a binocular treatment approach with the presence of stronger inhibition from the fellow to the amblyopic eye, but in a more passive way (Wang et al., 2018). Several studies showed that refractive correction alone successfully improved the amblyopic visual acuity in both children (Moseley et al., 2002; Cotter et al., 2006) and some adults (Gao et al., 2018a). A recent psychophysical study reported that refractive adaptation also reduced interocular suppression, suggesting that the corrected amblyopic eye gradually acquired enhanced competence in binocular vision, even with constant and high suppression from the fellow eye (Wang et al., 2018). In the current study, we developed a new dichoptic training paradigm (e.g., HNC) that maintained high-contrast noise stimuli in the fellow eye, aiming to practice the amblyopic eye in a more intensified condition. Since all our subjects wore appropriate glasses for at least 8 weeks before they participated in the experiment, our results demonstrated the extra benefits of active dichoptic training with sustained high suppression from the fellow to the amblyopic eye. Further improvements in both monocular and binocular functions after the second-phase HNC training in Group 2 also confirmed the efficacy of the HNC protocol.

We found that the magnitude of visual improvement, especially in binocular performance, following the new HNC training strategy was larger than the TNC strategy. Moreover, we observed pronounced further improvement in dichoptic masked CSF, dichoptic gain, visual acuity in the amblyopic eye, as well as stereoacuity in patients of Group 2 who had prior training experience with TNC. These results implied that although both strategies could help the amblyopic eye to exclude the masking effect from the fellow eye, training under a high and constant noise contrast (HNC) was probably more effective than training with progressive noise contrast (TNC) in the fellow eye. Gratings with gradually decreased contrast in the amblyopic eye and noise with high contrast in the fellow eye may better simulate the normal binocular viewing condition, in which the fellow eye exerts constant and stronger inhibition over the amblyopic eye (Huang et al., 2009, 2011). Our HNC approach may have encouraged the amblyopic eye to cooperate more actively with the fellow eye (Mitchell et al., 2003; Murphy et al., 2015).

Our results about TNC training differed from those of Zhang et al. in terms of improvement in stereoacuity, who found a significant (410.9″ ± 70.7″ to 152.7″ ± 35.9″) improvement in stereoacuity (Liu and Zhang, 2019). Although both studies exploited a similar strategy, the intensity of training was different, with more sessions of training (17 sessions) performed in Zhang et al., likely leading to larger visual improvements (Li R.W. et al., 2008). In addition, all our patients had received refractive correction and fellow eye patching therapy for more than 2 months, while most of the patients in the study of Zhang et al. were naive to clinical treatment, especially refractive correction (Gao et al., 2018a). Moreover, the extent of anisometropia was relatively larger (4.59 vs. 3.82 diopters), and the initial amblyopic visual acuity was better (0.45 vs. 0.63 logMAR) in our study, which may also contribute to the discrepancy in visual improvements (Zhou et al., 2006; Dobson et al., 2008).

Patients in Group 1 showed a significant but small improvement in monocular unmasked contrast sensitivity, while those in Group 2 showed no improvement. These results suggest that unlike monocular training (Zhou et al., 2006; Huang et al., 2008; Chen et al., 2016; Jia et al., 2018), dichoptic training might not relieve the intrinsic limitations of the amblyopic eye (Hess et al., 1978; Levi and Klein, 1985; Levi et al., 1999; Xu et al., 2006; Huang et al., 2007, 2009). One possibility is that relatively low training spatial frequency was used in our study (2–4 c/d), which has been proved to be less effective than high spatial frequency in recovering monocular functions (Zhou et al., 2006). Moreover, training under noise and clear display may involve asymmetric transfer characteristics, e.g., training at clear display can benefit performance in noise display but not vice versa, indicating different underlying mechanisms (Dosher and Lu, 2005; Xie and Yu, 2019). On the other hand, there was no significant correlation between all improvements in binocular and monocular vision after HNC training, similar to a previous study (Jia et al., 2018). Zhang et al. found that monocular training further reduced the contrast threshold of the amblyopic eye of patients with dichoptic TNC training experience (Liu and Zhang, 2019). Taken together, these results suggested that dichoptic and monocular training have (at least partially) different mechanisms of improving amblyopic vision. Joint application of monocular and dichoptic training protocols has great potential in amblyopia treatment and is worthy of future investigation (Levi and Li, 2009; Xi et al., 2014; Levi et al., 2015; Jia et al., 2018).

One may argue that our findings were related to the enhanced adaptation in the fellow eye due to continuous presentation of high-contrast noise image in it (Gardner et al., 2005; Kohn, 2007). We do not think it is possible. First, learning effects were found be more prominent with masked condition, indicating of specific learning effects. Second, we performed a retest on five patients 12 months post-training and found robust retention of the training effects (e.g., visual acuity and monocular unmasked CSF) following HNC training. On the contrary, our results suggested that dichoptic and monocular training may involve different mechanisms (e.g., bias the top–down attention toward the amblyopic eye) (Liu and Zhang, 2019). Another limitation for this study is the lack of a reversed crossover, i.e., HNC training followed by TNC training, without which we could not determine the exact interaction of the two training strategies. Our results, on the other hand, provided evidence that HNC training could bring extra benefits after intensive TNC training. We did not find significant difference in improvement after HNC training in Group 1 and after both TNC and HNC training in Group 2, in terms of visual acuity (t_{14} = 0.741, P = 0.483), stereopsis (t_{14} = 0.682, P = 0.544), AEM contrast sensitivity at the trained spatial frequency (t_{14} = 0.632, P = 0.548), and AEM AULCSF (t_{14} = 0.410, P = 0.694), lending further support to the existence of extra benefits from HNC training, as opposed to TNC training.

To our knowledge, this is the first study that made direct comparison between two possible strategies of dichoptic training in amblyopia. Our results favored the strategy with constant high-contrast noise in the fellow eye and progressive contrast reduction in the amblyopic eye, which might be different in nature from the dichoptic training paradigm that aimed to increase maximal tolerable noise in the fellow eye and better represented the normal binocular viewing conditions.

AUTHOR CONTRIBUTIONS

ZL, ZC, C-BH, and MY designed the study, contributed to the writing of the manuscript, analyzed the data, and prepared the figures. ZL, ZC, ML, and JY prepared the experiment. ZL, ZC, LG, YH, and LF tested the participants. All authors contributed to the article and approved the submitted version.

ACKNOWLEDGMENTS

We thank Prof. Robert Hess for his very kind help in giving advice to our experiment design.

REFERENCES

Astle, A. T., Webb, B. S., and McGraw, P. V. (2011). The pattern of learned visual improvements in adult amblyopia. *Invest. Ophthalmol. Vis. Sci.* 52, 7195–7204. doi: 10.1167/iovs.11-7584

Birch, E. E., Jost, R. M., De La Cruz, A., Kelly, K. R., Beauchamp, C. L., Dao, L., et al. (2019). Binocular amblyopia treatment with contrast-rebalanced movies. *J. AAPOS* 23, 160 e161–160 e165. doi: 10.1016/j.jaapos.2019.02.007

Birch, E. E., Li, S. L., Jost, R. M., Morale, S. E., De La Cruz, A., Stager, D., et al. (2015). Binocular iPad treatment for amblyopia in preschool children. *J. AAPOS* 19, 6–11. doi: 10.1016/j.jaapos.2014.09.009

Bossi, M., Tailor, V. K., Anderson, E. J., Bex, P. J., Greenwood, J. A., Dahlmann-Noor, A., et al. (2017). Binocular therapy for childhood amblyopia improves vision without breaking interocular suppression. *Invest. Ophthalmol. Vis. Sci.* 58, 3031–3043. doi: 10.1167/iovs.16-20913

Brainard, D. H. (1997). The psychophysics toolbox. *Spat. Vis.* 10, 433–436. doi: 10.1163/156856897X00357

Campana, G., Camilleri, R., Pavan, A., Veronese, A., and Lo Giudice, G. (2014). Improving visual functions in adult amblyopia with combined perceptual training and transcranial random noise stimulation (tRNS): a pilot study. *Front. Psychol.* 5:1402. doi: 10.3389/fpsyg.2014.01402

Chen, G., Hou, F., Yan, F. F., Zhang, P., Xi, J., Zhou, Y., et al. (2014). Noise provides new insights on contrast sensitivity function. *PLoS One* 9:e90579. doi: 10.1371/journal.pone.0090579

Chen, Z., Li, J., Liu, J., Cai, X., Yuan, J., Deng, D., et al. (2016). Monocular perceptual learning of contrast detection facilitates binocular combination in adults with anisometropic amblyopia. *Sci. Rep.* 6:20187. doi: 10.1038/srep20187

Cotter, S. A., Pediatric Eye Disease Investigator Group, Edwards, A. R., Wallace, D. K., Beck, R. W., Arnold, R. W., et al. (2006). Treatment of anisometropic amblyopia in children with refractive correction. *Ophthalmology* 113, 895–903. doi: 10.1016/j.ophtha.2006.01.068

Dobson, V., Miller, J. M., Clifford-Donaldson, C. E., and Harvey, E. M. (2008). Associations between anisometropia, amblyopia, and reduced stereoacuity in a school-aged population with a high prevalence of astigmatism. *Invest. Ophthalmol. Vis. Sci.* 49, 4427–4436. doi: 10.1167/iovs.08-1985

Dosher, B. A., and Lu, Z. L. (2005). Perceptual learning in clear displays optimizes perceptual expertise: learning the limiting process. *Proc. Natl. Acad. Sci. U.S.A.* 102, 5286–5290. doi: 10.1073/pnas.0500492102

Gao, T. Y., Anstice, N., Babu, R. J., Black, J. M., Bobier, W. R., Dai, S., et al. (2018a). Optical treatment of amblyopia in older children and adults is essential prior to enrolment in a clinical trial. *Ophthalm. Physiol. Opt.* 38, 129–143. doi: 10.1111/opo.12437

Gao, T. Y., Guo, C. X., Babu, R. J., Black, J. M., Bobier, W. R., Chakraborty, A., et al. (2018b). effectiveness of a binocular video game vs placebo video game for improving visual functions in older children, teenagers, and adults with amblyopia: a randomized clinical trial. *JAMA Ophthalmol.* 136, 172–181. doi: 10.1001/jamaophthalmol.2017.6090

Gardner, J. L., Sun, P., Waggoner, R. A., Ueno, K., Tanaka, K., and Cheng, K. (2005). Contrast adaptation and representation in human early visual cortex. *Neuron* 47, 607–620. doi: 10.1016/j.neuron.2005.07.016

Hess, R. F., and Bradley, A. (1980). Contrast perception above threshold is only minimally impaired in human amblyopia. *Nature* 287, 463–464. doi: 10.1038/287463a0

Hess, R. F., Campbell, F. W., and Greenhalgh, T. (1978). On the nature of the neural abnormality in human amblyopia; neural aberrations and neural sensitivity loss. *Pflugers. Arch.* 377, 201–207. doi: 10.1007/BF00584273

Hess, R. F., and Howell, E. R. (1977). The threshold contrast sensitivity function in strabismic amblyopia: evidence for a two type classification. *Vis. Res.* 17, 1049–1055. doi: 10.1016/0042-6989(77)90009-8

Hess, R. F., Mansouri, B., and Thompson, B. (2010). A new binocular approach to the treatment of amblyopia in adults well beyond the critical period of visual development. *Restor. Neurol. Neurosci.* 28, 793–802. doi: 10.3233/RNN-2010-0550

Holmes, J. M., and Clarke, M. P. (2006). Amblyopia. *Lancet* 367, 1343–1351. doi: 10.1016/S0140-6736(06)68581-4

Holmes, J. M., and Levi, D. M. (2018). Treatment of amblyopia as a function of age. *Vis. Neurosci.* 35:E015. doi: 10.1017/S0952523817000220

Holmes, J. M., Manh, V. M., Lazar, E. L., Beck, R. W., Birch, E. E., Kraker, R. T., et al. (2016). Effect of a binocular iPad game vs Part-time patching in children aged 5 to 12 years with Amblyopia: a randomized clinical trial. *JAMA Ophthalmol.* 134, 1391–1400. doi: 10.1001/jamaophthalmol.2016.4262

Holmes, J. M., Repka, M. X., Kraker, R. T., and Clarke, M. P. (2006). The treatment of amblyopia. *Strabismus* 14, 37–42. doi: 10.1080/09273970500536227

Hou, F., Huang, C. B., Tao, L., Feng, L., Zhou, Y., and Lu, Z. L. (2011). Training in contrast detection improves motion perception of sinewave gratings in amblyopia. *Invest. Ophthalmol. Vis. Sci.* 52, 6501–6510. doi: 10.1167/iovs.11-7541

Huang, C., Tao, L., Zhou, Y., and Lu, Z. L. (2007). Treated amblyopes remain deficient in spatial vision: a contrast sensitivity and external noise study. *Vis. Res.* 47, 22–34. doi: 10.1016/j.visres.2006.09.015

Huang, C. B., Zhou, J., Lu, Z. L., Feng, L., and Zhou, Y. (2009). Binocular combination in anisometropic amblyopia. *J. Vis.* 9, 11–16. doi: 10.1167/9.3.17

Huang, C. B., Zhou, J., Lu, Z. L., and Zhou, Y. (2011). Deficient binocular combination reveals mechanisms of anisometropic amblyopia: signal attenuation and interocular inhibition. *J. Vis.* 11:10.1167/11.6.44. doi: 10.1167/11.6.4

Huang, C. B., Zhou, Y., and Lu, Z. L. (2008). Broad bandwidth of perceptual learning in the visual system of adults with anisometropic amblyopia. *Proc. Natl. Acad. Sci. U.S.A.* 105, 4068–4073. doi: 10.1073/pnas.0800824105

Jia, W., Lan, F., Zhao, X., Lu, Z. L., Huang, C. B., Zhao, W., et al. (2018). The effects of monocular training on binocular functions in anisometropic amblyopia. *Vis. Res.* 152, 74–83. doi: 10.1016/j.visres.2017.02.008

Kelly, K. R., Jost, R. M., Dao, L., Beauchamp, C. L., Leffler, J. N., and Birch, E. E. (2016). Binocular iPad Game vs Patching for treatment of amblyopia in children: a randomized clinical trial. *JAMA Ophthalmol.* 134, 1402–1408. doi: 10.1001/jamaophthalmol.2016.4224

Kelly, K. R., Jost, R. M., Wang, Y. Z., Dao, L., Beauchamp, C. L., Leffler, J. N., et al. (2018). Improved binocular outcomes following binocular treatment for childhood Amblyopia. *Invest. Ophthalmol. Vis. Sci.* 59, 1221–1228. doi: 10.1167/iovs.17-23235

Kiorpes, L., Kiper, D. C., O'Keefe, L. P., Cavanaugh, J. R., and Movshon, J. A. (1998). Neuronal correlates of amblyopia in the visual cortex of macaque monkeys with experimental strabismus and anisometropia. *J. Neurosci.* 18, 6411–6424. doi: 10.1523/JNEUROSCI.18-16-06411.1998

Kiorpes, L., Tang, C., and Movshon, J. A. (1999). Factors limiting contrast sensitivity in experimentally amblyopic macaque monkeys. *Vis. Res.* 39, 4152–4160. doi: 10.1016/s0042-6989(99)00130-3

Knox, P. J., Simmers, A. J., Gray, L. S., and Cleary, M. (2012). An exploratory study: prolonged periods of binocular stimulation can provide an effective treatment for childhood amblyopia. *Invest. Ophthalmol. Vis. Sci.* 53, 817–824. doi: 10.1167/iovs.11-8219

Kohn, A. (2007). Visual adaptation: physiology, mechanisms, and functional benefits. *J. Neurophysiol.* 97, 3155–3164. doi: 10.1152/jn.00086.2007

Lesmes, L. A., Lu, Z. L., Baek, J., and Albright, T. D. (2010). Bayesian adaptive estimation of the contrast sensitivity function: the quick CSF method. *J. Vis.* 10, 17.1–1721. doi: 10.1167/10.3.17

Levi, D. M. (2006). Visual processing in amblyopia: human studies. *Strabismus* 14, 11–19. doi: 10.1080/09273970500536243

Levi, D. M., and Klein, S. A. (1985). Vernier acuity, crowding and amblyopia. *Vis. Res.* 25, 979–991. doi: 10.1016/0042-6989(85)90208-1

Levi, D. M., Klein, S. A., and Sharma, V. (1999). Position jitter and undersampling in pattern perception. *Vis. Res.* 39, 445–465. doi: 10.1016/s0042-6989(98)00125-4

Levi, D. M., Knill, D. C., and Bavelier, D. (2015). Stereopsis and amblyopia: a mini-review. *Vis. Res.* 114, 17–30. doi: 10.1016/j.visres.2015.01.002

Levi, D. M., and Li, R. W. (2009). Perceptual learning as a potential treatment for amblyopia: a mini-review. *Vis. Res.* 49, 2535–2549. doi: 10.1016/j.visres.2009.02.010

Levi, D. M., Polat, U., and Hu, Y. S. (1997). Improvement in Vernier acuity in adults with amblyopia. practice makes better. *Invest. Ophthalmol. Vis. Sci.* 38, 1493–1510.

Levitt, H. (1971). Transformed up-down methods in psychoacoustics. *J .Acoust. Soc. Am.* 49:467. doi: 10.1121/1.1912375

Li, J., Hess, R. F., Chan, L. Y., Deng, D., Yang, X., Chen, X., et al. (2013a). Quantitative measurement of interocular suppression in anisometropic amblyopia: a case-control study. *Ophthalmology* 120, 1672–1680. doi: 10.1016/j.ophtha.2013.01.048

Li, J., Thompson, B., Deng, D., Chan, L. Y., Yu, M., and Hess, R. F. (2013b). Dichoptic training enables the adult amblyopic brain to learn. *Curr. Biol.* 23, R308–R309. doi: 10.1016/j.cub.2013.01.059

Li, J., Spiegel, D. P., Hess, R. F., Chen, Z., Chan, L. Y., Deng, D., et al. (2015). Dichoptic training improves contrast sensitivity in adults with amblyopia. *Vis. Res.* 114, 161–172. doi: 10.1016/j.visres.2015.01.017

Li, S. L., Reynaud, A., Hess, R. F., Wang, Y. Z., Jost, R. M., Morale, S. E., et al. (2015). Dichoptic movie viewing treats childhood amblyopia. *J. AAPOS* 19, 401–405. doi: 10.1016/j.jaapos.2015.08.003

Li, J., Thompson, B., Lam, C. S., Deng, D., Chan, L. Y., Maehara, G., et al. (2011). The role of suppression in amblyopia. *Invest. Ophthalmol. Vis. Sci.* 52, 4169–4176. doi: 10.1167/iovs.11-7233

Li, R. W., Klein, S. A., and Levi, D. M. (2008). Prolonged perceptual learning of positional acuity in adult amblyopia: perceptual template retuning dynamics. *J. Neurosci.* 28, 14223–14229. doi: 10.1523/JNEUROSCI.4271-08.2008

Li, R. W., Young, K. G., Hoenig, P., and Levi, D. M. (2005). Perceptual learning improves visual performance in juvenile amblyopia. *Invest. Ophthalmol. Vis. Sci.* 46, 3161–3168. doi: 10.1167/iovs.05-0286

Liu, X. Y., and Zhang, J. Y. (2018). Dichoptic training in adults with amblyopia: additional stereoacuity gains over monocular training. *Vis. Res.* 152, 84–90. doi: 10.1016/j.visres.2017.07.002

Liu, X. Y., and Zhang, J. Y. (2019). Dichoptic de-masking learning in adults with Amblyopia and its mechanisms. *Invest. Ophthalmol Vis. Sci.* 60, 2968–2977. doi: 10.1167/iovs.18-26483

Lunghi, C., Morrone, M. C., Secci, J., and Caputo, R. (2016). Binocular rivalry measured 2 hours after occlusion therapy predicts the recovery rate of the amblyopic eye in anisometropic children. *Invest. Ophthalmol. Vis. Sci.* 57, 1537–1546. doi: 10.1167/iovs.15-18419

McKee, S. P., Levi, D. M., and Movshon, J. A. (2003). The pattern of visual deficits in amblyopia. *J. Vis.* 3, 380–405. doi: 10.1167/3.5.5

Mitchell, D. E., Kind, P. C., Sengpiel, F., and Murphy, K. (2003). Brief daily periods of binocular vision prevent deprivation-induced acuity loss. *Curr. Biol.* 13, 1704–1708. doi: 10.1016/j.cub.2003.09.026

Moseley, M. J., Neufeld, M., McCarry, B., Charnock, A., McNamara, R., Rice, T., et al. (2002). Remediation of refractive amblyopia by optical correction alone. *Ophthalm. Physiol. Opt.* 22, 296–299. doi: 10.1046/j.1475-1313.2002.00034.x

Mou, T. (2005). The 5-grade notation of the standard logarithmic visual acuity chart. *Chin. J. Optomet. Ophthalmol.* 7, 217–219. doi: 10.3760/cma.j.issn.1674-845X.2005.04.001

Murphy, K. M., Roumeliotis, G., Williams, K., Beston, B. R., and Jones, D. G. (2015). Binocular visual training to promote recovery from monocular deprivation. *J. Vis.* 15:15.1.2. doi: 10.1167/15.1.2

Ooi, T. L., Su, Y. R., Natale, D. M., and He, Z. J. (2013). A push-pull treatment for strengthening the 'lazy eye' in amblyopia. *Curr. Biol.* 23, R309–R310. doi: 10.1016/j.cub.2013.03.004

Pediatric Eye Disease Investigator Group,, J. M., Manny, R. E., Lazar, E. L., Birch, E. E., Kelly, K. R., et al. (2019). A Randomized trial of binocular dig rush game treatment for amblyopia in children aged 7 to 12 Years. *Ophthalmology* 126, 456–466. doi: 10.1016/j.ophtha.2018.10.032

Pelli, D. G. (1997). The VideoToolbox software for visual psychophysics: transforming numbers into movies. *Spat. Vis.* 10, 437–442. doi: 10.1163/156856897X00366

Polat, U., Ma-Naim, T., Belkin, M., and Sagi, D. (2004). Improving vision in adult amblyopia by perceptual learning. *Proc. Natl. Acad. Sci. U.S.A.* 101, 6692–6697. doi: 10.1073/pnas.0401200101

Polat, U., Ma-Naim, T., and Spierer, A. (2009). Treatment of children with amblyopia by perceptual learning. *Vis. Res.* 49, 2599–2603. doi: 10.1016/j.visres.2009.07.008

Shooner, C., Hallum, L. E., Kumbhani, R. D., Garcia-Marin, V., Kelly, J. G., Majaj, N. J., et al. (2017). Asymmetric dichoptic masking in visual cortex of amblyopic macaque monkeys. *J. Neurosci.* 37, 8734–8741. doi: 10.1523/JNEUROSCI.1760-17.2017

Sloper, J. (2016). New treatments for amblyopia-to patch or play? *JAMA Ophthalmol.* 134, 1408–1410. doi: 10.1001/jamaophthalmol.2016.4296

Subramanian, V., Jost, R. M., and Birch, E. E. (2013). A quantitative study of fixation stability in amblyopia. *Invest .Ophthalmol. Vis. Sci.* 54, 1998–2003. doi: 10.1167/iovs.12-11054

Tailor, V., Bossi, M., Greenwood, J. A., and Dahlmann-Noor, A. (2016). Childhood amblyopia: current management and new trends. *Br. Med. Bull.* 119, 75–86. doi: 10.1093/bmb/ldw030

Vedamurthy, I., Nahum, M., Bavelier, D., and Levi, D. M. (2015a). Mechanisms of recovery of visual function in adult amblyopia through a tailored action video game. *Sci. Rep.* 5:8482. doi: 10.1038/srep08482

Vedamurthy, I., Nahum, M., Huang, S. J., Zheng, F., Bayliss, J., Bavelier, D., et al. (2015b). A dichoptic custom-made action video game as a treatment for adult amblyopia. *Vis. Res.* 114, 173–187. doi: 10.1016/j.visres.2015.04.008

Wang, J., Feng, L., Wang, Y., Zhou, J., and Hess, R. F. (2018). Binocular benefits of optical treatment in anisometropic amblyopia. *J. Vis.* 18:6. doi: 10.1167/18.4.6

Xi, J., Jia, W. L., Feng, L. X., Lu, Z. L., and Huang, C. B. (2014). Perceptual learning improves stereoacuity in amblyopia. *Invest. Ophthalmol. Vis. Sci.* 55, 2384–2391. doi: 10.1167/iovs.13-12627

Xie, X. Y., and Yu, C. (2019). Perceptual learning of Vernier discrimination transfers from high to zero noise after double training. *Vis. Res.* 156, 39–45. doi: 10.1016/j.visres.2019.01.007

Xu, P., Lu, Z. L., Qiu, Z., and Zhou, Y. (2006). Identify mechanisms of amblyopia in Gabor orientation identification with external noise. *Vis. Res.* 46, 3748–3760. doi: 10.1016/j.visres.2006.06.013

Zhao, W., Jia, W. L., Chen, G., Luo, Y., Lin, B., He, Q., et al. (2017). A complete investigation of monocular and binocular functions in clinically treated amblyopia. *Sci. Rep.* 7:10682. doi: 10.1038/s41598-017-11124-0

Zhou, J., Reynaud, A., Yao, Z., Liu, R., Feng, L., Zhou, Y., et al. (2018). Amblyopic suppression: passive attenuation, enhanced Dichoptic masking by the fellow eye or reduced Dichoptic masking by the amblyopic eye? *Invest. Ophthalmol. Vis. Sci.* 59, 4190–4197. doi: 10.1167/iovs.18-24206

Zhou, Y., Huang, C., Xu, P., Tao, L., Qiu, Z., Li, X., et al. (2006). Perceptual learning improves contrast sensitivity and visual acuity in adults with anisometropic amblyopia. *Vis. Res.* 46, 739–750. doi: 10.1016/j.visres.2005.07.031

15

The Spatial Distribution of Relative Corneal Refractive Power Shift and Axial Growth in Myopic Children: Orthokeratology versus Multifocal Contact Lens

Fan Jiang[1], Xiaopeng Huang[1], Houxue Xia[1], Bingqi Wang[1], Fan Lu[1], Bin Zhang[2*] and Jun Jiang[1,3*]*

[1] School of Ophthalmology and Optometry, Wenzhou Medical University, Wenzhou, China, [2] College of Optometry, Nova Southeastern University, Fort Lauderdale, FL, United States, [3] Eye Hospital, Wenzhou Medical University, Wenzhou, China

Correspondence:
Fan Lu
lufan62@mail.eye.ac.cn
Bin Zhang
bz52@nova.edu
Jun Jiang
jjhsj@hotmail.com

Purpose: To determine if the spatial distribution of the relative corneal refractive power shift (RCRPS) explains the retardation of axial length (AL) elongation after treatment by either orthokeratology (OK) or multifocal soft contact lenses (MFCLs).

Methods: Children (8–14 years) were enrolled in the OK (n = 35) or MFCL (n = 36) groups. RCRPS maps were derived by computing the difference between baseline and 12-month corneal topography maps and then subtracting the apex values. Values at the same radius were averaged to obtain the RCRPS profile, from which four parameters were extracted: (1) Half_x and (2) Half_y, i.e., the x- and y-coordinates where each profile first reached the half peak; (3) Sum4 and (4) Sum7, i.e., the summation of powers within a corneal area of 4- and 7-mm diameters. Correlations between AL elongation and these parameters were analyzed by multiple linear regression.

Results: AL elongation in the OK group was significantly smaller than that in the MFCL group (p = 0.040). Half_x and Half_y were also smaller in the OK group than the MFCL group (p < 0.001 each). Half_x was correlated with AL elongation in the OK group (p = 0.005), but not in the MFCL group (p = 0.600). In an analysis that combined eyes of both groups, Half_x was correlated with AL elongation (β = 0.161, p < 0.001).

Conclusions: The OK-induced AL elongation and associated RCRPS Half_x were smaller than for the MFCL. Contact lenses that induce RCRPS closer to the corneal center may exert better myopia control.

Keywords: orthokeratology, multifocal soft contact lens, corneal refractive power, axial length, myopia

INTRODUCTION

The incidence of myopia has risen over the last several decades (Williams et al., 2015; Holden et al., 2016), particularly in East Asian countries where about 80% of the 18-year-olds are myopic (Rudnicka et al., 2016). Myopia is usually associated with excessive axial length (AL) elongation (Morgan et al., 2012), which increases the risk of ocular complications such as myopic maculopathy, retinal detachment, and glaucoma (Marcus et al., 2011; Flitcroft, 2012). Orthokeratology (OK) lenses and multifocal soft contact lenses (MFCLs) are the two most often used optical devices in the clinic to correct refractive error and to retard AL elongation (Huang et al., 2016; Kang, 2018). OK lenses have a reverse-geometry on the back surface that flattens the central zone of the cornea and steepens the mid-peripheral zone during overnight wear (Sridharan and Swarbrick, 2003). During the day, this altered corneal front surface induces myopic defocus on the peripheral retina (Charman et al., 2006; Queiros et al., 2010, 2018), and this may be a mechanism for myopia retardation (Smith et al., 2009; Benavente-Perez et al., 2014). In contrast, daytime MFCL wear directly imposes peripheral retinal myopic defocus when the lenses are worn (Sankaridurg et al., 2011; Allinjawi et al., 2016).

Recent studies suggested the importance of the spatial distribution of the peripheral myopic defocus in retarding axial growth. Liu and Wildsoet reported that two-zone bifocal spectacle lenses incorporating +5 diopter (D) of peripheral defocus, extending from 1.25 to 2.75 mm from the lens center to its periphery, were effective in retarding axial growth in chicks. However, more peripheral zones, beginning 3.25 mm from the lens center, had no effect (Liu and Wildsoet, 2011). A study in monkeys reported that lenses imposing myopic defocus close to the optic axis were more effective in inhibiting axial growth than those in which defocus was limited to the more peripheral regions, e.g., 20 degrees away from the optic axis (Smith et al., 2020).

In clinical studies of OK lenses, the change of corneal refractive power (CRP) could be captured by corneal topography. The difference in CRP before and after OK treatment was calculated as the CRP shift (CRPS). Subtracting the apex value from each point of the CRPS then derives the relative CRPS (RCRPS) that is related with the myopic shift in defocus on the peripheral retina (Kang and Swarbrick, 2013). Some studies have suggested that RCRPS is strongly associated with AL elongation (Zhong et al., 2014, 2015; Lee et al., 2018; Hu et al., 2019). However, existing studies used only simple measures, such as the maximum value of either the whole map (Lee et al., 2018) or along some axes (Zhong et al., 2014), or the summed value within a certain area (Zhong et al., 2015; Hu et al., 2019). Neither maximum nor summed value provides information on the spatial distribution of the RCRPS because lenses with different spatial distributions of RCRPS may have similar maximum and summed values. Therefore, in this study, we proposed a new index that we identify as "Half_x" to quantify the spatial distribution of the RCRPS. Furthermore, we then determine if variations in Half_x explain the variations in the retardation of AL elongation observed in children who underwent OK treatment.

Both OK lenses and MFCLs act by modifying the refractive power of the front optical surface. However, few studies have analyzed the axial retardation effect of MFCLs through the perspective of the RCRPS. Therefore, a second aim of the present study was to examine whether or not Half_x, the new index on RCRPS spatial distribution, could also be applied to MFCL wear. The analysis of such an index on OK and MFCL subjects as a combined group would provide a unified theoretic background to interpret the axial retardation effect. Moreover, the knowledge obtained from OK lens design could be utilized in MFCL design.

MATERIALS AND METHODS

Subjects

Thirty-seven MFCL subjects were enrolled in this registered clinical trial[1] (Registration number: ChiCTR-OOC-17012103). Thirty-seven OK subjects were from a previous study of OK lens safety. The inclusion criteria for both groups were as follows: 8 to 14 years of age, spherical equivalent (SE) from −1.00 D to −5.00 D, corneal astigmatism ≤1.50 D, best-corrected visual acuity greater than 20/25, no binocular vision dysfunction, no obvious angle kappa, no history of an OK lens or MFCL wear or any other myopia control treatments such as atropine, no application of atropine for cycloplegia during the past 30 days, no contact lens contraindications or related eye and systemic disease. All procedures complied with the Declaration of Helsinki, and the protocol was reviewed and approved by the Ethics Committee of the Eye Hospital of Wenzhou Medical University. All the examinations were conducted after the subjects, and their guardians fully understood and signed informed consent.

Refraction

Cycloplegic autorefraction was performed at baseline. One drop of 0.5% proparacaine was instilled. One minute later, this was followed by two drops of 1% cyclopentolate, administered 5 min apart. Refractive results were converted to SEs, which were calculated as the spherical power plus 1/2 cylindrical power.

Lens Fitting

In both groups, the lenses were fitted to both eyes according to the manufacturer's guidelines. For the OK group, a four-zone reverse geometry lens (Euclid Systems Corp., Herndon, VA, United States) is composed of oprifocon A [DK: 90×10^{-11} (cm^2/s) (mL O_2/mL*mmHg)] was used. The diameter of the lenses ranged from 10.2 to 10.6 mm. The lens consisted of a central base curve with a 6.2-mm optic zone, a 0.5-mm wide reverse curve, a 1.0 to 1.2-mm wide alignment curve, and a 0.5-mm wide peripheral curve. The subjects were instructed to wear them for at least 8 h every night. OK lens prescriptions were changed if the uncorrected visual acuity was less than 20/25 after regular wear for one month or unacceptable lens decentration was observed. For the MFCL group, a daily disposable soft contact lens (BioThin, Bio Optic Inc., Taiwan, China) made of ocufilcon D [DK: 19×10^{-11} (cm^2/s) (mL O_2/mL*mmHg)] with a diameter of 14.2 mm and a base curve of 8.6 mm was used. The lenses were designed to have the spherical distance power at the central treatment zone of 0–3 mm diameter and a myopic defocus zone of 3–6 mm diameter (Huang et al., 2020). Subjects were asked to wear the MFCL for at least 5 days/week, 8 h/day. MFCL

[1] http://www.chictr.org.cn/index.aspx

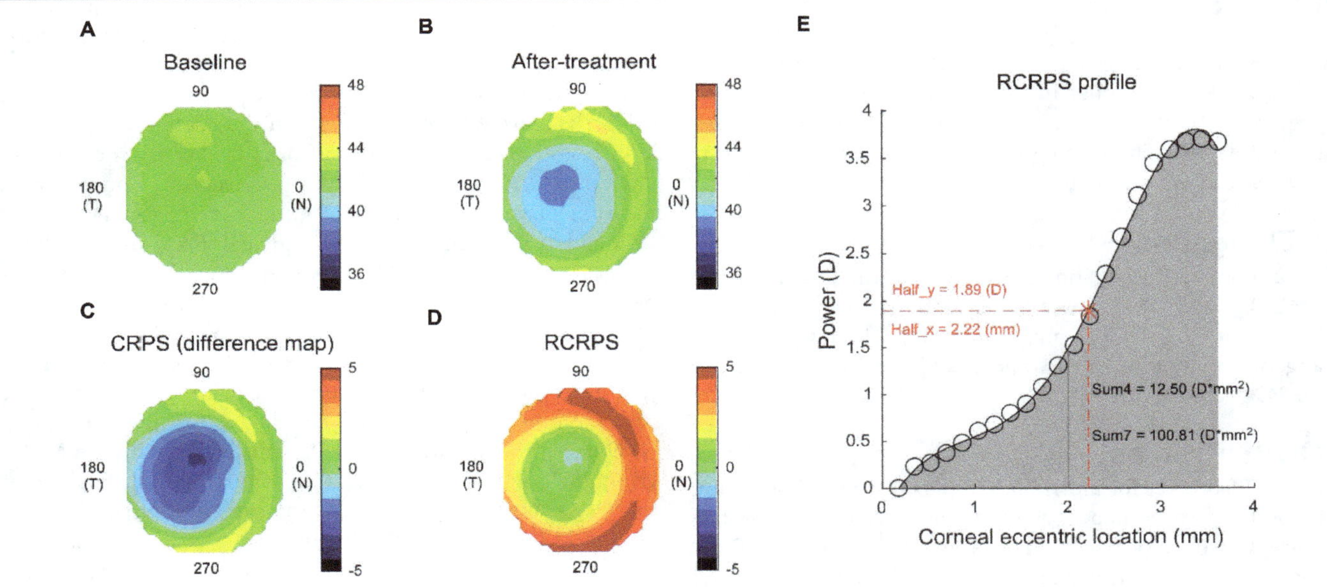

FIGURE 1 | Computation of the RCRPS for a representative eye. **(A)** An axial map at baseline. **(B)** An axial map at 12 months after treatment. **(C)** CRPS was derived by subtracting the baseline map from the after-treatment map. **(D)** RCRPS was derived by subtracting the center point value from each point on the CRPS. **(E)** RCRPS profile derived by taking the mean of each ring. Data are for an eye wearing the OK lens. Similar determinations were made for eyes wearing the MFCLs. RCRPS, relative corneal refractive power shift; CRPS, corneal refractive power shift; OK, orthokeratology; MFCL, multifocal soft contact lens; Half_x, the corneal eccentric location where RCRPS reached the half peak value; Half_y, half of the RCRPS peak value; Sum4, the integrated value of the RCRPS located within an area of 4-mm diameter; Sum7, the integrated value of the RCRPS located within an area of 7-mm diameter.

prescriptions were changed if the corrected visual acuity was less than 20/25, or the spherical over-refraction achieved −0.50 D in the follow-up visits.

Axial Length

AL was measured by the IOL-Master system (IOL-Master, Carl Zeiss, Jena, Germany) at baseline and at the 12-month follow-up visit. Measurements were performed by the same operator, and five reliable readings with a signal-to-noise ratio >2.1 were collected, of which the median value was used for analysis.

Corneal Topography

Corneal topography (Medmont E300; Medmont International Pty. Ltd., Victoria, Australia) was obtained at baseline and 12 months after lens wear was initiated to quantify RCRPS. For the OK group, the 12-month measurement was performed with the lens off, and for the MFCL group, it was done with the lens on. All measurements were conducted between 8 and 10 am to minimize the diurnal variation. Each exported axial map had 32 rings, each containing 300 data points. After preparing the baseline and the after-treatment topography maps (**Figures 1A,B** respectively), the CRPS map (**Figure 1C**) was obtained by subtracting the baseline map data from the after-treatment map data. Then, the apex value was subtracted from each point to derive the RCRPS map (**Figure 1D**). The profile of the RCRPS was calculated by taking the mean value of each ring and fitting a polynomial curve through them (**Figure 1E**). The point where RCRPS reached the half-peak value was identified, and the x-axis value of this point was defined as the Half_x, indicating how fast the RCRPS had risen. The y-axis value of the point was defined as the Half_y. Sum4 was defined as the integrated value of the RCRPS located within a corneal area of 4-mm diameter. Similarly, Sum7 was defined as the integrated value of the RCRPS located within a corneal area of 7-mm diameter. All calculations were conducted using the custom MATLAB function (MathWorks, Natick, WA, United States).

Pupil size was extracted from the topographic data obtained under ambient mesopic room illumination, but photopic conditions were still considered due to topographer intrinsic light level (Periman et al., 2003). Pupil radius was calculated by halving the average of horizontal and vertical pupil diameters.

Statistical Analyses

Only the right eyes were included in the analysis. The Schapiro-Wilk test was used to examine data distribution normality. For comparisons between the OK and MFCL groups, *t*-tests were used for normally distributed data, and Mann-Whitney *U* tests were used otherwise. Simple univariate regression was used first to explore the associations between AL elongation and baseline and RCRPS parameters. The parameters that showed significance were then further analyzed in a stepwise multivariate regression. Variable selection in the multivariable model was based on the Akaike Information Criterion (Akaike, 1974). All analyses were performed using the R programming package[2] (version 3.6.3), and $p < 0.05$ was defined as statistically significant.

[2]HTTP://www.r-project.org/

RESULTS

Two eyes of the OK group and one eye of the MFCL group were excluded due to poor measurement quality of the corneal topography. A total of 71 eyes were included in the analyses. There were no significant differences between the two groups in the baseline information (**Table 1**).

AL Elongation

The 12-month AL elongation for subjects in the OK group was 0.19 ± 0.20 mm, which was significantly smaller than in the MFCL group, 0.27 ± 0.15 mm (p = 0.040). The rate of the AL change was margin for the two groups (OK: 0.77%, MF: 1.12%, p = 0.049 (**Table 2**).

RCRPS Profiles

The RCRPS profiles for individuals in the OK and MFCL groups were both clearly S-shaped, as shown in representative profiles (**Figures 2A,B** respectively). However, there were significant differences between the two groups, as seen in the representative profiles. For instance, the profile for the OK subject (**Figure 2A**) reached the half peak at a relatively small corneal eccentric location (Half_x = 1.58 mm). At the 2.5 mm location, the value reached a plateau. In contrast, the profile for the MFCL subject (**Figure 2B**) remained low in the central region before it increased and reached the half peak farther from the center (Half_x = 2.56 mm) than for the OK subject. Consequently, the sum of values within the 4-mm diameter (Sum4 = 13.50 D*mm^2) for the OK subject was greater than for the MFCL subject (Sum4 = −1.65 D*mm^2), even though the two profiles had similar Sum7 values. Meanwhile, the AL elongation for the OK subject was much smaller than for the MFCL subject.

The RCRPS profile for the entire OK group started to rise at a location closer to the center than for the entire MFCL group (**Figure 3A**). The Half_x for the OK group (1.89 ± 0.45 mm) was significantly smaller than for the MFCL group (2.32 ± 0.28 mm; $p < 0.001$; **Figure 3B**). The Half_y for the OK group (1.15 ± 0.45 D) was significantly smaller than for the MFCL group (1.92 ± 0.66 D; $p < 0.001$; **Figure 3C**). The Sum4 in the OK group (8.77 ± 9.34 D*mm^2) was greater than for the MFCL group (4.01 ± 11.70 D*mm^2), but the difference was not significant (p = 0.063; **Figure 3D**). The Sum7

TABLE 1 | Baseline information for subjects.

Parameter	OK (n = 35)	MFCL (n = 36)	P value
Age (y)	10.5 ± 1.6	10.6 ± 1.4	0.953
Males (%)	12 (34%)	14 (39%)	0.876
SE (D)	−2.73 ± 0.99	−2.55 ± 0.86	0.515
Pupil radius (mm)	1.81 ± 0.48	1.83 ± 0.30	0.461

OK, orthokeratology; MFCL, multifocal contact lens; y, years old; SE, spherical equivalent; D, diopter.

TABLE 2 | Axial length and axial length change for subjects.

	OK	MFCL	P value
Baseline (mm)	24.63 ± 0.65	24.50 ± 0.63	0.366
12 months (mm)	24.82 ± 0.55	24.77 ± 0.64	0.723
Change (mm)	0.19 ± 0.20	0.27 ± 0.15	0.040
Rate of change (%)	0.77 ± 0.86	1.12 ± 0.60	0.049

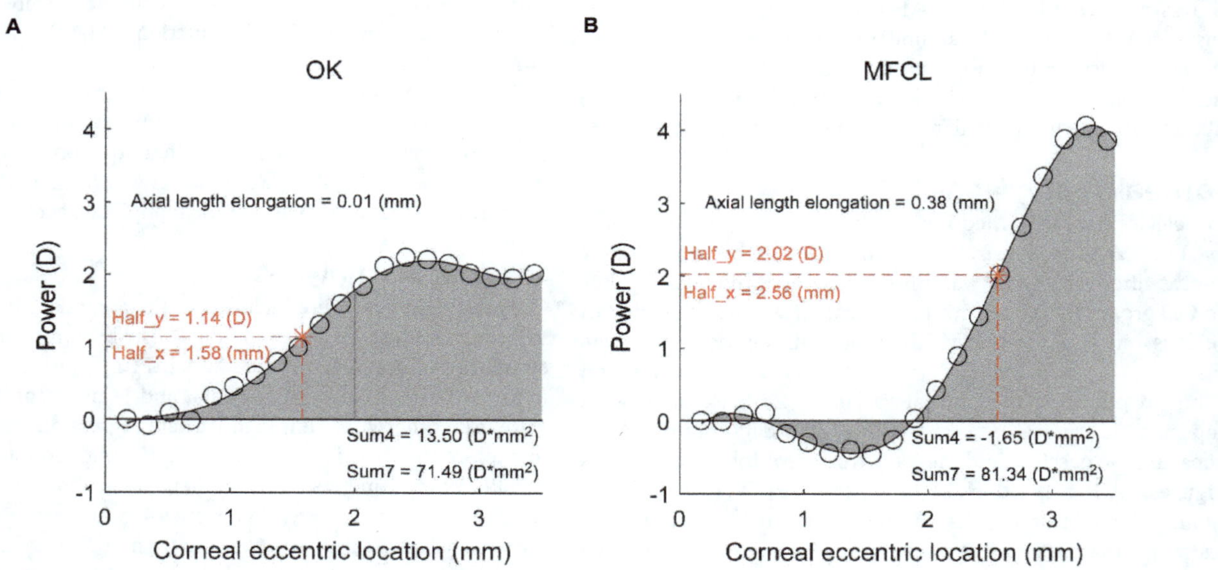

FIGURE 2 | Representative RCRPS profiles. **(A)** An eye in the OK group. **(B)** An eye from the MFCL group. RCRPS, relative corneal refractive power shift; D, diopter; OK, orthokeratology; MFCL, multifocal soft contact lens; Half_x, the corneal eccentric location where RCRPS reached the half peak value; Half_y, half of the RCRPS peak value; Sum4, the integrated value of the RCRPS located within an area of 4-mm diameter; Sum7, the integrated value of the RCRPS located within an area of 7-mm diameter.

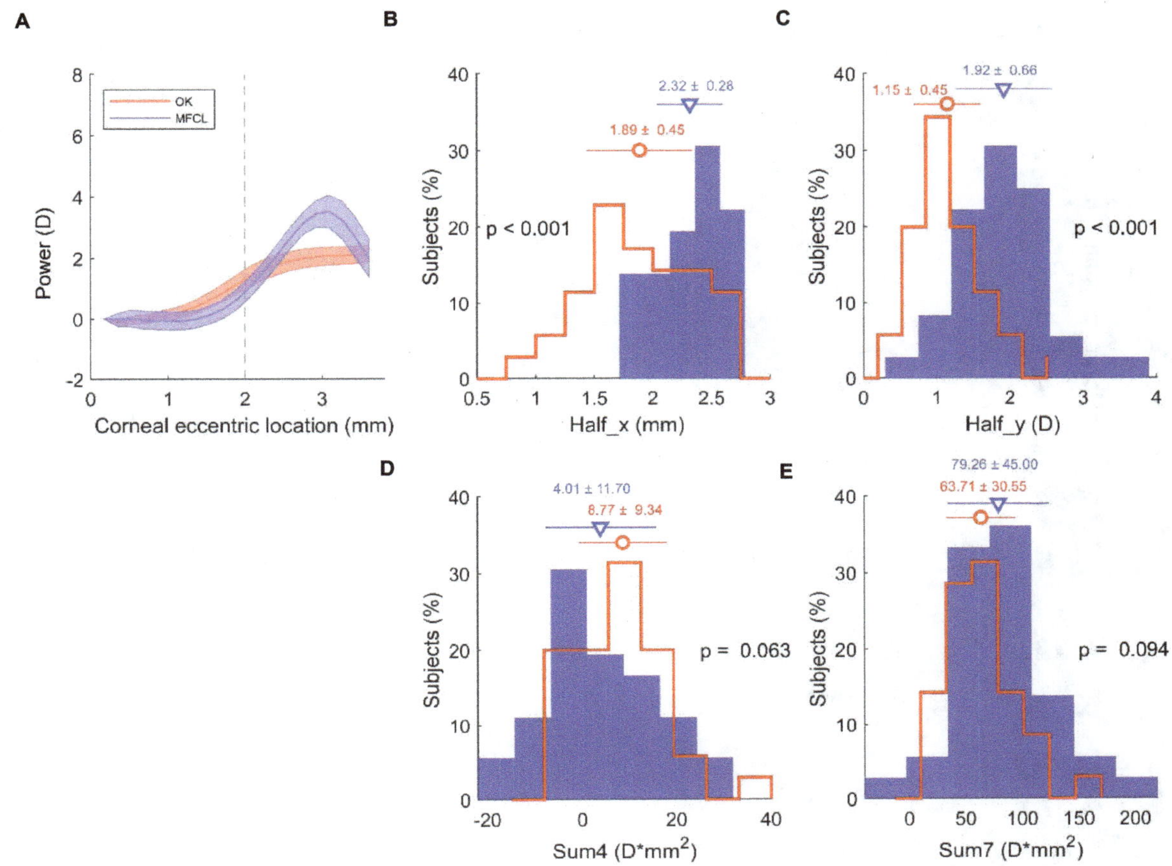

FIGURE 3 | RCRPS data from all subjects. **(A)** RCRPS profiles for the OK group (red) and MFCL group (blue). Solid line: mean value; shaded area: 95% confidence interval for the population means. **(B)** Half_x, **(C)** Half_y, **(D)** Sum4, and **(E)** Sum7. **(B–E)** OK group, red line; MFCL group, blue bars. RCRPS, relative corneal refractive power shift; D, diopter; OK, orthokeratology; MFCL, multifocal soft contact lens. Half_x, the corneal eccentric location where RCRPS reached the half peak value; Half_y, half of the RCRPS peak value; Sum4, the integrated value of the RCRPS located within an area of 4-mm diameter; Sum7, the integrated value of the RCRPS located within an area of 7-mm diameter.

was also not significantly different between the two groups (OK: 63.71 ± 30.55 D^*mm^2 vs MFCL: 79.26 ± 45.00 D^*mm^2, $p = 0.094$; **Figure 3E**).

In the OK group, all of the RCRPS parameters, including Half_x ($r = 0.428, p = 0.010$), Half_y ($r = -0.412, p = 0.014$), Sum4 ($r = -0.534, p < 0.001$), and Sum7 ($r = -0.477, p = 0.004$) were correlated with the baseline SE. None of these parameters were correlated with the baseline SE in MFCL subjects.

Association Between AL Elongation and RCRPS Parameters

The Half_x was positively correlated with AL elongation in the OK group and in the group formed by the combination of OK and MFCL subjects, but not the MFCL group (OK: $r = 0.610$, $p < 0.001$; MFCL: $r = 0.090, p = 0.600$; Combined data: $r = 0.497$, $p < 0.001$; **Figure 4A**). The Sum4 was negatively correlated with AL elongation in the OK group ($r = -0.491, p = 0.003$) and the combined group ($r = -0.351, p = 0.003$), but not the MFCL group MFCL group ($r = -0.146, p = 0.395$, **Figure 4B**). The difference between Half_x and pupil radius was positively correlated with AL elongation in the OK group ($r = 0.495$, $p = 0.002$) and the combined group ($r = 0.418$, $p < 0.001$), but not the MFCL group ($r = 0.102$, $p = 0.554$, **Figure 4C**). For both the OK and MFCL groups, the Half_y and Sum7 were not correlated with AL elongation (**Table 3**).

Regarding baseline parameters, age, AL, and SE were correlated with AL elongation in the OK group and the combined group, while only age was correlated with AL elongation in the MFCL group (**Table 3**). Stepwise multiple regression analyses showed that in the OK group and the combined group, only age and Half_x were significantly correlated with AL elongation. Decreasing Half_x by 1 mm was associated with a 0.161 mm reduction in 12-month AL elongation after optical interventions ($p < 0.001$).

DISCUSSION

In the present study, we found that AL elongation and the new index Half_x in the OK group were significantly smaller than

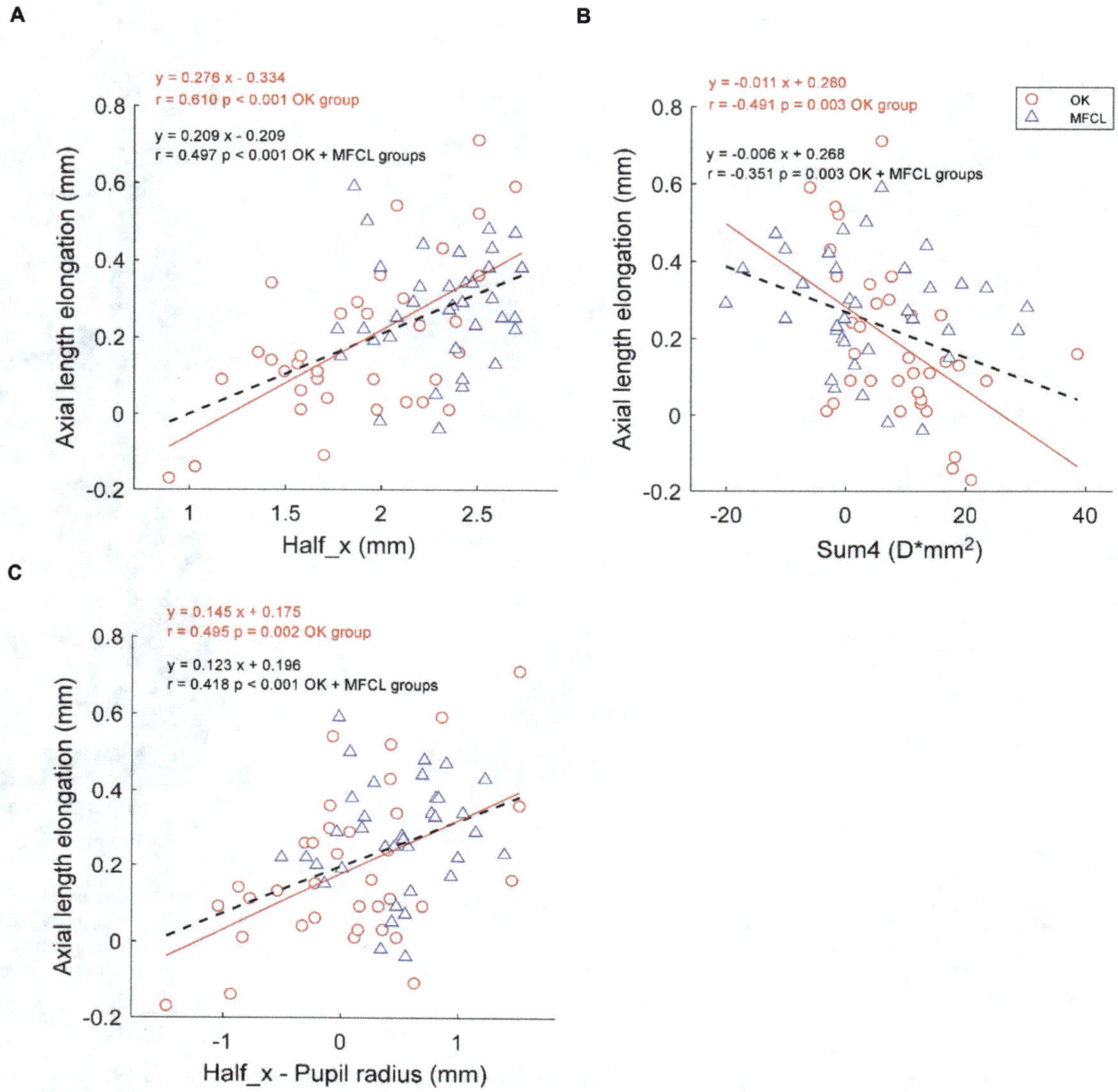

FIGURE 4 | Association between axial length elongation and RCRPS parameters **(A)** Half_x, **(B)** Sum4, **(C)** Half_x – Pupil radius for the OK group (red circles) and the MFCL group (blue triangles). The red solid line is the regression line of the OK data; the black dashed line is the regression line of the combined data. RCRPS, relative corneal refractive power shift; D, diopter; OK, orthokeratology; MFCL, multifocal soft contact lens; combined data: OK and MFCL; Half_x, the corneal eccentric location where RCRPS reached the half peak value; Sum4, the integrated value of the RCRPS located within an area of 4-mm diameter.

that in the MFCL group. More importantly, multiple regression analyses revealed that Half_x was significantly correlated with AL elongation in the OK group and in the combined OK and MFCL groups, but not the MFCL group alone.

The key difference in RCRPS profile could be explained by the differences in how MFCL and OK lenses alter the optical surfaces. For the MFCL, the changes in optical surfaces are mainly set by the lens design, which manifests as a sharply rising edge in the MFCL profile. For the OK lens, the changes in optical surfaces depend not only on lens design but also on the response of the cornea. With the optical zone pressing the central portion of the cornea and the alignment zone fitting closely to the peripheral corneal surface, a negative pressure forms in the reverse zone (VanderVeen et al., 2019). In the central portion of the cornea, the epithelial layer becomes significantly thinned while the stromal layer shows little change. Moving away from the center, the epithelial thinning gradually disappears while the stromal layer significantly thickens (Alharbi and Swarbrick, 2003; Lian et al., 2013). Such a gradual change from the center to mid-periphery was consistent with the RCRPS profile for the OK group in the current study, a gradient rising gradually from the center to the reverse zone. Because the RCRPS profile in OK subjects depends on the reaction of the cornea, all of the RCRPS parameters were correlated with baseline SE in the OK group but not in the MFCL group.

AL elongations of the OK and MFCL groups, 0.19 mm and 0.27 mm respectively, were consistent with the previous study (Paune et al., 2015). Our results suggest that the spatial distribution of the RCRPS, rather than the total amount (Zhong et al., 2015; Hu et al., 2019), is critical in slowing myopia progression. First, AL elongation was not related to the peak values, and the significantly greater peak values in MFCL subjects did not lead to smaller AL elongations. Second, the observation that Sum4 was correlated with AL elongation, while Sum7 was not, indicates that myopic defocus in the far periphery may not be as crucial as the myopic defocus in the paracentral periphery. Third, in the multiple regression analyses, the Half_x remained significant while Sum4 did not. The Half_x was correlated with AL elongation for the OK group but not for the MFCL group. One interpretation was that the RCRPS in the MFCL group was too far from corneal center to get into pupil region. Lights that originally could induce myopic defocus in the peripheral retina were partially blocked by iris. The other interpretation was the wearing time. OK lenses were used every night and the defocus treatments were in place all day long. MFCLs were requested to wear 5 days/week, 8 h/day, and the defocus treatments disappeared with the lenses off. Lam et al. reported that wearing time was a contribution factor to retardation effect of myopia progression with defocus incorporated soft contact lenses (Lam et al., 2014).

Previous studies have directly analyzed the summation of RCRPS components. Our results agreed with Hu et al., who reported that the area sum of RCRPS within a 4-mm diameter was correlated with AL elongation during OK lens wear (Hu et al., 2019). However, our study did not support previously identified predictive factors such as the maximal value and the sum of RCRPS within a 7.2-mm diameter (Zhong et al., 2015). Although there are no previous studies directly examining the spatial distribution of RCRPS, some studies did indicate an association between AL elongation and spatial distribution in an indirect way. A recent study showed that a smaller back optic zone diameter for the OK lens would produce a smaller plus power ring diameter on the cornea's front surface. When the plus power ring's horizontal sector was inside the pupil, the mean AL elongation

TABLE 3 | Linear regression analysis of AL elongation association with baseline data and RCRPS parameters.

Group	Parameter	Univariate model		Multivariate model	
		Beta (95% CI)	***P* value**	**Beta (95% CI)**	***P* value**
OK	Age (year)	−0.070 (−0.106 to −0.034)	**0.001**	−0.044 (−0.078 to −0.011)	**0.014**
	Gender (boys)	0.035 (−0.105 to 0.174)	0.628	\	\
	Baseline AL (mm)	−0.189 (−0.275 to −0.103)	**<0.001**	−0.066 (−0.161 to 0.029)	0.183
	Baseline SE (D)	0.072 (0.006 to 0.138)	**0.040**	Removed	
	Half_x (mm)	0.276 (0.154 to 0.398)	**<0.001**	0.186 (0.064 to 0.309)	**0.005**
	Half_y (D)	−0.037 (−0.189 to 0.116)	0.640	\	\
	Sum4 (D*mm^2)	−0.011 (−0.017 to −0.004)	**0.003**	Removed	
	Sum7 (D*mm^2)	−0.002 (−0.004 to 0.000)	0.114	\	\
	Half_x – PR (mm)	0.145 (0.058 to 0.231)	**0.002**	Removed	
MFCL	Age (year)	−0.045 (−0.076 to −0.014)	**0.008**	−0.045 (−0.076 to −0.014)	**0.008**
	Gender (boys)	0.016 (−0.086 to 0.118)	0.757	\	\
	Baseline AL (mm)	−0.015 (−0.092 to 0.062)	0.710	\	\
	Baseline SE (D)	0.013 (−0.044 to 0.069)	0.666	\	\
	Half_x (mm)	0.046 (−0.126 to 0.219)	0.600	\	\
	Half_y (D)	−0.014 (−0.087 to 0.060)	0.716	\	\
	Sum4 (D*mm^2)	−0.002 (−0.006 to 0.002)	0.395	\	\
	Sum7 (D*mm^2)	0.000 (−0.001 to 0.001)	0.453	\	\
	Half_x – PR (mm)	0.033 (−0.075 to 0.141)	0.554	\	\
Combined data	Age (year)	−0.058 (−0.083 to −0.034)	**<0.001**	−0.045 (−0.067 to −0.023)	**<0.001**
	Gender (boys)	0.019 (−0.069 to 0.107)	0.668	\	\
	Baseline AL (mm)	−0.109 (−0.171 to −0.048)	**0.001**	−0.047 (−0.102 to 0.007)	0.095
	Baseline SE (D)	0.050 (0.006 to 0.095)	**0.031**	Removed	
	Half_x (mm)	0.209 (0.123 to 0.295)	**<0.001**	0.161 (0.082 to 0.241)	**<0.001**
	Half_y (D)	0.022 (−0.040 to 0.084)	0.485	\	\
	Sum4 (D*mm^2)	−0.006 (−0.010 to −0.002)	**0.003**	Removed	
	Sum7 (D*mm^2)	−0.001 (−0.002 to 0.000)	0.290	\	\
	Half_x – PR (mm)	0.123 (0.060 to 0.186)	**<0.001**	Removed	

CI, confidence interval; AL, axial length; RCRPS, relative corneal refractive power shift; SE, spherical equivalent, D, diopter; OK, orthokeratology; MFCL, multifocal soft contact lens; Combined data, OK and MFCL groups together; Half_x, the corneal eccentric location where RCRPS reached the half peak value; Half_y, half of the RCRPS peak value; Sum4, the integrated value of the RCRPS located within an area of 4-mm diameter; Sum7, the integrated value of the RCRPS located within an area of 7-mm diameter; PR, pupil radius; Removed, Based on the Akaike Information Criterion, the factor was not selected for analysis in the multivariate model. Bolded values indicate $p < 0.05$.

of those subjects was 76% lesser than the subjects who had the plus power ring outside the pupil (Paune et al., 2021). Our study supported this result and found a linear correlation between AL elongation and the amount of Half_x inside the pupil. One study compared the reduction of the peripheral retinal hyperopic defocus in two different designs of progressive MFCLs. Only the lens with the additional power starting at the 3.5-mm diameter caused a significant reduction in the peripheral retinal hyperopic defocus, while the lens with the additional power starting at the 5.0-mm diameter did not (Allinjawi et al., 2016). Li et al. also reported that MFCLs with two concentric defocus rings in the periphery had better myopia control than MFCLs with a single peripheral defocus ring (Li et al., 2017). Due to the presence of the two concentric defocus rings in the periphery, the rising edge of the inner ring may be closer to the center than that in MFCLs with only one defocus ring. Smith et al. (2020) compared the treatment effects in infant monkeys with those in human clinical trials. They suggested that the relative effects on myopia control of the different optical treatments in both monkeys and humans were dependent on the eccentricity of the defocus.

The association between AL elongation and Half_x looks promising but should be taken with caution. First, in the current study, we only analyzed one design of MFCL. The effect of various optical designs of MFCLs on the spatial distribution of RCRPS should be compared in future studies. Second, other potentially influencing factors such as lens wearing time, and near-working time should be incorporated into the multiple regression analyses.

CONCLUSION

AL elongation in the OK group was significantly smaller than in the MFCL group over the 12-month study period. The difference in AL elongation may be attributed to the different RCRPS profiles induced by the two treatment modalities. Contact lenses with a smaller center treatment zone and closer adjacent additional power may lead to better myopia control.

AUTHOR CONTRIBUTIONS

FL, BZ, and JJ conceived the experiments and modified the manuscript. FJ and BZ determined the experimental methods, analyzed the data, and interpreted the data. XH, HX, and BW performed the experiments. FJ wrote the manuscript. All authors contributed to manuscript revision, read, and approved the submitted version.

ACKNOWLEDGMENTS

The authors thank Britt Bromberg, Ph.D., of Xenofile Editing (www.xenofileediting.com) for providing editing services for this manuscript.

REFERENCES

Akaike, H. (1974). A new look at the statistical model identification. *IEEE Trans. Automat. Contr.* 19, 716–723. doi: 10.1109/tac.1974.1100705

Alharbi, A., and Swarbrick, H. A. (2003). The effects of overnight orthokeratology lens wear on corneal thickness. *Invest. Ophthalmol. Vis. Sci.* 44, 2518–2523. doi: 10.1167/iovs.02-0680

Allinjawi, K., Sharanjeet-Kaur, S. K., Akhir, S. M., and Mutalib, H. A. (2016). Peripheral refraction with different designs of progressive soft contact lenses in myopes. *F1000Res.* 5:2742. doi: 10.12688/f1000research.9971.1

Benavente-Perez, A., Nour, A., and Troilo, D. (2014). Axial eye growth and refractive error development can be modified by exposing the peripheral retina to relative myopic or hyperopic defocus. *Invest. Ophthalmol. Vis. Sci.* 55, 6765–6773. doi: 10.1167/iovs.14-14524

Charman, W. N., Mountford, J., Atchison, D. A., and Markwell, E. L. (2006). Peripheral refraction in orthokeratology patients. *Optom. Vis. Sci.* 83, 641–648. doi: 10.1097/01.opx.0000232840.66716.af

Flitcroft, D. I. (2012). The complex interactions of retinal, optical and environmental factors in myopia aetiology. *Prog. Retin. Eye Res.* 31, 622–660. doi: 10.1016/j.preteyeres.2012.06.004

Holden, B. A., Fricke, T. R., Wilson, D. A., Jong, M., Naidoo, K. S., Sankaridurg, P., et al. (2016). Global prevalence of myopia and high myopia and temporal trends from 2000 through 2050. *Ophthalmology* 123, 1036–1042. doi: 10.1016/j.ophtha.2016.01.006

Hu, Y., Wen, C., Li, Z., Zhao, W., Ding, X., and Yang, X. (2019). Areal summed corneal power shift is an important determinant for axial length elongation in myopic children treated with overnight orthokeratology. *Br. J. Ophthalmol.* 103, 1571–1575. doi: 10.1136/bjophthalmol-2018-312933

Huang, J., Wen, D., Wang, Q., McAlinden, C., Flitcroft, I., Chen, H., et al. (2016). Efficacy comparison of 16 interventions for myopia control in children: a network meta-analysis. *Ophthalmology* 123, 697–708. doi: 10.1016/j.ophtha.2015.11.010

Huang, X., Wang, F., Lin, Z., He, Y., Wen, S., Zhou, L., et al. (2020). Visual quality of juvenile myopes wearing multifocal soft contact lenses. *Eye Vis. (Lond.)* 7:41. doi: 10.1186/s40662-020-00204-4

Kang, P. (2018). Optical and pharmacological strategies of myopia control. *Clin. Exp. Optom.* 101, 321–332. doi: 10.1111/cxo.12666

Kang, P., and Swarbrick, H. (2013). Time course of the effects of orthokeratology on peripheral refraction and corneal topography. *Ophthalmic Physiol. Opt.* 33, 277–282. doi: 10.1111/opo.12027

Lam, C. S., Tang, W. C., Tse, D. Y., Tang, Y. Y., and To, C. H. (2014). Defocus incorporated soft contact (DISC) lens slows myopia progression in Hong Kong Chinese schoolchildren: a 2-year randomised clinical trial. *Br. J. Ophthalmol.* 98, 40–45. doi: 10.1136/bjophthalmol-2013-303914

Lee, E. J., Lim, D. H., Chung, T. Y., Hyun, J., and Han, J. (2018). Association of axial length growth and topographic change in orthokeratology. *Eye Contact Lens* 44, 292–298. doi: 10.1097/ICL.0000000000000493

Li, S. M., Kang, M. T., Wu, S. S., Meng, B., Sun, Y. Y., Wei, S. F., et al. (2017). Studies using concentric ring bifocal and peripheral add multifocal contact lenses to slow myopia progression in school-aged children: a meta-analysis. *Ophthalmic Physiol. Opt.* 37, 51–59. doi: 10.1111/opo.12332

Lian, Y., Shen, M., Jiang, J., Mao, X., Lu, P., Zhu, D., et al. (2013). Vertical and horizontal thickness profiles of the corneal epithelium and Bowman's layer after orthokeratology. *Invest. Ophthalmol. Vis. Sci.* 54, 691–696. doi: 10.1167/iovs.12-10263

Liu, Y., and Wildsoet, C. (2011). The effect of two-zone concentric bifocal spectacle lenses on refractive error development and eye growth in young chicks. *Invest. Ophthalmol. Vis. Sci.* 52, 1078–1086. doi: 10.1167/iovs.10-5716

Marcus, M. W., de Vries, M. M., Junoy Montolio, F. G., and Jansonius, N. M. (2011). Myopia as a risk factor for open-angle glaucoma: a systematic review and meta-analysis. *Ophthalmology* 118, 1989–1994.e2. doi: 10.1016/j.ophtha.2011.03.012

Morgan, I. G., Ohno-Matsui, K., and Saw, S. M. (2012). Myopia. *Lancet* 379, 1739–1748. doi: 10.1016/S0140-6736(12)60272-4

Paune, J., Fonts, S., Rodriguez, L., and Queiros, A. (2021). The role of back optic zone diameter in myopia control with orthokeratology lenses. *J. Clin. Med.* 10:336. doi: 10.3390/jcm10020336

Paune, J., Morales, H., Armengol, J., Quevedo, L., Faria-Ribeiro, M., and Gonzalez-Meijome, J. M. (2015). Myopia control with a novel peripheral gradient soft lens and orthokeratology: a 2-year clinical trial. *Biomed. Res. Int.* 2015:507572. doi: 10.1155/2015/507572

Periman, L. M., Ambrosio, R. Jr., Harrison, D. A., and Wilson, S. E. (2003). Correlation of pupil sizes measured with a mesopic infrared pupillometer and a photopic topographer. *J. Refract. Surg.* 19, 555–559. doi: 10.3928/1081-597x-20030901-10

Queiros, A., Amorim-de-Sousa, A., Lopes-Ferreira, D., Villa-Collar, C., Gutierrez, A. R., and Gonzalez-Meijome, J. M. (2018). Relative peripheral refraction across 4 meridians after orthokeratology and LASIK surgery. *Eye Vis. (Lond.)* 5:12. doi: 10.1186/s40662-018-0106-1

Queiros, A., Gonzalez-Meijome, J. M., Jorge, J., Villa-Collar, C., and Gutierrez, A. R. (2010). Peripheral refraction in myopic patients after orthokeratology. *Optom. Vis. Sci.* 87, 323–329. doi: 10.1097/OPX.0b013e3181d951f7

Rudnicka, A. R., Kapetanakis, V. V., Wathern, A. K., Logan, N. S., Gilmartin, B., Whincup, P. H., et al. (2016). Global variations and time trends in the prevalence of childhood myopia, a systematic review and quantitative meta-analysis: implications for aetiology and early prevention. *Br. J. Ophthalmol.* 100, 882–890. doi: 10.1136/bjophthalmol-2015-307724

Sankaridurg, P., Holden, B., Smith, E. III, Naduvilath, T., Chen, X., de la Jara, P. L., et al. (2011). Decrease in rate of myopia progression with a contact lens designed to reduce relative peripheral hyperopia: one-year results. *Invest. Ophthalmol. Vis. Sci.* 52, 9362–9367. doi: 10.1167/iovs.11-7260

Smith, E. L. III, Arumugam, B., Hung, L. F., She, Z., Beach, K., and Sankaridurg, P. (2020). Eccentricity-dependent effects of simultaneous competing defocus on emmetropization in infant rhesus monkeys. *Vision Res.* 177, 32–40. doi: 10.1016/j.visres.2020.08.003

Smith, E. L. III, Hung, L. F., and Huang, J. (2009). Relative peripheral hyperopic defocus alters central refractive development in infant monkeys. *Vision Res.* 49, 2386–2392. doi: 10.1016/j.visres.2009.07.011

Sridharan, R., and Swarbrick, H. (2003). Corneal response to short-term orthokeratology lens wear. *Optom. Vis. Sci.* 80, 200–206. doi: 10.1097/00006324-200303000-00009

VanderVeen, D. K., Kraker, R. T., Pineles, S. L., Hutchinson, A. K., Wilson, L. B., Galvin, J. A., et al. (2019). Use of orthokeratology for the prevention of myopic progression in children: a report by the american academy of ophthalmology. *Ophthalmology* 126, 623–636. doi: 10.1016/j.ophtha.2018.11.026

Williams, K. M., Bertelsen, G., Cumberland, P., Wolfram, C., Verhoeven, V. J., Anastasopoulos, E., et al. (2015). Increasing prevalence of myopia in europe and the impact of education. *Ophthalmology* 122, 1489–1497. doi: 10.1016/j.ophtha.2015.03.018

Zhong, Y., Chen, Z., Xue, F., Miao, H., and Zhou, X. (2015). Central and peripheral corneal power change in myopic orthokeratology and its relationship with 2-year axial length change. *Invest. Ophthalmol. Vis. Sci.* 56, 4514–4519. doi: 10.1167/iovs.14-13935

Zhong, Y., Chen, Z., Xue, F., Zhou, J., Niu, L., and Zhou, X. (2014). Corneal power change is predictive of myopia progression in orthokeratology. *Optom. Vis. Sci.* 91, 404–411. doi: 10.1097/OPX.0000000000000183

16

Altered Spontaneous Brain Activity Patterns and Functional Connectivity in Adults with Intermittent Exotropia: A Resting-State fMRI Study

Xueying He[1†], Jie Hong[2†], Qian Wang[1], Yanan Guo[2], Ting Li[1], Xiaoxia Qu[1], Jing Liu[1], Wei Li[1], Lirong Zhang[1], Jing Fu[2] and Zhaohui Liu[1*]*

[1] Department of Radiology, Beijing Tongren Hospital, Capital Medical University, Beijing, China, [2] Department of Ophthalmology, Beijing Tongren Hospital, Capital Medical University, Beijing, China

***Correspondence:**
Zhaohui Liu
lzhtrhos@163.com
Jing Fu
fu_jing@126.com

† These authors have contributed equally to this work and share first authorship

The purpose of this study is to investigate brain functional changes in patients with intermittent exotropia (IXT) by analyzing the amplitude of low-frequency fluctuation (ALFF) of brain activity and functional connectivity (FC) using resting-state functional magnetic resonance imaging (rs-fMRI). There were 26 IXT patients and 22 age-, sex-, education-, and handedness-matched healthy controls (HCs) enrolled who underwent rs-fMRI. The ALFF, fractional ALFF (fALFF) values in the slow 4 and slow 5 bands, and FC values were calculated and compared. The correlations between ALFF/fALFF values in discrepant brain regions and clinical features were evaluated. Compared with HCs, ALFF/fALFF values were significantly increased in the right angular gyrus (ANG), supramarginal gyrus (SMG), inferior parietal lobule (IPL), precentral gyrus (PreCG), and the bilateral inferior frontal gyri (IFG), and decreased in the right precuneus gyrus (PCUN), left middle occipital gyrus (MOG), and postcentral gyrus (PoCG) in IXT patients. The Newcastle Control Test score was negatively correlated with ALFF values in the right IFG ($r = -0.738$, $p < 0.001$). The duration of IXT was negatively correlated with ALFF values in the right ANG ($r = -0.457$, $p = 0.049$). Widespread increases in FC were observed between brain regions, mainly including the right cuneus (CUN), left superior parietal lobule (SPL), right rolandic operculum (ROL), left middle temporal gyrus (MTG), left IFG, left median cingulate gyrus (DCG), left PoCG, right PreCG, and left paracentral gyrus (PCL) in patients with IXT. No decreased FC was observed. Patients with IXT exhibited aberrant intrinsic brain activities and FC in vision- and eye movement-related brain regions, which extend current understanding of the neuropathological mechanisms underlying visual and oculomotor impairments in IXT patients.

Keywords: intermittent exotropia, functional connectivity, amplitude of low-frequency fluctuations, resting-state functional MRI, spontaneous activity

INTRODUCTION

Comitant strabismus is a group of developmental diseases involving ocular motility impairment (Ouyang et al., 2017; Li et al., 2018). Intermittent exotropia (IXT) is the most common subtype of comitant strabismus, accounting for 58% of cases, with a prevalence ranging from 0.12 to 3.9% of the population worldwide (Chia et al., 2010; McKean-Cowdin et al., 2013; Fu et al., 2014; Pan et al., 2016). IXT manifests as intermittent squinting outward during distance fixation or inattention, which always gives rise to psychological problems and impaired social interaction (Brodsky and Jung, 2015; Yang et al., 2016; Zhu et al., 2018).

The precise pathological mechanisms underlying IXT remain unclear. Many authors proposed that IXT is caused by defective binocular fusion in the brain (Guyton, 2006; Brodsky and Jung, 2015). Abnormal fusion function leads to an inability to form normal stereoscopic vision. Li et al. (2016) found abnormal brain activity in binocular fusion-related cortices in IXT patients using task-based functional magnetic resonance imaging (fMRI). However, compared with task-fMRI, resting-state functional magnetic resonance imaging (rs-fMRI) requires minimal patient compliance, avoids potential performance confounders associated with cognitive activation paradigms in task-fMRI research, and is relatively easy to implement in clinical studies (Turner, 2013). Yang et al. (2014) and Tan et al. (2016) confirmed that the abnormal brain activity was exhibited in infantile esotropia and congenital comitant strabismus using rs-fMRI, which cannot totally represent the brain functional changes of IXT. Unfortunately, no study about IXT, a subtype of comitant exotropia, explores the spontaneous neural activity changes of attenuation of spontaneous blood oxygen level dependent (BOLD) fluctuations using rs-fMRI at present.

Analyses of the amplitude of low-frequency fluctuations (ALFF) and functional connectivity (FC) are two important methods used in rs-fMRI studies. ALFF is an rs-fMRI analysis technique used to measure spontaneous fluctuations of neural activities in BOLD signals, which has been reported to be a useful parameter by many authors (Logothetis et al., 2001; Biswal, 2012). Fractional ALFF (fALFF) is an index reflecting the relative contribution of specific low-frequency oscillations to the entire frequency range (Zhou et al., 2013). In previous rs-fMRI studies, the frequency band of 0.01 to 0.1 Hz most commonly revealed spontaneous oscillation activities, but lower frequency bands can better reflect local neural activity and reduce the influence of distant neural activity. The slow 4 (0.027–0.073 Hz) band and slow 5 (0.01–0.027 Hz) band in fALFF were deemed to be more sensitive and specific frequency bands for intrinsic brain activity to analyze alterations in neural activity (Han et al., 2012; Zhou et al., 2013). A combination of the two parameters can be used to acquire more information about the brain in IXT patients and verify abnormal functional activity (Li et al., 2014). FC analysis is an effective method with which to estimate spontaneous functional activity and it measures temporal relevance between the BOLD signals of two brain areas that occur in turn (Tomasi and Volkow, 2010). Analyses of ALFF, fALFF, and FC simultaneously allow researchers to explore the synchronization between brain regions and the activation of each brain region.

In this study, we investigated the ALFF, fALFF, and FC value changes of the whole brain using rs-fMRI in IXT patients and explored the correlation between the ALFF/fALFF value changes and clinical features, including the duration and severity of IXT. In accord with previous studies of strabismus, we hypothesized that IXT patients would exhibit aberrant intrinsic spontaneous brain activity and FC.

MATERIALS AND METHODS

Subjects

A total of 26 IXT patients (14 male individuals, 12 female individuals, age = 28.23 ± 8.14 years) were enrolled in this study. In addition, we recruited 24 healthy control subjects (HCs) (14 male individuals, 10 female individuals, age = 28.82 ± 6.48 years) from the local community, matched with IXT patients in terms of gender, age, education, and right or left handedness. All participants underwent MR examination and a series of ophthalmological examinations, including measurement of best corrected visual acuity, fundus examination, synoptophore, alternate cover test, and the Newcastle Control Test (NCT). This study was approved by the medical research ethics committee and institutional review board of Capital Medical University, Beijing Tongren Hospital, and written informed consent was obtained from all participants.

The IXT patients were recruited based on the following criteria: (1) evidence of IXT on the basis of history and clinical examination (loss of stereoscopic vision detected by synoptophore and/or deflection time accounted for more than half of waking time, and exotropia deviation $< -15\Delta$), (2) best-corrected visual acuity (VA) ≥ 1.0, (3) adults over 18 years old, (4) no ongoing amblyopia treatment, and (5) ability to understand and cooperate with inspection, and voluntarily provide written informed consent. The inclusion criteria of HCs included the (2)–(5) of the above standards and free of any ocular diseases. The exclusion criteria included: (1) other kinds of strabismus, such as constant exotropia, esotropia, or incomitant strabismus, (2) ocular diseases (e.g., amblyopia, cataract, glaucoma, optic neuritis, and macular degeneration), (3) accompanied by vertical strabismus, (4) previous eye surgery history, (5) history of diseases involving psychiatric, cardiovascular, or cerebral disease, (6) drug or alcohol addiction, and (7) contraindication for MRI examination (treatable or accidental magnetizable metal in cardiac pacemaker or prosthesis, or previous head or spinal trauma requiring neurosurgery), (8) head motion larger than 2 mm maximum displacement in any direction or an angular rotation greater than 2° throughout the scan. According to these criteria, 26 IXT patients and 22 HCs were enrolled in this study.

Magnetic Resonance Imaging Data Acquisition

Images were acquired using a 3.0 T MRI scanner (Discovery MR750; General Electric, Milwaukee, WI, United States). A matched eight-channel phased array coil was used with earplugs and foam padding to reduce scanner noise and head motion. The images were parallel to the anterior commissure (AC)-posterior commissure (PC) line and covered the whole brain. Resting-state fMRI was obtained using an echo planar imaging (EPI) pulse sequence with the following parameters: repetition time (TR)/echo time (TE) = 2000/35 ms, flip angle = 90°, field of view (FOV) = 240 mm × 240 mm, matrix = 64 × 64, voxel size = 3.75 mm × 3.75 mm × 4.0 mm, and 180 time points. Axial slices were obtained with 5 mm thickness. The pulse duration of each fMRI session was 400 s. The three-dimensional brain volume (3D-BRAVO) sequences were used to acquire high-resolution structural images (TR = 8.16 ms, TE = 3.18 ms, TI = 450 ms, matrix = 256 × 256, FOV = 240 mm × 240 mm, slice thickness = 1.0 mm without gap, flip angle = 12°, gap = 0 mm, 188 slices, and voxel size = 1 mm × 1 mm × 1 mm). The total scan duration of the 3-dimensional brain volume sequence was 259 s. During scanning, subjects were asked to remain motionless, to stay awake, and not to think of anything specific until the scan was over.

Data Preprocessing

Preprocessing was carried out using Data Processing Assistant for Resting-State fMRI (DPARSF 4.2; State Key Laboratory of Cognitive Neuroscience and Learning, Beijing Normal University, Beijing, China[1]) and CONN functional connectivity toolbox (Whitfield-Gabrieli and Nieto-Castanon, 2012) based on Statistical Parametric Mapping (SPM12)[2] running under MATLAB R2013b (The MathWorks, Natick, United States). The first 10 volumes were removed to allow participants to adapt to the scanning noise and the signal equilibrium was measured after converting DICOM files to NIFTI images. Slice timing, head motion correction, spatial normalization to the Montreal Neurological Institute (MNI) template (resampling voxel size = 3 mm × 3 mm × 3 mm) were then performed. We used a linear regression process to remove the effects of head motion and other possible sources of artifacts: (1) six motion parameters, (2) whole-brain signal averaged over the entire brain, (3) white matter signal, and (4) cerebrospinal fluid signal. In addition, the linear trend of time courses was removed. Preprocessing of voxel-based morphometry (VBM) was carried out using DPARSF 4.2. The imaging of 3D-BROVA was converted from DICOM files to NIFTI images. Then segmentation and spatial normalization were performed to extract the gray matter volume (GMV). After that the images were smoothed by a Gaussian kernel (full width at half-maximum of 8 mm).

Voxel-Wise Amplitude of Low-Frequency Fluctuations/Fractional Amplitude of Low-Frequency Fluctuation Analysis

DPARSF 4.2 was performed to calculate the ALFF and fALFF values. Briefly, the time courses were first transformed to the frequency domain using Fast Fourier Transform (FFT) (parameters: FFT length = shortest, taper percent = 0). The square root of the power spectrum obtained by FFT was computed, then averaged across 0.01–0.08 Hz at each voxel, which was taken as ALFF. Fractional ALFF is the fraction of amplitude of low-frequency fluctuation in a given frequency band over the entire frequency range. The low-frequency range was further disassembled into a slow 4 (0.027–0.073 Hz) and a slow 5 (0.01–0.027 Hz) band for the BOLD signal, to make the data more robust against physiological noise. The fALFF values were then calculated for slow 4 and slow 5 bands. The ALFF/fALFF value for each voxel was divided by the global mean ALFF/fALFF value for each participant to reduce the global effects of variability. Finally, the ALFF/fALFF images were smoothed by a Gaussian kernel (full width at half-maximum of 6 mm).

Voxel-Wise Functional Connectivity Analysis

Before FC analysis, a temporal bandpass filter (0.01–0.08 Hz) was used to minimize the effects of low frequency drift and high frequency noise. Then FC analysis was performed using the CONN toolbox. Based on the ALFF result, the region that showed significant difference between the IXT patient and HCs was defined as the region of interest (ROI) using DPARSF 4.2. After that, we performed a voxel-wise FC analysis by computing the temporal correlation between the mean time series of the ROI and the time series of each voxel within the brain. The data were transformed using Fisher r-to-z transformation to improve normality of the correlation coefficients. Meanwhile, the FC images were smoothed by a Gaussian kernel (full width at half-maximum of 6 mm).

Validation Analysis

Given that GMV atrophy may affect the ALFF/fALFF and FC changes, we analyzed intergroup differences in both GMV to evaluate whether any significant gray matter (GM) changes were significant in IXT patients. We compared GMV between the IXT and HC groups using a two-sample t-test in SPSS and applied a voxel-wise comparison to identify structures that differed significantly in volume between the two groups. There was no report about GM atrophy previously in IXT patients, however, we investigated the ALFF/fALFF comparisons with GMV as an additional covariate to exclude the effect of GM atrophy.

Statistical Analysis

To examine the demographic data, clinical features, and head motion parameters, a two-sample t-test was used for normally distributed data, and the Mann–Whitney U test was used for non-normally distributed data. Statistical significance was set at $p < 0.05$. A one-sample t-test ($p < 0.05$, Gaussian random field (GRF)-corrected) was used to extract ALFF results across subjects within each group. A two-sample t-test was used to compare the ALFF and fALFF values for the slow 4 and slow 5 bands differences between groups, while age, gender, and education were included as covariates. The statistical threshold was set at a voxel level of $p < 0.001$ and a cluster level of $p < 0.05$, GRF-corrected. Pearson correlation analysis was performed using SPSS to explore the relationships between mean ALFF/fALFF and

[1] http://restfmri.net/forum/DPARSF

[2] http://www.fil.ion.ucl.ac.uk/spm/

mean FC values of discrepant brain regions and NCT scores, IXT duration in the patient group with a $p < 0.05$. A two-sample, two-tailed t-test was performed to compare the FC maps between IXT patients and HCs, while age, gender, and education were included as covariates. The statistical threshold was set at a voxel level of $p < 0.001$ and a cluster level of $p < 0.05$, GRF-corrected.

RESULTS

Demographics and Clinical Features

Clinical characteristics of enrolled 26 IXT patients and 22 HCs are listed in **Table 1**. There was no significant difference in age ($p = 0.786$), sex ($p = 0.572$), education ($p = 0.726$), handedness ($p > 0.999$), and the best-corrected VA(R/L) (right: $p = 0.160$; left: $p = 0.094$). Head motion parameters did not differ significantly between groups ($p = 0.231$).

Voxel-Wise Amplitude of Low-Frequency Fluctuations and Fractional Amplitude of Low-Frequency Fluctuation Differences

Altered ALFF values across all subjects in the two groups during the resting state are shown in **Figure 1**. The general trend of regional brain activity was similar between the two groups and some regions exhibited significantly higher ALFF values than other brain regions during the resting state, including the bilateral middle temporal gyrus (MTG) and inferior parietal lobule (IPL). Bilateral precuneus gyrus (PCUN) showed lower ALFF values than other regions.

Compared with HCs, IXT patients had significant ALFF values increase the right angular gyrus (ANG), supramarginal gyrus (SMG), IPL, the bilateral inferior frontal gyri (IFG), and a decrease in the right PCUN (**Figure 2**, and **Table 2**). Meanwhile, in the IXT group, the fALFF values were significantly increased in the right SMG and right precentral gyrus (PreCG) and decreased in the left middle occipital gyrus (MOG) and postcentral gyrus (PoCG) for the slow 4 band (**Figure 3**, and **Table 3**). Increased fALFF values were found in the left IFG for the slow 5 band (**Figure 3**, and **Table 3**).

TABLE 1 | Demographics and clinical measurements of IXT patients and HCs.

	IXT (n = 26)	HC (n = 22)	t-value	P-value
Sex, male/female	14/12	10/12	0.569	0.572*
Age (years)	28.23 ± 8.14	28.82 ± 6.48	−0.273	0.786†
Handedness	26R	22R	N/A	>0.999*
Education (years)	15.38 ± 2.93	16.59 ± 2.72	−1.484	0.726†
Duration (years)	10.33 ± 9.12	N/A	N/A	N/A
Newcastle control test	5.25 ± 1.87	N/A	N/A	N/A
The best-corrected VA (R)	0.98 ± 0.11	1.02 ± 0.07	−1.433	0.160†
The best-corrected VA (L)	0.98 ± 0.11	1.04 ± 0.13	−1.720	0.094†
Prism diopter/near	−73.26 ± 34.43	N/A	N/A	N/A
Prism diopter/distance	−69.57 ± 35.32	N/A	N/A	N/A
Mean fd-power	0.11 ± 0.04	0.10 ± 0.03	1.213	0.231†

Data are presented as mean ± SD; HC, healthy control; IXT, intermittent exotropia; N/A, not applicable; VA, visual acuity; R, right; L, left.
**Chi-square test.*
†Two-sample t-test.

Voxel-Wise Functional Connectivity Analysis

Among the intergroup comparisons, we found four ROIs with significantly increased FC with other brain clusters in the IXT group (**Figure 4** and **Table 4**). Compared with HCs, IXT patients showed increased FC between right ANG and right cuneus (CUN), left superior parietal lobule (SPL). The FC between right IPL and right CUN were increased. The FC between right PreCG and right rolandic operculum (ROL), left MTG, left IFG, and left median cingulate gyrus (DCG) were increased. The FC between right SMG and left PoCG, right PreCG and left paracentral gyrus (PCL) was also increased. No decreased FC was observed.

Correlation Between Amplitude of Low-Frequency Fluctuations/Fractional Amplitude of Low-Frequency Fluctuation, Functional Connectivity Values, and Clinical Characteristics

The NCT score was negatively correlated with ALFF values in the right IFG ($r = -0.738$, $p < 0.001$). The duration of IXT was negatively correlated with ALFF values the right ANG ($r = -0.457$, $p = 0.049$) (**Figure 5**). There is no correlation found between fALFF and FC values and clinical characteristics.

Validation Analysis

Global GMV is $(0.697 \pm 0.053) \times 10^6$ mm^3 in IXT patients and $(0.678 \pm 0.067) \times 10^6$ mm^3 in HCs. No significant difference was found in global GMV between groups ($t = 1.080$, $p = 0.286$). There were no clusters survived after correction for multiple comparisons in voxel-based analysis between the two groups, corrected for GRF.

After correction with GMV as an additional covariate of no interest, the brain regions with altered ALFF/fALFF values showed the same distributions to those observed without GMV correction. The results suggested that most of the ALFF/fALFF value changes were independent of GMV atrophy in IXTs.

DISCUSSION

Compared with HCs, the IXT patients showed significantly decreased ALFF/fALFF values in the right PCUN and increased in the bilateral IFG, the right ANG, right SMG gyrus, right IPL, right PreCG, and decreased in the left MOG, PoCG, which are associated with fusion, stereoscopic vision, and eye position control. Then we analyzed the FC of these activity-altered brain regions. Increased FC was found between these areas and other brain regions. These results prove that the neurological activity changes of IXT involve vision- and oculomotor-related brain regions. Furthermore, we found a negative correlation between the duration of IXT, the NCT scores, and ALFF values in part of the brain regions. The previous studies have suggested that the ALFF and FC could

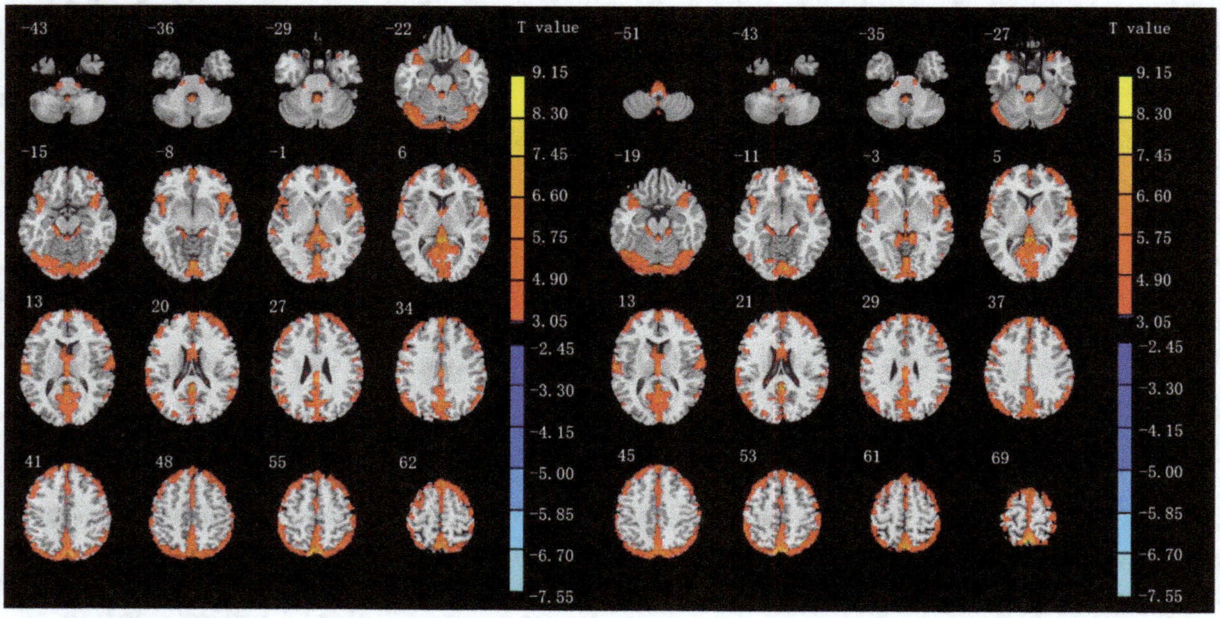

FIGURE 1 | Results of ALFF values of IXT patients **(left)** and HCs **(right)** in the rs-fMRI using one-sample *t*-test. ($P < 0.05$, GRF correction).

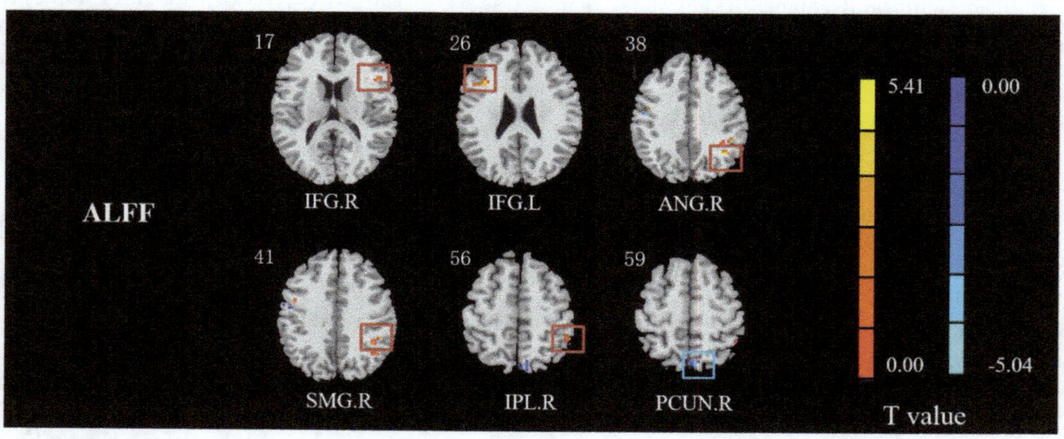

FIGURE 2 | The different ALFF regions between IXT patients and HCs. ALFF values in IXT patients increased in the right ANG, SMG, IPL, and the bilateral IFG, and decreased in the right PCUN. (GRF corrected, $P < 0.05$.) ANG: angular gyrus; SMG: supramarginal gyrus; IPL: inferior parietal lobule; IFG: inferior frontal gyrus; PCUN: precuneus.

be influenced by regional GM atrophy which may lead to artificial reduction in regional ALFF and FC results (Oakes et al., 2007). In addition, ametropia may lead to changes in regulatory function and then affect the results (Kim and Kim, 2017). In this study, the differences of GMV and bilateral best-corrected VA between IXTs and HCs were not significant, which confirmed the results of ALFF and fALFF changes in IXTs are credible.

In the current study, the ALFF values of MOG were decreased. The MOG participates the stereovision function which also plays an important role in the category-selective attention-modulated unconscious face/tool processing and spatial processing (Fortin et al., 2002; Tu et al., 2013). Zhu et al. (2018) found that the FC values of MOG were significantly decreased in patients with concomitant exotropia, while IXT is a subtype of concomitant exotropia. Consistently, we demonstrated that the decreased brain function of MOG reflects the defects in the stereovision function in IXT patients. However, before IXT developed into constant exotropia, part of stereovision function still existed, suggesting that some stereopsis related brain regions might have compensatory functions. Increased ALFF/fALFF values were found in the right ANG, right SMG, and right IPL, which supported stereoscopic vision impaired in IXT. The main visual

TABLE 2 | Regions revealing significant ALFF differences between IXT patients and HCs ($P < 0.05$, corrected for GRF).

Brain region	Peak MNI, mm			Peak T value	Number of voxels
	x	y	z		
R IFG	51	21	58	5.0795	17
L IFG	−36	21	24	5.2910	17
R ANG	39	−57	36	5.4563	19
R SMG	48	−42	36	5.0933	40
R IPL	48	−42	36	5.0933	40
R PCUN	6	−72	57	−4.4851	19

R: right; L: left; MNI: Montreal Neurological Institute; IFG: inferior frontal gyrus; ANG: angular gyrus; SMG: supramarginal gyrus; IPL: inferior parietal lobule; PCUN: precuneus.

pathways include the ventral and dorsal streams (Lee et al., 2000). The dorsal visual pathway originates from the V1, passes through V2 and middle temporal areas, and arrives at the IPL. This pathway primarily takes part in the processing of spatial position information and eye movement (Merigan and Maunsell, 1993; Tootell et al., 1998). The ANG and SMG occupy a part of the IPL. The IPL extracts information about depth from motion to form stereoscopic vision, and is involved in the dynamic display of objects, providing immediate instructions to induce attentional shifts from one object to another (Yang et al., 2014). In patients with IXT, stereoscopic vision is damaged to varying degrees. To produce effective stereoscopic vision, IXT patients may require more neural activity in the dorsal visual pathway. Previous studies of strabismus and its subtype, including infantile esotropia, have found increased spontaneous activities in the ANG (Yang et al., 2014; Tan et al., 2016). A previous task-fMRI study reported that the IPL exhibited increased activation intensity in IXT patients (Li et al., 2016), which are similar to the current findings. Therefore, the increased ALFF/fALFF values of brain regions in dorsal visual pathway may be a compensatory process of stereoscopic vision.

Meanwhile, IXT patients showed increased FC between right ANG and right CUN, left SPL and the FC between right IPL and right CUN, between right SMG and left PoCG, right PreCG and left PCL was also increased. The CUN plays an important role in spatial processing, which is in charge of modifying and transmitting visual information to the extrastriate cortex (Daw, 1998). The SPL is responsible for transmitting visual information to the frontal lobe to control visuomotor integration and encode visual and proprioceptive targets, which plays a vital role in body position (Caminiti et al., 1996; Felician et al., 2004; Iacoboni and Zaidel, 2004; McGuire and Sabes, 2011). The PoCG, PreCG, and PCL belong to the motor and sensory networks, which is related to the ocular movement. The strengthening of the FC between the region of dorsal visual pathway and CUN, SPL further suggests that this is a compensatory effect for impaired stereoscopic vision.

Amplitude of low-frequency fluctuations values of the right PCUN in IXT patients were lower than those of HCs, which indicated the underlying mechanism of IXT should be defective binocular fusion proposed by many neurologists and pathologists (Pettigrew et al., 1968; Poggio and Fischer, 1977). A well-coordinated binocular fusion function is required before normal stereoscopic vision can be formed. The PCUN is crucial to visual processing, belonging to the occipital cortex and participating in both the dorsal and ventral visual pathways (Nagahama et al., 1999; Cavanna and Trimble, 2006; Tan et al., 2016; Hensch and Quinlan, 2018). Given fusion-related stimulation by task-based fMRI, Li et al., 2016 also found BOLD signals increased in the bilateral PCUN and concluded that the PCUN was associated with binocular fusion (Fu et al., 2014). Meanwhile, the PCUN is believed to play an important role in the visuomotor coordination (Nagahama et al., 1999; Cavanna and Trimble, 2006;

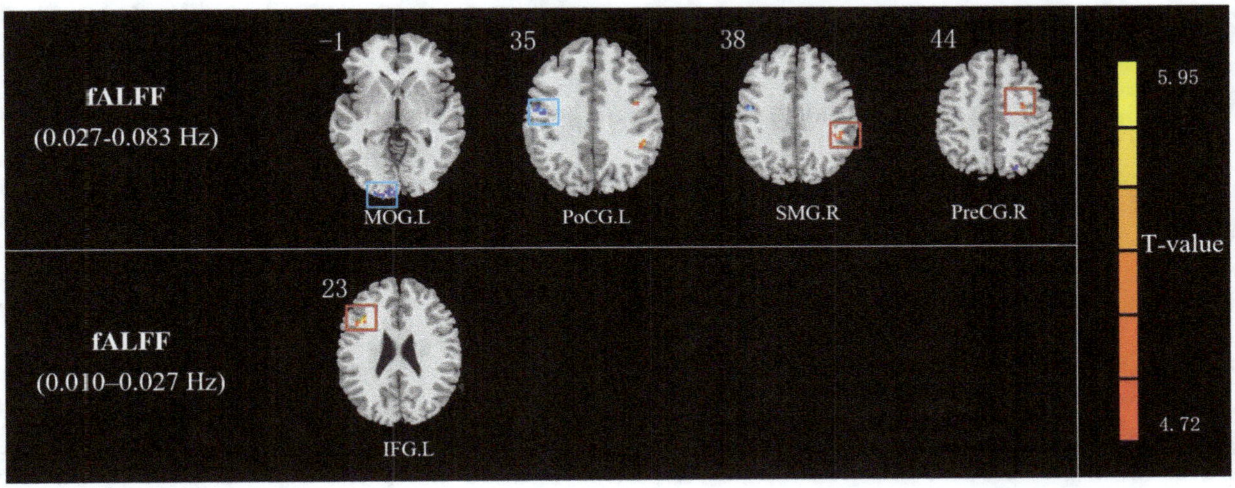

FIGURE 3 | The different fALFF values of brain regions between IXT patients and HCs. The fALFF values in slow 4 (0.027–0.073 Hz) band increased in the right SMG and right PreCG and decreased in the left MOG and PoCG in IXT patients. The fALFF values in slow 5 (0.01–0.027 Hz) band increased in the left IFG in IXT patients. (GRF corrected, $P < 0.05$). SMG: supramarginal gyrus; PreCG: precentral gyrus; IFG: inferior frontal gyrus; MOG: middle occipital lobe gyrus; PoCG: postcentral gyrus.

TABLE 3 | Regions revealing significant fALFF differences between IXT patients and HCs ($P < 0.05$, corrected for GRF).

fALFF	Brain region	Peak MNI, mm			Peak T value	Number of voxels
		x	y	z		
Slow 5 band	L IFG	−39	18	24	5.5655	14
Slow 4 band	R PreCG	36	−3	42	4.2404	14
	R SMG	48	−42	39	4.8967	14
	L PoCG	−48	−9	36	−4.6384	19
	L MOG	−27	−102	3	−4.6430	39

R: right; L: left; MNI: Montreal Neurological Institute; IFG: inferior frontal gyrus; PreCG: precentral gyrus; SMG: supramarginal gyrus; MOG: middle occipital lobe gyrus; PoCG: postcentral gyrus.

TABLE 4 | The peak MNI coordinates and intensity of brain clusters with significant intergroup differences in voxel-wise FC values ($P < 0.05$, corrected for GRF).

ROI	Brain region	Peak MNI, mm			Peak T value	Number of voxels
		x	y	z		
R ANG	L SPL	−24	−66	48	4.7865	23
	R CUN	12	−78	28	4.6788	14
R IPL	R CUN	10	−79	30	5.0084	38
R PreCG	R ROL	50	−2	15	5.3324	311
	L MTG	−54	−34	−2	4.0213	30
	L IFG	−54	9	15	5.3297	309
	L DCG	−7	4	46	4.7603	122
R SMG	L PoCG	−44	−26	59	4.7762	44
	R PreCG	9	−16	67	4.6095	82
	L PCL	−7	−29	69	5.6774	63

R: right; L: left; MNI: Montreal Neurological Institute; ANG: angular gyrus; SPL: superior parietal lobule; CUN: cuneus; IPL: inferior parietal lobule; PreCG: precentral gyrus; ROL: rolandic operculum; MTG: middle temporal gyrus; IFG: inferior frontal gyrus; DCG: median cingulate gyrus; SMG: supramarginal gyrus; PoCG: postcentral gyrus; PCL: paracentral gyrus.

Hensch and Quinlan, 2018). The decreased PCUN activities in patients with IXT may have caused the decreased fusion and visuomotor coordination.

In addition to the PCUN, we also found abnormal spontaneous brain activity in PreCG, PoCG, and IFG. As mentioned above, the PreCG and PoCG belong to the motor and sensory networks, which are related to the ocular movement. A previous study demonstrated that the PreCG is involved in the encoding of oculomotor (Iacoboni et al., 1997). Moreover, another research showed that stimulating the PreCG controls eye movement (Blanke et al., 2000). Zhu et al. (2018) reported that neural activity in the left PreCG was decreased in patients with comitant exotropia. The frontal lobe serves a vital role in visual processing and associated eye movements (Shao et al., 2019). It is well established that the IFG is critical for response inhibition as a part of the frontal cortex and may be involved in the suppression of eye movement (Aron et al., 2003). The lower regional homogeneity (Reho) values were observed in IFG

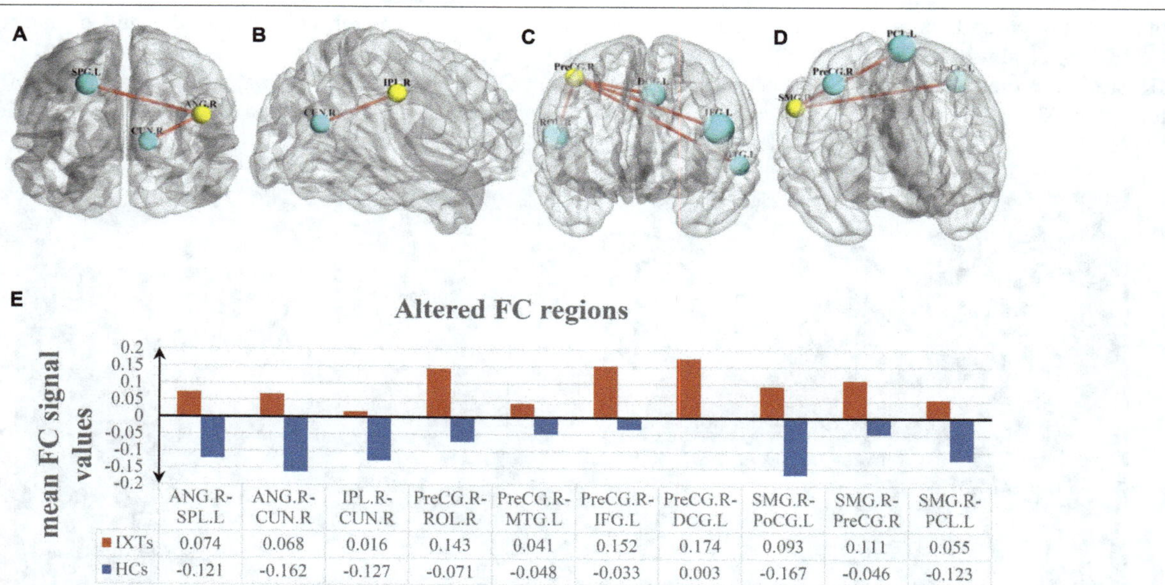

FIGURE 4 | Intergroup comparison of voxel-wise FC between the IXT patient and HCs. FC between the right ANG and right CUN, left SPL was significantly increased **(A)**. FC between the right IPL and right CUN was significantly increased **(B)**. FC between the right PreCG and right ROL, left MTG, left IFG, and left DCG was significantly increased **(C)**. FC between the right SMG and left PoCG, right PreCG and left PCL was significantly increased **(D)**. The yellow balls indicate the seed ROI, while the cyan balls indicate the ROIs with significantly different FC values. The size of the cyan balls corresponds to the *t*-values from the two-sample *t*-tests. The mean FC values of altered brain region is shown in **(E)** and the details of the negative regions can be found in **Table 4**. ANG: angular gyrus; SPL: superior parietal lobule; CUN: cuneus; IPL: inferior parietal lobule; PreCG: precentral gyrus; ROL: rolandic operculum; MTG: middle temporal gyrus; IFG: inferior frontal gyrus; DCG: median cingulate gyrus; SMG: supramarginal gyrus; PoCG: postcentral gyrus; PCL: paracentral gyrus.

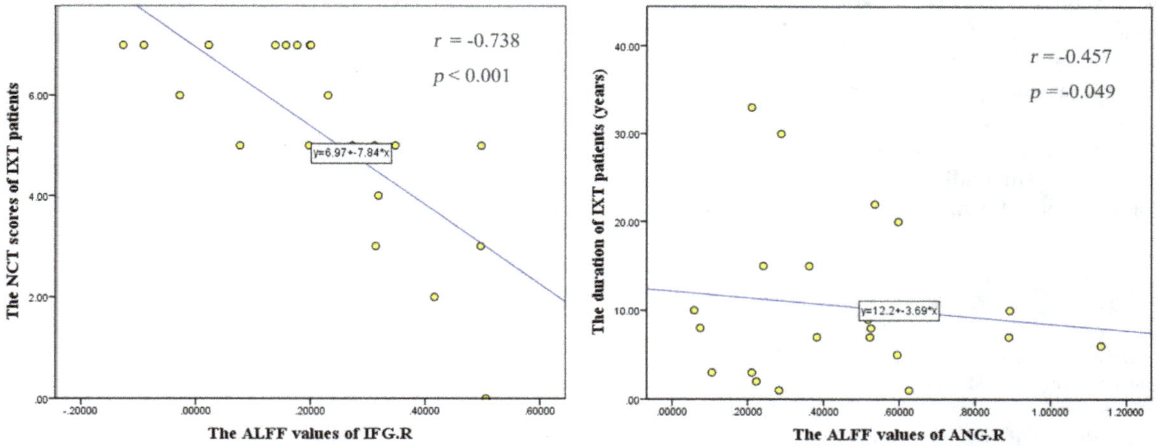

FIGURE 5 | Correlations between the ALFF values and behavioral performance in IXT patients. The NCT scores were negatively correlated with ALFF values in the right IFG ($r = -0.738$, $p < 0.001$). The duration of IXT was negatively correlated with ALFF values of the right ANG ($r = -0.457$, $p = 0.049$). IFG: inferior frontal gyrus; ANG: angular gyrus.

of patients with strabismus and amblyopia (Shao et al., 2019). However, our study found increased ALFF/fALFF values in the PreCG and IFG, which is different from previous studies. We speculated IXT, as a transitional stage to constant exotropia, still has a part of function to control eye position. The increased FC was found between right PreCG and right ROL, left MTG, left IFG, and left DCG. Roker reported the activation of MTG with the fusion stimulus, and MTG is a region responsible for 3D surface orientation and retinal image velocities (Nguyenkim and DeAngelis, 2003; Rokers et al., 2009). The DCG is an important element of visual cortices, where it helps control visual attention and the encoding of visual information (Hickey et al., 2010). The increased ALFF/fALFF values in the PreCG, IFG, and increased FC between these regions and brain areas related to the ocular movement indicates a compensation and devotion to remaining in the normal eye position. Some scholars believe that ROL is associated with self-rating affective and apathetic depressive symptoms, which may indicate symptoms of depression of IXT patients (Sutoko et al., 2020).

In the IXT, abnormal spontaneous neural activities were mainly located in the right hemisphere, especially dorsal spatial processing pathway (Kwee et al., 1999; Nishida et al., 2001; Fortin et al., 2002). Consistent with our results, Yan et al. (2010) suggested that the dorsal visual pathway was abnormal or impaired in patients with comitant exotropia, combining VBM and voxel-based analysis of DTI results. Interestingly, utilizing fMRI and PET, many studies also found that the stereopsis areas were in the right parietal lobule and its surrounding areas (Kwee et al., 1999; Nishida et al., 2001). In our study, these stereopsis areas of the right hemisphere are likely to be impaired in IXT patients, leading to impaired stereopsis. The NCT scores are the standard measure for evaluating the function of eye position control of IXT. The higher NCT scores represent more severity of IXT. The activities in the IFG were lower with increased severity of IXT in the study, which suggest decreased compensation with the progression of IXT. When IXT evolves into constant exotropia, decompensation will occur at the end, which is supported by Shao et al. They found the Reho values in IFG are lower in patients with strabismus and amblyopia (Aron et al., 2003). Furthermore, we found a negative correlation between the ALFF values of the right ANG and duration. The ANG is involved in the formation of stereoscopic vision, and with the prolongation of duration of disease, the impaired stereoscopic vision of patients is aggravated, then the activity of ANG maybe decreased.

In conclusion, changed ALFF/fALFF values and FC values are found in vision- and eye movement-related regions in IXT patients. In addition, the changes in activity of certain brain regions are associated with duration and the severity of the disease.

LIMITATIONS

The current study involved several limitations that should be considered. First, despite us investigating the brain function changes of IXT, we did not carry on the study on the different subtypes of IXT. Second, we did not consider psychological problems of IXT patients. Meanwhile, the sample size of the study is not very large, studying a larger sample would be useful to allow more detailed neurophysiological and neuroimaging investigations. In the future, we will continue to expand the sample size and gather neuropsychological assessment data for deeper and more detailed study.

CONCLUSION

The patients with IXT showed widespread ALFF/fALFF changes of neural activity and FC changes, which were located in the fusion-, stereopsis-, and oculomotor-related regions. These results indicated that the IXT is a complex central nervous system disease affecting multiple brain regions. Moreover, abnormal spontaneous neural activities in the right IFG and the right ANG are correlated with the progression of IXT, suggesting that ALFF and fALFF might be useful complementary indicators for the disease. The current findings extend understanding of the neuropathological mechanisms of IXT.

AUTHOR CONTRIBUTIONS

XH, ZL, and JF contributed to conception and design of the study. YG, JH, and XH organized the database. XH, WL, and JL performed the statistical analysis. XH wrote the first draft of the manuscript. XH and QW wrote sections of the manuscript. XQ, TL, and LZ provide technological support. All authors contributed to manuscript revision, read, and approved the submitted version.

REFERENCES

Aron, A. R., Fletcher, P. C., Bullmore, E. T., Sahakian, B. J., and Robbins, T. W. (2003). Stop-signal inhibition disrupted by damage to right inferior frontal gyrus in humans. *Nat. Neurosci.* 6, 115–116. doi: 10.1038/nn1003

Biswal, B. B. (2012). Resting state fMRI: a personal history. *Neuroimage* 62, 938–944.

Blanke, O., Spinelli, L., Thut, G., Michel, C. M., Perrig, S., Landis, T., et al. (2000). Location of the human frontal eye field as defined by electrical cortical stimulation: anatomical, functional and electrophysiological characteristics. *Neuroreport* 11, 1907–1913. doi: 10.1097/00001756-200006260-00021

Brodsky, M. C., and Jung, J. (2015). Intermittent exotropia and accommodative esotropia: distinct disorders or two ends of a spectrum? *Ophthalmology* 122, 1543–1546. doi: 10.1016/j.ophtha.2015.03.004

Caminiti, R., Ferraina, S., and Johnson, P. B. (1996). The sources of visual information to the primate frontal lobe: a novel role for the superior parietal lobule. *Cereb. Cortex* 6, 319–328. doi: 10.1093/cercor/6.3.319

Cavanna, A. E., and Trimble, M. R. (2006). The precuneus: a review of its functional anatomy and behavioural correlates. *Brain* 129(Pt 3), 564–583. doi: 10.1093/brain/awl004

Chia, A., Dirani, M., Chan, Y., Gazzard, G., Au Eong, K., Selvaraj, P., et al. (2010). Prevalence of amblyopia and strabismus in young Singaporean Chinese children. *Invest. Ophthalmol. Vis. Sci.* 51, 3411–3417. doi: 10.1167/iovs.09-4461

Daw, N. W. (1998). Critical periods and amblyopia. *Arch. Ophthalmol.* 116, 502–505. doi: 10.1001/archopht.116.4.502

Felician, O., Romaiguère, P., Anton, J. L., Nazarian, B., Roth, M., Poncet, M., et al. (2004). The role of human left superior parietal lobule in body part localization. *Ann. Neurol.* 55, 749–751. doi: 10.1002/ana.20109

Fortin, A., Ptito, A., Faubert, J., and Ptito, M. (2002). Cortical areas mediating stereopsis in the human brain: a PET study. *Neuroreport* 13, 895–898. doi: 10.1097/00001756-200205070-00032

Fu, J., Li, S. M., Liu, L. R., Li, J. L., Li, S. Y., Zhu, B. D., et al. (2014). Prevalence of amblyopia and strabismus in a population of 7th-grade junior high school students in Central China: the Anyang Childhood Eye Study (ACES). *Ophthalmic Epidemiol.* 21, 197–203. doi: 10.3109/09286586.2014.904371

Guyton, D. L. (2006). The 10th Bielschowsky Lecture. Changes in strabismus over time: the roles of vergence tonus and muscle length adaptation. *Binocul. Vis. Strabismus Q.* 21, 81–92.

Han, Y., Lui, S., Kuang, W., Lang, Q., Zou, L., and Jia, J. (2012). Anatomical and functional deficits in patients with amnestic mild cognitive impairment. *PLoS One* 7:e28664. doi: 10.1371/journal.pone.0028664

Hensch, T. K., and Quinlan, E. M. (2018). Critical periods in amblyopia. *Vis. Neurosci.* 35, E014. doi: 10.1017/S0952523817000219

Hickey, C., Chelazzi, L., and Theeuwes, J. (2010). Reward changes salience in human vision via the anterior cingulate. *J. Neurosci.* 30, 11096–11103. doi: 10.1523/JNEUROSCI.1026-10.2010

Iacoboni, M., Woods, R. P., Lenzi, G. L., and Mazziotta, J. C. (1997). Merging of oculomotor and somatomotor space coding in the human right precentral gyrus. *Brain* 120 (Pt 9), 1635–1645. doi: 10.1093/brain/120.9.1635

Iacoboni, M., and Zaidel, E. (2004). Interhemispheric visuo-motor integration in humans: the role of the superior parietal cortex. *Neuropsychologia* 42, 419–425. doi: 10.1016/j.neuropsychologia.2003.10.007

Kim, W. J., and Kim, M. M. (2017). Variability of preoperative measurements in intermittent exotropia and its effect on surgical outcome. *J AAPOS* 21, 210–214. doi: 10.1016/j.jaapos.2017.05.006

Kwee, I. L., Fujii, Y., Matsuzawa, H., and Nakada, T. (1999). Perceptual processing of stereopsis in humans: high-field (3.0-tesla) functional MRI study. *Neurology* 53, 1599–1601. doi: 10.1212/wnl.53.7.1599

Lee, H. W., Hong, S. B., Seo, D. W., Tae, W. S., and Hong, S. C. (2000). Mapping of functional organization in human visual cortex: electrical cortical stimulation. *Neurology* 54, 849–854. doi: 10.1212/wnl.54.4.849

Li, D., Li, S., and Zeng, X. (2018). Analysis of alterations in white matter integrity of adult patients with comitant exotropia. *J. Int. Med. Res.* 46, 1963–1972. doi: 10.1177/0300060518763704

Li, Q., Bai, J., Zhang, J., Gong, Q., and Liu, L. (2016). Assessment of cortical dysfunction in patients with intermittent exotropia: an fMRI study. *PLoS One* 11:e0160806. doi: 10.1371/journal.pone.0160806

Li, T., Liu, Z., Li, J., Liu, Z., Tang, Z., Xie, X., et al. (2014). Altered amplitude of low-frequency fluctuation in primary open-angle glaucoma: a resting-state FMRI study. *Invest. Ophthalmol. Vis. Sci.* 56, 322–329. doi: 10.1167/iovs.14-14974

Logothetis, N. K., Pauls, J., Augath, M., Trinath, T., and Oeltermann, A. (2001). Neurophysiological investigation of the basis of the fMRI signal. *Nature* 412, 150–157. doi: 10.1038/35084005

McGuire, L. M., and Sabes, P. N. (2011). Heterogeneous representations in the superior parietal lobule are common across reaches to visual and proprioceptive targets. *J. Neurosci.* 31, 6661–6673. doi: 10.1523/JNEUROSCI.2921-10.2011

McKean-Cowdin, R., Cotter, S. A., Tarczy-Hornoch, K., Wen, G., Kim, J., Borchert, M., et al. (2013). Prevalence of amblyopia or strabismus in asian and non-Hispanic white preschool children: multi-ethnic pediatric eye disease study. *Ophthalmology* 120, 2117–2124. doi: 10.1016/j.ophtha.2013.03.001

Merigan, W. H., and Maunsell, J. H. (1993). How parallel are the primate visual pathways? *Annu. Rev. Neurosci.* 16, 369–402. doi: 10.1146/annurev.ne.16.030193.002101

Nagahama, Y., Okada, T., Katsumi, Y., Hayashi, T., Yamauchi, H., Sawamoto, N., et al. (1999). Transient neural activity in the medial superior frontal gyrus and precuneus time locked with attention shift between object features. *Neuroimage* 10, 193–199. doi: 10.1006/nimg.1999.0451

Nguyenkim, J. D., and DeAngelis, G. C. (2003). Disparity-based coding of three-dimensional surface orientation by macaque middle temporal neurons. *J. Neurosci.* 23, 7117–7128. doi: 10.1523/JNEUROSCI.23-18-07117.2003

Nishida, Y., Hayashi, O., Iwami, T., Kimura, M., Kani, K., Ito, R., et al. (2001). Stereopsis-processing regions in the human parieto-occipital cortex. *Neuroreport* 12, 2259–2263. doi: 10.1097/00001756-200107200-00043

Oakes, T. R., Fox, A. S., Johnstone, T., Chung, M. K., Kalin, N., and Davidson, R. J. (2007). Integrating VBM into the General Linear Model with voxelwise anatomical covariates. *Neuroimage* 34, 500–508. doi: 10.1016/j.neuroimage.2006.10.007

Ouyang, J., Yang, L., Huang, X., Zhong, Y. L., Hu, P. H., Zhang, Y., et al. (2017). The atrophy of white and gray matter volume in patients with comitant strabismus: evidence from a voxel-based morphometry study. *Mol. Med. Rep.* 16, 3276–3282. doi: 10.3892/mmr.2017.7006

Pan, C. W., Zhu, H., Yu, J. J., Ding, H., Bai, J., Chen, J., et al. (2016). Epidemiology of intermittent exotropia in preschool children in China. *Optom. Vis. Sci.* 93, 57–62. doi: 10.1097/OPX.0000000000000754

Pettigrew, J. D., Nikara, T., and Bishop, P. O. (1968). Responses to moving slits by single units in cat striate cortex. *Exp. Brain Res.* 6, 373–390. doi: 10.1007/BF00233185

Poggio, G. F., and Fischer, B. (1977). Binocular interaction and depth sensitivity in striate and prestriate cortex of behaving rhesus monkey. *J. Neurophysiol.* 40, 1392–1405. doi: 10.1152/jn.1977.40.6.1392

Rokers, B., Cormack, L. K., and Huk, A. C. (2009). Disparity- and velocity-based signals for three-dimensional motion perception in human MT+. *Nat. Neurosci.* 12, 1050–1055 doi: 10.1038/nn.2343

Shao, Y., Li, Q. H., Li, B., Lin, Q., Su, T., Shi, W. Q., et al. (2019). Altered brain activity in patients with strabismus and amblyopia detected by analysis of regional homogeneity: a resting-state functional magnetic resonance imaging study. *Mol. Med. Rep.* 19, 4832–4840. doi: 10.3892/mmr.2019.10147

Sutoko, S., Atsumori, H., Obata, A., Funane, T., Kandori, A., Shimonaga, K., et al. (2020). Lesions in the right Rolandic operculum are associated with self-rating affective and apathetic depressive symptoms for post-stroke patients. *Sci. Rep.* 10:20264. doi: 10.1038/s41598-020-77136-5

Tan, G., Huang, X., Zhang, Y., Wu, A. H., Zhong, Y. L., Wu, K., et al. (2016). A functional MRI study of altered spontaneous brain activity pattern in patients with congenital comitant strabismus using amplitude of low-frequency fluctuation. *Neuropsychiatr. Dis. Treat.* 12, 1243–1250. doi: 10.2147/NDT.S104756

Tomasi, D., and Volkow, N. D. (2010). Functional connectivity density mapping. *Proc. Natl. Acad. Sci. U. S. A.* 107, 9885–9890.

Tootell, R. B., Hadjikhani, N. K., Mendola, J. D., Marrett, S., and Dale, A. M. (1998). From retinotopy to recognition: fMRI in human visual cortex. *Trends Cogn. Sci.* 2, 174–183. doi: 10.1016/s1364-6613(98)01171-1

Tu, S., Qiu, J., Martens, U., and Zhang, Q. L. (2013). Category-selective attention modulates unconscious processes in the middle occipital gyrus. *Conscious Cogn.* 22, 479–485. doi: 10.1016/j.concog.2013.02.007

Turner (2013). "R: functional magnetic resonance imaging (fMRI)," in *Encyclopedia of Sciences and Religions*, eds A. L. C. Runehov and L. Oviedo. 35.

Whitfield-Gabrieli, S., and Nieto-Castanon, A. (2012). Conn: a functional connectivity toolbox for correlated and anticorrelated brain networks. *Brain Connect.* 2, 125–141. doi: 10.1089/brain.2012.0073

Yan, X., Lin, X., Wang, Q., Zhang, Y., Chen, Y., Song, S., et al. (2010). Dorsal visual pathway changes in patients with comitant extropia. *PLoS One* 5:e10931. doi: 10.1371/journal.pone.0010931

Yang, M., Chen, J., Shen, T., Kang, Y., Deng, D., Lin, X., et al. (2016). Clinical characteristics and surgical outcomes in patients with intermittent exotropia: a large sample study in South China. *Medicine (Baltimore)* 95:e2590. doi: 10.1097/MD.0000000000002590

Yang, X., Zhang, J., Lang, L., Gong, Q., and Liu, L. (2014). Assessment of cortical dysfunction in infantile esotropia using fMRI. *Eur. J. Ophthalmol.* 24, 409–416. doi: 10.5301/ejo.5000368

Zhou, G., Liu, P., Wang, J., Wen, H., Zhu, M., Zhao, R., et al. (2013). Fractional amplitude of low-frequency fluctuation changes in functional dyspepsia: a resting-state fMRI study. *Magn. Reson. Imaging* 31, 996–1000. doi: 10.1016/j.mri.2013.03.019

Zhu, P. W., Huang, X., Ye, L., Jiang, N., Zhong, Y. L., Yuan, Q., et al. (2018). Altered intrinsic functional connectivity of the primary visual cortex in youth patients with comitant exotropia: a resting state fMRI study. *Int. J. Ophthalmol.* 11, 668–673. doi: 10.18240/ijo.2018.04.22

17

Evaluating the Performance of qVFM in Mapping the Visual Field of Simulated Observers with Eye Diseases

*Pengjing Xu[1,2,3], Luis Andres Lesmes[4], Deyue Yu[1] and Zhong-Lin Lu[5,6,7]**

[1] College of Optometry, The Ohio State University, Columbus, OH, United States, [2] Shanghai Technology Development Co., Ltd., Shanghai, China, [3] Shanghai-Warsaw Joint Laboratory on Artificial Intelligence, Shanghai, China, [4] Adaptive Sensory Technology, Inc., San Diego, CA, United States, [5] Division of Arts and Sciences, NYU Shanghai, Shanghai, China, [6] Center for Neural Science, Department of Psychology, New York University, New York, NY, United States, [7] NYU-ECNU Institute of Cognitive Neuroscience at NYU Shanghai, Shanghai, China

***Correspondence:**
Zhong-Lin Lu
zhonglin@nyu.edu

Purpose: Recently, we developed a novel active learning framework, qVFM, to map visual functions in the visual field. The method has been implemented and validated in measuring light sensitivity and contrast sensitivity visual field maps (VFMs) of normal observers. In this study, we evaluated the performance of the qVFM method in mapping the light sensitivity VFM of simulated patients with peripheral scotoma, glaucoma, age-related macular degeneration (AMD), and cataract.

Methods: For each simulated patient, we sampled 100 locations (60 × 60 degrees) of the visual field and compared the performance of the qVFM method with a procedure that tests each location independently (the qYN method) in a cued Yes/No task. Two different switch modules, the distribution sampling method (DSM) and parameter delivering method (PDM), were implemented in the qVFM method. Simulated runs of 1,200 trials were used to compare the accuracy and precision of the qVFM-DSM, qVFM-PDM and qYN methods.

Results: The qVFM method with both switch modules can provide accurate, precise, and efficient assessments of the light sensitivity VFM for the simulated patients, with the qVFM-PDM method better at detecting VFM deficits in the simulated glaucoma.

Conclusions: The qVFM method can be used to characterize residual vision of simulated ophthalmic patients. The study sets the stage for further investigation with real patients and potential translation of the method into clinical practice.

Keywords: Bayesian adaptive testing, active learning, perimetry, visual-field map, scotoma, glaucoma, age-related macular degeneration, cataract

INTRODUCTION

Standard automated perimetry (SAP) (Goldmann, 1945a,b; Harms, 1952; Aulhorn and Harms, 1972; Lachenmayr et al., 1994; Rogers and Landers, 2005; Milner and Goodale, 2006; Strasburger et al., 2011) is used to assess the light sensitivity visual field map (VFM) in routine clinical eye exams to detect and manage a number of eye diseases that cause visual field deficits, including glaucoma (Caprioli, 1991; Smith et al., 1996; Ng et al., 2012), peripheral scotoma caused by a number of

TABLE 1 | Parameters of the normal observer: EPA (unit: degree/$\sqrt{dB}$), EPB (unit: degree/$\sqrt{dB}$), EPZ (unit: dB), SLA (unit: dB/degree), SLB (unit: dB/degree), and λ.

Parameters	EPA	EPB	EPZ	SLA	SLB	λ
Value	81.0	41.1	24.3	0.020	0.032	1.20
SD	2.4	2.9	0.62	0.035	0.045	0.14

In this study, the dB values were calculated as −10 × log10[luminance (in asb)/10000].

pathogenesis (Portney and Krohn, 1978; Fendrich et al., 1992), age-related macular degeneration (AMD) (Anderson et al., 2011; Luu et al., 2013), cataract (Radius, 1978; Lam et al., 1991), retinitis pigmentosa (Jacobson et al., 1986; Iannaccone et al., 1995), cytomegalovirus retinitis (Bachman et al., 1992; Thorne et al., 2011), stroke (Townend et al., 2007), and other neurological deficits (Papageorgiou et al., 2007). However, the assessment of VFM based on SAP is very noisy (Heijl et al., 1989). To improve

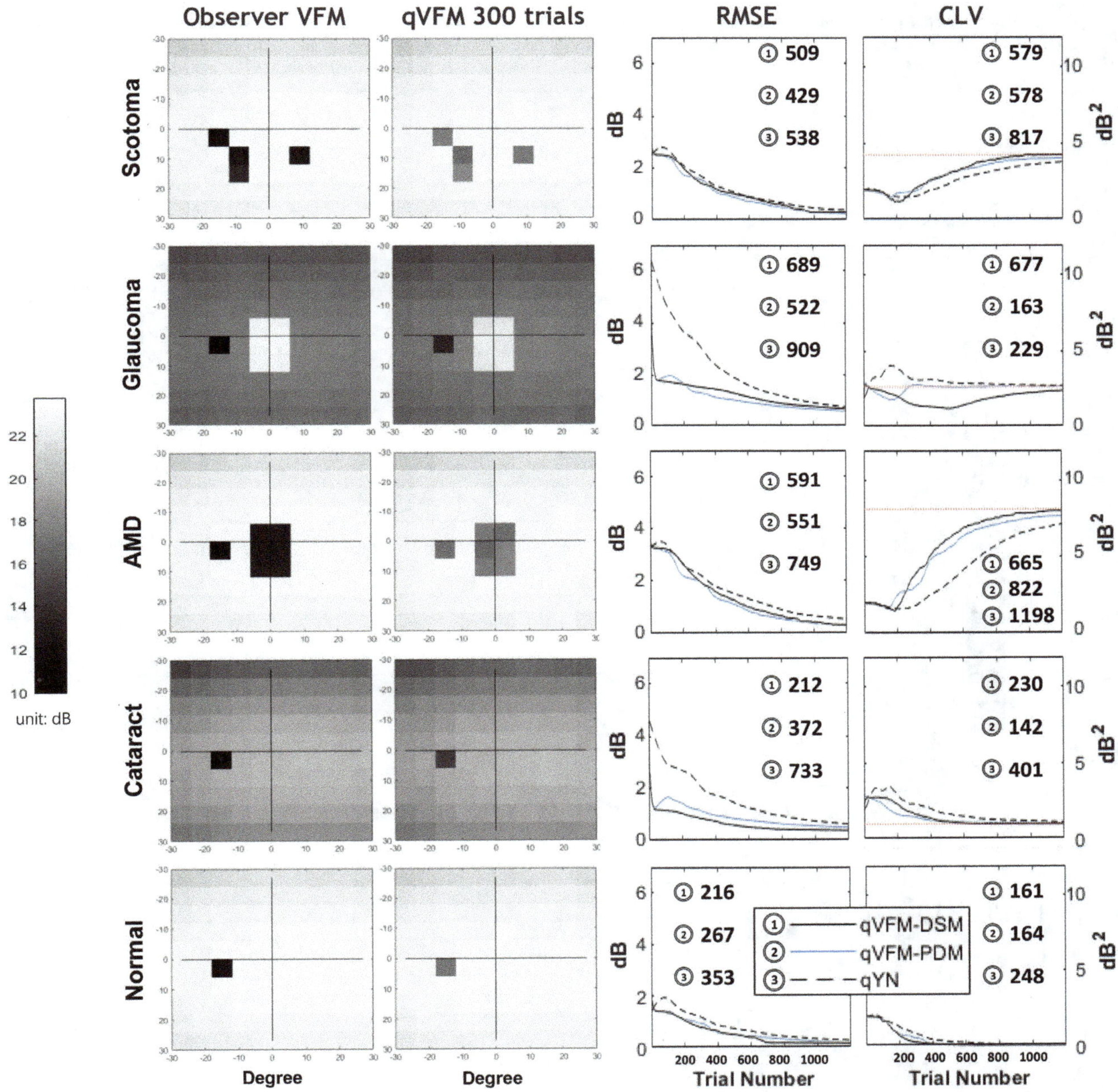

FIGURE 1 | Summary results from the five simulated observers across 200 runs. The true VFM of each simulated observer (monocular) is presented in the first column with an achromatic colormap. The estimated VFMs obtained with the qVFM-PDM method after 300 trials are presented in the second column. The corresponding root mean squared error (RMSE) and corrected loss variance (CLV) of the estimates as functions of trial number are shown in the third and fourth columns. The trial numbers needed to achieve 1 dB RMSE and 1 dB^2 within CLV are shown in the corresponding subplots for the three methods.

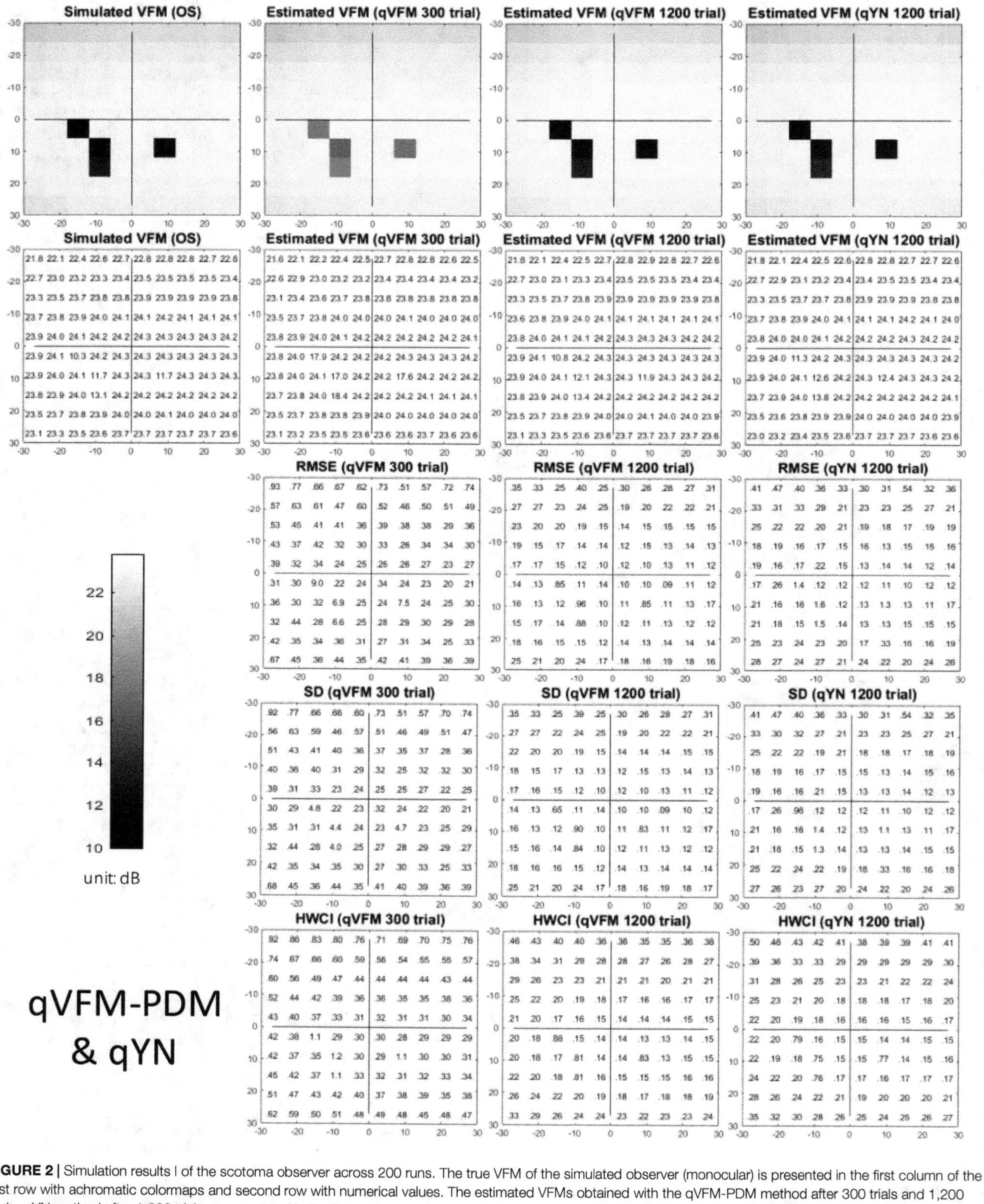

FIGURE 2 | Simulation results I of the scotoma observer across 200 runs. The true VFM of the simulated observer (monocular) is presented in the first column of the first row with achromatic colormaps and second row with numerical values. The estimated VFMs obtained with the qVFM-PDM method after 300 trials and 1,200 trials, qYN method after 1,200 trials are presented in the first and second rows, respectively. The corresponding RMSE, SD, and 68.2% HWCI of the estimates are in the third, fourth, and fifth rows.

the precision of light sensitivity VFM in automated perimetry and enable assessments of other visual functions, we recently developed a novel active learning framework, the qVFM method, that combines a global module for preliminary assessment of the shape of the VFM and a local module for assessing visual function at individual visual field locations (Xu et al., 2018, 2019a,b, 2020). Both computer simulations and psychophysical validation studies that tested the light sensitivity VFM of 12 eyes of six normal observers (Xu et al., 2019a) and contrast sensitivity VFM of 10 eyes of five normal observers (Xu et al., 2020) showed that

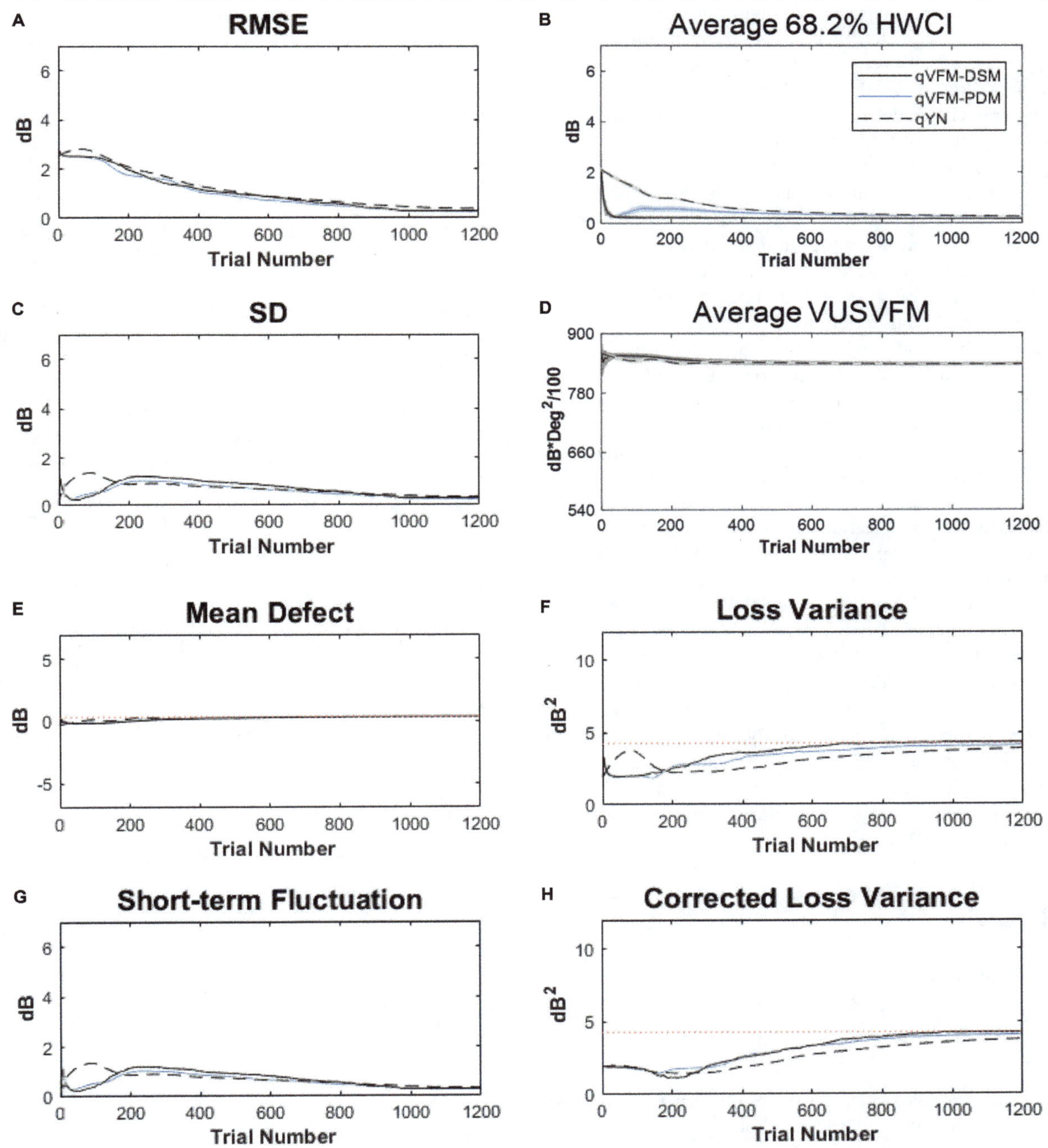

FIGURE 3 | Performance I of the qVFM-DSM, qVFM-PDM and qYN methods in estimating VFM of the simulated scotoma observer across 200 runs. **(A)** Average root mean squared error, **(B)** Average 68.2% HWCI of the estimated VFM, **(C)** Average standard deviation, **(D)** Average volume under the surface of the VFM (VUSVFM), **(E)** Mean defect, **(F)** Short-term fluctuation, **(G)** Loss variance, and **(H)** Corrected loss variance. Results from the qVFM-DSM and qVFM-PDM methods are shown in solid black and blue lines, and results from the qYN method are shown in dashed lines. The true values of the global indices are shown in red dotted lines. For panels **(B,D)**, shaded regions represent ± 1 SD of the corresponding value.

the qVFM method could provide accurate, precise and efficient VFM assessments.

In Xu et al. (2019a), we compared the qVFM method with the conventional staircase-based SAP methods. We showed that the conventional staircase-based SAP methods exhibited considerable larger biases and variabilities than the qVFM. The focus of the current study is to evaluate the potential of the qVFM method in mapping the light sensitivity VFM of simulated patients with peripheral scotoma, glaucoma, AMD, and cataract. Specifically, we simulated a scotoma observer with three scotomas located in the periphery, a glaucoma observer with peripheral vision deficits outside of the fovea, an AMD observer with deficits at the fovea, and a cataract observer with lower light sensitivity across the entire visual field. This is the first step in our attempt toward evaluating the qVFM method in clinical populations. We plan to further evaluate and translate the qVFM method into clinical practice in the future.

The qVFM method consists of three modules, a preliminary assessment of the general shape of the VFM (the global module), an assessment of visual functions at each individual visual field location (the local module), and a switch module that determines when to switch from the global module to the local module. The global module is used to estimate the overall shape of the visual field in the beginning of the assessment, and the local module is used to provide a detailed location-by-location characterization of the VFM based on priors generated from the global module. Given that the goal of clinical VFM assessment is to detect deviations from the normal VFM, it is essential to assess the performance of the qVFM method in measuring pathological visual fields with characteristic patterns that deviate severely from the normal VFM. Our hypothesis is that even though the global module does not provide a complete model of the detailed structure of the VFM in some severe cases, it still provides a reasonable approximation, and then the local module can swiftly take over to measure the detailed local structure of the VFM. We also compared two different switching methods in this study, one based on a distribution sampling method (DSM) (Xu et al., 2018, 2019a), and the other a newly developed procedure based on a parameter delivering method (PDM).

METHODS

qVFM Implementation

Developed in Xu et al. (2019a,b, 2020), the qVFM method consists of three major modules (see **Supplementary Appendix B** for more details):

(1) The global module, which measures the shape of the VFM modeled as a tilted elliptic paraboloid function (TEPF) with five parameters (Eq. 1). The score at each visual field location represents a measure of visual function (e.g., light sensitivity, contrast sensitivity) at that location.
(2) The switch module, which evaluates the rate of information gain in the global module and determines when to switch to the local module. At the switching point, the module generates a prior distribution of the measure of visual function at each visual field location based on the posterior distribution from the global module.
(3) The local module, which uses the prior generated by the switch module to provide assessment of visual function at each visual field location. It uses another Bayesian adaptive procedure that determines the order and test stimulus based on the relative information gain across locations.

The global module models and assesses the global shape of light sensitivity VFM as a TEPF:

$$\tau\left(x,y\right)=EPZ-\left(\frac{x}{EPA}\right)^2-\left(\frac{y}{EPB}\right)^2+SLA*x+SLB*y, \tag{1}$$

where EPZ (unit: dB) is the light sensitivity at the fovea, EPA (unit: degree/$\sqrt{dB}$) is the root bandwidth in the horizontal direction of the light sensitivity VFM, EPB (unit: degree/$\sqrt{dB}$) is the root bandwidth in the vertical direction, SLA (unit: dB/degree) is the horizontal tilt level of the light sensitivity VFM, and SLB (unit: dB/degree) is the vertical tilt level. The height of the TEPF, $\tau(x,\ y)$, is the light sensitivity (unit: dB) at visual field location (x, y) at $d' = 1.0$.

A Yes/No (YN) task was adapted in this study, which means that the probability of reporting target presence is determined by both the light sensitivity and decision criterion. After introducing

TABLE 2 | RMSE, SD, average 68.2% HWCI, mean defect, loss variance and corrected loss variance of the estimated VFM from the qVFM-DSM, qVFM-PDM and qYN methods in the beginning (0 trial), after 300 and 1,200 trials are listed for the simulated scotoma observer.

Scotoma	Trial number	0	300	1,200	True value	1 dB/dB^2 threshold
RMSE (dB)	qVFM-DSM	2.54	1.42	0.29		509 ± 70
	qVFM-PDM	2.54	1.57	0.25		429 ± 40
	qYN	2.54	1.71	0.37		538 ± 33
SD (dB)	qVFM-DSM	0	1. 15	0. 29		
	qVFM-PDM	0	0.99	0. 24		
	qYN	0	0.89	0. 33		
HWCI (dB)	qVFM-DSM	2.12	0. 22	0.17		
	qVFM-PDM	2.12	0. 48	0.24		
	qYN	2.12	0. 73	0.26		
Mean defect (dB)	qVFM-DSM	−0.26	0.20	0.36	0.36	
	qVFM-PDM	−0.26	0.19	0.36	0.36	
	qYN	−0.26	0.26	0.36	0.36	
Loss variance (dB^2)	qVFM-DSM	1.95	3.27	4.33	4.28	
	qVFM-PDM	1.95	2.84	4.15	4.28	
	qYN	1.95	2.31	3.89	4.28	
Corrected loss variance (dB^2)	qVFM-DSM	1.95	1.94	4.24	4.28	579 ± 68
	qVFM-PDM	1.95	1.86	4.15	4.28	578 ± 61
	qYN	1.95	1.50	3.79	4.28	817 ± 69

The corresponding true values are listed in the sixth column. Trial numbers needed to achieve 1 dB RMSE and 1 dB^2 within the corrected loss variance are listed with their SD in the last column.

the sixth parameter λ for decision criterion, the global model can predict the overall probability of light detection across the visual field $p(\vec{\theta})$, where $\vec{\theta}$ = (*EPZ*, *EPA*, *EPB*, *SLA*, *SLB*, λ), with a fixed slope of the psychometric function. A prior distribution $p_{t=0}(\vec{\theta})$ is defined based on *a priori* knowledge of the VFM before any data collection. In addition, all possible stimulus intensities and stimulus locations *(x, y)* are included in the stimulus space. The optimal stimulus in the next trial, which would generate the maximum expected information gain, is determined *via* a one-step-ahead search strategy. After receiving the response from the observer, the posterior distribution of the parameters is updated using Bayes rule (Kontsevich and Tyler, 1999; Lesmes et al., 2006, 2010, 2015).

Since the global module cannot estimate the detailed structure of the VFM, a local module is necessary for a more detailed assessment. The switch module determines the switching point and also sets the prior distributions for the local module. Two different switch methods were implemented in this study, the DSM (Xu et al., 2018, 2019a) and the newly developed PDM. In this study, the prior distribution in the local module was defined with a two-dimensional probability distribution of light sensitivity and decision criterion at each visual field location. The DSM and PDM used the same trend of expected information gain in the global model to determine the switching point, but different procedures to generate the prior distributions for the local module from the six-dimensional posterior distribution in the global module.

The DSM samples the posterior distribution in the global module repeatedly to generate the prior distributions at each visual location in the local module, with 1,600 samples per location. The PDM computes the means of the marginal posterior distributions of the five parameters (EPZ, EPA, EPB, SLA, and SLB) of the TEPF model, and sets the expected value of the prior for light sensitivity, τ(x,y), at each visual field location based on the TEPF model. It also sets the expected value of the prior of decision criterion λ at each visual field location, using its mean of the marginal posterior distribution from the global module. It then uses the average 68.2% half width of the credible interval (HWCI) of the posterior distributions of the estimated light sensitivities and decision criterions across all visual field locations to set the variability of the prior distributions in the local module. Specifically, a hyperbolic secant (sech) function (King-Smith and Rose, 1997) is used to set up the prior distributions. For each parameter θ_i (i = 1, 2), the mode of the marginal prior $p(\theta_i)$ is

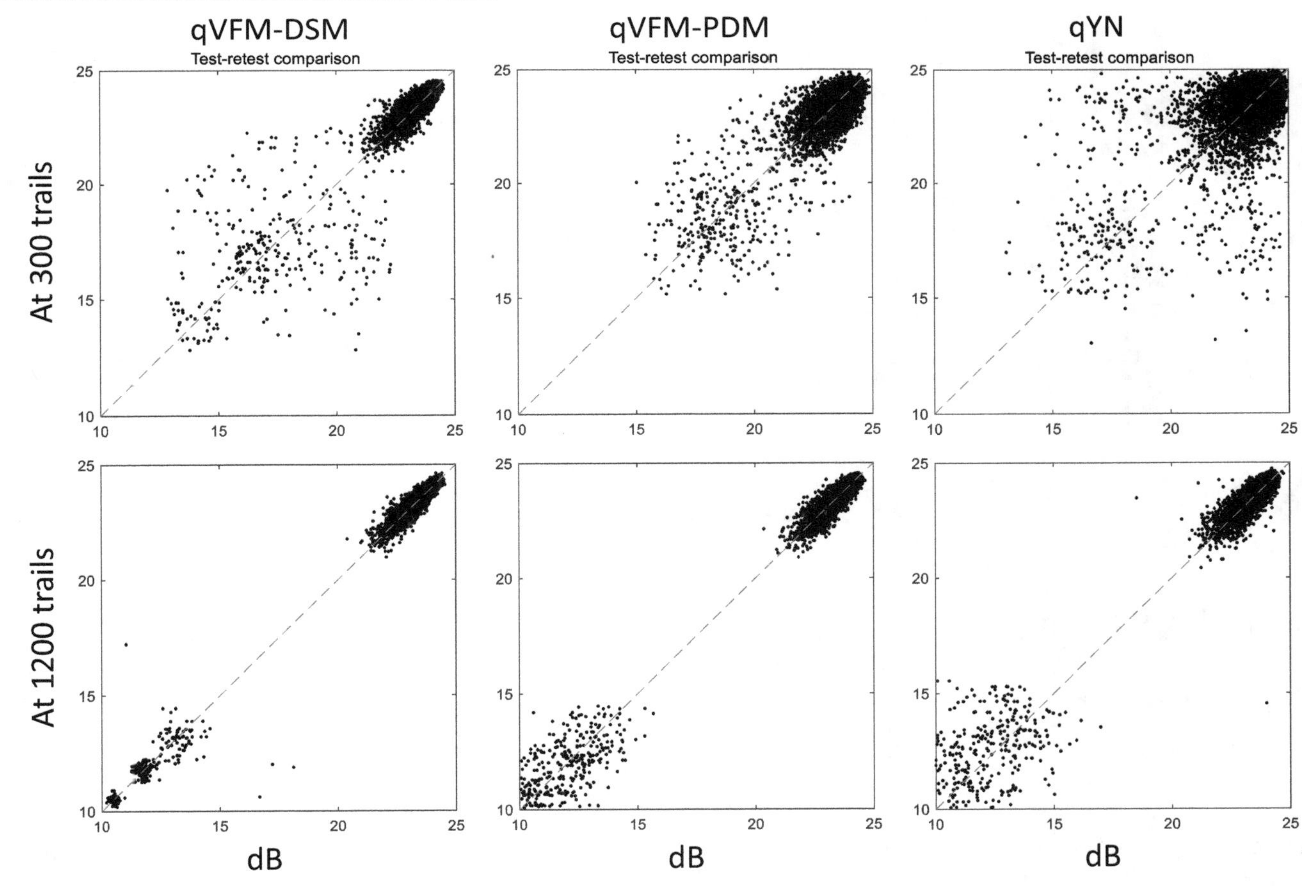

FIGURE 4 | Performance II of the qVFM-DSM, qVFM-PDM, and qYN methods in estimating VFM of the simulated scotoma observer. Test-retest comparison of the estimated light sensitivities from repeated 200 runs at 300 and 1,200 trials.

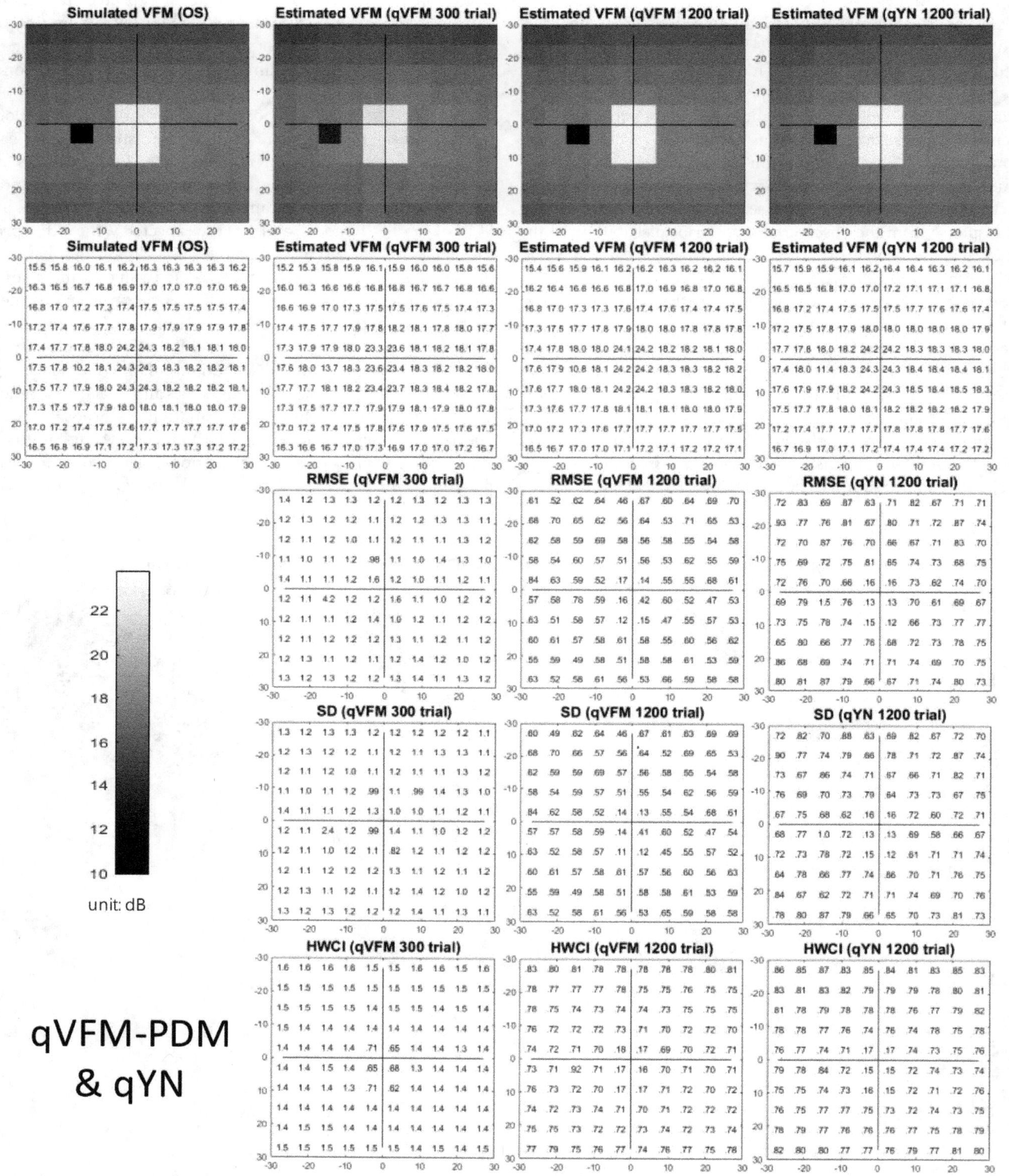

FIGURE 5 | Simulation results I of the glaucoma observer across 200 runs. The true VFM of the simulated observer (monocular) is presented in the first column of the first row with achromatic colormaps and second row with numerical values. The estimated VFMs obtained with the qVFM-PDM method after 300 trials and 1,200 trials, qYN method after 1,200 trials are presented in the first and second rows, respectively. The corresponding RMSE, SD, and 68.2% HWCI of the estimates are shown in the third, fourth, and fifth rows.

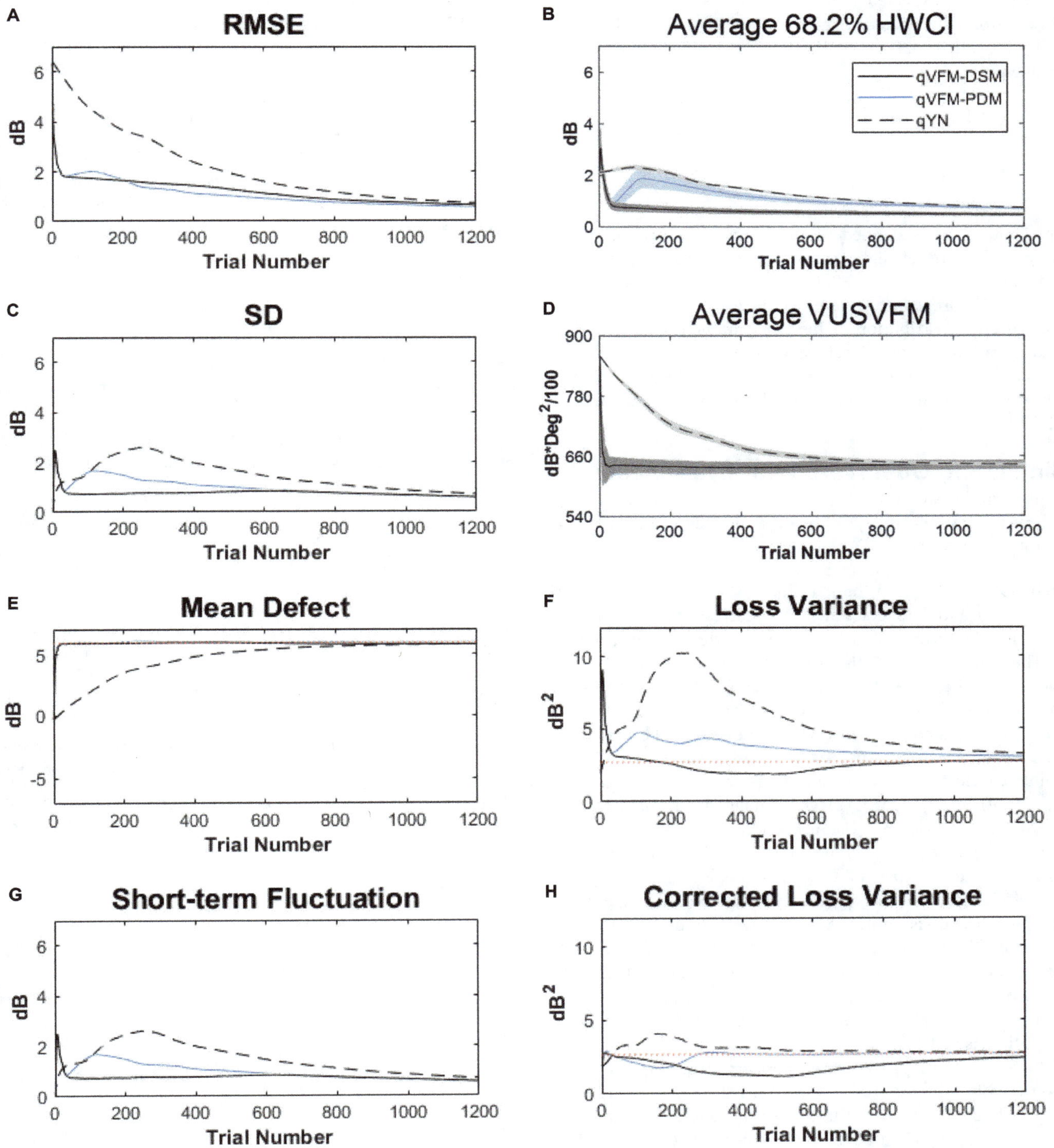

FIGURE 6 | Performance I of the qVFM-DSM, qVFM-PDM and qYN methods in estimating VFM of the simulated glaucoma observer across 200 runs. **(A)** Average root mean squared error, **(B)** Average 68.2% HWCI of the estimated VFM, **(C)** Average standard deviation, **(D)** Average volume under the surface of the VFM (VUSVFM), **(E)** Mean defect, **(F)** Short-term fluctuation, **(G)** Loss variance, and **(H)** Corrected loss variance. Results from the qVFM-DSM and qVFM-PDM methods are shown in solid black and blue lines, and results from the qYN method are shown in dashed lines. The true values of the global indices are shown in red dotted lines. For panels **(B,D)**, shaded regions represent ± 1 SD of the corresponding value.

defined by the expected value of the corresponding parameter, $\theta_{i,guess}$, from the posterior distributions of the global module, and the width is defined by the 68.2% credible interval of that parameter.

$$P(\theta_i) = \text{sech}[\theta_{i,confidence} \times (\theta_i - \theta_{i,\,guess})], \quad (2)$$

where:

$$\text{sech}(z) = \frac{2}{e^z + e^{-z}}. \quad (3)$$

The joint prior is defined as the normalized product of the marginal priors of light sensitivity and decision criterion, generated for each visual field location in the local module.

The qYN procedure (Lesmes et al., 2015) is used to estimate the posterior distribution of the two parameters at each visual field location in the local module. It is also used as a reduced qVFM procedure that has only the local module for performance comparison with the full qVFM procedure that has all three modules.

Simulating Observers With Eye Diseases

In this study, we simulated the VFM of the OS eye of five observers: one normally sighted, and four with peripheral scotoma, glaucoma, AMD, or cataract.

The parameters of the normal observer were the same as those used in Xu et al. (2019a). **Table 1** lists the values of EPA, EPB, EPZ, SLA, SLB, λ and the average SDs of the corresponding parameters from the 12 eyes of six normal observers tested in that study.

The blind spot of the simulated OS eye was at 15 degrees left and three degrees below the fovea, i.e., (−15, 3). At the stated coordinate, each point represented a 6-degree square region. For the four simulated observers with eye diseases, the parameters were modified from those of the normal observer: (1) The simulated scotoma observer had three scotomas, located at (9, 9), (−9, 9), and (−9, 15). (2) The simulated glaucoma observer had defective peripheral vision outside of the central 12 × 15 degrees rectangle area from the upper-left (−6, −6) to the lower-right (6, 9), in which light sensitivity was 2.5 times lower than that of the normal observer. (3) The simulated AMD observer had poor foveal vision in the central 12 × 15 degrees rectangle area from the upper-left (−6, −6) to the lower-right (6, 9), in which light sensitivity was 12.3 dB, about 12 dB lower than that of the normal observer. (4) The simulated cataract observer had 1.7 times lower light sensitivity than the normal observer across the entire visual field.

In the simulations, observers performed the light detection task described in Xu et al. (2019a). Briefly, the test target was a small light disc with a 0.43-degree diameter with luminance between 31.5 and 950 asb (corresponding to 10.2–25.0 dB). Each trial began with a potential 150-ms target at one of the 100 cued visual field locations. Simulated observers were asked to indicate the presence or absence of the target, with the luminance of the target determined by an adaptive procedure in each trial. Their response in each trial was determined by their light sensitivity VFM defined by the simulation procedure, which was unknown to the qVFM procedure that was used to estimate their light sensitivity VFM. The performance of the full qVFM procedure, with both the DSM and PDM switch modules, was compared with that of the qYN procedure, which assessed light sensitivity at each location independently, in 200 repeated simulations of 1,200 trials each.

Evaluation Metrics

We quantified the accuracy of the estimated VFMs using the root mean squared error (RMSE) of the estimated sensitivities across all 100 visual field locations. RMSE after the i-th trial can be calculated as:

$$\text{RMSE}_i = \sqrt{\frac{\sum_k \sum_j \left(\tau_{ijk} - \tau_k^{true}\right)^2}{J \times K}}, \quad (4)$$

where τ_{ijk} is the estimated sensitivity at the k-th visual field location after the i-th trial in the j-th run, and $\tau_k{}^{true}$ is the true sensitivity at that location.

Two methods were used to assess the precision of the qVFM procedure. The first is based on the standard deviation (SD) of repeated measures:

$$\text{SD}_i = \sqrt{\frac{\sum_k \sum_j [\tau_{ijk} - mean(\tau_{ijk})]^2}{J \times K}}. \quad (5)$$

TABLE 3 | RMSE, SD, average 68.2% HWCI, mean defect, loss variance and corrected loss variance of the estimated VFM from the qVFM-DSM, qVFM-PDM and qYN methods in the beginning (0 trial), after 300 and 1,200 trials are listed for the simulated glaucoma observer.

Glaucoma	Trial number	0	300	1,200	True value	1 dB/dB^2 threshold
RMSE (dB)	qVFM-DSM	6.40	1.52	0.65		689 ± 35
	qVFM-PDM	6.40	1.30	0.58		522 ± 21
	qYN	6.40	3.13	0.73		909 ± 26
SD (dB)	qVFM-DSM	0	0.76	0.58		
	qVFM-PDM	0	1.23	0.57		
	qYN	0	2.45	0.71		
HWCI (dB)	qVFM-DSM	2.12	0.63	0.46		
	qVFM-PDM	2.12	1.44	0.71		
	qYN	2.12	1.68	0.74		
Mean defect (dB)	qVFM-DSM	−0.26	5.92	5.79	5.91	
	qVFM-PDM	−0.26	5.99	5.91	5.91	
	qYN	−0.26	4.22	5.79	5.91	
Loss variance (dB^2)	qVFM-DSM	1.95	2.01	2.73	2.67	
	qVFM-PDM	1.95	4.43	3.02	2.67	
	qYN	1.95	9.23	3.22	2.67	
Corrected loss variance (dB^2)	qVFM-DSM	1.95	1.43	2.38	2.67	677 ± 46
	qVFM-PDM	1.95	2.79	2.69	2.67	163 ± 15
	qYN	1.95	3.17	2.72	2.67	229 ± 26

The corresponding true values are listed in the sixth column. Trial numbers needed to achieve 1 dB RMSE and 1 dB^2 within the corrected loss variance are listed with their SD in the last column.

The second is the HWCI of the posterior distributions of the estimated sensitivities. The 68.2% credible interval represents the range within which the actual value lies with 68.2% probability, representing an interval that contains the true value of the parameter in 68.2% of unlimited repetitions.

Global indices on the estimated VFMs were also adapted and calculated for each method, including mean defect, loss variance, short-term fluctuation and corrected loss variance (Flammer et al., 1985). These metrics are used in the clinic to quantify diffuse depression, local defects, and scatter observed during VFM tests as well as local inhomogeneity of visual field defects.

The mean defect (MD) of the estimated sensitivities across all 100 visual field locations after the i-th trial is calculated as:

$$\mathrm{MD}_i = \frac{\sum_k \sum_j \left(\tau_k^{true} - \tau_{\mathrm{ijk}}\right)}{J \times K}, \tag{6}$$

The loss variance (LV) is calculated as:

$$\mathrm{LV}_i = \frac{\sum_k \sum_j \left(\tau_{\mathrm{ijk}} - \tau_k^{true} + \mathrm{MD}_i\right)^2}{J \times (K-1)}. \tag{7}$$

The short-term fluctuation (SF) is calculated as:

$$\mathrm{SF}_i = \sqrt{\frac{\sum_k \sum_j \left(\tau_{ijk} - mean(\tau_{ijk})\right)^2}{(J-1) \times K}}. \tag{8}$$

The corrected loss variance (CLV) is calculated as:

$$CLV_i = \mathrm{LV}_i - \mathrm{SF}_i{}^2. \tag{9}$$

RESULTS

We present the simulation results for the scotoma, glaucoma, AMD, cataract, and normal observers in the following sections. **Figure 1** provides a summary of the major results.

Simulated Scotoma Observer

The estimated light sensitivity VFMs, the corresponding RMSE, standard deviation and average 68.2% HWCI for the simulated scotoma observer, obtained from the qVFM-PDM methods are shown in **Figure 2**, along with results from the qYN method. The corresponding results from the qVFM-DSM are shown in **Supplementary Figure A1**.

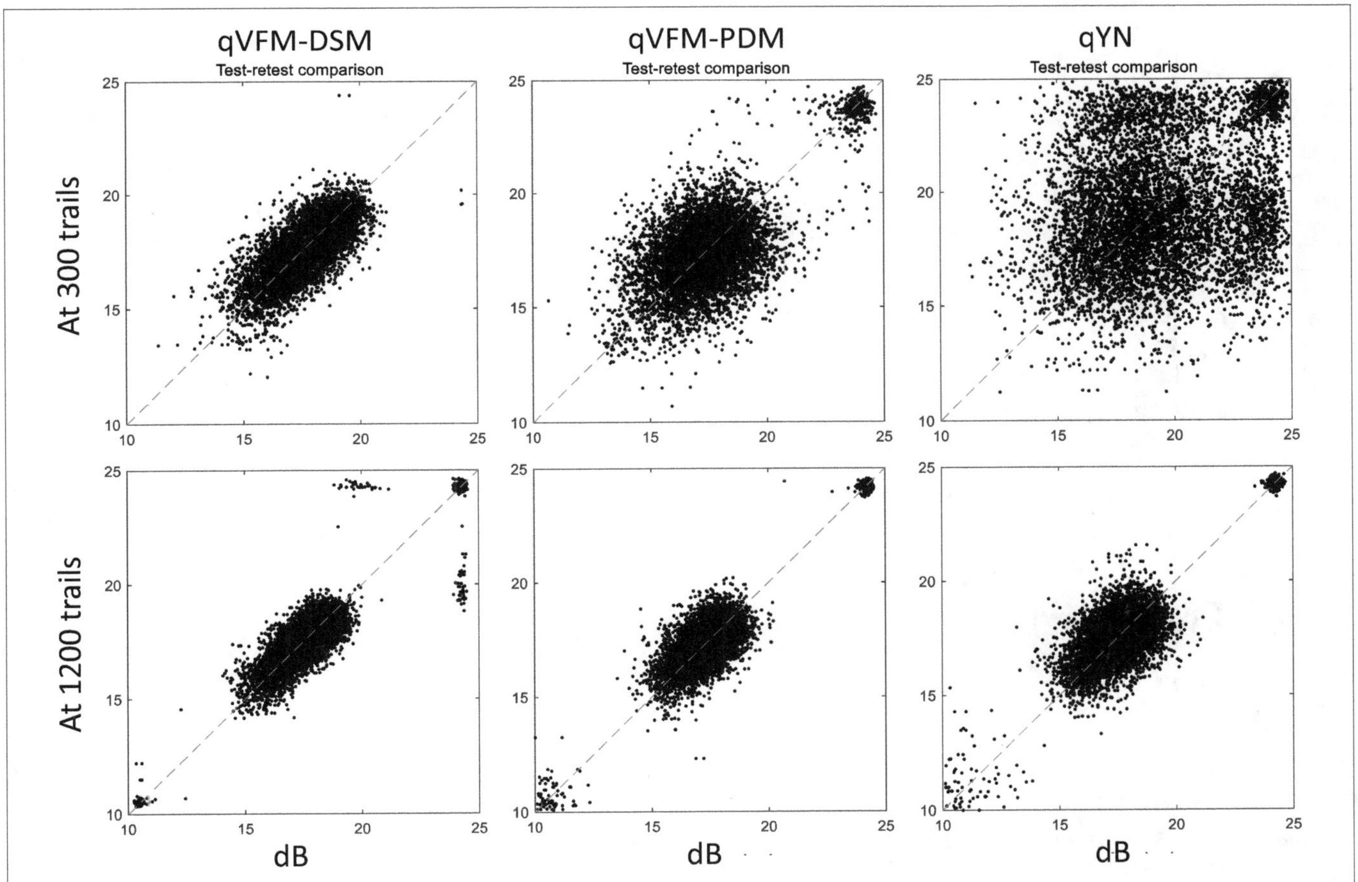

FIGURE 7 | Performance II of the three methods in estimating VFM of the simulated glaucoma observer. Test-retest comparison of the estimated light sensitivities from repeated 200 runs at 300 and 1,200 trials.

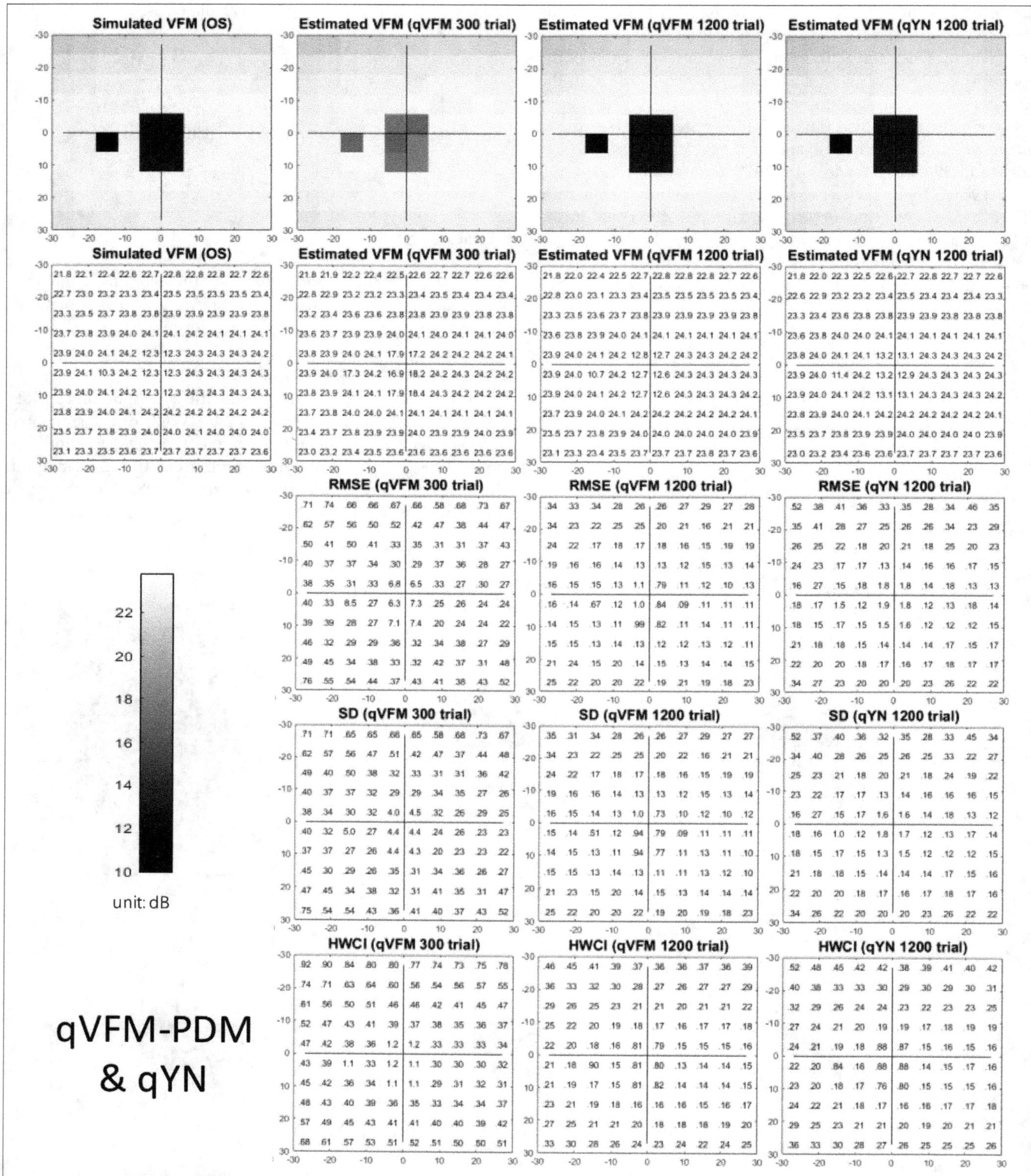

FIGURE 8 | Simulation results I of the AMD observer across 200 runs. The true VFM of the simulated observer (monocular) is presented in the first column of the first row with achromatic colormaps and second row with numerical values. The estimated VFMs obtained with the qVFM-PDM method after 300 trials and 1,200 trials, qYN method after 1,200 trials are presented in the first and second rows, respectively. The corresponding RMSE, SD, and 68.2% HWCI of the estimates are shown in the third, fourth, and fifth rows.

Compared with the simulated normal observer, the average light sensitivity deficit across the three scotoma locations is 12.0 dB for the simulated scotoma observer. Across the three scotoma locations, the average estimated deficits are 7.79 ± 5.70 dB and 11.9 ± 1.21 dB after 300 and 1,200 trials with the qVFM-DSM method, 6.53 ± 4.43 dB and 11.8 ± 0.86 dB after 300 and 1,200 trials with the qVFM-PDM method, and 11.3 ± 1.34 dB after 1,200 trials with the qYN method.

For the trial-by-trial performance, the RMSE, the average 68.2% HWCI, SD, the mean defect, the loss variance, the

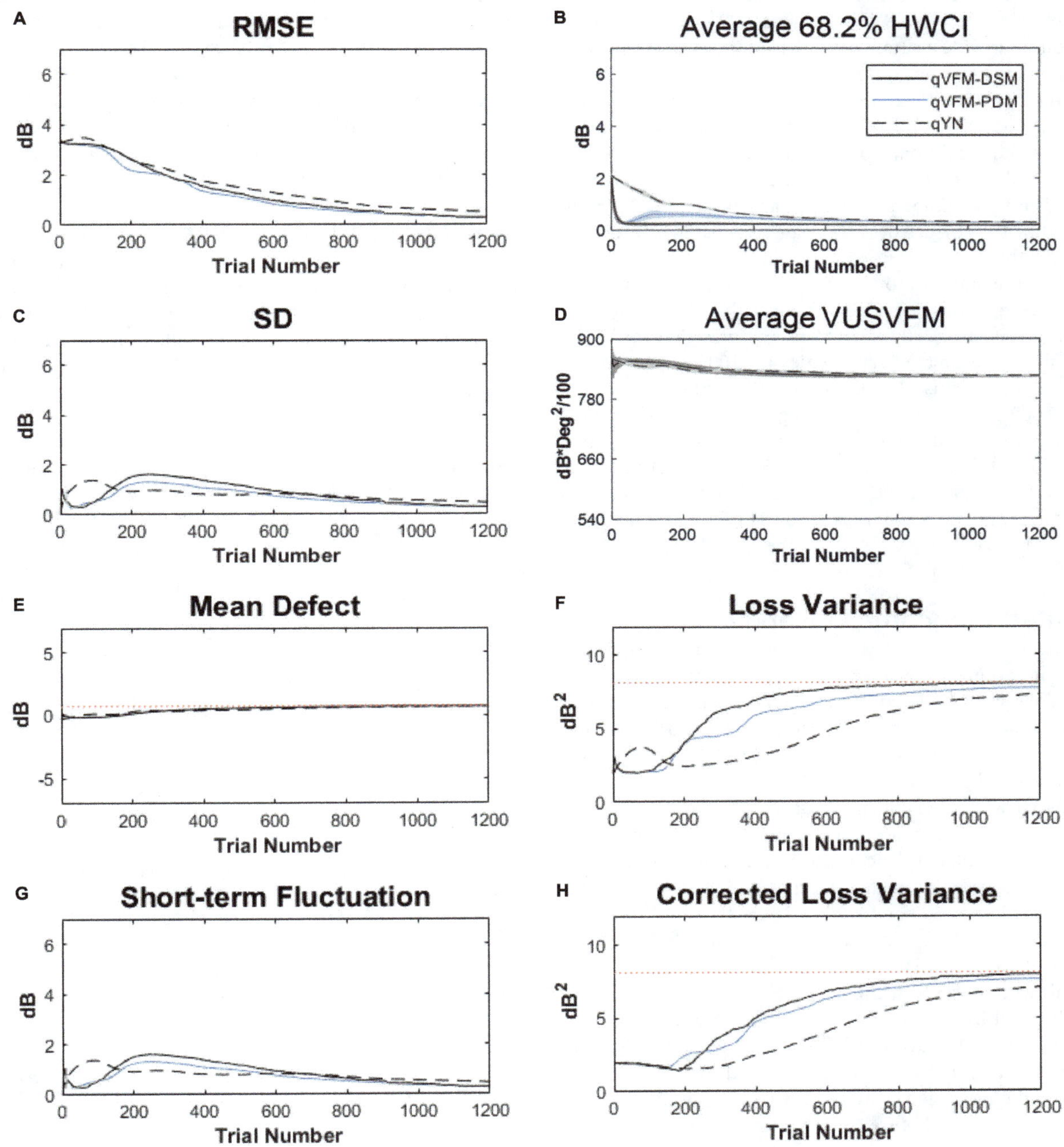

FIGURE 9 | Performance I of the three methods in estimating VFM of the simulated AMD observer across 200 runs. **(A)** Average root mean squared error, **(B)** Average 68.2% HWCI of the estimated VFM, **(C)** Average standard deviation, **(D)** Average volume under the surface of the VFM (VUSVFM), **(E)** Mean defect, **(F)** Short-term fluctuation, **(G)** Loss variance, and **(H)** Corrected loss variance. Results from the qVFM-DSM and qVFM-PDM methods are shown in solid black and blue lines, and results from the qYN method are shown in dashed lines. The true values of the global indices are shown in red dotted lines. For panels **(B,D)**, shaded regions represent ± 1 SD of the corresponding value.

short-term fluctuation and the corrected loss variance of the estimated light sensitivity VFM from the qVFM-DSM, qVFM-PDM, and qYN methods are shown in **Figures 3A–C,E–H**, with numerical results listed in **Table 2**.

In characterizing spatial vision, the area under the log contrast sensitivity function is often used as a summary metric (Applegate et al., 1998, 2000; Oshika et al., 1999, 2006; van Gaalen et al., 2009). In **Figure 3D**, we show the average volume under the surface of the VFM (VUSVFM) across 200 iterations of the simulation to provide a summary metric of the entire visual field for the simulated scotoma observer.

For the simulated scotoma observer, the results show that the qVFM-DSM and qVFM-PDM methods have similar performance. In addition, both the qVFM-DSM and qVFM-PDM methods demonstrate better efficiency than the qYN method. The trial numbers needed to achieve 1 dB RMSE and 1 dB^2 within the corrected loss variance are shown in the last column of **Table 2**.

For the simulated scotoma observer, test–retest reliabilities of the three methods are assessed through analysis of VFM estimates at 300 and 1,200 trials across 200 runs (**Figure 4**). Each subplot displays estimated sensitivities (at 100 VFM locations) of the 100 paired runs (100 locations × 100 random pairs of runs = 10,000 data points). The average test–retest correlations for the paired VFM estimates at 300 trials are 0.909 (SD = 0.002) for the qVFM-DSM, 0.842 (SD = 0.003) for the qVFM-PDM and 0.592 (SD = 0.008) for the qYN methods, respectively. The average correlations at 1,200 trials are 0.994 (SD = 0.0001) for the qVFM-DSM, 0.99 (SD = 0.0003) for the qVFM-PDM and 0.98 (SD = 0.0005) for the qYN methods, respectively.

Simulated Glaucoma Observer

The estimated light sensitivity VFMs, the corresponding RMSE, standard deviation and average 68.2% HWCI for the simulated glaucoma observer, obtained from the qVFM-PDM methods are shown in **Figure 5**, along with the results from the qYN method. The corresponding results from the qVFM-DSM are shown in **Supplementary Figure A2**.

Compared with the simulated normal observer, the average light sensitivity deficit across all glaucoma damaged locations is 6.28 dB for the simulated glaucoma observer. Across the damaged locations, the average estimated deficits are 5.99 ± 0.77 dB and 6.13 ± 0.51 dB after 300 and 1,200 trials with the qVFM-DSM method, 6.32 ± 1.24 dB and 6.28 ± 0.59 dB after 300 and 1,200 trials with the qVFM-PDM method, and 6.16 ± 0.73 dB after 1,200 trials with the qYN method.

For the trial-by-trial performance, the RMSE, the average 68.2% HWCI, SD, the average VUSVFM, the mean defect, the loss variance, the short-term fluctuation, and the corrected loss variance of the estimated light sensitivity VFM from the three methods are shown in **Figure 6**, with numerical results listed in **Table 3**.

For this simulated glaucoma observer, the qVFM-PDM method exhibited better performance than the qVFM-DSM method after 300 trials. The SD and short-term fluctuation of the estimated VFM obtained from the qVFM-PDM method are smaller, with the corrected loss variance approaching to the true value faster, compared with the qVFM-DSM method. Both qVFM methods demonstrated better efficiency than the qYN method. The trial numbers needed to achieve 1 dB RMSE and 1 dB^2 within the corrected loss variance are shown in **Table 3** for the three methods.

For the simulated glaucoma observer, test–retest reliabilities of the three methods are assessed through analysis of VFM estimates at 300 and 1,200 trials across 200 runs (**Figure 7**). The average test–retest correlations for the paired VFM estimates at 300 trials are 0.725 (SD = 0.006) for the qVFM-DSM, 0.694 (SD = 0.006) for the qVFM-PDM and 0.274 (SD = 0.01) for the qYN methods, respectively. The average correlations at 1,200 trials are 0.917 (SD = 0.002) for the qVFM-DSM, 0.917 (SD = 0.002) for the qVFM-PDM and 0.875 (SD = 0.003) for the qYN methods, respectively.

Simulated AMD Observer

The estimated light sensitivity VFMs, the corresponding RMSE, standard deviation and average 68.2% HWCI for the simulated AMD observer, obtained from the qVFM-PDM methods are shown in **Figure 8**, along with the results from the qYN method. The corresponding results from the qVFM-DSM are in shown in **Supplementary Figure A3**.

TABLE 4 | RMSE, SD, average 68.2% HWCI, mean defect, loss variance and corrected loss variance of the estimated VFM from the qVFM-DSM, qVFM-PDM and qYN methods in the beginning (0 trial), after 300 and 1,200 trials are listed for the simulated AMD observer.

AMD	Trial number	0	300	1,200	True value	1 dB/dB^2 threshold
RMSE (dB)	qVFM-DSM	3.26	1.98	0.30		591 ± 62
	qVFM-PDM	3.26	1.95	0.30		551 ± 18
	qYN	3.26	2.23	0.52		749 ± 28
SD (dB)	qVFM-DSM	0	1.55	0.30		
	qVFM-PDM	0	1.24	0.28		
	qYN	0	0.95	0.47		
HWCI (dB)	qVFM-DSM	2.12	0.24	0.19		
	qVFM-PDM	2.12	0.53	0.27		
	qYN	2.12	0.76	0.29		
Mean defect (dB)	qVFM-DSM	−0.26	0.40	0.71	0.72	
	qVFM-PDM	−0.26	0.40	0.71	0.72	
	qYN	−0.26	0.37	0.69	0.72	
Loss variance (dB^2)	qVFM-DSM	1.95	6.18	8.08	8.11	
	qVFM-PDM	1.95	4.50	7.71	8.11	
	qYN	1.95	2.65	7.32	8.11	
Corrected loss variance (dB^2)	qVFM-DSM	1.95	3.74	7.99	8.11	665 ± 66
	qVFM-PDM	1.95	2.93	7.63	8.11	822 ± 65
	qYN	1.95	1.74	7.10	8.11	1,198 ± 24

The corresponding true values are listed in the sixth column. Trial numbers needed to achieve 1 dB RMSE and 1 dB^2 within the corrected loss variance are listed with their SD in the last column.

Compared with the simulated normal observer, the average light sensitivity deficit across all AMD damaged VF locations is 12.0 dB for the simulated AMD observer. Across all the damaged locations, the average estimated deficits are 7.60 ± 5.69 dB and 11.8 ± 1.64 dB after 300 and 1,200 trials with the qVFM-DSM method, 6.52 ± 4.38 dB and 11.6 ± 0.87 dB after 300 and 1,200 trials with the qVFM-PDM method, and 11.2 ± 1.64 dB after 1,200 trials with qYN method.

For the trial-by-trial performance, the RMSE, the average 68.2% HWCI, SD, the average VUSVFM, the mean defect, the loss variance, the short-term fluctuation, and the corrected loss variance of the estimated VFM from the three methods are shown in **Figure 9**, with numerical values listed in **Table 4**.

For the simulated AMD observer, the results showed that the qVFM-DSM and qVFM-PDM methods have similar performance. Both qVFM-DSM and qVFM-PDM methods demonstrated better efficiency than the qYN method. The trial numbers needed to achieve 1 dB RMSE and 1 dB^2 within the corrected loss variance are shown in **Table 4** for the three methods.

For the simulated AMD observer, test–retest reliabilities of the three methods are assessed through analysis of VFM estimates at 300 and 1,200 trials across 200 runs (**Figure 10**). The average test–retest correlations for the paired VFM estimates at 300 trials are 0.868 (SD = 0.003) for the qVFM-DSM, 0.876 (SD = 0.003) for the qVFM-PDM and 0.585 (SD = 0.008) for the qYN method, respectively. The average correlations at 1,200 trials are 0.994 (SD = 0.0001) for the qVFM-DSM, 0.991 (SD = 0.0002) for the qVFM-PDM and 0.974 (SD = 0.001) for the qYN methods, respectively.

Simulated Cataract Observer

The estimated light sensitivity VFMs, the corresponding RMSE, standard deviation and average 68.2% HWCI for the simulated cataract observer, obtained from the qVFM-PDM methods are shown in **Figure 11**, along with the results from the qYN method. The corresponding results from the qVFM-DSM are shown in **Supplementary Figure 4**.

For the trial-by-trial performance, the RMSE, the average 68.2% HWCI, SD, the average VUSVFM, the mean defect, the loss variance, the short-term fluctuation, and the corrected loss variance of the estimated VFM from the three methods are shown in **Figure 12**, with some numerical values listed in **Table 5**.

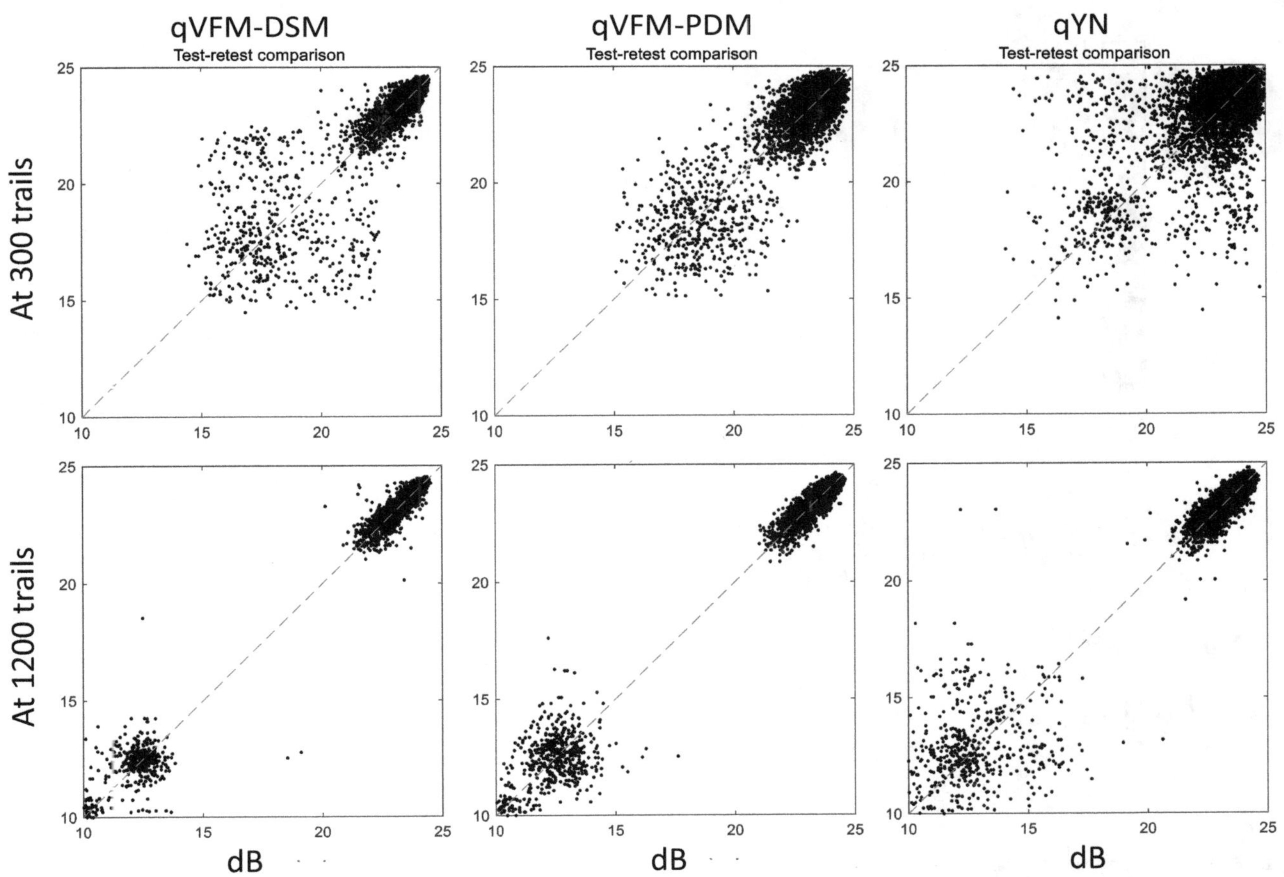

FIGURE 10 | Performance II of the qVFM-DSM, qVFM-PDM and qYN methods in estimating VFM of the simulated AMD observer. Test-retest comparison of the estimated light sensitivities from repeated 200 runs at 300 and 1,200 trials.

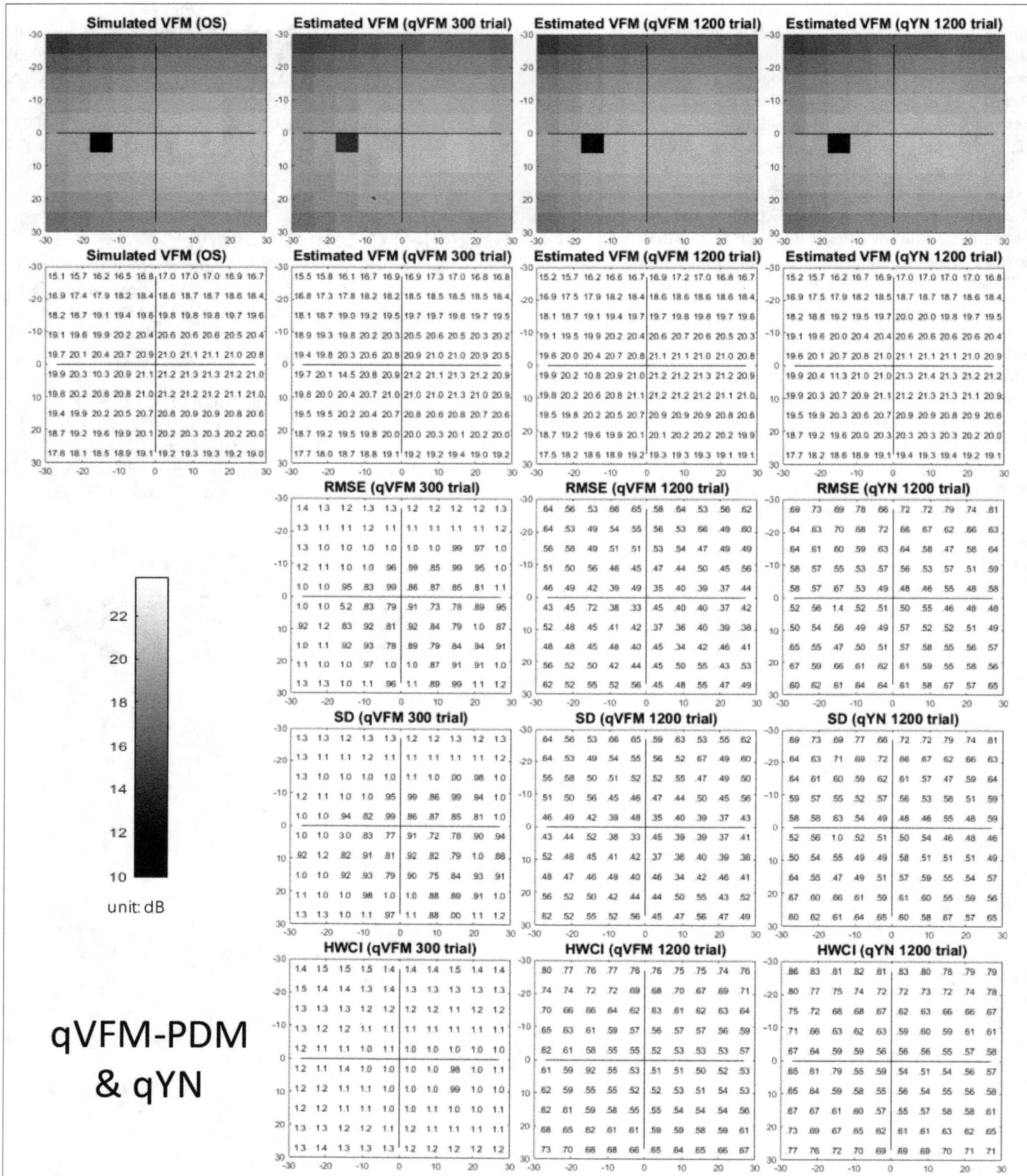

FIGURE 11 | Simulation results I of the cataract observer across 200 runs. The true VFM of the simulated observer (monocular) is presented in the first column of the first row with achromatic colormaps and second row with numerical values. The estimated VFMs obtained with the qVFM-PDM method after 300 trials and 1,200 trials, qYN method after 1,200 trials are presented in the first and second rows, respectively. The corresponding RMSE, SD, and 68.2% HWCI of the estimates are in the third, fourth, and fifth rows.

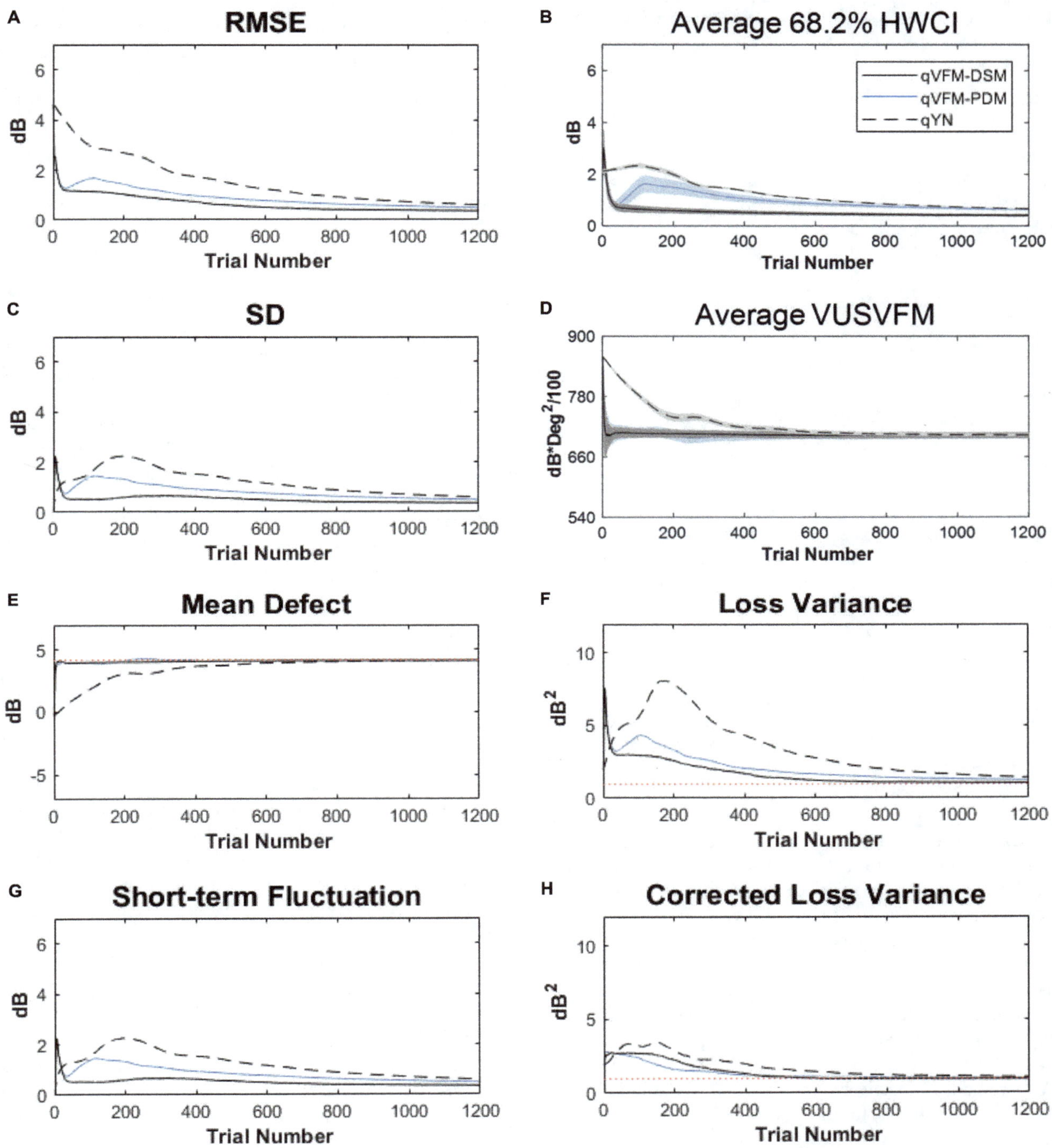

FIGURE 12 | Performance I of the three methods in estimating VFM of the simulated cataract observer across 200 runs. **(A)** Average root mean squared error, **(B)** Average 68.2% HWCI of the estimated VFM, **(C)** Average standard deviation, **(D)** Average volume under the surface of the VFM (VUSVFM), **(E)** Mean defect, **(F)** Short-term fluctuation, **(G)** Loss variance, and **(H)** Corrected loss variance. Results from the qVFM-DSM and qVFM-PDM methods are shown in solid black and blue lines, and results from the qYN method are shown in dashed lines. The true values of the global indices are shown in red dotted lines. For panels **(B,D)**, shaded regions represent ± 1 SD of the corresponding value.

For the simulated cataract observer, the results showed that the qVFM-DSM and qVFM-PDM methods had similar performance. The RMSE of the estimated VFM from qVFM-DSM method is lower than that from the qVFM-PDM method, while the SD and short-term fluctuation from the qVFM-PDM are smaller than those from the qVFM-DSM method. Both qVFM methods

TABLE 5 | RMSE, SD, average 68.2% HWCI, mean defect, loss variance and corrected loss variance of the estimated VFM from the qVFM-DSM, qVFM-PDM and qYN methods in the beginning (0 trial), after 300 and 1,200 trials are listed for the simulated cataract observer.

Cataract	Trial number	0	300	1,200	True value	1 dB/dB² threshold
RMSE (dB)	qVFM-DSM	4.63	0.85	0.37		212 ± 22
	qVFM-PDM	4.63	1.17	0.49		372 ± 27
	qYN	4.63	2.15	0.61		733 ± 29
SD (dB)	qVFM-DSM	0	0.65	0.36		
	qVFM-PDM	0	1.08	0.49		
	qYN	0	1.77	0.60		
HWCI (dB)	qVFM-DSM	2.12	0.55	0.40		
	qVFM-PDM	2.12	1.23	0.62		
	qYN	2.12	1.51	0.66		
Mean defect (dB)	qVFM-DSM	−0.26	4.04	4.12	4.16	
	qVFM-PDM	−0.26	4.20	4.18	4.16	
	qYN	−0.26	3.26	4.10	4.16	
Loss variance (dB²)	qVFM-DSM	1.95	2.04	1.07	0.98	
	qVFM-PDM	1.95	2.63	1.26	0.98	
	qYN	1.95	5.44	1.43	0.98	
Corrected loss variance (dB²)	qVFM-DSM	0	1.61	0.94	0.98	230 ± 24
	qVFM-PDM	0	1.45	1.01	0.98	142 ± 14
	qYN	0	2.27	1.07	0.98	401 ± 31

The corresponding true values are listed in the sixth column. Trial numbers needed to achieve 1 dB RMSE and 1 dB² within the corrected loss variance are listed with their SD in the last column.

demonstrated better efficiency than the qYN method. The trial numbers needed to achieve 1 dB RMSE and 1 dB² within the corrected loss variance are shown in **Table 5** for the three methods.

For the simulated cataract observer, test–retest reliabilities of the three methods are assessed through analysis of VFM estimates at 300 and 1,200 trials across 200 runs (**Figure 13**). The average test–retest correlations for the paired VFM estimates at 300 trials are 0.89 (SD = 0.002) for the qVFM-DSM, 0.667 (SD = 0.007) for the qVFM-PDM and 0.389 (SD = 0.01) for the qYN methods, respectively. The average correlations at 1,200 trials are 0.96 (SD = 0.001) for the qVFM-DSM, 0.92 (SD = 0.002) for the qVFM-PDM and 0.881 (SD = 0.003) for the qYN method, respectively.

Simulated Normal Observer

The estimated light sensitivity VFMs, the corresponding RMSE, standard deviation and average 68.2% HWCI for the simulated normal observer, obtained from the qVFM-PDM methods are shown in **Figure 14**, along with the results from the qYN method. The corresponding results from the qVFM-DSM are shown in **Supplementary Figure 5**.

The RMSE, the average 68.2% HWCI, SD, the average VUSVFM, the mean defect, the loss variance, the short-term fluctuation, and the corrected loss variance of the estimated light sensitivity VFM from the three methods are shown in **Supplementary Figure 6**, with some numerical values listed in **Table 6**.

For the simulated normal observer, the performance of the qVFM-DSM and qVFM-PDM methods is similar. The RMSE and loss variance of both qVFM-DSM and qVFM-PDM methods drop quickly below those of the qYN method from the beginning, while those of the qYN method exhibit fluctuations. The trial numbers, needed to achieve 1 dB RMSE and 1 dB² within the corrected loss variance, are shown in **Table 6** for the three methods.

For the simulated normal observer, test–retest reliabilities of the three methods are assessed through analysis of VFM estimates at 300 and 1,200 trials across 200 runs (**Supplementary Figure 7**). The average test–retest correlations for the paired VFM estimates at 300 trials are 0.901 (SD = 0.002) for the qVFM-DSM, 0.784 (SD = 0.005) for the qVFM-PDM and 0.507 (SD = 0.009) for the qYN methods, respectively. The average correlations at 1,200 trials are 0.99 (SD = 0.001) for the qVFM-DSM, 0.983 (SD = 0.0004) for the qVFM-PDM and 0.969 (SD = 0.001) for the qYN methods, respectively.

DISCUSSION

In this study, we tested the performance of the qVFM method with two different switch modules, the DSM and PDM, along with the qYN method, in estimating the light sensitivity VFM of simulated observers with peripheral scotoma, glaucoma, AMD, cataract and normal vision. The results show that, whereas all three methods could provide accurate and precise assessment of VFM deficits, the qVFM method with both switch modules were more efficient than the qYN method. The qVFM-DSM and qVFM-PDM methods exhibited comparable performance in most cases, but the qVFM-PDM method was better at detecting vision loss in the simulated glaucoma. The results demonstrated the potential of the qVFM method in clinical applications.

Comparison With Staircase-Based and SITA Algorithms

Most of the existing algorithms for static automated perimetry (SAP) are based on the staircase strategy (Weijland et al., 2004). In these algorithms, stimulus intensities are varied according to an up-and-down bracketing procedure in each location. The threshold values are estimated directly or scaled from the last seen stimulus intensity or the average of the last seen and unseen stimulus intensities in each location. In addition, the test procedures usually start from measuring thresholds at four primary points, one in each quadrant of the visual field, and followed by measurements of thresholds in the rest of the visual field with initial values based on the results at the primary points.

The conventional method with the Humphrey Field Analyzer is "Full Threshold," which is currently regarded as the standard technique in SAP. With initial stimulus intensity levels

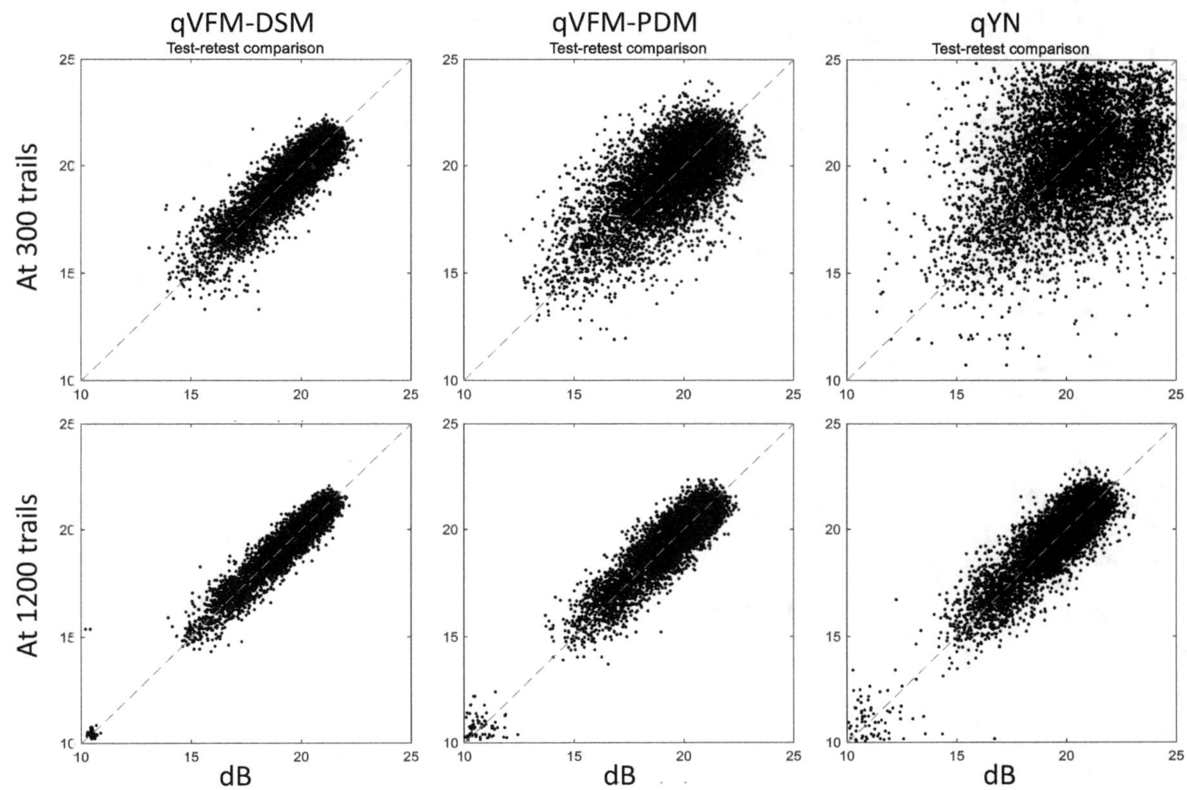

FIGURE 13 | Performance II of the qVFM-DSM, qVFM-PDM and qYN methods in estimating VFM of the simulated cataract observer. Test-retest comparison of the estimated light sensitivities from repeated 200 runs at 300 and 1,200 trials.

determined from a normative data set, the stimulus intensity at each test location is varied in steps of 4 dB until the first response reversal occurs and then subsequently varied in steps of 2 dB, referred as the 4-2 dB staircase procedure. The stimulus intensity of the last-seen presentation is taken as the final threshold estimate, after a second response reversal has occurred at a given location (Artes et al., 2002). The other conventional method implemented in OCTOPUS perimeters uses a 4-2-1 dB staircase procedure, which further reduces the step size to 1 dB after two reversals. The mean value of the dimmest stimulus seen and the brightest stimulus not seen is defined as the threshold (Morales et al., 2000).

In our previous study (Xu et al., 2019a), we compared the performance of the qVFM method and the staircase procedures, including both the 4-2 and 4-2-1 algorithms. The simulation results showed that, even with the initial stimulus intensity at each location matched with the true threshold of the simulated observer in staircase procedures, the staircase algorithms used in conventional SAP procedures still led to obvious biases and variabilities (**Figure 15**).

Another test algorithm, SITA (Swedish Interactive Thresholding Algorithm), can produce the same quality of test results as the Full Threshold strategy with considerable reduction of test time. However, it can only be used with the Goldmann III size stimulus of the Humphrey perimeter, and was only released for glaucomatous patients because it's *a priori* threshold distribution was based on glaucoma (Bengtsson and Heijl, 1998; Artes et al., 2002). In our previous study (Xu et al., 2019a), we compared the SITA family, including SITA standard, SITA Fast and SITA Faster, with the qVFM method. Although both the SITA and the qVFM methods are based on the Bayesian adaptive testing framework, the qVFM is quite different from the SITA:

(1) Stimulus selection in the SITA family follows the conventional up-down staircase algorithm in each location with the stepsize no smaller than 2 dB, and the test follows the "grown pattern" procedure across the visual field (Bengtsson et al., 1997). In the qVFM method, the stepsize in the stimulus space can be as small as 0.12 dB. Both the global and local modules use the one-step-ahead search strategy across the entire visual field to determine the optimal stimulus in the next trial that would lead to the minimum expected entropy, equivalent to maximizing information gain on the next trial. More precise stimulus intensity and location selection in the qVFM method potentially leads to more accurate threshold estimation.
(2) The frequency-of-seeing curves (FOS-curves, a YN psychometric function) in the SITA is not adjusted with the observer's decision criterion (Bengtsson et al., 1997).

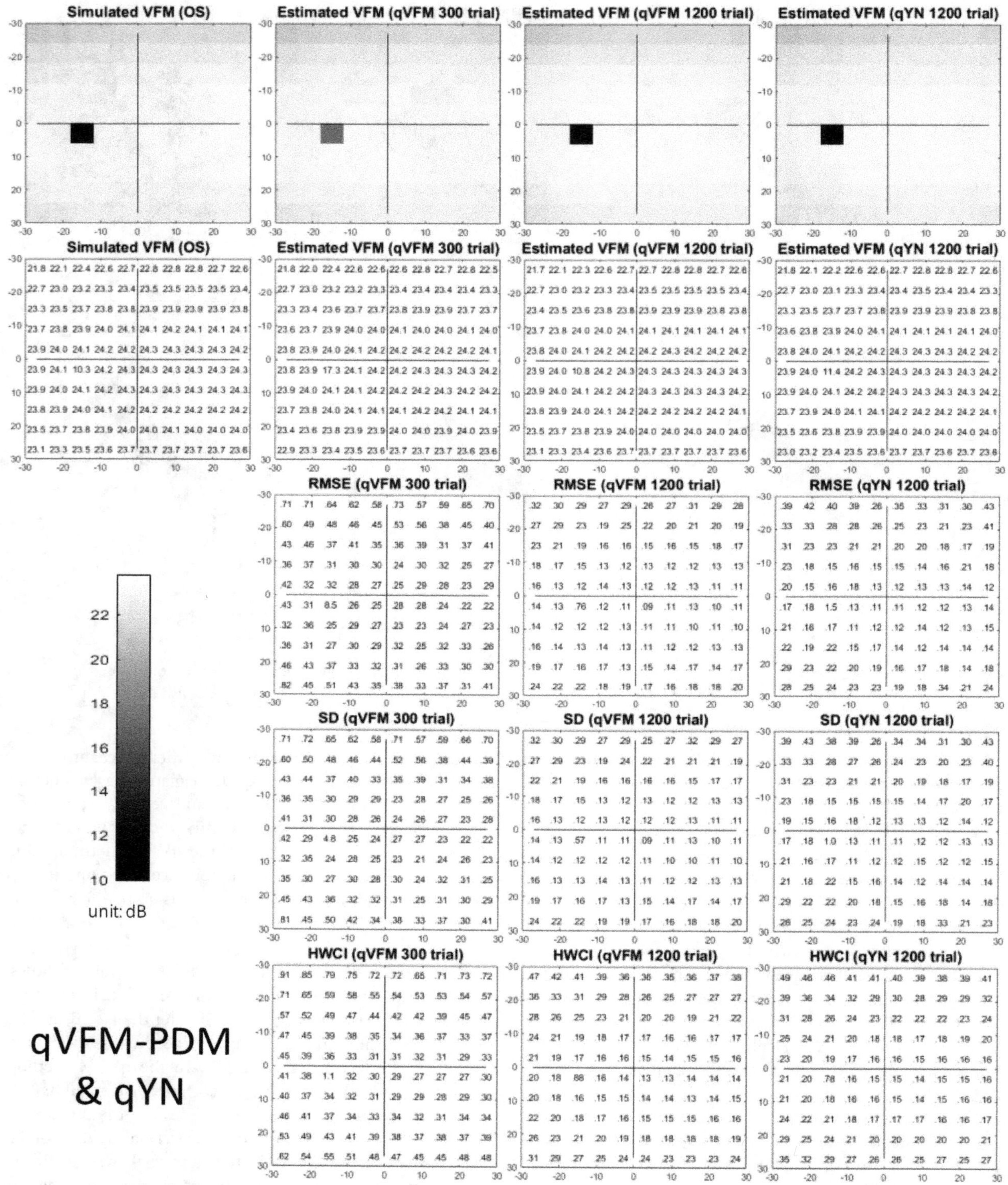

FIGURE 14 | Performance I of the qVFM-DSM, qVFM-PDM and qYN methods in estimating VFM of the simulated normal observer across 200 runs. **(A)** Average root mean squared error, **(B)** Average 68.2% HWCI of the estimated VFM, **(C)** Average standard deviation, **(D)** Average volume under the surface of the VFM (VUSVFM), **(E)** Mean defect, **(F)** Short-term fluctuation, **(G)** Loss variance, and **(H)** Corrected loss variance. Results from the qVFM-DSM and qVFM-PDM methods are shown in solid black and blue lines, and results from the qYN method are shown in dashed lines. The true values of the global indices are shown in red dotted lines. For panels **(B,D)**, shaded regions represent ± 1 SD of the corresponding value.

TABLE 6 | RMSE, SD, average 68.2% HWCI, mean defect, loss variance and corrected loss variance of the estimated VFM from the qVFM-DSM, qVFM-PDM and qYN methods in the beginning (0 trial), after 300 and 1,200 trials are listed for the simulated normal observer.

Normal	Trial number	0	300	1,200	True value	1 dB/dB^2 threshold
RMSE (dB)	qVFM-DSM	1.41	0.77	0.15		216 ± 28
	qVFM-PDM	1.41	0.94	0.19		267 ± 35
	qYN	1.41	1.16	0.27		353 ± 16
SD (dB)	qVFM-DSM	0	0.63	0.15		
	qVFM-PDM	0	0.62	0.18		
	qYN	0	0.75	0.24		
HWCI (dB)	qVFM-DSM	2.12	0.20	0.15		
	qVFM-PDM	2.12	0.45	0.22		
	qYN	2.12	0.70	0.24		
Mean defect (dB)	qVFM-DSM	−0.26	−0.05	0	0	
	qVFM-PDM	−0.26	0	0.01	0	
	qYN	−0.26	0.12	0.02	0	
Loss variance (dB^2)	qVFM-DSM	1.95	0.60	0.02	0	
	qVFM-PDM	1.95	0.89	0.04	0	
	qYN	1.95	1.35	0.07	0	
Corrected loss variance (dB^2)	qVFM-DSM	1.95	0.19	0	0	161 ± 19
	qVFM-PDM	1.95	0.50	0	0	164 ± 16
	qYN	1.95	0.79	0.01	0	248 ± 32

The corresponding true values are listed in the sixth column. Trial numbers needed to achieve 1 dB RMSE and 1 dB^2 within the corrected loss variance are listed with their SD in the last column.

Previous studies showed that the conventional YN threshold estimates exhibit approximately 25–50% more variability (i.e., standard deviation) than the criterion-free forced-choice threshold estimates (McKee et al., 1985; King-Smith et al., 1994). In this study, we implemented the qVFM method based on the qYN procedure, which combines elements of Signal Detection Theory (SDT) and Bayesian adaptive inference to concurrently estimate thresholds associated with a d' level (rather than a percent yes level) and decision criterion (Lesmes et al., 2015). Our study showed this method can deliver criterion-free thresholds on the light detection YN perimetric task with significant performance improvements.

(3) The prior distribution in the SITA is only optimized for normal and glaucoma observers, not for patients with other eye diseases (Bengtsson and Heijl, 1998). In the qVFM, the global module performs an individualized test that takes into account of the population properties in its prior but continues to optimize the test for each individual, including patients with abnormal VFMs. Because the method is completely systematic and not oriented toward any particular pathological pattern, the qVFM is not limited to a specific eye disease.

(4) Because locations with defective visual sensitivity tend to appear in clusters in glaucomatous visual fields, the prior threshold distribution in each test location in the SITA is calculated with inter-location correlations (Bengtsson et al., 1997). Such correlations may not be present in other eye diseases. In the qVFM, the local module is used to estimate visual threshold in each visual field location independently, making it possible to detect steep visual sensitivity changes in the visual field, such as scotoma resulting from optic neuropathies or visual field islands in retinitis pigmentosa.

(5) Since the age corrected normal and glaucomatous priors need enormous data collection to generate, the development of the SITA has so far been focused on light sensitivity maps with Goldmann III size stimulus for the 30-2, 24-2, 10-2 test patterns in the Humphrey Field Analyzer (Bengtsson et al., 1997; Phu et al., 2017). Whereas the test area in the SITA is limited to the central 30 degrees of the visual field with less than 76 test locations, the qVFM can map larger areas of the visual field with different type of stimulus and a flexible number of test locations, without restricts from prior knowledge as SITA.

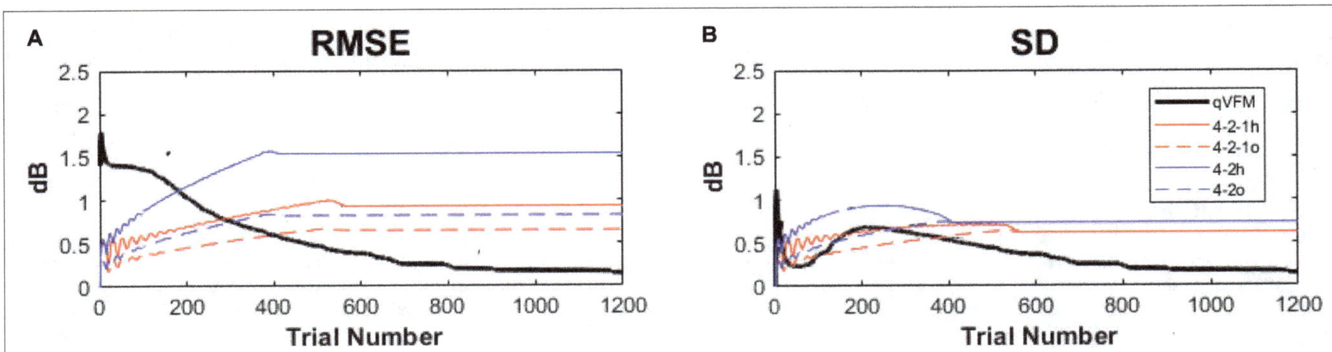

FIGURE 15 | Performance comparison between the qVFM method and staircase procedures in simulation tests across 1,000 runs. **(A)** Average root mean squared error, **(B)** Average standard deviation. Results from the qVFM are shown in black solid lines. Results from the staircase 4-2-1 algorithm of h and o methods are shown in red solid and dashed lines. Results from the staircase 4-2 algorithm of h and o methods are shown in blue solid and dashed lines. The h method uses the last seen stimulus intensity as the estimated threshold, the o method uses the average of the last seen and unseen stimulus intensities as the estimated threshold.

Alternative Methods for the Switch Module

In previous studies (Xu et al., 2018, 2019a,b, 2020), we generated the prior distributions in the local module by sampling the posterior from the global module using the qVFM-DSM method. The method was used to effectively transmit information obtained from the global module to the local module. However, it might generate priors that are too strong and hinder the detection of local VF deficits by the local module. In this study, we developed a new switch model, the qVFM-PDM mothed. It marginalizes the posterior distributions of the six parameters from the global module, and uses the average 68.2% HWCI of the estimated sensitivities and decision criterion across all VF locations to assign priors in the local module. By averaging estimated variabilities across all the VF locations to generate the prior distribution for each location in the local module, the qVFM-PDM is more robust and better enables the local module to detect local VF deficits. Our results showed that, although both the qVFM-DSM and qVFM-PDM methods performed well in estimating the VFM of the simulated observes, the qVFM-PDM method exhibited better performance in detecting VF loss in the simulated glaucoma in this study.

In these implementations, the rate of information gain in the global module was used to compute the switching point. Alternative methods could be used to determine the switching point, such as the relative amount of information gain from the global and local modules, a criterion based on the HWCI of the estimated VFM, or the convergence of parameters in the global module. Constrained by the amount of computation required to maintain and update the various probability distributions in both the global and local modules, we only performed a one-way switch from the global module to the local module in the current study. With additional computing power or better algorithms, we might be able to switch between the two modules multiple times if necessary.

Paths for Potential Extension

In this study, we took a very conservative approach in setting the prior for all the simulated observers. The prior was in fact mis-informative for the simulated observers with peripheral scotoma, glaucoma, AMD, and cataract. As a result, the qVFM method exhibited worse performance in the beginning of the estimating process. A hierarchical Bayes extension of qVFM could be developed to provide a judicious way to derive informative priors for different patient populations (Kim et al., 2014; Gu et al., 2016): An incoming patient is assigned to some possible disease categories, each with its own prior distributions. The hierarchical qVFM would update both category probabilities and the distribution of the VFM parameters during the test, and update the prior of each disease category after testing each patient. Alternatively, or jointly within the hierarchical framework, the prior in the qVFM could be informed by knowledge obtained from each patient's pervious diagnoses.

The qVFM method provides a general framework for mapping many other visual functions, such as visual acuity, CSF, color, stereo vision, reading speed, motion sensitivity, temporary sensitivity, and crowding. Once developed, measurements of the multiple VFMs would allow us to analyze and model the relationships among multiple visual functions as well as performance in everyday visual tasks, and identify the core metrics of functional vision deficits in patients with eye disease.

The broad adoption of the qVFM method would also require development of less expensive and integrated devices. Given the current development of cost-effective eye trackers and rapid improvement of consumer technology, we are optimistic that this could be accomplished in the near future.

CONCLUSION

In this study, we showed that the qVFM method can be used to characterize residual vision of simulated ophthalmic patients. It sets the stage for further investigation with real patients. We anticipate that the qVFM method, with additional tests on real patients, can be potentially translated into clinical practice in the future.

AUTHOR CONTRIBUTIONS

Z-LL, PX, LL, and DY designed the qVFM algorithms. PX performed simulations and analyzed the data. PX and Z-LL wrote the manuscript with input from all authors. Z-LL and DY supervised the project. All authors contributed to the article and approved the submitted version.

REFERENCES

Anderson, A. J., Johnson, C. A., and Werner, J. S. (2011). Measuring visual function in AMD with frequency-doubling (Matrix) perimetry. *Optom. Vis. Sci.* 88, 806–815. doi: 10.1097/opx.0b013e31821861bd

Applegate, R. A., Hilmantel, G., Howland, H. C., Tu, E. Y., Starck, T., and Zayac, E. J. (2000). Corneal first surface optical aberrations and visual performance. *J. Refract. Surg.* 16, 507–514. doi: 10.3928/1081-597x-20000901-04

Applegate, R. A., Howland, H. C., Sharp, R. P., Cottingham, A. J., and Yee, R. W. (1998). Corneal aberrations and visual performance after radial keratotomy. *J. Refract. Surg.* 14, 397–407. doi: 10.3928/1081-597x-19980701-05

Artes, P. H., Iwase, A., Ohno, Y., Kitazawa, Y., and Chauhan, B. C. (2002). Properties of perimetric threshold estimates from full threshold, SITA standard, and SITA fast strategies. *Invest. Ophthalmol. Vis. Sci.* 43, 2654–2659.

Aulhorn, E., and Harms, H. (1972). "Visual perimetry," in *Visual Psychophysics Handbook of Sensory Physiology*, eds M. Alpern, E. Aulhorn, H. B. Barlow, E. Baumgardt, H. R. Blackwell, D. S. Blough, et al. (Berlin: Springer Berlin Heidelberg), 102–145. doi: 10.1007/978-3-642-88658-4_5

Bachman, D. M., Bruni, L. M., DiGioia, R. A., Harris, P. J., McMackin, C. M., Pistole, M. C., et al. (1992). Visual field testing in the management of cytomegalovirus retinitis. *Ophthalmology* 99, 1393–1399. doi: 10.1016/s0161-6420(92)31803-2

Bengtsson, B., and Heijl, A. (1998). Evaluation of a new perimetric threshold strategy, SITA, in patients with manifest and suspect glaucoma. *Acta Ophthalmol.* 76, 268–272. doi: 10.1034/j.1600-0420.1998.760303.x

Bengtsson, B., Olsson, J., Heijl, A., and Rootzén, H. (1997). A new generation of algorithms for computerized threshold perimetry, SITA. *Acta Ophthalmol. Scand.* 75, 368–375. doi: 10.1111/j.1600-0420.1997.tb00392.x

Caprioli, J. (1991). Automated perimetry in glaucoma. *Am. J. Ophthalmol.* 111, 235–239.

Fendrich, R., Wessinger, C. M., and Gazzaniga, M. S. (1992). Residual vision in a scotoma: implications for blindsight. *Science* 258, 1489–1491. doi: 10.1126/science.1439839

Flammer, J., Drance, S. M., Augustiny, L., and Funkhouser, A. (1985). Quantification of glaucomatous visual field defects with automated perimetry. *Invest. Ophthalmol. Vis. Sci.* 26, 176–181.

Goldmann, H. (1945a). Ein selbstregistrierendes Projektionskugelperimeter. *Ophthalmologica* 109, 71–79. doi: 10.1159/000300225

Goldmann, H. (1945b). Grundlagen exakter perimetrie. *Ophthalmologica* 109, 57–70. doi: 10.1159/000300224

Gu, H., Kim, W., Hou, F., Lesmes, L. A., Pitt, M. A., Lu, Z.-L., et al. (2016). A hierarchical Bayesian approach to adaptive vision testing: a case study with the contrast sensitivity function. *J. Vis.* 16:15. doi: 10.1167/16.6.15

Harms, H. (1952). Die praktische Bedeutung quantitativer perimetrie. *Klin. Monbl. Augenheilkd. Augenarztl. Fortbild.* 121, 683–692.

Heijl, A., Lindgren, A., and Lindgren, G. (1989). Test-retest variability in glaucomatous visual fields. *Am. J. Ophthalmol.* 108, 130–135. doi: 10.1016/0002-9394(89)90006-8

Iannaccone, A., Rispoli, E., Vingolo, E. M., Onori, P., Steindl, K., Rispoli, D., et al. (1995). Correlation between Goldmann perimetry and maximal electroretinogram response in retinitis pigmentosa. *Doc. Ophthalmol.* 90, 129–142. doi: 10.1007/bf01203333

Jacobson, S. G., Voigt, W. J., Parel, J.-M., Apathy, P. P., Nghiem-Phu, L., Myers, S. W., et al. (1986). Automated light-and dark-adapted perimetry for evaluating retinitis pigmentosa. *Ophthalmology* 93, 1604–1611. doi: 10.1016/s0161-6420(86)33522-x

Kim, W., Pitt, M. A., Lu, Z.-L., Steyvers, M., and Myung, J. I. (2014). A hierarchical adaptive approach to optimal experimental design. *Neural Comput.* 26, 2465–2492. doi: 10.1162/NECO_a_00654

King-Smith, P. E., Grigsby, S. S., Vingrys, A. J., Benes, S. C., and Supowit, A. (1994). Efficient and unbiased modifications of the QUEST threshold method: theory, simulations, experimental evaluation and practical implementation. *Vis. Res.* 34, 885–912. doi: 10.1016/0042-6989(94)90039-6

King-Smith, P. E., and Rose, D. (1997). Principles of an adaptive method for measuring the slope of the psychometric function. *Vis. Res.* 37, 1595–1604. doi: 10.1016/s0042-6989(96)00310-0

Kontsevich, L. L., and Tyler, C. W. (1999). Bayesian adaptive estimation of psychometric slope and threshold. *Vis. Res.* 39, 2729–2737. doi: 10.1016/s0042-6989(98)00285-5

Lachenmayr, B. J., Kojetinsky, S., Ostermaier, N., Angstwurm, K., Vivell, P. M., and Schaumberger, M. (1994). The different effects of aging on normal sensitivity in flicker and light-sense perimetry. *Invest. Ophthalmol. Vis. Sci.* 35, 2741–2748.

Lam, B. L., Alward, W. L., and Kolder, H. E. (1991). Effect of cataract on automated perimetry. *Ophthalmology* 98, 1066–1070. doi: 10.1016/s0161-6420(91)32175-4

Lesmes, L. A., Jeon, S.-T., Lu, Z.-L., and Dosher, B. A. (2006). Bayesian adaptive estimation of threshold versus contrast external noise functions: the quick TvC method. *Vis. Res.* 46, 3160–3176. doi: 10.1016/j.visres.2006.04.022

Lesmes, L. A., Lu, Z.-L., Baek, J., and Albright, T. D. (2010). Bayesian adaptive estimation of the contrast sensitivity function: the quick CSF method. *J. Vis.* 10:17.

Lesmes, L. A., Lu, Z.-L., Baek, J., Tran, N., Dosher, B. A., and Albright, T. D. (2015). Developing Bayesian adaptive methods for estimating sensitivity thresholds (d') in Yes-No and forced-choice tasks. *Front. Psychol.* 6:1070. doi: 10.3389/fpsyg.2015.01070

Luu, C. D., Dimitrov, P. N., Wu, Z., Ayton, L. N., Makeyeva, G., Aung, K.-Z., et al. (2013). Static and flicker perimetry in age-related macular degeneration. *Invest. Ophthalmol. Vis. Sci.* 54, 3560–3568.

McKee, S. P., Klein, S. A., and Teller, D. Y. (1985). Statistical properties of forced-choice psychometric functions: implications of probit analysis. *Percept. Psychophys.* 37, 286–298. doi: 10.3758/bf03211350

Milner, D., and Goodale, M. (2006). *The Visual Brain in Action*. Oxford: OUP.

Morales, J., Weitzman, M. L., and González de la Rosa, M. (2000). Comparison between tendency-oriented perimetry (TOP) and octopus threshold perimetry. *Ophthalmology* 107, 134–142. doi: 10.1016/S0161-6420(99)00026-3

Ng, M., Sample, P. A., Pascual, J. P., Zangwill, L. M., Girkin, C. A., Liebmann, J. M., et al. (2012). Comparison of visual field severity classification systems for glaucoma. *J. Glaucoma* 21, 551–561. doi: 10.1097/ijg.0b013e31821dac66

Oshika, T., Klyce, S. D., Applegate, R. A., and Howland, H. C. (1999). Changes in corneal wavefront aberrations with aging. *Invest. Ophthalmol. Vis. Sci.* 40, 1351–1355.

Oshika, T., Okamoto, C., Samejima, T., Tokunaga, T., and Miyata, K. (2006). Contrast sensitivity function and ocular higher-order wavefront aberrations in normal human eyes. *Ophthalmology* 113, 1807–1812. doi: 10.1016/j.ophtha.2006.03.061

Papageorgiou, E., Hardiess, G., Schaeffel, F., Wiethoelter, H., Karnath, H.-O., Mallot, H., et al. (2007). Assessment of vision-related quality of life in patients with homonymous visual field defects. *Graefes Arch. Clin. Exp. Ophthalmol.* 245, 1749–1758. doi: 10.1007/s00417-007-0644-z

Phu, J., Khuu, S. K., Zangerl, B., and Kalloniatis, M. (2017). A comparison of Goldmann III, V and spatially equated test stimuli in visual field testing: the importance of complete and partial spatial summation. *Ophthalmic Physiol. Opt.* 37, 160–176. doi: 10.1111/opo.12355

Portney, G. L., and Krohn, M. A. (1978). The limitations of kinetic perimetry in early scotoma detection. *Ophthalmology* 85, 287–293. doi: 10.1016/s0161-6420(78)35666-9

Radius, R. L. (1978). Perimetry in cataract patients. *Arch. Ophthalmol.* 96, 1574–1579. doi: 10.1001/archopht.1978.03910060208004

Rogers, T. J., and Landers, D. M. (2005). Mediating effects of peripheral vision in the life event stress/athletic injury relationship. *J. Sport Exerc. Psychol.* 27, 271–288. doi: 10.1123/jsep.27.3.271

Smith, S. D., Katz, J., and Quigley, H. A. (1996). Analysis of progressive change in automated visual fields in glaucoma. *Invest. Ophthalmol. Vis. Sci.* 37, 1419–1428.

Strasburger, H., Rentschler, I., and Jüttner, M. (2011). Peripheral vision and pattern recognition: a review. *J. Vis.* 11:13. doi: 10.1167/11.5.13

Thorne, J. E., Van Natta, M. L., Jabs, D. A., Duncan, J. L., Srivastava, S. K., and Studies of Ocular Complications of Aids Research Group (2011). Visual field loss in patients with cytomegalovirus retinitis. *Ophthalmology* 118, 895–901. doi: 10.1016/j.ophtha.2010.09.017

Townend, B. S., Sturm, J. W., Petsoglou, C., O'Leary, B., Whyte, S., and Crimmins, D. (2007). Perimetric homonymous visual field loss post-stroke. *J. Clin. Neurosci.* 14, 754–756. doi: 10.1016/j.jocn.2006.02.022

van Gaalen, K. W., Jansonius, N. M., Koopmans, S. A., Terwee, T., and Kooijman, A. C. (2009). Relationship between contrast sensitivity and spherical aberration: comparison of 7 contrast sensitivity tests with natural and artificial pupils in healthy eyes. *J. Cataract Refract. Surg.* 35, 47–56. doi: 10.1016/j.jcrs.2008.09.016

Weijland, A., Fankhauser, F., Bebie, H., and Flammer, J. (2004). *Automated Perimetry: Visual Field Digest*. Köniz, Switzerland: Haag-Streit AG.

Xu, P., Lesmes, L. A., Yu, D., and Lu, Z.-L. (2018). A novel Bayesian adaptive method for mapping the visual field. *Invest. Ophthalmol. Vis. Sci.* 59, 1266–1266.

Xu, P., Lesmes, L. A., Yu, D., and Lu, Z.-L. (2019a). A novel Bayesian adaptive method for mapping the visual field. *J. Vis.* 19:16. doi: 10.1167/19.14.16

Xu, P., Lesmes, L. A., Yu, D., and Lu, Z.-L. (2019b). Mapping contrast sensitivity of visual field with Bayesian adaptive qVFM method. *Invest. Ophthalmol. Vis. Sci.* 60:4377.

Xu, P., Lesmes, L. A., Yu, D., and Lu, Z.-L. (2020). Mapping the contrast sensitivity of the visual field with bayesian adaptive qVFM. *Front. Neurosci.* 14:665. doi: 10.3389/fnins.2020.00665

18

Decline of Orientation and Direction Sensitivity in the Aging Population

*Lin Xia[1,2], He Chen[3], Jiong Dong[1,2], Sha Luo[1,2] and Lixia Feng[1,2]**

[1] Department of Ophthalmology, First Affiliated Hospital of Anhui Medical University, Hefei, China, [2] Anhui Branch of National Clinical Research Center for Ocular Diseases, Hefei, China, [3] Hefei National Laboratory for Physical Sciences at Microscale, School of Life Sciences, University of Science and Technology of China, Hefei, China

Correspondence:
Lixia Feng
lixiafeng@163.com

While the aging population is growing, our knowledge regarding age-related deterioration of visual perception remains limited. In the present study, we investigated the effects of aging on orientation and direction sensitivity in a healthy population using a weighted up–down adaptive method to improve the efficiency and reliability of the task. A total of 57 healthy participants aged 22–72 years were included and divided into old and young groups. Raw experimental data were processed using a psychometric method to determine the differences between the two groups. In the orientation task, the threshold of the discrimination angle and bias (i.e., the difference between the perceived midpoint from the logistic function and the reference point) was increased, while the lapsing rate (i.e., 1 − the maximum logistic function) did not significantly change in the old group compared with the young group. In the motion direction task, the threshold, bias, and lapsing rate were significantly increased in the old group compared with the young group. These results suggest that the decreased ability of old participants in discrimination of stimulus orientation and motion direction could be related to the impaired function of visual cortex.

Keywords: vision, orientation, motion direction, aging, perception deficits, psychometric function

INTRODUCTION

Vision and other sensory organs deteriorate with aging, thereby decreasing the quality of life of the aging population (Andersen, 2012). Due to ocular changes, lens opacification and reduced ocular size limit light transmittance and increase scattering (van de Kraats and van Norren, 2007; Petrash, 2013; Guillon et al., 2016), resulting in impaired quality of light projected to the retina (Weale, 1988; IJspeert et al., 1990). However, decreased optical quality does not account for all aging-associated changes in the visual sensory system; microstructural changes and aging central nervous system also play a role in visual sensory dysfunction. For example, certain photoreceptor and retina ganglion cells are lost during aging (Panda-Jonas et al., 1995; Harman et al., 2000; Jackson et al., 2002), while cognitive aging influences age-related vision dysfunction (Bennett et al., 1999; Hedden and Gabrieli, 2005; Loerch et al., 2008), and contrast sensitivity and spatial learning are affected by aging (Faubert, 2002; Betts et al., 2007; Yamamoto and Degirolamo, 2012).

Visual information from the binocular retina is transmitted to the primary visual cortex, responsible for visual perception of objects' movement, size, and color, which is located in the occipital lobe. The visual information stream is then transmitted to other cortex for stereopsis, depth perception, and other advanced visual function. Neurons in the primary visual cortex are responsible for orientation, while middle temporal (MT) functions for motion direction of objects (Gold and Ding, 2013; Patten et al., 2017).

During psychometric tasks, choosing between two alternative forced choices is a common method for vision quantification, where participants rely on a neural decoding process to select an option (Gold and Ding, 2013). During the judgment process of the orientation or motion direction, neurons in the visual cortex responsible for the same orientation are activated, while those responsible for the opposite orientation are suppressed (Wang, 2008; Gold and Ding, 2013). The cortex integrates different types of neuronal signals and produces a decision only when the integral signal reaches a threshold. Hence, reduced neuronal inhibition contributes to false selections in orientation and motion direction discrimination tasks, which are thought to be a marker of aging. However, most previous alternative forced-choice psychophysics tasks are coarse with two opposite directions of motion (Snowden and Kavanagh, 2006; Allen et al., 2010), while fine tasks that require participants to discriminate between two similar directions of motion are rare (Ball and Sekuler, 1986; Pilz et al., 2017).

Although previous studies have shown that orientation sensitivity decreases with age in human and macaque monkeys (Schmolesky et al., 2000; Betts et al., 2007; Govenlock et al., 2009; McKendrick et al., 2018), the perceptual orientation tuning curve did not significantly change in aged participants when using a sine-wave raster in various orientations, despite significant differences in the contrast sensitivity between the young and aged groups were observed (Delahunt et al., 2008). To date, the effects of aging on the visual sensory system remain unclear.

In this study, we used MATLAB software to create two different types of new tasks to determine the visual sensory ability, including orientation and motion direction discrimination, during aging. In both tasks, the discrimination threshold, bias of the perceived midpoint, and lapsing rate in participants of different ages were recorded and calculated based on a previous method (Tzvetanov, 2012). For the orientation tasks, we measured discrimination ability using Gabor patches placed at different angles, while for motion direction tasks, we measured discrimination capacity using several random dots moving in different directions. Our new tasks are suitable for a broader age range and could be used to determine potential visual perception alterations in aging (Casco et al., 2017; Pilz et al., 2017).

MATERIALS AND METHODS

Participants

A total of 57 healthy adults aged 22–72 years were recruited through annual physical examinations and were divided into two groups: young [n = 28, age (mean ± SEM): 29.04 ± 1.40 years] and old (n = 28, age: 57.29 ± 1.08 years) groups. All participants underwent a complete binocular health examination by an experienced ophthalmologist for visual diseases, such as strabismus, amblyopia, cataract, and macular degeneration. Participants' binocular best-corrected visual acuity was not greater than 0.2 logMAR, and all had participated with their best-corrected visual acuity. Participants with the following conditions were excluded: strabismus, anisometropia, diabetes mellitus, history of eye pathology or operations, or central system diseases. All participants were instructed and trained on similar tasks to familiarize themselves with the tasks and the definition of left and right of stimuli before formal testing. This study was approved by the local ethics committee.

Stimulus

All participants were tested in a dark room, where the screen was the only light source. A 21-inch CRT monitor (Sony Corporation, Japan) was used as the displayer for all tasks, which has 1,024 × 768 pixel resolution with an 85-Hz refresh rate. The environment was silent and tidy, with only a participant and a researcher in the room. The monitor screen was turned on 30 min before the tasks for stabilization. The screen luminance was calibrated to control display contrast. Stimuli were generated using MATLAB Version R2016a with the Psychophysics toolbox (Brainard, 1997; Pelli, 1997). A chin forehead rest was used to stabilize the eyes at 1,500 mm in front of the screen.

In the orientation discrimination task, a Gabor patch was produced, which illustrated a circular sine-wave raster without background noise and had a gradual Gaussian blur edge. The frequency and contrast of Gabor patches were constant, while the spatial frequency of the Gabor patch was 3 cyc/deg. The Gabor patch was presented at different angles relative to the vertical axis for 150 ms in each trial. Representative stimuli are shown in **Figures 1A,B**. In the motion direction discrimination task, 80 random dots were randomly allocated to the center circle area of the displayer. All the dots moved in the same direction inside the circle. If a dot moved out of the circle, it disappeared and reappeared at the opposite edge of the circle to continue moving. The dots were presented for 200 ms in each trial. The representative stimulus is shown in **Figures 1C,D**.

Procedure

During the experiment, the participants completed an orientation discrimination task and a motion direction discrimination task independently. All responses were inputted using a standard keyboard. In each trial, participants were asked to stare at the center of the black dot/red square of the screen binocularly and to press the space button to present the stimulus and the left/right button to submit responses. For the orientation task, participants were required to indicate the orientation of the static Gabor patch (counterclockwise deviation versus clockwise deviation from the vertical). For the motion direction task, participants were required to indicate the direction of the moving dots (counterclockwise deviation versus clockwise deviation from the upward). There were 100 trials in the orientation task and 80 in the motion direction task. The repeating procedure is illustrated in **Figure 2**.

The psychophysical task measurements were performed using a weighted up–down adaptive method to improve the efficiency and reliability of the task (Treutwein and Strasburger, 1999). The orientation task included two staircases that started from -21° and +21°, respectively. The presented stimuli were alternately

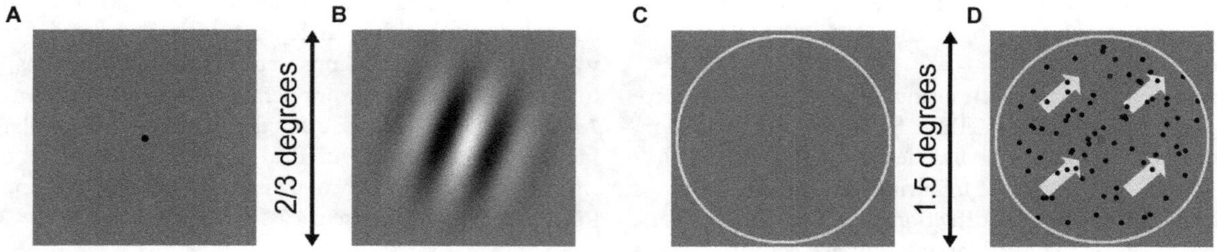

FIGURE 1 | Example stimuli for orientation and motion direction tasks. **(A)** The fixation dot for orientation was presented at first while waiting for the participants to prepare. **(B)** When participants pressed the space button, the fixation dot disappeared, and the Gabor patches were presented for 150 ms. The spatial frequency of the Gabor patch was 3 cyc/deg and filtered with a gradual Gaussian blur from the center to the edge and a circle mask. The visual angle of the Gabor patch was 2/3° when participants sit 1,500 mm in front of the screen. **(C)** The fixation square and circle for motion direction were presented at first while waiting for the participants to prepare. **(D)** When the participants pressed the space button, the moving dots moved in the same direction for 200 ms. The visual angle of the white circle was 1.5° for the participants when 1,500 mm in front of the screen.

from the staircases. The two staircases were assigned up/down steps of 5/2° and 2/5°, with convergence points of 71.43 and 28.57%, respectively. In both staircases, the next stimulus would increase the number of steps if the current answer were correct, and *vice versa*. Each staircase consisted of 50 trials. Representative psychometric curves are shown in **Figures 4A,B**. The motion direction task also included two staircases that started at -15° and +15°, respectively. The presented stimuli were from the staircases alternately. The two staircases were assigned up/down steps of 3/1° and 1/3°, with convergence points of 75 and 25%, respectively. Each staircase consisted of 40 trials. Representative psychometric curves are shown in **Figures 6A,B**. No feedback on the answer correctness was provided to the participants.

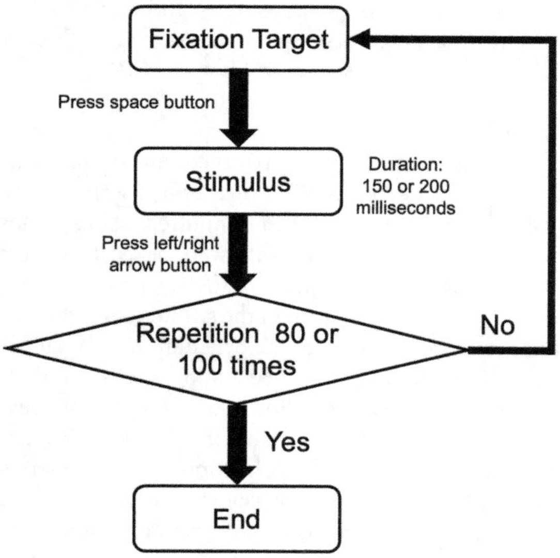

FIGURE 2 | The procedure of a single task in orientation and motion directions. Participants performed a two-alternative forced-choice task. After pressing the space button, participants pressed the left or right button according to the orientation of Gabor patches or the motion direction of random dots. Then, the procedure was repeated 80 times for orientation task and 100 times for motion direction task.

Data Analysis

All participants' responses to the respective stimulus degrees were analyzed, as described previously (27, 31). Briefly, for each task, data were analyzed by calculating the proportion of clockwise responses at each deviation degree x: $p_x = y_x / n_x$. For the orientation task, y_x is the count of clockwise responses from the vertical direction at the deviation degree x (or the upward motion direction for the motion direction task), and n_x is the total number of trails at the deviation degree x. For degree x, a negative value indicates counterclockwise, while a positive value indicates clockwise. This experimental dataset $\{x_i, p_i\}$ is modeled as a logistic function:

$$p(x) = l + \frac{1 - 2l}{1 + \exp\left(-\frac{\ln(21/4)}{\sigma} \times (x - \mu)\right)}$$

where l is the lapsing rate of the participant, μ is the perceived midpoint or the reference point of the participant, and σ is the discrimination threshold around the midpoint. This function was adjusted based on the data using Bayesian fitting (Treutwein and Strasburger, 1999). In this study, we extracted the threshold, bias, and lapsing rate of each participant in the orientation and motion direction tasks. The threshold (equal to σ) refers to the minimum angles from the vertical or upward motion direction; the bias (equal to the absolute value of μ) represents the difference between the perceived participant's midpoint and the vertical or upward motion direction; the lapsing rate (i.e., 1-the maximum of the logistic function) indicates that of the participant. To better understand the parameters, we constructed a diagram to show an example of psychometric curve and the meaning of the threshold, bias, and lapsing rate (**Figure 3**).

To assess discrimination ability differences in orientation and motion direction tasks between the young and old groups, GraphPad Prism 9.0 (GraphPad Software, United States) was used to perform the Mann–Whitney test for abnormal distribution data. For correlation analysis of age and threshold, bias, and lapsing rate, Spearman's rank correlation was performed using GraphPad Prism 9.0. A p-value of <0.05 was considered statistically significant.

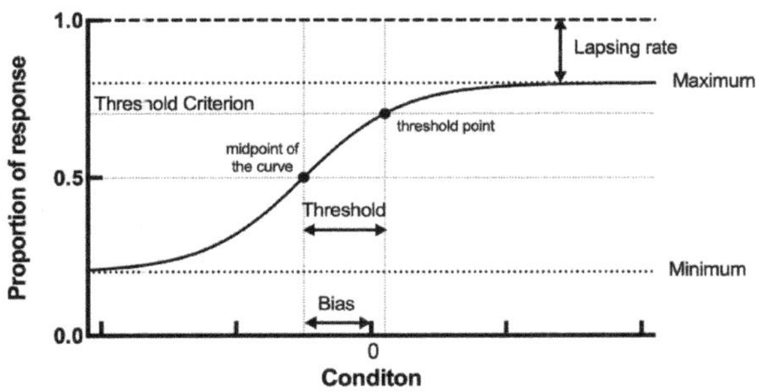

FIGURE 3 | Example plots of a young participant and an old participant showing the raw data analysis in the orientation task. **(A,B**, respectively) Examples of the staircase plots showing the within-staircase trail number *versus* the orientation angles in Gabor patches for a young participant and an old participant. Open symbols are for convergence point of 28.57% and filled symbols for convergence points of 71.43%. The negative angles represent counterclockwise relative to the vertical, and *vice versa*. **(C)** Examples of the plots showing the proportion of the clockwise responses *versus* the orientation angles in Gabor patches and the respective psychometric functions. The black X shape, rhombus, and curve (function parameters: l = 0.0072, μ = 1.5518, and σ = 2.4718) for an old participant. The blue dots, rhombus, and curve for a young participant (function parameters: l = 0.0028, μ = 0.0782, and σ = 0.9106). Rhombus is the midpoint of the curve.

RESULTS

Clinical Details of Participants

All participants enrolled in this study were healthy adults. A total of 56 participants performed the assigned two tasks. Before the experiment, all participants underwent thorough physical and eye examinations. **Table 1** summarizes the clinical information of participants.

TABLE 1 | Clinical information of both groups, including age, sex, best-corrected visual acuity, and education background.

Clinical details	Young group	Old group
Number	28	28
Age, years		
Mean ± SD	29.04 ± 7.42	57.29 ± 5.72
Median, *n* (range)	25.5 (22–49)	56 (50–72)
Sex		
Female	21	18
Male	7	10
Best corrected visual acuity, logMAR		
OD, Mean ± SD	0.025 ± 0.065	0.046 ± 0.074
OS, Mean ± SD	0.025 ± 0.075	0.025 ± 0.070
Education background		
Primary school	2	10
Middle school	2	17
College and above	24	1

Orientation Discrimination

In the orientation discrimination experiment, both young and old participants were required to indicate the orientation of the static Gabor patch (left versus right). Each response was recorded as staircase plots according to the convergence point. Example plots are shown for a young participant and an old participant in **Figures 4A,B**, respectively. For the young participant, the staircase was straight to the midpoint and formed a zigzag around the vertical direction (0°), while for the old participant, the staircase plots were wider and repeated irregularly, suggesting that the old participant could not discriminate the small angles clearly in the experiment.

Example plots are shown for a young participant with the following parameters: l = 0.0028, μ = 0.0782, and σ = 0.9106 and an old participant with the following parameters: l = 0.0072, μ = 1.5518, and σ = 2.4718 in **Figure 4C**. The threshold, bias, and lapsing rate of all participants were used for further statistical analysis. The shapes of psychometric curves vary in slope, horizontal shift, and height with different parameters, which can be used to compare the performance between young and old participants directly. Compared with the old participant, the young participant's datasets were nearly located on the respective curve having a larger slope and height and a smaller horizontal shift (**Figure 4C**). These results suggest that old participants had decreased ability and increased error rate in the discrimination of fine orientation difference.

The results for both young and old participants are summarized in **Figure 5**. Compared with the young group, the old group had a higher threshold of orientation discrimination (**Figure 5A**), an increased bias of the perceived midpoint of orientation (**Figure 5B**), and a larger lapsing rate in the orientation task (**Figure 5C**); the differences in the threshold and bias between the two groups were significant. This result suggests that in fine orientation discrimination, aging participants need stronger stimuli to discriminate clearly. In addition, the vertical orientation judged by aging participants was more oblique, suggesting an imbalance of neural mechanisms specialized for orientation discrimination in aging.

Motion Direction Discrimination

In the motion direction discrimination experiment, both young and old participants were required to indicate the motion direction of the dots (leftward versus rightward). Each response was recorded as staircase plots based on the convergence point. Example plots are shown for a young participant and an old participant in **Figures 6A,B**, respectively. Similarly, for the young participant, the staircase was straight to the midpoint and formed a zigzag around the upward motion direction (0°). However, the staircase plots in the old participant were wider and repeated irregularly, suggesting that the old participant could not discriminate moving dots with small motion direction difference well in the experiment.

The data analysis process in the motion direction discrimination task was similar to that in the orientation discrimination task. Example plots are shown for a young participant with the following parameters: l = 0.0049, μ = 0.7850, and σ = 0.4270 and an old participant with the following parameters: l = 0.0124, μ = 2.1248, and σ = 3.8050 in **Figure 6C**. The psychometrics curve difference between young and old participants can also be used to compare their performance directly. Compared with the old participant, the young participant's datasets were nearly located on the respective curve, and the curve had a larger slope and height and a smaller horizontal shift (**Figure 6C**). These results suggest that old participants had impaired ability in discriminating stimuli with fine motion directions.

The results for both young and old participants are summarized in **Figure 7**. Older participants had a higher threshold of motion direction discrimination than young participants (**Figure 7A**). In addition, old participants had an increased bias of the perceived midpoint in motion direction discrimination (**Figure 7B**), and significantly higher lapsing rate than that of young participants (**Figure 7C**).

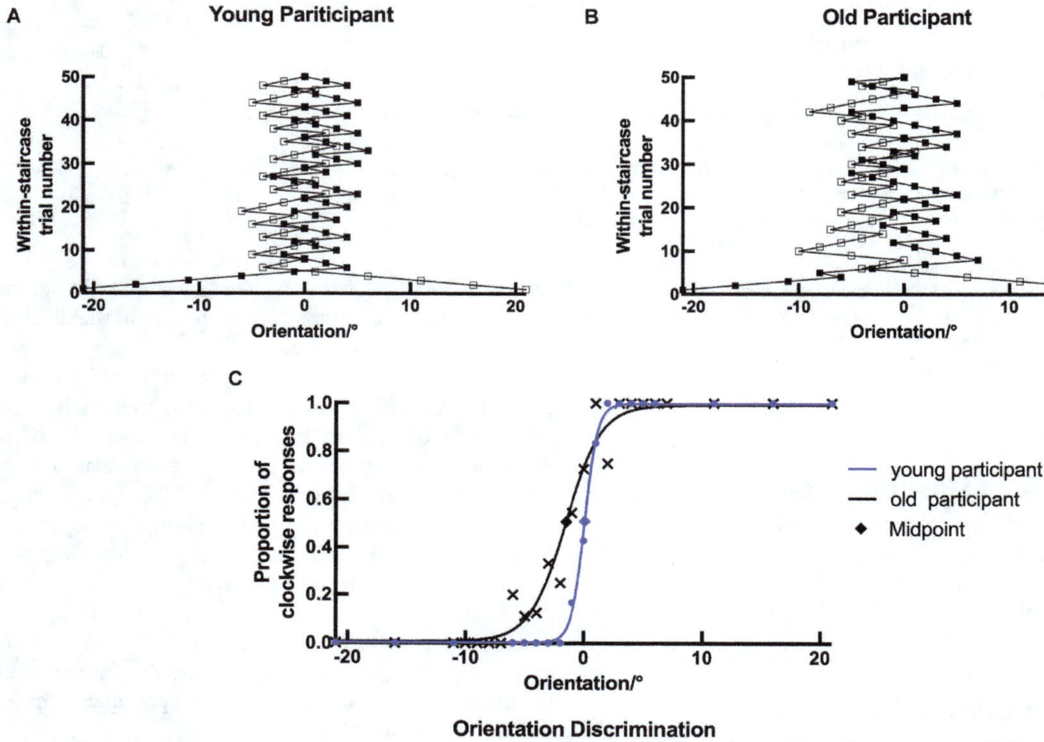

FIGURE 4 | The discrimination ability difference of orientation between the young and old groups. **(A)** Statistical results showing the threshold differences between the young (n = 26) and old (n = 26) groups. **(B)** Statistical results showing the bias differences between the young (n = 28) and old (n = 27) groups. **(C)** Statistical results showing the lapsing rate differences between the young (n = 28) and old (n = 25) groups. Data are expressed as mean ± SEM. $^{*}p < 0.05$ for the young group and the old group in the threshold and bias. ns indicates no significant difference between the young and old group in the lapsing rate analysis.

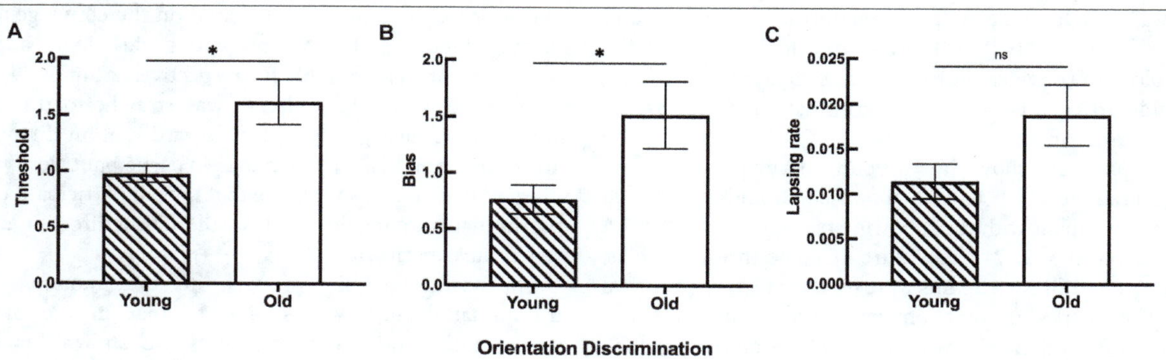

FIGURE 5 | A diagram of psychometric curve and meaning of threshold, bias, and lapsing rate. The threshold represents the horizontal distance between the threshold point and midpoint of the curve. The bias represents the horizontal distance between the midpoint and x = 0. The lapsing rate represents the vertical distance between the maximum of the curve and y = 1.

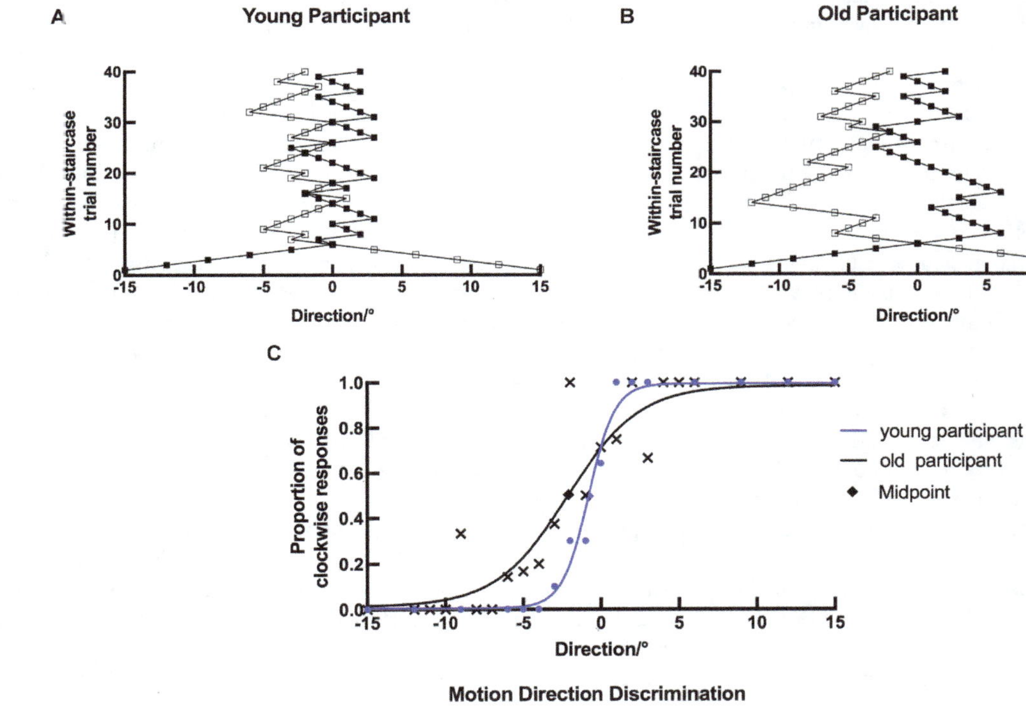

FIGURE 6 | Example plots of a young participant and an old participant showing the raw data analysis in the motion direction task. **(A,B**, respectively) Examples of the staircase plots showing the within-staircase trail number *versus* the motion direction angles for a young participant and an old participant. Open symbols are for convergence point of 25%, and filled symbols are for convergence points of 75%. The negative angles represent counterclockwise relative to the upward motion direction, and *vice versa*. **(C)** Examples of the plots showing the proportion of the clockwise responses *versus* the angles in motion direction and the respective psychometric function. The black X, rhombus shape, and curve (function parameters: l = 0.0124, μ = 2.1248, and σ = 3.8050) for an old participant. The blue dots, rhombus, and curve for a young participant (function parameters: l = 0.0049, μ = 0.7850, and σ = 0.4270). Rhombus is the midpoint of the curve.

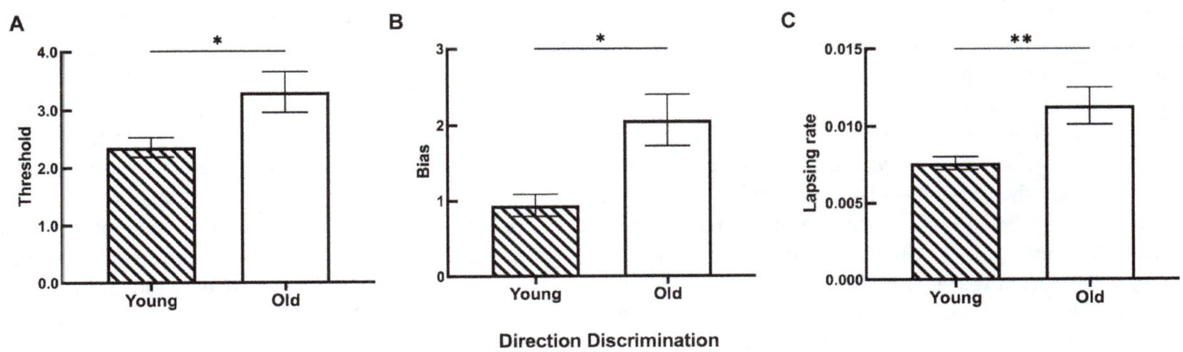

FIGURE 7 | The discrimination ability difference of motion direction between the young and old groups. **(A)** Statistical results showing the threshold differences between the young (n = 26) and old (n = 27) groups. **(B)** Statistical results showing the bias differences between the young (n = 23) and old (n = 26) groups. **(C)** Statistical results showing the lapsing rate differences between the young (n = 27) and old (n = 24) groups. Data are expressed as mean ± SEM. $^{*}p < 0.05$ for the young group and the old group in the threshold and bias analyses. $^{**}p < 0.01$ for the young group and the old group in the lapsing rate analysis.

DISCUSSION

In this study, we used two new tasks to investigate changes in fine visual perception in a normal aging population and compared the discrimination ability of micro-angle changes between young and old participants. The results showed that (1) compared with young adults, aging adults had a higher threshold, an increased bias, and a higher lapsing rate in the orientation task, although some differences were not statistically significant; (2) in the motion direction task, old participants had a higher threshold, an increased bias, and a significantly higher lapsing rate than young participants. These findings suggest that old adults have an altered visual perception. We also analyzed the correlation of age and threshold, bias, and lapsing rate in orientation and motion direction discrimination tasks. In the orientation discrimination task, the log threshold was significantly correlated with age (regression coefficient $r = 0.3199$, $p < 0.05$); the log bias (regression coefficient $r = 0.2386$, $p = 0.0793$) and log lapsing rate (regression coefficient $r = 0.1374$, $p = 0.3267$) showed an increased trend with age, although not significant (**Supplementary Figure 1**). In the motion direction task, the log threshold (regression coefficient $r = 0.3221$, $p < 0.05$), log bias (regression coefficient $r = 0.3365$, $p < 0.05$), and log lapsing rate (regression coefficient $r = 0.3698$, $p < 0.01$) were all correlated with age (**Supplementary Figure 2**). However, the increasing trend of these parameters might be not accordant with different age ranges. A previous study has reported piecewise linear functions between age and contrast sensitivity (Tang and Zhou, 2009), while another has also showed similar sensitivity to motion in participants with lower age ranges (Bennett et al., 2007). This might be attributed to the stable discrimination ability in young adults. Only when the visual function impaired beyond compensatory ability with aging, the abnormal discrimination ability could be detected.

In the orientation discrimination tasks, a higher threshold among aged participants indicated that old individuals might have worse orientation discrimination ability of small angle changes, although their visual acuity might be normal. The bias of the aged participants was increased, suggesting an imbalance of neurons responsible for different orientations in the visual cortex. In addition, old participants had a relatively high lapsing rate in the orientation task, partially due to a limited number of participants and the fact that the static sine wave raster tasks are relatively easy for aging individuals compared with the motion direction task.

In the motion direction discrimination tasks, old participants required stronger stimuli to make a correct judgment, suggesting a decreased discrimination ability of motion dots. Furthermore, participants in both groups had a higher threshold in motion direction tasks than in orientation tasks, suggesting a higher sensitivity of the motion direction task in aging. This result may be explained by the different visual process streams in the visual cortex for the two stimuli. Meanwhile, receiving visual information is an "encoding" procedure to extract motion features, while discrimination is the "decoding" procedure to make a judgment regarding the moving direction (Graham, 1989). This complex task involving multiple visual areas could show clearer vision perception changes in healthy aging.

In addition, previous studies have found that the discrimination ability difference of motion direction tasks between young and old participants increased when the dots moved at lower speeds (Snowden and Kavanagh, 2006). In this study, the stimuli dots moved at 8°/s, similar to that in a previous study, and our results are in line with that of Snowden and Kavanagh (2006). Moreover, the effect of stimulus size on discrimination remains controversial. When the stimulus size increases, the number of dots also increases to maintain the density; the increased size may activate the cortex responsible for both the central and peripheral visual fields; reduced peripheral suppression was reported in older participants (Mapstone et al., 2008; Betts et al., 2009). Meanwhile, the number of dots can influence discrimination ability (Betts et al., 2005). In our study, the stimulus size was only 1.5°, a small central circle in the vision field, which was associated with the central visual field and less affected by the surrounding area.

Both anatomy and neurophysiology studies on aging have shown that impaired visual perception might be correlated with brain deterioration in older population. Myelinated fibers and synapses in the brain regions, including the V1 area, are degraded in aging monkeys (Peters et al., 2001; Peters, 2009). These anatomical changes may be partially responsible for the increased response time and decreased vision perception. In this study, higher lapsing rate and increased bias of older participants were observed in the motion direction tasks, which is in line with previous findings (Wang et al., 2005).

In addition to structural changes in aging brains, decreased selectivity and increased spontaneous brain activity have also been demonstrated in senescent mammals (Delahunt et al., 2008). Studies have suggested that orientation and direction selectivity are reduced in aging monkeys and cats (Wang et al., 2006; Yu et al., 2006), and that acetylcholine and GABAergic neurotransmitters are important for orientation selectivity, indicating that insufficient inhibition of cortical neurons may contribute to age-related vision impairment (Schmolesky et al., 2000; Andersen and Ni, 2008; Edden et al., 2009; McKendrick et al., 2018). In addition, it has also been reported that reduction of orientation selectivity is reversed by local administration of GABA agonists (Leventhal et al., 2003), and downregulation of inhibitory neurotransmitters in aging contributes to hyperactivity of the visual cortex (Delahunt et al., 2008). A previous study has also found that orientation detection thresholds were significantly negatively correlated with visual cortex GABA levels for obliquely oriented patterns, and gamma oscillation frequency was positively correlated with GABA levels in the primary visual cortex, suggesting that visual perception is impaired in the healthy aging population (Edden et al., 2009). In this study, the bias of old participants in both tasks was nearly double than that of the young participants, which may partially be due to the GABAergic neurotransmitter level change or the increased brain activity and background noise in the visual cortex.

A contrast, which is the basis of visual perception, is the difference between light and dark conditions. In macaque brains, the primary visual cortex (V1) is involved in contrast perception (Ruiz and Paradiso, 2012). V1 activity is also associated with the contrast stimuli (Niemeyer and Paradiso, 2017). Studies have shown that the contrast of a target could influence the discrimination ability of healthy participants, especially aging participants (Allen et al., 2010). In this study, the orientation discrimination tasks were dependent on the contrast sensitivity and spatial frequency selectivity to excite orientation-tuned neurons and recognize Gabor patches. As the contrast decreases, the accuracy also decreases, and participants' discrimination becomes less reliable with increased variability (Tzvetanov, 2012). Hence, in this study, the target contrast was 0.9 in the orientation tasks and 1.0 in motion direction tasks to ensure reliability and efficiency. Our results illustrated the discrimination ability changes of small angles among older participants, even with sufficient contrast stimuli.

Notably, the motion direction task primarily evaluates the visual cortex neurons' ability to process moving objects. The analysis mechanism of motion direction in visual cortex differs from that of static contrast stimuli. Different neurons in the visual cortex can be activated by different directions of stimuli; this phenomenon is referred to as direction selectivity (Tzvetanov, 2012; Chaplin et al., 2018). However, only a small number of neurons in the V1 area exhibit direction selectivity, although visual information from both eyes is transmitted to V1 at the first stage in primates (Davies et al., 2016). Most neurons in the MT show a strong directional selectivity, which might be associated with the motion direction discrimination task (Albright, 1984; Elston and Rosa, 1997). An fMRI study reported functional changes in the MT area in response to stimuli of drifting Gabor patches in different sizes and contrasts, suggesting that the MT area might be involved in the direction-selectivity process (Turkozer et al., 2016). In this study, the motion direction tasks adopted a random-dot pattern without orientation cues. Based on our findings and those of previous studies, the decreased discrimination of motion direction may demonstrate the aging effect on the visual cortex, especially in the MT area. Meanwhile, the increased bias in the motion direction task may suggest an imbalance of direction-selectivity neurons in aging.

CONCLUSION

In this study, we have developed two new psychometric tasks to investigate fine orientation and motion direction discrimination in young and old adults with normal visual acuity. Our results illustrated that aging participants exhibited increased threshold and bias in both tasks, and a higher lapsing rate in the motion direction task. Compared with previous orientation and motion direction tasks, our tasks are more rapid and simpler for fine visual perception in older individuals (Pilz et al., 2017). Although visual acuity remains to be examined clinically, other psychometric examinations or treatment methods need to be developed to prevent or delay visual perception in aging.

AUTHOR CONTRIBUTIONS

LF designed the research. LX, JD, and SL performed the tasks for subjects. HC wrote the Matlab programs. LX and HC wrote the article. All authors contributed to the article and approved the submitted version.

ACKNOWLEDGMENTS

The authors thank Huan Wang for providing some of the programs. The authors are grateful to all study participants.

REFERENCES

Albright, T. D. (1984). Direction and orientation selectivity of neurons in visual area MT of the macaque. *J. Neurophysiol.* 52, 1106–1130. doi: 10.1152/jn.1984.52.6.1106

Allen, H. A., Hutchinson, C. V., Ledgeway, T., and Gayle, P. (2010). The role of contrast sensitivity in global motion processing deficits in the elderly. *J. Vis.* 10:15. doi: 10.1167/10.10.15

Andersen, G. J. (2012). Aging and vision: changes in function and performance from optics to perception. *Wiley Interdiscip. Rev. Cogn. Sci.* 3, 403–410. doi: 10.1002/wcs.1167

Andersen, G. J., and Ni, R. (2008). Aging and visual processing: declines in spatial not temporal integration. *Vis. Res.* 48, 109–118. doi: 10.1016/j.visres.2007.10.026

Ball, K., and Sekuler, R. (1986). Improving visual perception in older observers. *J. Gerontol.* 41, 176–182. doi: 10.1093/geronj/41.2.176

Bennett, P. J., Sekuler, A. B., and Ozin, L. (1999). Effects of aging on calculation efficiency and equivalent noise. *J. Opt. Soc. Am. A Opt. Image Sci. Vis.* 16, 654–668. doi: 10.1364/josaa.16.000654

Bennett, P. J., Sekuler, R., and Sekuler, A. B. (2007). The effects of aging on motion detection and direction identification. *Vis. Res.* 47, 799–809. doi: 10.1016/j.visres.2007.01.001

Betts, L. R., Sekuler, A. B., and Bennett, P. J. (2007). The effects of aging on orientation discrimination. *Vis. Res.* 47, 1769–1780. doi: 10.1016/j.visres.2007.02.016

Betts, L. R., Sekuler, A. B., and Bennett, P. J. (2009). Spatial characteristics of center-surround antagonism in younger and older adults. *J. Vis.* 9, 25.1–15. doi: 10.1167/9.1.25

Betts, L. R., Taylor, C. P., Sekuler, A. B., and Bennett, P. J. (2005). Aging reduces center-surround antagonism in visual motion processing. *Neuron* 45, 361–366. doi: 10.1016/j.neuron.2004.12.041

Brainard, D. H. (1997). The psychophysics toolbox. *Spat Vis.* 10, 433–436. doi: 10.1163/156856897x00357

Casco, C., Barollo, M., Contemori, G., and Battaglini, L. (2017). The effects of aging on orientation discrimination. *Front. Aging Neurosci.* 9:45. doi: 10.3389/fnagi.2017.00045

Chaplin, T. A., Rosa, M. G. P., and Lui, L. L. (2018). Auditory and visual motion processing and integration in the primate cerebral cortex. *Front. Neural Circuits* 12:93. doi: 10.3389/fncir.2018.00093

Davies, A. J., Chaplin, T. A., Rosa, M. G., and Yu, H. H. (2016). Natural motion trajectory enhances the coding of speed in primate extrastriate cortex. *Sci. Rep.* 6:19739. doi: 10.1038/srep19739

Delahunt, P. B., Hardy, J. L., and Werner, J. S. (2008). The effect of senescence on orientation discrimination and mechanism tuning. *J. Vis.* 8, 5.1–9. doi: 10.1167/8.3.5

Edden, R. A., Muthukumaraswamy, S. D., Freeman, T. C., and Singh, K. D. (2009). Orientation discrimination performance is predicted by GABA concentration and gamma oscillation frequency in human primary visual cortex. *J. Neurosci.* 29, 15721–15726. doi: 10.1523/jneurosci.4426-09.2009

Elston, G. N., and Rosa, M. G. (1997). The occipitoparietal pathway of the macaque monkey: comparison of pyramidal cell morphology in layer III of functionally related cortical visual areas. *Cereb. Cortex* 7, 432–452. doi: 10.1093/cercor/7.5.432

Faubert, J. (2002). Visual perception and aging. *Can. J. Exp. Psychol.* 56, 164–176.

Gold, J. I., and Ding, L. (2013). How mechanisms of perceptual decision-making affect the psychometric function. *Prog. Neurobiol.* 103, 98–114. doi: 10.1016/j.pneurobio.2012.05.008

Govenlock, S. W., Taylor, C. P., Sekuler, A. B., and Bennett, P. J. (2009). The effect of aging on the orientational selectivity of the human visual system. *Vis. Res.* 49, 164–172. doi: 10.1016/j.visres.2008.10.004

Graham, N. V. S. (1989). *Visual Pattern Analyzers*. New York, NY: Oxford University Press.

Guillon, M., Dumbleton, K., Theodoratos, P., Gobbe, M., Wooley, C. B., and Moody, K. (2016). The effects of age, refractive status, and luminance on pupil size. *Optom. Vis. Sci.* 93, 1093–1100. doi: 10.1097/opx.0000000000000893

Harman, A., Abrahams, B., Moore, S., and Hoskins, R. (2000). Neuronal density in the human retinal ganglion cell layer from 16-77 years. *Anat. Rec.* 260, 124–131. doi: 10.1002/1097-0185(20001001)260:2<124::Aid-ar20<3.0.Co;2-d

Hedden, T., and Gabrieli, J. D. (2005). Healthy and pathological processes in adult development: new evidence from neuroimaging of the aging brain. *Curr. Opin. Neurol.* 18, 740–747. doi: 10.1097/01.wco.0000189875.29852.48

Jackson, G. R., Owsley, C., and Curcio, C. A. (2002). Photoreceptor degeneration and dysfunction in aging and age-related maculopathy. *Ageing Res. Rev.* 1, 381–396. doi: 10.1016/s1568-1637(02)00007-7

IJspeert, J. K., de Waard, P. W., van den Berg, T. J., and de Jong, P. T. (1990). The intraocular straylight function in 129 healthy volunteers; dependence on angle, age and pigmentation. *Vis. Res.* 30, 699–707. doi: 10.1016/0042-6989(90)90096-4

Leventhal, A. G., Wang, Y., Pu, M., Zhou, Y., and Ma, Y. (2003). GABA and its agonists improved visual cortical function in senescent monkeys. *Science* 300, 812–815. doi: 10.1126/science.1082874

Loerch, P. M., Lu, T., Dakin, K. A., Vann, J. M., Isaacs, A., Geula, C., et al. (2008). Evolution of the aging brain transcriptome and synaptic regulation. *PLoS One* 3:e3329. doi: 10.1371/journal.pone.0003329

Mapstone, M., Dickerson, K., and Duffy, C. J. (2008). Distinct mechanisms of impairment in cognitive ageing and Alzheimer's disease. *Brain* 131(Pt 6), 1618–1629. doi: 10.1093/brain/awn064

McKendrick, A. M., Chan, Y. M., and Nguyen, B. N. (2018). Spatial vision in older adults: perceptual changes and neural bases. *Ophthalmic Physiol. Opt.* 38, 363–375. doi: 10.1111/opo.12565

Niemeyer, J. E., and Paradiso, M. A. (2017). Contrast sensitivity, V1 neural activity, and natural vision. *J. Neurophysiol.* 117, 492–508. Epub 2016/11/11. doi: 10.1152/jn.00635.2016.,

Panda-Jonas, S., Jonas, J. B., and Jakobczyk-Zmija, M. (1995). Retinal photoreceptor density decreases with age. *Ophthalmology* 102, 1853–1859. doi: 10.1016/s0161-6420(95)30784-1

Patten, M. L., Mannion, D. J., and Clifford, C. W. G. (2017). Correlates of perceptual orientation biases in human primary visual cortex. *J. Neurosci.* 37, 4744–4750. doi: 10.1523/jneurosci.3511-16.2017

Pelli, D. G. (1997). The videotoolbox software for visual psychophysics: transforming numbers into movies. *Spat Vis.* 10, 437–442. doi: 10.1163/156856897x00366

Peters, A. (2009). The effects of normal aging on myelinated nerve fibers in monkey central nervous system. *Front. Neuroanat.* 3:11. doi: 10.3389/neuro.05.011.2009

Peters, A., Moss, M. B., and Sethares, C. (2001). The effects of aging on layer 1 of primary visual cortex in the rhesus monkey. *Cereb. Cortex* 11, 93–103. doi: 10.1093/cercor/11.2.93

Petrash, J. M. (2013). Aging and age-related diseases of the ocular lens and vitreous body. *Invest. Ophthalmol. Vis. Sci.* 54, ORSF54–ORSF59. doi: 10.1167/iovs.13-12940

Pilz, K. S., Miller, L., and Agnew, H. C. (2017). Motion coherence and direction discrimination in healthy aging. *J. Vis.* 17:31. doi: 10.1167/17.1.31

Ruiz, O., and Paradiso, M. A. (2012). Macaque V1 representations in natural and reduced visual contexts: spatial and temporal properties and influence of saccadic eye movements. *J. Neurophysiol.* 108, 324–333. doi: 10.1152/jn.00733.2011

Schmolesky, M. T., Wang, Y., Pu, M., and Leventhal, A. G. (2000). Degradation of stimulus selectivity of visual cortical cells in senescent rhesus monkeys. *Nat. Neurosci.* 3, 384–390. doi: 10.1038/73957

Snowden, R. J., and Kavanagh, E. (2006). Motion perception in the ageing visual system: minimum motion, motion coherence, and speed discrimination thresholds. *Perception* 35, 9–24. doi: 10.1068/p5399

Tang, Y., and Zhou, Y. (2009). Age-related decline of contrast sensitivity for second-order stimuli: earlier onset, but slower progression, than for first-order stimuli. *J. Vis.* 9:18. doi: 10.1167/9.7.18

Treutwein, B., and Strasburger, H. (1999). Fitting the psychometric function. *Percept. Psychophys* 61, 87–106. doi: 10.3758/bf03211951

Turkozer, H. B., Pamir, Z., and Boyaci, H. (2016). Contrast affects fMRI activity in middle temporal cortex related to center-surround interaction in motion perception. *Front. Psychol.* 7:454. doi: 10.3389/fpsyg.2016.00454

Tzvetanov, T. (2012). A single theoretical framework for circular features processing in humans: orientation and direction of motion compared. *Front. Comput. Neurosci.* 6:28. doi: 10.3389/fncom.2012.00028

van de Kraats, J., and van Norren, D. (2007). Optical density of the aging human ocular media in the visible and the UV. *J. Opt. Soc. Am. A. Opt. Image Sci. Vis.* 24, 1842–1857. doi: 10.1364/josaa.24.001842

Wang, H., Xie, X., Li, X., Chen, B., and Zhou, Y. (2006). Functional degradation of visual cortical cells in aged rats. *Brain Res.* 1122, 93–98. doi: 10.1016/j.brainres.2006.09.010

Wang, X. J. (2008). Decision making in recurrent neuronal circuits. *Neuron* 60, 215–234. doi: 10.1016/j.neuron.2008.09.034

Wang, Y., Zhou, Y., Ma, Y., and Leventhal, A. G. (2005). Degradation of signal timing in cortical areas V1 and V2 of senescent monkeys. *Cereb. Cortex* 15, 403–408. doi: 10.1093/cercor/bhh143

Weale, R. A. (1988). Age and the transmittance of the human crystalline lens. *J. Physiol.* 395, 577–587. doi: 10.1113/jphysiol.1988.sp016935

Yamamoto, N., and Degirolamo, G. J. (2012). Differential effects of aging on spatial learning through exploratory navigation and map reading. *Front. Aging Neurosci.* 4:14. doi: 10.3389/fnagi.2012.00014

Yu, S., Wang, Y., Li, X., Zhou, Y., and Leventhal, A. G. (2006). Functional degradation of extrastriate visual cortex in senescent rhesus monkeys. *Neuroscience* 140, 1023–1029. doi: 10.1016/j.neuroscience.2006.01.015

19

Impact of Temporal Visual Flicker on Spatial Contrast Sensitivity in Myopia

Jie Ye[1], Pawan Sinha[2], Fang Hou[1], Xianghang He[1,3], Meixiao Shen[1], Fan Lu[1]* and Yilei Shao[1]**

[1] School of Ophthalmology and Optometry, Wenzhou Medical University, Wenzhou, China, [2] Department of Brain and Cognitive Sciences, Massachusetts Institute of Technology, Cambridge, MA, United States, [3] Fuzhou Aier Eye Hospital, Fuzhou, China

***Correspondence:**
Yilei Shao
magic_shao@163.com
Fan Lu
lufan@mail.eye.ac.cn
Pawan Sinha
psinha@mit.edu

Purpose: To investigate whether short-term exposure to high temporal frequency full-field flicker has an impact on spatial visual acuity in individuals with varying degrees of myopia.

Methods: Thirty subjects (evenly divided between control and experimental groups) underwent a 5-min exposure to full-field flicker. The flicker rate was lower than critical flicker frequency (CFF) for the experimental group (12.5 Hz) and significantly higher than CFF for the controls (60 Hz). Spatial contrast sensitivity function (CSF) was measured before and immediately after flicker exposure. We examined whether the post flicker CSF parameters were different from the pre-exposure CSF values in either of the subject groups. Additionally, we examined the relationship between the amount of CSF change from pre to post timepoints and the degree of subjects' myopia. The CSF parameters included peak frequency, peak sensitivity, bandwidth, truncation, and area under log CSF (AULCSF).

Results: There was no significant difference of all five pre-exposure CSF parameters between the two groups at baseline ($P = 0.333 \sim 0.424$). Experimental group subjects exhibited significant ($P < 0.005$) increases in peak sensitivity and AULCSF, when comparing post-exposure results to pre-exposure ones. Controls showed no such enhancements. Furthermore, the extent of these changes in the experimental group was correlated significantly with the participants' refractive error ($P = 0.005$ and 0.018, respectively).

Conclusion: Our data suggest that exposure to perceivable high-frequency flicker (but, not to supra-CFF frequencies) enhances important aspects of spatial contrast sensitivity, and these enhancements are correlated to the degree of myopia. This finding has implications for potential interventions for cases of modest myopia.

Keywords: visual plasticity, myopia, spatial contrast sensitivity, temporal visual flicker, flicker adaptation

INTRODUCTION

Myopia is one of the foremost causes of visual impairment around the world (Wong et al., 2014; Ohno-Matsui et al., 2016). Although the exact etiology of myopia is still unknown, genetic as well as environmental factors are implicated. One such environmental factor is exposure to visual flicker. High-frequency flicker has been found to suppress the axial elongation of animal eyes

(Shih et al., 1997; Li et al., 2012). The secretion of compounds such as dopamine (DA) and crystallin proteins, are believed to be involved in linking flicker and myopia (Shih et al., 1997; Li et al., 2012).

From the perspective of neurophysiology, the influence of flicker on myopia is puzzling. The mammalian visual pathway is generally divided into two major streams of processing, parvocellular and magnocellular. The former has sensitivity to high spatial frequency stimuli while the latter is sensitive to high temporal frequencies (Burr and Ross, 1982; Livingstone and Hubel, 1987; Lee et al., 1990; Geisler et al., 2001). Given that the most evident impact of myopia is on spatial contrast sensitivity, especially in the high spatial frequency regime, the parvocellular pathway is believed to be more strongly involved in the genesis of myopia (Oen et al., 1994; Hashemi et al., 2012). The reduction of high spatial frequency details in the retinal image, especially during near-work with accommodation lag, would be expected to lead to axial elongation and further myopic development (Woodman et al., 2011; Hughes and Read, 2020). The magnocellular pathway's involvement in myopia remains unclear. Probing the effect of temporal flicker, which is the purview of the magnocellular system, on myopia, can help reveal whether this pathway does in fact play a role in the condition.

Studies with non-human subjects have provided initial evidence for the influence of flicker on myopia. Given these results, it is important to explore how this factor impacts human vision; the results can have implications for our basic understanding of myopia as well as for the design of practical interventions for this condition. The objective of the current study was to investigate the effect of short-term flicker on human spatial visual acuity and, especially, its correlation with myopia.

MATERIALS AND METHODS

Subjects

Thirty young adult subjects from Wenzhou Medical University were enrolled in the study and were randomly assigned to equal-sized control and experimental groups. All subjects had a comprehensive primary eye examination including measurements of the refractive error and best-corrected visual acuity (BCVA), slit-lamp examinations, axial length (AL, measured by IOL-master 500; IOLMaster, Carl Zeiss Meditec, Dublin, CA, United States), and so on. The BCVA was recorded as the logarithm of minimal angle resolution (LogMAR). The inclusion criteria were as follows: age between 20 and 30 years old, refractive error range from -8.0 diopter (D) to $+0.5$ D with astigmatism less than -1.5 D, and BCVA ≤ 0. None of the subjects had any systemic disease, ocular pathology, history of laser treatment, trauma, or eye surgery. All subjects who participated in this study signed consent forms and were treated in accordance with the tenets of the Declaration of Helsinki. This study was approved by the Ethics Committee of Wenzhou Medical University and all subjects were naïve as to the specific purpose of this experiment.

Spatial Contrast Sensitivity Function Test

A custom-built quick contrast sensitivity function (qCSF) system with digit stimuli was used to test the spatial contrast sensitivity function (CSF). Details of qCSF software have been reported in our previous study (Zheng et al., 2018). Briefly, the qCSF software was run in MATLAB (MathWorks, Natick, MA, United States) on an Apple Mac mini-computer (Model No. A1347; Apple Inc., Cupertino, CA, United States) with a 60 Hz refresh rate and mean luminance of 91.2 cd/m^2. The CSF test was conducted binocularly with the subject's best refractive error correction. Contrast sensitivity thresholds for spatial frequencies ranging from 0.50 to 15.8 cycle per degree (cpd) were measured. The bandpass-filtered digits were used as the visual stimuli to measure the contrast sensitivity thresholds (**Figure 1A**). The center frequency of the filter was designed to be three cycles per object, with one-octave full bandwidth at half height (Zheng et al., 2018). Each digit visual stimulus duration was 133 ms, which reduced the likelihood of saccade execution during stimulus presentation and was suitable for the temporal integration (Breitmeyer and Ganz, 1977; Legge, 1978; Purves et al., 2001). Each experimental session comprised 100 trials of two consecutive qCSF runs (50 trials $\times$ 2 runs). The subjects responded with what digit they saw at each trial. The measurement duration of the CSF test was approximately 2–3 min. From the test results, we derived the peak sensitivity (the peak gain), peak frequency (the spatial frequency corresponding to peak gain), bandwidth (the function's full width at half peak sensitivity), truncation (the distance between the peak sensitivity and plateau), and the area under log CSF (AULCSF) by CSF curve fitting (**Figure 1B**). The accuracy and repeatability of the qCSF system have been demonstrated in our previous paper (Zheng et al., 2019).

Process

To have all subjects start from a comparable baseline, they were dark-adapted for a period of 10-min. The subsequent test process for the control and experimental groups differed in the following way: After dark adaptation, **control** subjects were assessed via qCSF system and then asked to view for a period of 5 min full-field flicker with a temporal frequency of 60 Hz square-wave with an equal duty cycle [which, by virtue of being significantly higher than human critical flicker frequency (CFF)], was perceived as a steady field. They were then retested using the qCSF system. The **experimental group** also underwent baseline CSF assessment after the 10-min dark adaptation. Subsequently, they viewed full-field flicker with a temporal frequency of 12.5 Hz square-wave with an equal duty cycle for 5-min. They were then retested using the qCSF system. The full-field flicker was presented as a Ganzfeld setup. A pair of safety-goggles with the transparent surface filling the entire visual field and lined with translucent vellum was used. A flickering light observed while wearing these goggles was experienced as a full-field flicker. The full-field flicker stimuli that the control and experimental subjects viewed were matched in their mean luminance (91.2 cd/m^2). All subjects viewed the stimuli with best refractive error corrections by wearing glasses while positioned in a chin rest to avoid the movement of the position and distance from the stimuli (1.34 m).

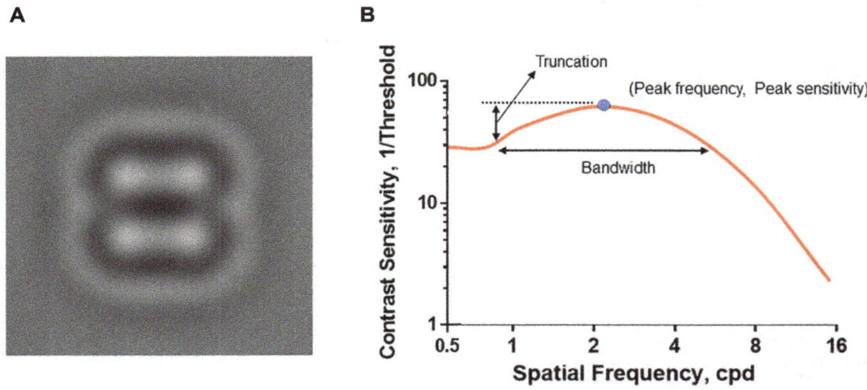

FIGURE 1 | Introduction of qCSF visual stimuli and CSF curve. **(A)** The representative visual stimuli sample. The bandpass-filtered digits were used as the visual stimuli to measure the contrast sensitivity thresholds. **(B)** The CSF curve. Peak sensitivity, peak gain; Peak frequency, the spatial frequency corresponding to peak gain; Bandwidth, the function's full-width at half peak sensitivity; Truncation, the distance between the peak sensitivity and plateau.

None of the subjects reported experiencing any discomfort during the session.

Statistical Analysis

All data were analyzed with SPSS software (version 22.0; SPSS, Inc., Chicago, IL, United States). All continuous variables were calculated as means ± standard deviations (SDs). The refractive error was transformed in the form of the spherical equivalent comprising the spherical diopter plus half of the cylindrical diopter. Only the refractive error of the dominant eye was used for further comparison and correlation analysis. The dominant eye was determined by the Hole-in-card test (Seijas et al., 2007). The post alterations in the CSF parameters from baseline were analyzed. Paired *t*-tests were used to compare the differences between the two groups and the two measurement points (baseline and post). The repeated measures analysis of variance (ANOVA) was also used to compare the differences of five CSF parameters with the two-measurement points as the within-subjects variables and groups as between-subjects factors. The general estimating equation was used to adjust the influence of baseline CSF parameters on the comparisons of the post alteration of the CSF parameters between the two groups. Pearson and partial correlation were used to analyze the correlation between the alteration magnitudes and refractive error. The $P < 0.05$ was considered as the statistical significance.

RESULTS

Basic Patients Characteristics

There were 15 subjects (Female: Male = 11:4) in the control group and 15 (Female: Male = 11:4) in the experimental group, respectively. Control and experimental groups did not differ significantly in age (25.8 ± 1.9 years vs. 26.2 ± 2.1 years, $P = 0.327$). There was no significant difference in refractive error between the control and experimental group (−5.86 ± 1.73 D vs. −6.01 ± 1.76 D, $P = 0.413$). The axial length of control group was similar with experimental group (25.32 ± 0.62 mm vs. 25.30 ± 0.63 mm, $P = 0.442$).

Differences in CSF Alteration in the Two Groups

There was no significant difference between control and experimental groups for any of the five CSF parameters at baseline ($P = 0.333 \sim 0.424$, **Table 1**). However, post-flicker exposure CSF measurements revealed notable differences between the groups.

Figure 2 shows the CSF curves of six representative subjects (three control and the other three experimental) at baseline and post-flicker. **Figure 3** shows the average CSF curves in the control and experimental groups with their standard deviation values. Control group participants exhibited no significant changes in their CSF parameters from before to after flicker exposure (**Figure 4**). However, significant changes of peak sensitivity and AULCSF were evident in the data from the experimental group (**Figures 4A,E**). For the post five CSF parameters, a repeated measures ANOVA showed that the flicker exposures have a significant effect in peak sensitivity [$F(1,28) = 11.291$, $P = 0.002$] and AULCSF [$F(1,28) = 11.022$, $P = 0.003$]. There was a significant interaction between group and flicker exposure in peak sensitivity [$F(1,28) = 4.180$, $P = 0.049$] and AULCSF [$F(1,28) = 5.088$, $P = 0.032$]. **Figure 5** plots the data in terms of changes from the baseline, and highlights the significant differences of two parameters (peak sensitivity: Control group 1.552 ± 5.570 vs. Experimental group 6.374 ± 7.241, $P = 0.025$; AULCSF: Control group 0.685 ± 2.452 vs. Experimental group 3.588 ± 3.595, $P = 0.016$; **Figure 5**, Paired *t*-tests).

Correlation Between the CSF Alteration and Refractive Error

We computed the correlation between the post-flicker alteration of CSF parameters and magnitude of refractive error in the experimental group. We found peak sensitivity ($r = 0.675$, $P = 0.003$) and AULCSF ($r = 0.579$, $P = 0.012$) to be correlated

TABLE 1 | Summary of mean qCSF parameters at baseline, post alteration from baseline in two groups.

	Peak sensitivity	Peak frequency	Bandwidth	Truncation	AULCSF
Baseline					
Control group (*N* = 15)	54.882 ± 11.360	1.317 ± 0.411	3.107 ± 0.461	0.139 ± 0.044	15.667 ± 6.920
Experimental group (*N* = 15)	53.087 ± 11.230	1.347 ± 0.425	3.071 ± 0.455	0.136 ± 0.033	15.001 ± 6.213
P	0.333	0.424	0.415	0.421	0.392
Post Alteration from Baseline					
Control group (*N* = 15)	1.552 ± 5.570	−0.111 ± 0.339	0.134 ± 0.423	−0.003 ± 0.045	0.685 ± 2.452
Experimental group (*N* = 15)	6.374 ± 7.241	−0.029 ± 0.446	0.150 ± 0.459	−0.011 ± 0.044	3.588 ± 3.595
P	**0.025 (0.017)**	0.287 (0.278)	0.462 (0.461)	0.321 (0.314)	**0.016 (0.010)**

AULCSF, the area under log CSF; P-value between the control and experimental groups.
Values in parentheses were the p-values after the adjustment for the corresponding data at baseline by the general estimating equation. The bold values just means the P-value less than 0.05.

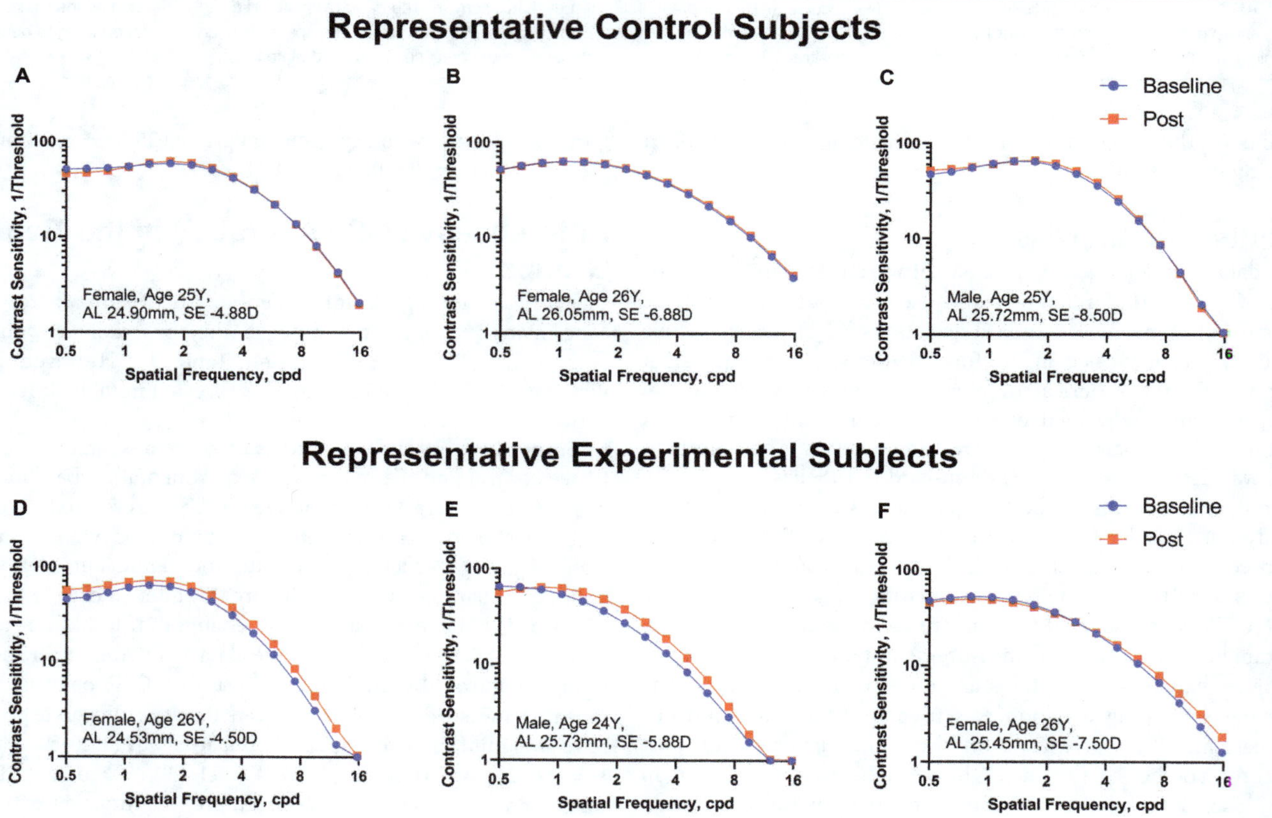

FIGURE 2 | The CSF curves in six representative cases from the control and experimental groups. **(A–C)** Control group. **(D–F)** Experimental group. Cpd, cycle per degree.

with the refractive error (**Figure 6** and **Table 2**). These significant correlations still existed after adjusting the corresponding baseline CSF parameters (**Table 2**) in the experimental group. There was no statistically significant association of the refractive error with post-flicker alteration of peak frequency, bandwidth, and truncation in the experimental group ($r = -0.200 \sim 0.025$, $P = 0.237 \sim 0.465$, **Figure 6** and **Table 2**). In the control group, there were no significant correlations between CSF parameters alteration and refractive error ($r = -0.277 \sim 0.444$, $P = 0.097 \sim 0.845$).

DISCUSSION

We evaluated the impact on spatial contrast sensitivity of short-term exposure to perceivable high-frequency flicker, in myopic patients. Our data revealed that the peak sensitivity and AULCSF increased significantly after exposure to merely 5 min of perceivable high-frequency flicker, but not to flicker with a frequency greater than CFF. Furthermore, since the refractive error increased with negative numbers, the magnitude of increase in these parameter values was significantly negatively correlated

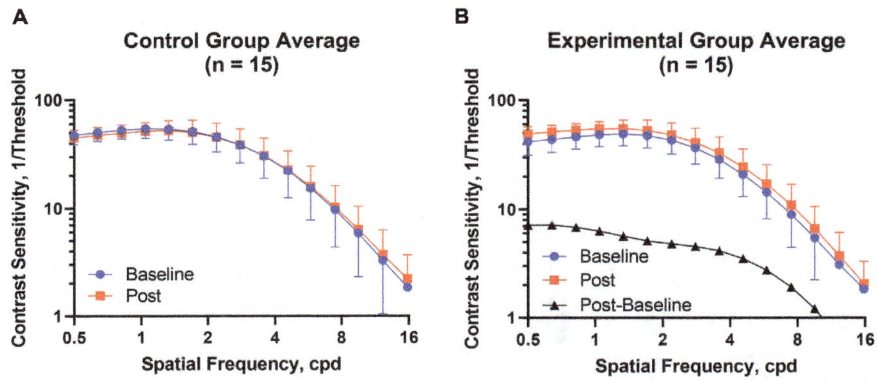

FIGURE 3 | The CSF curves in the control and experimental groups with average CSF and standard deviation value. **(A)** Control group. **(B)** Experimental group. Cpd, cycle per degree.

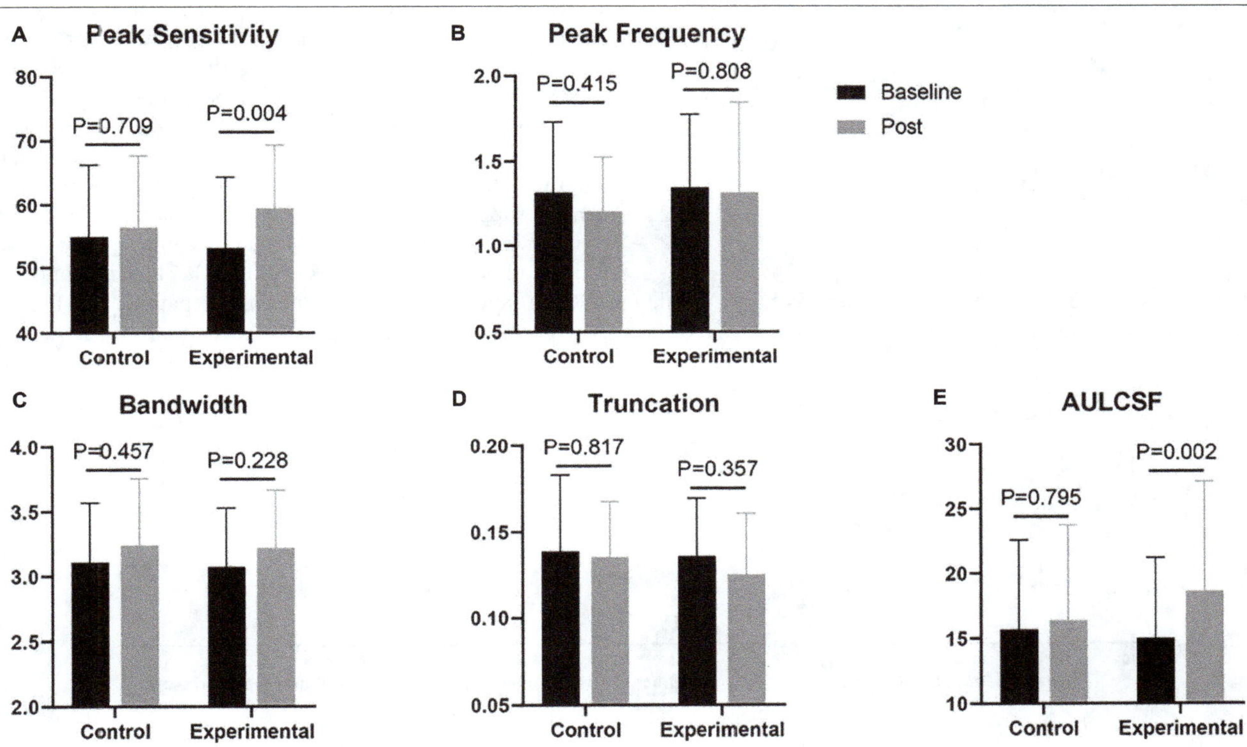

FIGURE 4 | Comparisons of CSF parameters between baseline and post. **(A)** Peak sensitivity; **(B)** Peak frequency; **(C)** Bandwidth; **(D)** Truncation; **(E)** AULCSF. The *p*-value shown in each panel corresponds to the result of a *t*-test.

to the severity of myopia with greater changes associated with less degree of myopia.

Previous work has reported that flicker adaptation raises spatial frequency of "coarse" test gratings, but does not yield any improvements with finer gratings (Kaneko et al., 2015). However, Arnold et al. (2016) have reported improvements in the ability to see fine facial details after flicker exposure. In the present study, we used digit stimuli (as a finer test method) (Zheng et al., 2019) to detect the effect of flicker exposure on high spatial frequency perception, and the results demonstrate significant improvements. It is worth noting that although the CSF value was lower with our qCSF system than traditional method, it would be similar to traditional value when converted into the root mean square contrast, as has been verified in our previous paper (Zheng et al., 2019).

The rapid alteration of the CSF curve following brief flicker exposure indicates plasticity of the mechanisms underlying fine spatial acuity in adults. What is notable is that the manipulation (temporal flicker) is designed to impact the magnocellular pathway, while the consequence (changes in fine spatial contrast

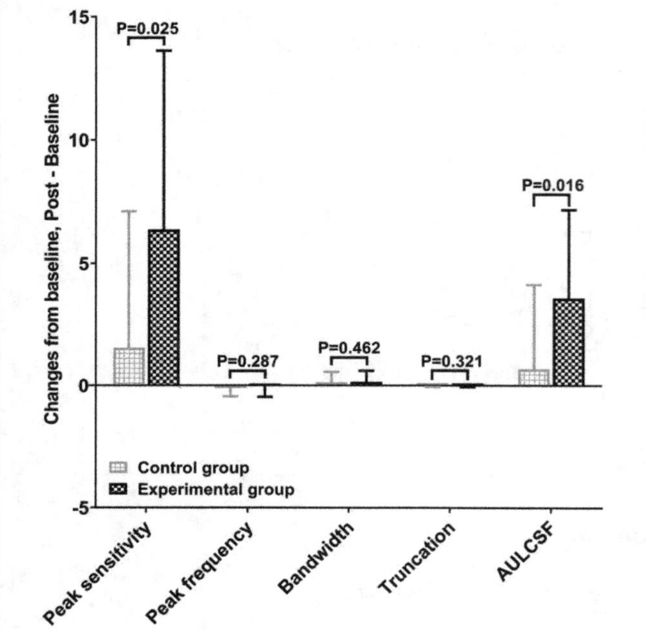

FIGURE 5 | Mean changes of post CSF parameters from baseline in control and experimental group.

TABLE 2 | The correlation between the post alteration CSF parameters from baseline and the refractive error in the experimental group.

	r	*P*	*P**
Peak sensitivity	0.675	**0.003**	**0.005**
Peak frequency	0.025	0.465	0.358
Bandwidth	−0.081	0.388	0.360
Truncation	−0.200	0.237	0.069
AULCSF	0.579	**0.012**	**0.018**

**The P-value of the correlation between the post alteration CSF parameters from baseline and the refractive error after adjusting the corresponding baseline CSF parameters. The bold values just means the P-value less than 0.05.*

sensitivity) is associated with the parvocellular pathway. While the precise mechanisms by which this cross-pathway effect is obtained are yet unclear, we speculate that the shape of the CSF curve, especially the peak spatial frequency and AULCSF, are jointly governed by the parvocellular and magnocellular pathways rather than by the former alone (Kaneko et al., 2015). Short-term perceivable high-frequency flicker may lead to adaptation of the magnocellular pathway and a corresponding reduction in its contribution to spatial CSF relative to that of the parvocellular pathway. This parvo-favoring imbalance may lead to improving the acuity of spatial vision (Kitterle and Beard, 1983; Zhuang et al., 2015). Prior work suggests that the interaction between the two pathways may take the form of suppression, with the magnocellular pathway exerting a suppressive influence on the parvocellular pathway under normal photopic conditions (Smith, 1971; Cass and Alais, 2006). Adaptation of the magnocellular pathway by the short-term perceivable high-frequency flicker may lift some of this

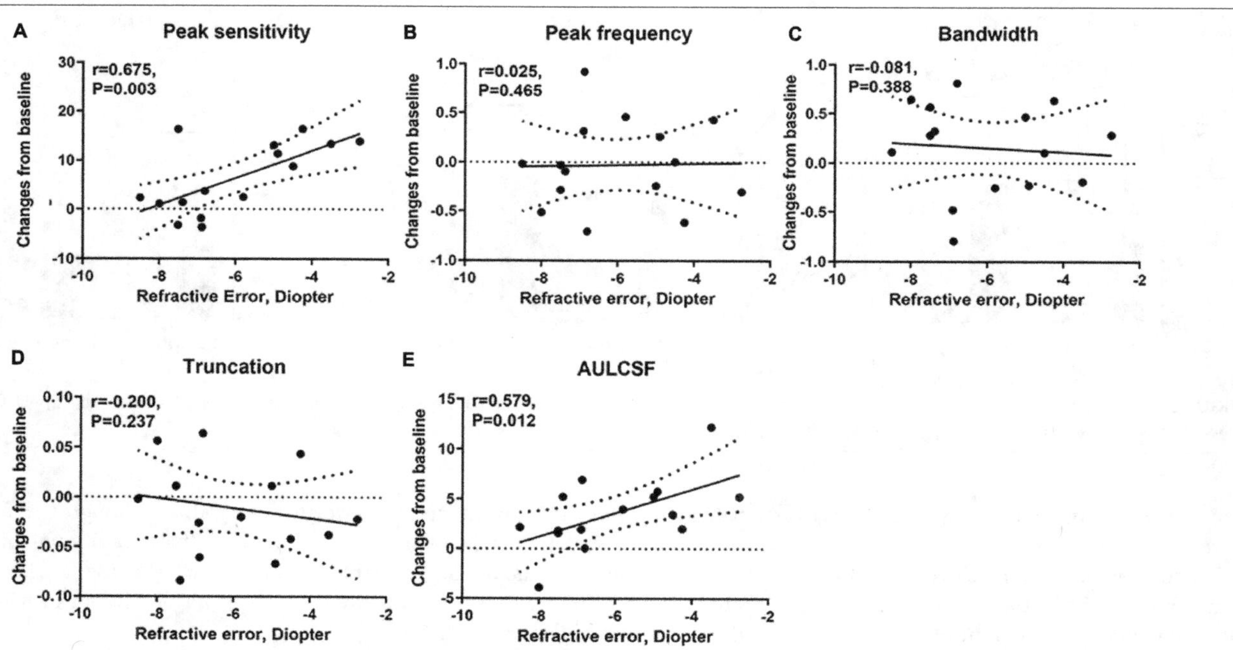

FIGURE 6 | The correlation of the changes in CSF parameters from baseline and refractive error in the experimental group. **(A)** The correlation of the changes in peak sensitivity from baseline and refractive error. **(B)** The correlation of the changes in peak frequency from baseline and refractive error. **(C)** The correlation of the changes in bandwidth from baseline and refractive error. **(D)** The correlation of the changes in truncation from baseline and refractive error. **(E)** The correlation of the changes in AULCSF from baseline and refractive error.

suppression of the parvocellular pathway, with a consequent improvement of high-spatial frequency visual perception.

One important doubt for us now is whether 0.5 cpd was low enough to be mainly within the purview of the magnocellular pathway, as the qCSF software in the current study measured CSF from 0.5 to 15.8 cpd. Previous study showed that after adaption to the flicker could knock out the transient channels, and then (by implication) reduce the sensitivity to low spatial frequencies (Kaneko et al., 2015), which might be different from the **Figure 3** curve in our study. Kaneko et al. (2015) considered the 3 cpd as the cutoff spatial frequency for the transient and sustained channels. While, past work suggested that in macaque monkeys, 2 cpd was still mainly modulated by parvocellular pathway (Merigan et al., 1991). In our previous study, we already found that the congenital cataract children with serious impaired spatial visual function but not temporal visual function were with peak sensitivity at around and even less than 0.5 cpd after surgery (Ye et al., 2021). Hence, the range of the spatial frequencies we measured in the current study might still be mainly subserved by the parvocellular pathway. We acknowledged the puzzlement regarding the observed differences in the contrast sensitivity at low and high spatial frequencies after flicker experience. We believe that future studies with larger sample sizes are needed to pursue this potentially interesting finding.

In the current study, subjects were asked to gaze at the full-field flicker stimulus without any specific accommodation stimuli. The data revealed that this effect was flicker-specific and not simply the outcome of prolonged light stimulation (Riddell, 1935; Ginsburg, 1966) since it was found to occur when subjects were exposed to a perceivable flicker but not a seemingly steady light (Riddell, 1935; Ginsburg, 1966). Additionally, the flicker effect was not related to the spatial extent of the stimuli (Zhuang et al., 2015). The flicker stimuli were much easier than pattern stimuli to be recognized (Kitterle and Beard, 1983). These results have implications for understanding spatial acuity outcomes following treatment for congenital cataracts. Severe congenital cataract patients have access to full-field flicker despite being unable to resolve any spatial forms. This temporal experience may facilitate the development of spatial function, and thus potentially account for the observed spatial acuity outcomes in such individuals (Kalia et al., 2014).

The mechanistic underpinnings for explaining the association between high-frequency flicker and myopia are yet unclear. At the same time, the perceptual learning produces roles in myopia is under popular discussion. It had been reported the perceptual learning with longer duration and even for several days would improve the visual function in myopia by improving neural procession (Camilleri et al., 2014, 2016; Yan et al., 2015). The flicker effect in our current study might not produce improvements comparable with those obtained with perceptual learning on visual function due to different mechanisms or short flicker duration. We still need to consider the underpinning of the flicker effect on myopia. In non-human animal models, it has been reported that deprivation and defocus induced myopia is inhibited by flicker of frequency 6 Hz or above (Gottlieb et al., 1991; Li et al., 2012). This may be because high-frequency flicker causes a hypermetropic shift, leads to hyperactivity of ganglion cells, and stimulates the release of DA from the retina, thereby reducing receptive field sizes, which may play a role in CSF, and even suppress myopic development (Shih et al., 1997; Crewther et al., 2006; Zhang et al., 2011). There may also be flicker-induced arrest of axial elongation and a corresponding reduction in myopic progression. Myopia has previously been shown to be strongly associated with axial elongation (Schwahn and Schaeffel, 1997; Read et al., 2010) perhaps as a consequence of the blurry retinal images with higher internal noise, especially during the near-work with accommodation lag (Yan et al., 2015). With the perceivable high-frequency flicker role on the improved spatial visual acuity, even might be with reduced internal noise, we speculated the effect of the axial elongation would be reduced. Interestingly, it has been reported that children with form-deprivation myopia induced by severe congenital cataracts do not exhibit large axial elongation, compared to age-matched normally sighted children to some extent (Kun et al., 2018). This axial elongation may be prevented by the access the children have to full-field flicker without the accompanying spatial signal that may, on its own, induce elongation. Although this potential link between flicker and myopia, through the intermediary of axial length deserves further exploration, its use as an explanatory mechanism for our results is probably potentially meaningful, given the rapidity with which flicker is found to alter spatial function.

Our results reveal that the effect of flicker on myopia is related to the degree of myopia. The higher the degree of myopia, the less the flicker effect on spatial visual function. What might account for this negative correlation? We offer a tentative hypothesis. High myopia might impact parvocellular and magnocellular pathways. The retinal nerve fiber layer (RNFL), the origination of the parvocellular and magnocellular pathways, is reported to be thinner in high myopia, especially in the peripheral area (Wang et al., 2018; Lee et al., 2019). This is especially evident in the RNFL of the magnocellular pathway in the peripheral retina. Hence, the significant decrease of RNFL thickness in high myopia might lead to a reduced sensitivity of the magnocellular pathway to flicker stimuli, which in turn reduces the pathway's impact on spatial function.

We note some limitations in our current study. Our sample size is modest, especially from the perspective of assessing correlations between CSF parameters and refractive error. Although previous psychophysical and neurophysiological studies have demonstrated the usefulness of small samples (Anderson and Vingrys, 2001), the current results need to be verified with larger cohort sizes for us to be able to repose confidence in their replicability. We have also not systematically varied the duration of the flicker exposure to probe how it modulates the impact on spatial CSF, though it had been reported that the contrast sensitivity alteration was unrelated to a further longer duration (Kitterle and Beard, 1983). The persistence of the results also needs further research to determine how long-lasting the effects are and how they are influenced by the duration of flicker exposure. Finally, future work can derive correlation values not just between dominant eye refractive error and CSF parameter change (as we have done here), but also non-dominant eye error, with both binocular and monocular CSF values. In this context, it is worth noting that the flicker effect is consistent between monocular and binocular presentations (Zhuang and Shevell, 2015).

In summary, we have found that perceivable high-frequency flicker enhances the acuity of spatial vision in myopic individuals, and this enhancement is negatively correlated with the degree of myopia. The mechanisms underlying this influence are not definitively established yet, but may involve reduced suppressive interactions between magnocellular and parvocellular pathways and, over longer timescales, arrest of axial elongation by flicker. If these results are corroborated in future studies with more participants, we expect them to have important implications for the design of interventions of cases of moderate myopia.

AUTHOR CONTRIBUTIONS

JY, PS, and FL contributed to the conception and design of the study. JY and FH determined the experimental methods. JY performed the experiments. JY and XH analyzed and interpreted the data. JY, MS, and YS wrote and modified the manuscript. All authors contributed to manuscript revision, read, and approved the submitted version.

REFERENCES

Anderson, A. J., and Vingrys, A. J. (2001). Small samples: does size matter? *Invest. Ophthalmol. Vis. Sci.* 42, 1411–1413.

Arnold, D. H., Williams, J. D., Phipps, N. E., and Goodale, M. A. (2016). Sharpening vision by adapting to flicker. *Proc. Natl. Acad. Sci. U.S.A.* 113, 12556–12561. doi: 10.1073/pnas.1609330113

Breitmeyer, B. G., and Ganz, L. (1977). Temporal studies with flashed gratings: inferences about human transient and sustained channels. *Vis. Res.* 17, 861–865. doi: 10.1016/0042-6989(77)90130-4

Burr, D. C., and Ross, J. (1982). Contrast sensitivity at high velocities. *Vis. Res.* 22, 479–484. doi: 10.1016/0042-6989(82)90196-1

Camilleri, R., Pavan, A., and Campana, G. (2016). The application of online transcranial random noise stimulation and perceptual learning in the improvement of visual functions in mild myopia. *Neuropsychologia* 89, 225–231. doi: 10.1016/j.neuropsychologia.2016.06.024

Camilleri, R., Pavan, A., Ghin, F., and Campana, G. (2014). Improving myopia via perceptual learning: is training with lateral masking the only (or the most) efficacious technique? *Atten. Percept. Psychophys.* 76, 2485–2494. doi: 10.3758/s13414-014-0738-8

Cass, J., and Alais, D. (2006). Evidence for two interacting temporal channels in human visual processing. *Vis. Res.* 46, 2859–2868.

Crewther, S. G., Barutchu, A., Murphy, M. J., and Crewther, D. P. (2006). Low frequency temporal modulation of light promotes a myopic shift in refractive compensation to all spectacle lenses. *Exp. Eye Res.* 83, 322–328. doi: 10.1016/j.exer.2005.12.016

Geisler, W. S., Albrecht, D. G., Crane, A. M., and Stern, L. (2001). Motion direction signals in the primary visual cortex of cat and monkey. *Vis. Neurosci.* 18, 501–516. doi: 10.1017/s0952523801184014

Ginsburg, N. (1966). Local adaptation to intermittent light as a function of frequency and eccentricity. *Am. J. Psychol.* 79, 296–300.

Gottlieb, M. D., Marran, L., Xu, A. M., Nickla, D. L., and Wallman, J. (1991). The EMM etropization process in chicks is compromised by dim light. *Invest. Ophthalmol. Vis. Sci.* 32:1203.

Hashemi, H., Khabazkhoob, M., Jafarzadehpur, E., Emamian, M. H., Shariati, M., and Fotouhi, A. (2012). Contrast sensitivity evaluation in a population-based study in Shahroud. *Iran. Ophthalmol.* 119, 541–546. doi: 10.1016/j.ophtha.2011.08.030

Hughes, R. P. J., and Read, S. A. (2020). Changes in ocular biometry during short-term accommodation in children. *Ophthal. Physiol. Opt.* 40, 584–594. doi: 10.1111/opo.12711

Kalia, A., Lesmes, L. A., Dorr, M., Gandhi, T., Chatterjee, G., Ganesh, S., et al. (2014). Development of pattern vision following early and extended blindness. *Proc. Natl. Acad. Sci. U.S.A.* 111, 2035–2039. doi: 10.1073/pnas.1311041111

Kaneko, S., Giaschi, D., and Anstis, S. (2015). Flicker adaptation or superimposition raises the apparent spatial frequency of coarse test gratings. *Vis. Res.* 108, 85–92. doi: 10.1016/j.visres.2015.01.005

Kitterle, F. L., and Beard, B. L. (1983). The effects of flicker adaptation upon temporal contrast enhancement. *Percept. Psychophys.* 33, 75–78. doi: 10.3758/bf03205868

Kun, L., Szigeti, A., Bausz, M., Nagy, Z. Z., and Maka, E. (2018). Preoperative biometry data of eyes with unilateral congenital cataract. *J. Cataract. Refract. Surg.* 44, 1198–1202. doi: 10.1016/j.jcrs.2018.06.054

Lee, B. B., Pokorny, J., Smith, V. C., Martin, P. R., and Valberg, A. (1990). Luminance and chromatic modulation sensitivity of macaque ganglion cells and human observers. *J. Opt. Soc. Am. A* 7, 2223–2236. doi: 10.1364/josaa.7.002223

Lee, M. W., Kim, J. M., Shin, Y. I., Jo, Y. J., and Kim, J. Y. (2019). Longitudinal changes in peripapillary retinal nerve fiber layer thickness in high myopia: a prospective, observational study. *Ophthalmology* 126, 522–528. doi: 10.1016/j.ophtha.2018.07.007

Legge, G. E. (1978). Sustained and transient mechanisms in human vision: temporal and spatial properties. *Vis. Res.* 18, 69–81. doi: 10.1016/0042-6989(78)90079-2

Li, S., Wu, J., Ding, H., Liao, A., He, H., Stell, W. K., et al. (2012). Flicker downregulates the content of crystallin proteins in form-deprived C57BL/6 mouse retina. *Exp. Eye Res.* 101, 1–8. doi: 10.1016/j.exer.2012.05.003

Livingstone, M. S., and Hubel, D. H. (1987). Psychophysical evidence for separate channels for the perception of form, color, movement, and depth. *J. Neurosci.* 7, 3416–3468. doi: 10.1523/jneurosci.07-11-03416.1987

Merigan, W. H., Katz, L. M., and Maunsell, J. H. (1991). The effects of parvocellular lateral geniculate lesions on the acuity and contrast sensitivity of macaque monkeys. *J. Neurosci.* 11, 994–1001. doi: 10.1523/JNEUROSCI.11-04-00994.1991

Oen, F. T., Lim, T. H., and Chung, M. P. (1994). Contrast sensitivity in a large adult population. *Ann. Acad. Med. Singap.* 23, 322–326.

Ohno-Matsui, K., Lai, T. Y., Lai, C. C., and Cheung, C. M. (2016). Updates of pathologic myopia. *Prog. Retin. Eye Res.* 52, 156–187. doi: 10.1016/j.preteyeres.2015.12.001

Purves, D., Augustine, G. J., Fitzpatrick, D., Hall, W. C., Lamantia, A. S., Mcnamara, J. O., et al. (2001). *Neuroscience*. Sunderland: Sinauer Associates.

Read, S. A., Collins, M. J., and Sander, B. P. (2010). Human optical axial length and defocus. *Invest. Ophthalmol. Vis. Sci.* 51, 6262–6269. doi: 10.1167/iovs.10-5457

Riddell, L. A. (1935). Local adaptation to flicker and its relation to light adaptation. *J. Physiol.* 84, 111–120. doi: 10.1113/jphysiol.1935.sp003260

Schwahn, H. N., and Schaeffel, F. (1997). Flicker parameters are different for suppression of myopia and hyperopia. *Vis. Res.* 37, 2661–2673. doi: 10.1016/s0042-6989(97)00114-4

Seijas, O., Gómez de Liaño, P., Gómez de Liaño, R., Roberts, C. J., Piedrahita, E., and Diaz, E. (2007). Ocular dominance diagnosis and its influence in monovision. *Am. J. Ophthalmol.* 144, 209–216. doi: 10.1016/j.ajo.2007.03.053

Shih, Y. F., Lin, S. Y., Huang, J. K., Jian, S. W., Lin, L. L., and Hung, P. T. (1997). The choroidal blood flow response after flicker stimulation in chicks. *J. Ocul. Pharmacol. Ther.* 13, 213–218. doi: 10.1089/jop.1997.13.213

Smith, R. A. Jr. (1971). Studies of temporal frequency adaptation in visual contrast sensitivity. *J. Physiol.* 216, 531–552. doi: 10.1113/jphysiol.1971.sp009539

Wang, C. Y., Zheng, Y. F., Liu, B., Meng, Z. W., Hong, F., Wang, X. X., et al. (2018). Retinal nerve fiber layer thickness in children: the gobi desert children eye study. *Invest. Ophthalmol. Vis. Sci.* 59, 5285–5291. doi: 10.1167/iovs.18-25418

Wong, T. Y., Ferreira, A., Hughes, R., Carter, G., and Mitchell, P. (2014). Epidemiology and disease burden of pathologic myopia and myopic choroidal neovascularization: an evidence-based systematic review. *Am. J. Ophthalmol.* 157, 9–25. doi: 10.1016/j.ajo.2013.08.010

Woodman, E. C., Read, S. A., Collins, M. J., Hegarty, K. J., Priddle, S. B., Smith, J. M., et al. (2011). Axial elongation following prolonged near work in myopes and emmetropes. *Br. J. Ophthalmol.* 95, 652–656. doi: 10.1136/bjo.2010.180323

Yan, F. F., Zhou, J., Zhao, W., Li, M., Xi, J., Lu, Z. L., et al. (2015). Perceptual learning improves neural processing in myopic vision. *J. Vis.* 15:12. doi: 10.1167/15.10.12

Ye, J., Gupta, P., Shah, P., Tiwari, K., Gandhi, T., Ganesh, S., et al. (2021). Resilience of temporal processing to early and extended visual deprivation. *Vis. Res.* 186, 80–86. doi: 10.1016/j.visres.2021.05.004

Zhang, A. J., Jacoby, R., and Wu, S. M. (2011). Light- and dopamine-regulated receptive field plasticity in primate horizontal cells. *J. Comp. Neurol.* 519, 2125–2134. doi: 10.1002/cne.22604

Zheng, H., Shen, M., He, X., Cui, R., Lesmes, L. A., Lu, Z. L., et al. (2019). Comparing spatial contrast sensitivity functions measured with digit and grating stimuli. *Transl. Vis. Sci. Technol.* 8:16. doi: 10.1167/tvst.8.6.16

Zheng, H., Wang, C., Cui, R., He, X., Shen, M., Lesmes, L. A., et al. (2018). Measuring the contrast sensitivity function using the qCSF method with 10 digits. *Transl. Vis. Sci. Technol.* 7:9. doi: 10.1167/tvst.7.6.9

Zhuang, X., Pokorny, J., and Cao, D. (2015). Flicker adaptation desensitizes the magnocellular but not the parvocellular pathway. *Invest. Ophthalmol. Vis. Sci.* 56, 2901–2908. doi: 10.1167/iovs.14-16067

Zhuang, X., and Shevell, S. K. (2015). Monocular and binocular mechanisms mediating flicker adaptation. *Vis. Res.* 117, 41–48. doi: 10.1016/j.visres.2015.08.020

20

Cataract Surgery in Dry Eye Disease: Visual Outcomes and Complications

Pragnya R. Donthineni[1], *Anthony V. Das*[2], *Swapna S. Shanbhag*[1] *and Sayan Basu*[1,3*]

[1] The Cornea Institute, L V Prasad Eye Institute, Hyderabad, India, [2] Department of eyeSmart EMR & AEye, L V Prasad Eye Institute, Hyderabad, India, [3] Center for Ocular Regeneration (CORE), L V Prasad Eye Institute, Hyderabad, India

***Correspondence:**
Sayan Basu
sayanbasu@lvpei.org

Purpose: To describe the visual outcomes and complications following cataract surgery in dry eye disease (DED).

Methods: This retrospective study included 668 eyes of 399 patients with DED, who underwent cataract surgery between 2011 and 2019 at our multi-tier ophthalmology hospital network. Based on etiology, they were divided into three groups: cicatrizing conjunctivitis (CC), meibomian gland dysfunction (MGD), and Sjogren's syndrome (SS). The data on demographics, visual impairment, surgical technique, visual outcomes, and complications were collected using an electronic medical record system. Median LogMAR best corrected visual acuity (BCVA) with interquartile range (IQR) was compared using Wilcoxon's rank sum test.

Results: The median age at which cataract surgery was performed was 58 (IQR: 47–65) years. Etiology of DED was CC in 279, MGD in 255, and SS in 134 eyes. Most (471) eyes underwent phacoemulsification, under peribulbar anesthesia (548) through a temporal clear corneal incision (209) with foldable intraocular lens implantation (417). The overall median LogMAR BCVA improved from 1.1 (IQR: 0.6–2.1) at baseline to 0.3 (IQR: 0.1–0.7) and 0.1 (IQR: 0–0.65) at 1 and 6 weeks ($p < 0.0001$) post-operatively. The median 6 weeks post-operative BCVA was 0.3, 0.1, and 0.1 in CC, MGD, and SS, respectively, and significantly better than at baseline ($p < 0.0001$). The leading cause of sub-optimal vision was corneal scarring (44; 9%), and the most common complication was posterior capsular rupture with vitreous loss (23; 3%).

Conclusion: Cataract surgery has good visual outcomes in patients with DED, without any disconcerting rate of complications. Pre-existing keratopathy is the main determinant of the extent of post-operative visual recovery.

Keywords: dry eye disease (DED), cataract surgery, Stevens–Johnson syndrome (SJS), Sjogren's syndrome, electronic medical records (EMR)

INTRODUCTION

Dry eye disease (DED) comprises a spectrum of disorders which cause tear film instability, hyperosmolarity, chronic inflammation, and neurosensory abnormalities, all of which lead to chronic ocular surface dysfunction (1). In addition to causing keratopathy, preexisting DED poses challenges during cataract surgery, especially in the presence of chronic inflammation, cicatrizing changes, lid abnormalities, and compromised media clarity (2).

It is also known to worsen following cataract surgery leading to a higher rate of complications and compromised visual outcomes (3–6). This is probably due to increased inflammation, toxicity from eye drops containing preservatives like benzalkonium chloride (BAK), and corneal nerve damage from limbal incisions. Besides, phacoemulsification, by itself, has been reported to cause a reduction in tear film breakup time, tear meniscus height, and corneal sensitivity post-operatively (7).

Studies done in larger cohorts in India have reported an increased incidence of DED with age, which is also the pattern seen with cataract (8, 9). It is hence not uncommon to encounter situations where we need to either simultaneously or sequentially manage both dry eye and cataract. In order to achieve successful results, the need to understand the various factors governing the outcomes of cataract surgery in eyes with pre-existing DED cannot be overemphasized. Most studies in the existing literature have looked at outcomes of cataract surgery in specific disorders causing severe DED in smaller cohorts (10–12). Thus, in the current study, the authors have attempted to study the etiology-based visual outcomes and complications of cataract surgery in a larger cohort of patients with DED.

MATERIALS AND METHODS

Study Design, Period, Location, and Approval

This was a retrospective study that included 668 eyes of 399 patients diagnosed with dry eye disease who underwent cataract surgery between August 2010 and May 2019 at a multi-tier ophthalmology hospital network in India (13). The study was approved by the Institutional Ethics Committee and adhered to the Declaration of Helsinki. A standard consent form including consent for electronic data privacy was obtained from all the patients. The clinical data of each patient who underwent a comprehensive ophthalmic examination was entered into a browser-based electronic medical records system (eyeSmart EMR) by uniformly trained ophthalmic personnel and supervised by an ophthalmologist using a standardized template (14).

Cases, Data Retrieval, and Classification

The eyeSmart EMR was screened for patients with symptoms, signs, referral, or final diagnosis or management suggestive of DED. The detailed process of identifying patients with a diagnosis of DED has been described (8). Among these patients, only those with both symptoms and signs of DED were included in the study as per the recommendations of the tear film and ocular surface dry eye workshop (TFOS DEWS) II (15). Complaints of dryness, grittiness, irritation, foreign body sensation, or discomfort, not associated with severe pain, sudden vision loss, itching, discharge or signs of allergy, contact lens wear, or recent systemic infection were considered positive for DED symptoms. Those with fluorescein breakup time (FBUT) <10 s, corneal fluorescein staining of >5 spots, Schirmer's test $I \leq 10$ mm/5 min, abnormal meibomian gland function (poor expressibility, blockage, or atrophy) were considered as positive for signs of DED.

Among these patients with preexisting DED, those who underwent cataract surgery during the study period were included in this study. These patients were classified into evaporative dry eye disease (MGD) and aqueous deficiency dry eye (ADDE) based on TFOS DEWS II classification (15). All the patients with ADDE underwent an evaluation by the internist to diagnose the underlying systemic association. Based on etiology, they were further divided into three groups as (i) meibomian gland dysfunction (MGD), (ii) Sjogren's syndrome (SS), and (iii) cicatrizing conjunctivitis (CC). Those with systemic examination and serology suggestive of Sjogren's syndrome (primary or secondary) were included in group SS. All patients of ADDE with signs of conjunctival cicatrization were diagnosed and included into CC group based on an algorithmic approach including a detailed history, clinical examination, and diagnostic workup that has been described (16, 17). The data on age, gender, best corrected visual acuity (BCVA) at presentation, type of cataract surgery performed, complications, and post-operative BCVA at 1 and 6 weeks were documented and extracted using the eyeSmart EMR. The main outcome measures considered were post-operative distance BCVA as per WHO guidelines (18) and the rate and type of complication post-cataract surgery.

Interventions and Post-operative Follow-Up

All the patients were taken up for cataract surgery after optimization of the ocular surface. The standard criteria considered to decide on the type of anesthesia were (i) age of the patient, (ii) patient cooperation, (iii) pupillary dilatation, (iv) corneal clarity, (v) ability to tolerate microscopic light (vi), grade of cataract, and (vii) presence of symblepharon. In cooperative patients with good media clarity and pupillary dilatation, topical anesthesia was administered. Peribulbar blocks were administered in patients with compromised media clarity, poor pupillary dilatation, inability to cooperate, hard cataracts, and when long surgical time was anticipated. A mixture of 4–5 mL lidocaine hydrochloride (2%) and 2–3 mL bupivacaine hydrochloride (0.5%) were used for peribulbar injection. Intraocular lens (IOL) power calculation was done using laser interferometric biometry (LENSTAR). Keratometry (K) readings from corneal topography were used in case of steep corneas, and standard K readings were used when they could not be captured. The cases with advanced keratopathy, who were already scleral contact lens users with unreliable keratometry and IOL power calculation, were left aphakic, and the residual refractive error was subsequently incorporated into the scleral contact lens.

Abbreviations: DED, dry eye disease; BAK, benzalkonium chloride; EMR, electronic medical record system; FBUT, fluorescein breakup time; MGD, meibomian gland disease; SS, Sjogren's syndrome; CC, chronic cicatrizing conjunctivitis; BCVA, best corrected visual acuity; WHO, World Health Organization; K, keratometry readings; HPMC, hydroxy-propyl methylcellulose; PMMA, Polymethyl methacrylate; BCL, bandage contact lens; IQR, inter-quartile range; SJS, Stevens-Johnson syndrome; OCP, ocular cicatricial pemphigoid; GVHD, graft-versus-host disease; MSICS, manual small incision cataract surgery; ECCE, extracapsular cataract extraction; ICCE, intracapsular cataract extraction; PCR, posterior capsular rupture; DMD, Descemet's membrane detachment; ZD, zonular dialysis; IOL, intraocular lens; NSAID, non-steroidal anti-inflammatory drugs; NITBUT, non-invasive tear breakup time.

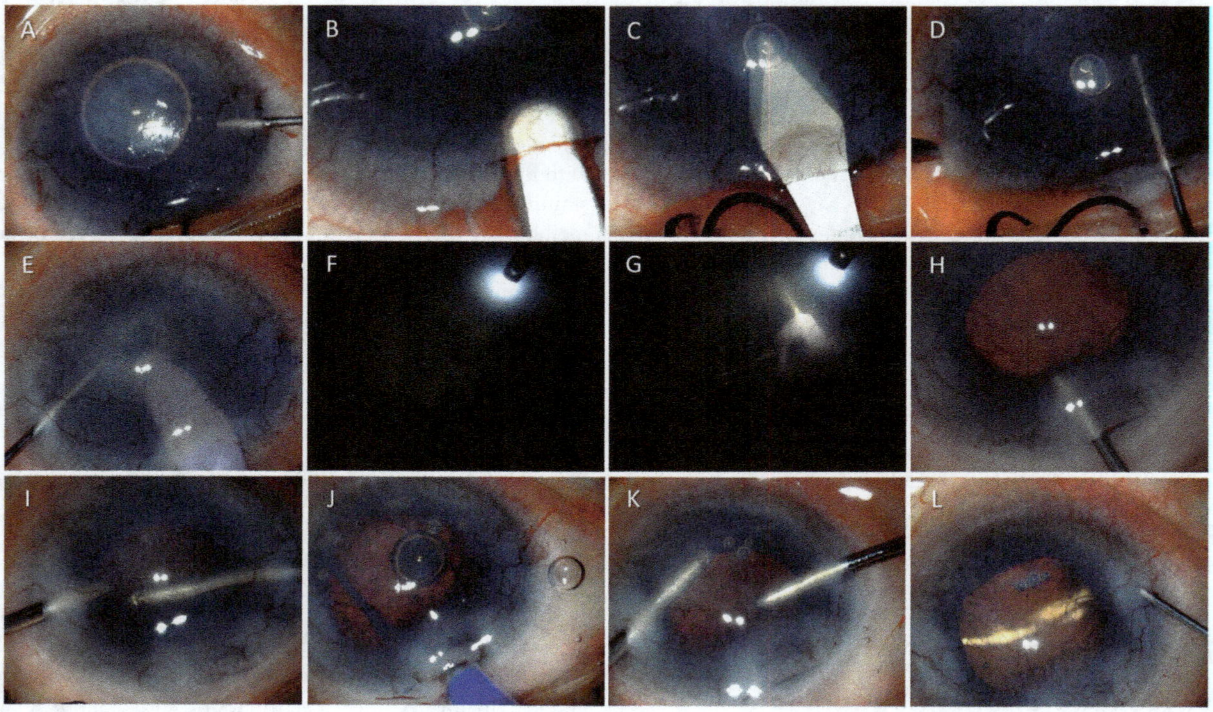

FIGURE 1 | Surgical technique of phacoemulsification in a case of dry eye disease due to ocular cicatrizing pemphigoid. The figure shows serial photomicrographs demonstrating the steps of cataract surgery in a 54-year-old patient with ocular cicatrizing pemphigoid (OCP). Image **(A)** shows injection of Trypan blue through a paracentesis at 10 o'clock position during cataract surgery to enhance visualization of the anterior capsule, followed by a 2.8 mm superior clear corneal incision using a crescent blade **(B)** and anterior chamber entry using a 2.8 mm keratome knife **(C)**. Continuous curvilinear capsulorhexis is being performed using a cystitome **(D)** followed by nucleus management using stop and chop technique **(E)** under endoilluminator assistance **(F)** and **(G)**. Image **(H)** shows injection of viscoelastic into the anterior chamber and clear visualization of the posterior capsule under retro illumination. The bottom row shows cortical aspiration using a bimanual irrigation aspiration cannula **(I)**, foldable intraocular lens implantation **(J)**, and removal of viscoelastic from the anterior chamber **(K)** prior to wound hydration and closure **(L)**.

Prior to surgery, povidone iodine (5%) was used to disinfect conjunctiva and the skin around the eye. Phacoemulsification was performed in eyes with adequate media clarity, good pupillary dilatation, and even in eyes with moderate to severe keratopathy with the assistance of an endoilluminator (**Figure 1**). In eyes with significant corneal scarring, hard cataracts, significant symblepharon, a manual small incision cataract surgery (MSICS) with Blumenthal technique was performed. Extracapsular cataract extraction (ECCE) was performed in eyes with very poor media clarity. Scleral incisions were taken in eyes with peripheral corneal thinning and temporal approach and lateral canthotomy, or lid sutures were taken in cases with poor exposure. Special intraoperative precautions for dry eyes like (i) liberal application of dispersive viscoelastic in the form of 2% hydroxy-propyl methylcellulose (HPMC) on the ocular surface, after speculum application and throughout surgery, (ii) incisions avoiding areas of corneal scarring and thinning, (iii) coaxial illumination/red reflex enhancer, (iv) use of trypan blue (0.06%) for capsulorhexis, and (v) therapeutic bandage contact lens (BCL) at the end of the surgery (which was removed at 1 week) were undertaken based on the severity of keratopathy due to DED. Wound closure was done in all cases with irregular or thin corneas with interrupted 10-0 monofilament nylon sutures.

Post-operative regimen included prednisolone acetate (1%) eye drops six times a day, tapered by one drop each week for 6 weeks, and moxifloxacin hydrochloride (0.5%) four times a day for 1 week. Other medications like topical lubricants, cyclosporine, and systemic medications that were being used pre-operatively were continued. Patients were seen on post-operative day 1, week 1, and 6 weeks.

Statistical Analysis

Descriptive statistics using mean (± standard deviation) and median with inter-quartile range (IQR) were used to elucidate the demographic data. All tables for age, gender, etiological diagnosis, and outcomes were drawn and analyzed using Microsoft Excel (Microsoft Corporation, Redmond, USA). Median distance LogMAR BCVA with IQR was calculated for each group and post-operative visit and compared using Wilcoxon's signed-rank test for paired samples.

RESULTS

Demographics and Etiology of DED

The median age of DED patients undergoing cataract surgery was 58 years (IQR: 47–65). Among the 399 cases, 265 (66.42%)

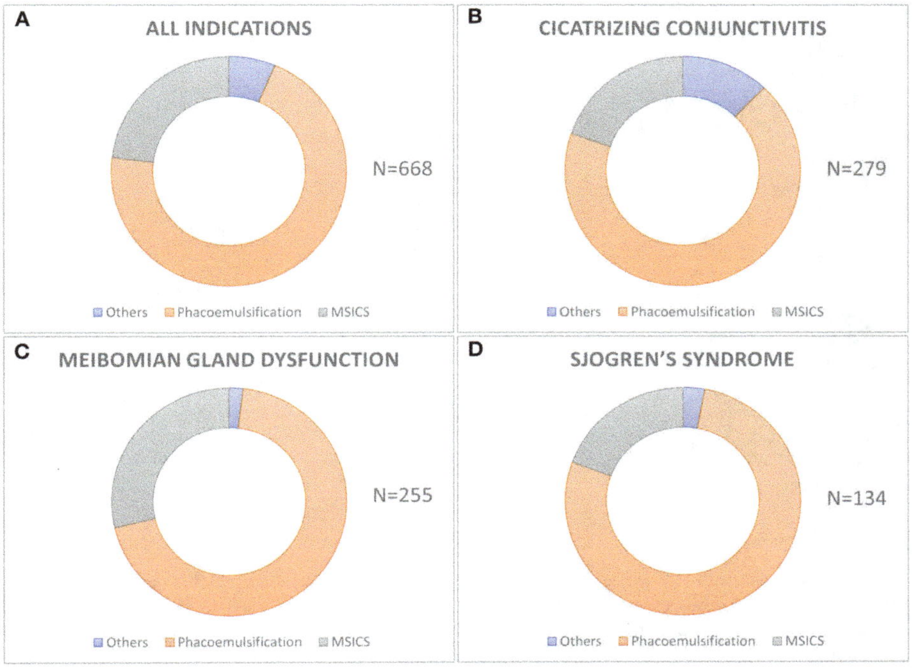

FIGURE 2 | Techniques of cataract surgery used in different etiologies of dry eye disease. The donut graph shows the distribution of various techniques of cataract surgery in the entire cohort **(A)** and in different etiologies of dry eye like cicatrizing conjunctivitis **(B)**, meibomian gland disease **(C)**, and Sjogren's syndrome **(D)**. Phacoemulsification is the most common technique of cataract surgery performed in all the three groups and also in the entire cohort.

and 134 (33.58%) were females and males, respectively. Of the 668 eyes included in the study, CC was the most common cause of DED seen in 279 (41.77%) eyes followed by MGD and SS, which were seen in 255 (38.17%) and 134 (20.06%) eyes, respectively. Of the 279 eyes with CC, Stevens–Johnson syndrome (SJS) was the leading cause seen in 209 (31.29%) eyes followed by ocular cicatricial pemphigoid (OCP) and graft-versus-host disease (GVHD) in 59 (8.8%) and 1 (0.15%) eye. The cause of cicatrization was unknown in 10 (1.5%) eyes. Among the 134 (20.06%) eyes with SS, primary and secondary SS was diagnosed in 19 (2.84%) and 115 (17.22%) eyes, respectively.

Technique and Details of Cataract Surgery

Of the 668 eyes, phacoemulsification was the most common surgical procedure performed in 471 (70.5%) eyes followed by manual small incision cataract surgery (MSICS) in 154 (23.05%), extracapsular cataract extraction (ECCE) in 42 (6.3%), and intracapsular cataract extraction (ICCE) in 1 (0.15%) eye (**Figure 2**). Peribulbar anesthesia was used in 548 (82.04%), topical in 105 (15.87%), and general anesthesia was required in 14 (2.1%) cases. Of the 471 eyes which underwent phacoemulsification, it was performed through a 2.8 mm clear corneal incision in 304 (64.5%; 209/68.75% of which were temporal), limbal incision in 35 (7.4%), and scleral incision in 132 (28.1%) eyes, while all MSICS and ECCE surgeries were done through (5–8 mm) superior scleral incisions. A continuous curvilinear capsulotomy was used in 512 (76.65%, 6/1.2% of which were femtosecond laser-assisted), can-opener in 151 (22.6%), and envelope in 5 (0.75%) eyes. The nucleotomy technique in 471 eyes undergoing phacoemulsification was stop and chop in 257 (54.6%), direct vertical chop in 121 (25.7%), divide and conquer in 36 (7.64%), phaco-aspiration in 51 (10.8%), chip and flip in 3 (0.63%), and phaco plow in 3 (0.63%). All MSICS surgeries were performed using the Blumenthal technique. The irrigating solution used was ringer lactate in 493 (73.8%) and balanced salt solution in 175 (26.2%) eyes. The intra-ocular visco-surgical devices used were 2% hydroxy-propyl methylcellulose (HPMC) in 552 (82.63%) eyes and hyaluronic acid 10 mg/mL in the remaining 116 (17.37%) eyes. There were 44 (6.5%) eyes that were left aphakic, while 417 (62.43%) eyes were implanted with a foldable acrylic IOL, and 207 (30.99%) eyes had a rigid Polymethyl methacrylate (PMMA) IOL implanted. Among the 417 eyes with foldable acrylic IOLs implanted, 374 were non-aspheric monofocal (89.7%), 25 (5.99%) were aspheric monofocal, 14 (3.36%) were aspheric multifocal, 2 (0.48%) were aspheric toric, and 2 (0.48%) were aspheric toric-multifocals.

Visual Outcomes

The overall median pre-operative LogMAR BCVA was 1.1 (IQR: 0.6–2.1). The BCVA improved to a median of 0.3 (IQR: 0.1–0.7) at post-operative 1 week (**Figure 3**). Further improvement was seen at the final post-operative visit at 6 weeks (**Figure 3**), with a median of 0.1 (IQR: 0–0.65). To put this in Snellen equivalents, the overall median BCVA

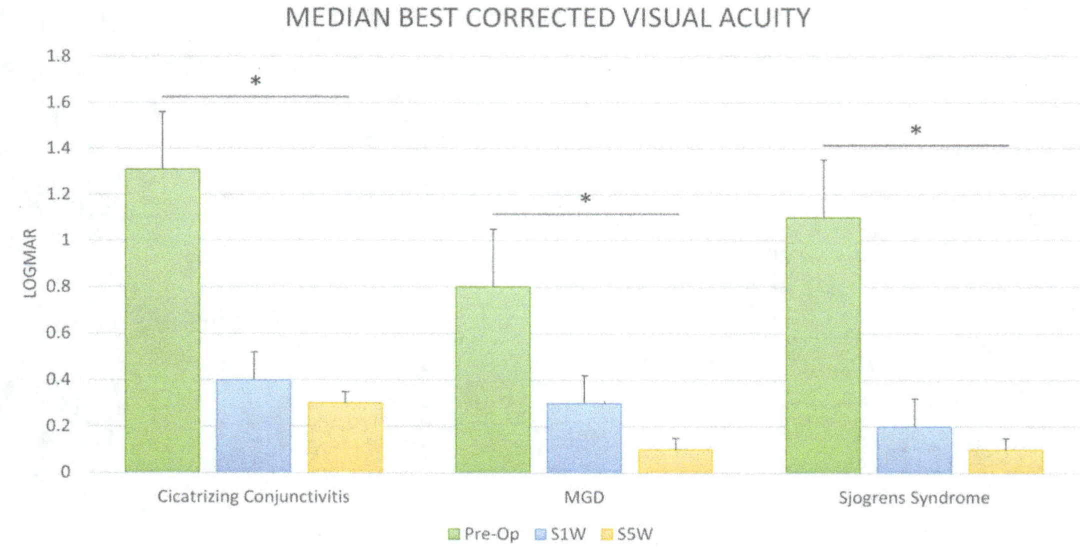

FIGURE 3 | Visual outcomes after cataract surgery in dry eye disease. The bar diagram shows the median LogMAR corrected distance visual acuity (BCVA) prior to cataract surgery (Pre-op) and at 1 (S1W) and 6 weeks (S6W) post-surgery in cicatrizing conjunctivitis (CC), meibomian gland disease (MGD), and Sjogren's syndrome (SS). The visual improvement was significant and gradually increased up to 6 weeks post-surgery from baseline in all the three groups. *Statistically significant difference (Wilcoxon's signed-rank test).

improved from 20/250 pre-operatively to 20/25 at 6 weeks post-operatively ($p < 0.0001$).

Complications

Surgical complications occurred in 43 (6.44%) of the 668 eyes (**Figure 4**). Intra-operative complications included posterior capsular rupture (PCR) with vitreous loss in 23 (3.44%), zonular dehiscence (ZD) in 4 (0.6%), and iridodialysis in 2 (0.3%) eyes. Post-operative complications included Descemet's membrane detachment (DMD) in 6 (0.9%), wound dehiscence/leakage in 4 (0.6%), corneal epithelial defect in 2 (0.3%), and intraocular lens (IOL) malposition in 2 (0.3%) eyes. There were no cases of immediate or late onset surgical site infection or endophthalmitis noted in this cohort.

Causes of Sub-optimal Visual Recovery

Of the 668 eyes that underwent cataract surgery, low vision (≤20/80) was seen in 61 (9.13%) eyes, all of which were related to keratopathy. The most common cause was preexisting corneal scarring in 44 (72.13%) eyes followed by corneal decompensation, epithelial irregularities, keratinization of the corneal surface, and corneal vascularization seen in 5 (8.2%), 4 (6.56%), 2 (3.28%), and 1 (1.63%) eye, respectively. The cause for low vision was not discernable in 5 (8.2%) eyes.

Cicatrizing Conjunctivitis ($n = 279$)

Phacoemulsification was the most common surgical procedure, performed in 190 (68.1%) eyes, followed by MSICS in 55 (19.71%), ECCE in 33 (11.83%), and ICCE in 1 (0.36%) case. The median pre-operative LogMAR BCVA was 1.31 (IQR: 0.8–2.8). The median LogMAR BCVA at post-operative 1 week was 0.4 (IQR: 0.1–1) and at 6 weeks post-operative was 0.3 (IQR: 0–1). To put this in Snellen equivalents, the overall median BCVA improved from 20/400 pre-operatively to 20/40 at 6 weeks post-operatively ($p < 0.0001$). Surgical complications were encountered in 22 (7.89%) eyes. PCR with vitreous loss was the most common complication seen in 13 (4.65%) eyes followed by wound dehiscence, DMD, ZD, IOL malposition, and iridodialysis seen in 3 (1.08%), 2 (0.72%), 2 (0.72%), 1(0.36%), and 1(0.36) eyes, respectively.

Meibomian Gland Dysfunction ($n = 255$)

Phacoemulsification was the most common surgical procedure performed in 177 (69.4%) eyes followed by MSICS in 73 (28.63%) and ECCE in 5 (1.96%) cases. The median pre-operative LogMAR BCVA was 0.8 (IQR: 0.5–1.5). The corresponding median LogMAR BCVA at post-operative 1 week was 0.3 (IQR: 0.1–0.6), and that at surgical 6 weeks was 0.1 (IQR: 0–0.3). To put this in Snellen equivalents, the overall median BCVA improved from 20/125 pre-operatively to 20/25 at 6 weeks post-operatively ($p < 0.0001$). The surgical complications were encountered in 17 (6.67%) eyes. PCR with vitreous loss was the most common complication seen in 7 (2.74%) eyes followed by DMD, corneal epithelial defect, wound dehiscence, ZD, IOL malposition, and iridodialysis seen in 3 (1.18%), 2 (0.78%), 2 (0.78%), 1 (0.36%), 1 (0.36%), and 1 (0.36) eyes, respectively.

Sjogren's Syndrome ($n = 134$)

Phacoemulsification was the most common surgical procedure performed in 104 (77.61%) eyes followed by MSICS in 26 (19.4%) and ECCE in 4 (2.99%) cases. The median pre-operative

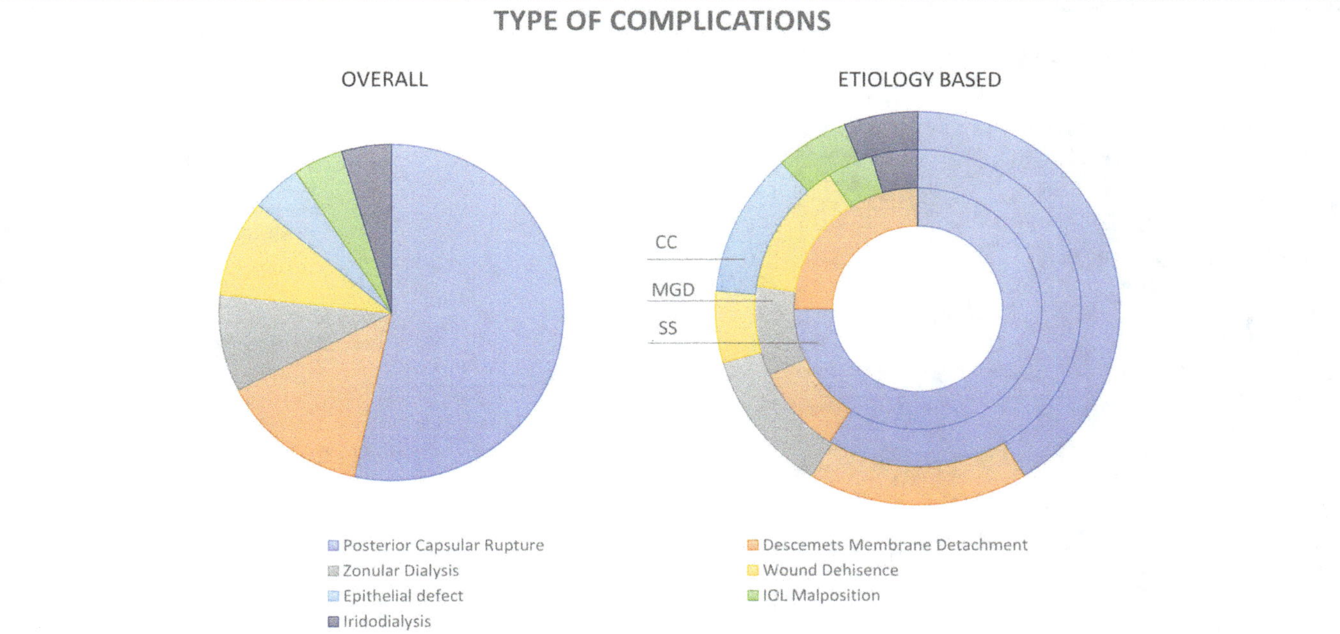

FIGURE 4 | Complications of cataract surgery in dry eye disease. Pie diagram showing the distribution of various types of complications in the entire study cohort (image on the left). The distribution within the groups; i.e., cicatrizing conjunctivitis (CC), meibomian gland dysfunction (MGD), and Sjogren's syndrome (SS) are depicted in the donut graph (image to the right).

LogMAR BCVA was 1.1 (IQR: 0.65–1.9). The median LogMAR BCVA at post-operative 1 week was 0.2 (IQR: 0–0.5) and at post-operative 6-weeks was 0.1 (IQR: 0–0.4). To put this in Snellen equivalents, the overall median BCVA improved from 20/250 pre-operatively to 20/25 at 6 weeks post-operatively ($p < 0.0001$). The surgical complications were encountered in 4 (2.98%) eyes. PCR with vitreous loss was the most common complication seen in 3 (2.24%) eyes followed by DMD seen in 1 (0.75%) eye.

DISCUSSION

In the presence of DED, where there is loss of homeostasis with a hostile environment, an otherwise routinely performed intervention like cataract surgery becomes quite challenging (19). Thus, in the current study the authors aimed to look at the etiology-based visual outcomes and complications following cataract surgery in eyes with preexisting DED. This study found that overall, the visual outcomes of cataract surgery, irrespective of the etiology of DED, were good and without any alarming rate of post-operative complications. All cases of sub-optimal visual recovery had some degree of keratopathy, particularly corneal scarring, although the degree of keratopathy could not be quantified and correlated with the visual outcomes.

The mean age at which patients with DED underwent cataract surgery was found to be 55 years, which was much early as compared to 70–75 years reported for most routine cataract surgeries (20–22). This is not surprising and is because of associated chronic inflammation, long-term and/or frequent use of topical or even systemic steroids, early presentation due to keratopathy, or early surgical planning for ease of surgery (23). Early surgical intervention after stabilizing the ocular surface is preferred especially in patients with SJS and OCP; as both the density of cataract and keratopathy progress with time making surgical intervention more onerous (11, 23). Phacoemulsification was the most common type of surgery performed in all the three categories of DED and is a feasible option when planned before media clarity gets significantly compromised (10, 23, 24). While phacoemulsification can still be performed in eyes with significant keratopathy with the assistance of an endoilluminator (10, 25), ECCE needs to be performed in the presence of severe keratopathy (23). Two thirds of the eyes which needed ECCE in our cohort had dry eye associated with CC, which implies a higher level of surgical complexity. Posterior capsular rupture with vitreous loss was the most common complication noted in all the three groups, which is expected in a setting of compromised media clarity. Thus, judicious use of viscoelastic and trypan blue to enhance visualization of the anterior capsule may help minimize this complication (26). DMD was noted in 0.9% of the operated eyes, which was limited to the incision sites and resolved without any surgical interventions. Though noted in a small proportion of patients, it should be watched for cautiously intraoperatively, to avoid the need for surgical intervention in these eyes which are at high risk for failure following corneal transplant (27). Though corneal melt following cataract surgery has been reported in some studies, especially with use of

TABLE 1 | Overview of literature on visual outcomes and complications following cataract surgery in dry eye disease (DED).

References	No of eyes (*n*)	Diagnosis	Mean age (years)	Type of surgery	Pre-op mean LogMAR BCVA	Post-op mean LogMAR BCVA	Complications (*n*; %)
Narang et al. (23)	40	SJS	–	Phaco ECCE	1.61	1 month–0.30 LFU–0.48	PCR (2/40; 5%) Ocular surface breakdown (4/40; 10%)
Sharma et al. (10)	21	SJS	32 ± 12	Phaco	2.29	1 month: 0.84	CED (2/21; 9.5%) and filamentary keratitis (2/21; 9.5%)
de Melo et al. (24)	72	GVHD	56	Phaco	0.39	1 year: 0.08	CME (4/72; 5.5), keratitis with perforation (2/72; 2.7%)
Puranik et al. (30)	9	OCP	60 ± 2	ECCE Phaco	–	>2 lines improvement in 6 of 9 eyes at 1 year	SPK (1/9; 11%), CED (1/9; 11%), CME (1/9; 11%)
Ram et al. (6)	25	Non-specific	59 ± 10	Phaco	–	0 (13 eyes) 0.2–0.5 (8 eyes) 0.5–1 (4 eyes)	SPK (8/25; 32%) and CED (8/25; 32%)
Geerling et al. (31)	15	OCP	73	Phaco ECCE ICCE	–	0.5 (1 month to 1 year)	Perforation (2/15; 13.3%), progressive surface disease (6/15; 40%)
Ram et al. (12)	21	SS	Group 1: 61 ± 8 Group 2: 61 ± 10	ECCE and ICCE	CFCF-1.3	Group 1: 0.5 Group 2: 0.3	Group 1: post-operative endophthalmitis (3/21; 14.2%), peripheral keratolysis (4/21; 19%) Group 2: filamentary keratitis (6/21; 28.5%) peripheral keratolysis (2/21; 9.5%)

BCVA, best corrected visual acuity; SJS, Stevens-Johnson syndrome; CED, corneal epithelial defect; Phaco, phacoemulsification; ECCE, extracapsular cataract extraction; PCR, posterior capsular rupture; GVHD, graft-versus-host disease; CME, cystoid macular edema; OCP, ocular cicatricial pemphigoid; SPK, superficial punctate keratitis; SS, Sjogren's syndrome; ICCE, intracapsular cataract extraction.

non-steroidal anti-inflammatory drug (NSAIDs) eye drops, we did not encounter this complication in any of the eyes that were treated with them (3, 28, 29).

Another interesting finding noted in this study was the pattern of visual recovery at first and sixth weeks following cataract surgery. While the BCVA improved gradually up to 6 weeks post-surgery in MGD and SS; in eyes with CC, the visual recovery was similar at 1 and 6 weeks post-surgery. This was consistent with the characteristic pattern of visual recovery reported previously in patients with SJS (23). Most findings in this study like mean age at surgery, choice of surgical technique, and complications corroborated with that reported in smaller cohorts of either SJS/OCP or SS, and an overview of literature on visual outcomes and complications following cataract surgery in DED is described in **Table 1**.

The main strength of the study lies in its sample size and the standardized and digitized way of data entry. The main limitation of the study is its retrospective design and the lack of data on scores based on questionnaires and objective tests like tear osmolarity and non-invasive tear breakup time (NITBUT), which could help correlate the severity of DED preoperatively to visual outcomes following cataract surgery. Also, inclusion of a control group comprising eyes that underwent routine cataract surgery without pre-existing DED or other ocular surface co-morbidities would have added value to this study. However, the lack of such a control group is another limitation of this study. It would be interesting to plan a prospective study in the future including the subjective and objective assessment of DED both before and after cataract surgery to understand the impact of cataract surgery on pre-existing DED and vice versa.

In conclusion, this study found that the visual outcomes after cataract surgery in DED were satisfactory, across different etiologies. Pre-existing keratopathy, specifically corneal scarring, was the main determinant of sub-optimal visual outcomes. The study also found that there were no alarmingly high rates of intra- or post-operative complications and no sight-threatening issues with cataract surgery in DED. The findings of this study will not only help cataract surgeons in better prognostication for their patients but will also help patients in avoiding delaying cataract surgery because of the unreasonable fear of complications.

AUTHOR CONTRIBUTIONS

PD, AD, and SB: concept and design of study or acquisition of data or analysis and interpretation of data. PD, AD, SS, and SB: drafting the article or revising it critically for important intellectual content and final approval of the version to be published. All authors contributed to the article and approved the submitted version.

ACKNOWLEDGMENTS

The authors wish to acknowledge the support of our Department of eyeSmart EMR and AEye team specially Mr. Ranganath Vadapalli and Mr. Mohammad Pasha.

REFERENCES

Craig JP, Nichols KK, Akpek EK, Caffery B, Dua HS, Joo CK, et al. TFOS DEWS II definition and classification report. *Ocul Surf.* (2017) 15:276– 83. doi: 10.1016/j.jtos.2017.05.008

Sangwan VS, Gupta S, Das S. Cataract surgery in ocular surface diseases: clinical challenges and outcomes. *Curr Opin Ophthalmol.* (2018) 29:81– 7. doi: 10.1097/ICU.0000000000000441

Ting DSJ, Ghosh S. Acute corneal perforation 1 week following uncomplicated cataract surgery: the implication of undiagnosed dry eye disease and topical NSAIDs. *Ther Adv Ophthalmol.* (2019) 11. doi: 10.1177/25158414198 69508

Harada K, Mohamed YH, Uematsu M, Inoue D, Ueki R, Harada S, et al. Three cases of acute sterile corneal melt after cataract surgery. *Am J Ophthalmol Case Rep.* (2018) 13: 62–5. doi: 10.1016/j.ajoc.2018.12.004

Bloomfield SE, Becker CG, Christian CL, JS Nauheim. Bilateral necrotizing scleritis with marginal corneal ulceration after cataract surgery in a patient with vasculitis. *Br J Ophthalmol.* (1980) 64:170–4. doi: 10.1136/bjo.64.3.170

Ram J, Gupta A, Brar G, Kaushik S, Gupta A. Outcomes of phacoemulsification in patients with dry eye. *J Cataract Refract Surg.* (2002) 28:1386–9. doi: 10.1016/S0886-3350(02)01387-1

Khanal S, Tomlinson A, Esakowitz L, Bhatt P, Jones D, Nabili S, et al. Changes in corneal sensitivity and tear physiology after phacoemulsification. *Ophthalmic Physiol Opt.* (2008) 28:127–34. doi: 10.1111/j.1475-1313.2008.00539.x

Donthineni PR, Kammari P, Shanbhag SS, Singh V, Das AV, Basu S. Incidence, demographics, types and risk factors of dry eye disease in India: electronic medical records driven big data analytics report I. *Ocul Surf.* (2019) 17:250– 6. doi: 10.1016/j.jtos.2019.02.007

Donthineni PR, Das AV, Basu S. Dry eye disease in children and adolescents in India. *The Ocul Surf.* (2020) 18:777–82. doi: 10.1016/j.jtos.2020.07.019

Sharma N, Aron N, Venugopal R, Sangwan S, Titiyal JS, Agarwal T. New surgical approach in cases of cataract with ocular Stevens–Johnson syndrome. *J Cataract Refract Surg.* (2016) 42:1549–55. doi: 10.1016/j.jcrs.2016. 09.012

Sangwan VS, Burman S. Cataract surgery in Stevens–Johnson syndrome. *J Cataract Refract Surg.* (2005) 31:860–2. doi: 10.1016/j.jcrs.2004.07.023

Ram J, Sharma A, Pandav SS, A Gupta, P Bambery. Cataract surgery in patients with dry eyes. *J Cataract Refract Surg.* (1998) 24:1119– 24. doi: 10.1016/S0886-3350(98)80107-7

Rao GN, Khanna RC, Athota SM, Rajshekar V, Rani PK. Integrated model of primary and secondary eye care for underserved rural areas: the L V Prasad Eye Institute experience. *Indian J Ophthalmol.* (2012) 60:396– 400. doi: 10.4103/0301-4738.100533

Das AV, Kammari P, Vadapalli R, Basu S. Big data and the eyeSmart electronic medical record system—an 8-year experience from a three- tier eye care network in India. *Indian J Ophthalmol.* (2020) 68:427– 32. doi: 10.4103/ijo.IJO_710_19

Wolffsohn JS, Arita R, Chalmers R, Djalilian A, Dogru M, Dumbleton K, et al. TFOS DEWS II Diagnostic Methodology report. *Ocul Surf.* (2017) 15:539–74. doi: 10.1016/j.jtos.2017.05.001

Shanbhag SS, Chanda S, Donthineni PR, Sane SS, Priyadarshini SR, Basu S. Clinical clues predictive of Stevens-Johnson syndrome as the cause of chronic cicatrising conjunctivitis. *Br J Ophthalmol.* (2020) 104:1005–09. doi: 10.1136/bjophthalmol-2019-314928

Vazirani J, Donthineni PR, Goel S, Mahuvakar S, Narang P, et al. Chronic cicatrizing conjunctivitis: a review of the differential diagnosis and algorithmic approach to management. *Indian J Ophthalmol.* (2020) [in press].

World Health Organization. *Change the Definition of Blindness.* (2008). Available online at: https://www.who.int/blindness/Change%20the %20Definition%20 of%20Blindness.pdf (accessed September 23, 2020).

Rolando M, Zierhut M. The ocular surface and tear film and their dysfunction in dry eye disease. *Surv Ophthalmol.* (2001) 45(Suppl. 2):S203– 10. doi: 10.1016/S0039-6257(00)00203-4

O'Reilly P, Mahmoud U, Hayes P, Tormey P, Beatty P. Age and sex profile of patients having cataract surgery between 1986 and 2003. *J Cataract Refract Surg.* (2005) 31:2162–6. doi: 10.1016/j.jcrs.2005.08.044

Erie JC, Baratz KH, Hodge DO, Schleck CD, Burke JP. Incidence of cataract surgery from 1980 through 2004: 25-year population-based study. *J Cataract Refract Surg.* (2007) 33:1273–7. doi: 10.1016/j.jcrs.2007.03.053

Behndig A, Montan P, Stenevi U, Kugelberg M, Lundström M. One million cataract surgeries: Swedish National Cataract Register 1992–2009. *J Cataract Refract Surg.* (2011) 37:1539–45. doi: 10.1016/j.jcrs.2011.05.021

Narang P, Mohamed A, Mittal V, Sangwan VS. Cataract surgery in chronic Stevens-Johnson syndrome: aspects and outcomes. *Br J Ophthalmol.* (2016) 100:1542–1546. doi: 10.1136/bjophthalmol-2015-308041

de Melo Franco R, Kron-Gray MM, De la Parra-Colin P, He Y, Musch DC, Mian SI, et al. Outcomes of cataract surgery in graft-versus-host disease. *Cornea.* (2015) 34:506–11. doi: 10.1097/ICO.0000000000000395

Nishimura A, Kobayashi A, Segawa Y, Sugiyama K. Endoillumination-assisted cataract surgery in a patient with corneal opacity. *J Cataract Refract Surg.* (2003) 29:2277–80. doi: 10.1016/S0886-3350(03)00493-0

Bhartiya P, Sharma N, Ray M, Sinha R, Vajpayee RB. Trypan blue assisted phacoemulsification in corneal opacities. *Br J Ophthalmol.* (2002) 86:857– 9. doi: 10.1136/bjo.86.8.857

Al-Swailem S. Graft failure: II. Ocular surface complications. *Int Ophthalmol.* (2007) 28:175–89. doi: 10.1007/s10792-007-9127-9

Wolf EJ, Kleiman LZ, Schrier A. Nepafenac associated corneal melt. *J Cataract Refract Surg.* (2007) 33:1974–5. doi: 10.1016/j.jcrs.2007.06.043

Bekendam PD, Narváez J, Agarwal M. Case of corneal melting associated with the use of topical nepafenac. *Cornea.* (2007) 26:1002–3. doi: 10.1097/ICO.0b013e3180cfe626

Puranik CJ, Murthy SI, Taneja M, Sangwan VS. Outcomes of cataract surgery in ocular cicatricial pemphigoid. *Ocul Immunol Inflamm.* (2013) 21:449– 54. doi: 10.3109/09273948.2013.819106

Geerling G, Dart JK. Management and outcome of cataract surgery in ocular cicatricial pemphigoid. *Graefes Arch Clin Exp Ophthalmol.* (2000) 238:112– 8. doi: 10.1007/PL00007877

21

Nc2Eye: A Curated ncRNAomics Knowledgebase for Bridging Basic and Clinical Research in Eye Diseases

Yan Zhang†, Zhengbo Xue†, Fangjie Guo†, Fulong Yu, Liangde Xu and Hao Chen**

School of Biomedical Engineering, School of Ophthalmology and Optometry and Eye Hospital, Wenzhou Medical University, Wenzhou, China

***Correspondence:**
Liangde Xu
xuld@eye.ac.cn
Hao Chen
chenhao@mail.eye.ac.cn

†These authors share first authorship

Eye diseases (EDs) represent a group of disorders affecting the visual system, most of which can lead to visual impairment and blindness. Accumulating evidence reveals that non-coding RNAs (ncRNAs) are closely associated with a wide variety of EDs. However, abundant associations between ncRNAs and EDs are scattered across the published literature, obstructing a global view of ncRNA-ED associations. A public resource of high-quality manually curated ncRNAomics knowledge associated with EDs remains unavailable. To address this gap, we thus developed Nc2Eye (http://nc2eye.bio-data.cn/), which is the first knowledgebase dedicated to providing a comprehensive ncRNAomics resource for bridging basic and clinical research in EDs. Through a comprehensive review of more than 2400 published papers, Nc2Eye catalogs 7088 manually curated ncRNA-ED associations involving 4363 ncRNAs across eight species. We also provide detailed descriptions and annotation information for each ncRNA-disease association such as ncRNA categories, experimental methods, expression pattern and related clinical drugs. To further expand the pathogenic ncRNAs, we also collected more than 90 high-throughput EDs-related transcriptome datasets. Furthermore, a user-friendly interface was constructed for convenient and flexible data browsing, querying, and retrieving. We believe that Nc2Eye is a timely and valuable knowledgebase for significantly improving and useful for discovery of new diagnostic and therapeutic biomarkers.

Keywords: eye diseases, non-coding RNAs, knowledgebase, epigenomics, website

INTRODUCTION

Eye diseases (EDs) represent a group of disorders affecting the visual system. It was estimated that 217 million people (3.1% of the world population) suffered from moderate to severe visual disturbance in the world in 2015, while 36 million were blind (Bourne et al., 2017). There are more than 150 kinds of EDs recorded in medical subject headings (MeSH) (Bhattacharya et al., 2011), most of which can lead to visual impairment and blindness, such as cataract, age-related macular degeneration (AMD), diabetic retinopathy (DR), retinoblastoma (RB), and degenerative myopia, etc. The pathogenesis of EDs at the molecular level remains poorly understood.

Non-coding RNAs (ncRNAs), such as microRNA (miRNA), long non-codingRNA (lncRNA) and circlar RNA (circRNA), are a large category of functional RNA molecules involved in regulating many biological processes (Esteller, 2011). Numerous studies demonstrated that ncRNAs play important roles in various EDs (Li et al., 2016; Rassi et al., 2017; Zhang et al., 2017). For example, the lncRNA *PVT1* is up-regulated in RB tissues and silencing *PVT1* can suppress the tumor growth (Wu et al., 2019). Overexpression of circRNA *cPWWP2A* was reported to alleviate retinal vascular dysfunction in DR by inhibiting *miR-579* activity (Liu et al., 2019). *miR-27a* is up-regulated in uveal melanoma cell lines (Venza et al., 2014) and Sun et al. (2009) found that genistein inhibited uveal melanoma cell proliferation in part through decreasing *miR-27a* expression. These studies suggested that ncRNAs not only contribute to the understanding of the molecular mechanisms of EDs, but also have important implications for the development of new therapeutic targets.

With the progression of disease-related ncRNA study, some disease-associated ncRNA resources were constructed, such as LncRNADisease (Chen et al., 2013), miR2Disease (Jiang et al., 2009), and MNDR (Cui et al., 2018). These databases contained a wide variety of human diseases and there were only a few ncRNAs involved in EDs. Subsequently, several ophthalmology-related databases were built recently. For example, KmeyeDB (Kawamura et al., 2010) and RetinoGenetics (Ran et al., 2014) provided gene mutations in EDs. miRNeye (Karali et al., 2010) focused on the differentially expressed miRNAs in ocular tissues. iSyTE (Kakrana et al., 2018) integrated all publicly available lens gene expression data. However, there is still no an ED-specialized database that provides the comprehensive resource on diverse types of ncRNAs across various EDs.

To fill the gap, we constructed Nc2Eye, a manually curated database, to provide experimentally validated ncRNA-ED associations. The current version of Nc2Eye contains 7088 associations between 104 EDs and 4363 ncRNAs in eight species, through a comprehensive review of more than 2400 published papers. To investigate the underlying molecular mechanism of EDs, Nc2Eye gathered more than 90 high-throughput transcriptome datasets in EDs, and normal controls. In addition, Nc2Eye provided a user-friendly interface for convenient and flexible data browsing, querying, retrieving and submitting. Nc2Eye is a timely and valuable resource to significantly improve our understanding of ncRNA dysfunction in EDs.

DATA COLLECTION AND DATABASE CONTENT

Experimentally Supported ncRNA-ED Associations

To ensure the accuracy and reliability in the data collection process, we manually curated all Nc2Eye entries by the following steps. First, we searched the PubMed database (Sayers et al., 2019) with the MeSH term "EDs" and a list of keywords about ncRNAs, including "ncRNA," "non-coding RNA," "non-coding," "lncRNA," "long non-coding RNA," "miRNA," "microRNA," "siRNA," "shRNA," "snoRNA," "piRNA," "circular RNA," "circRNA," "miR-," "and "let-." Considering that some papers have not been assigned MeSH term, we chose the eye disease names from MeSH term as keywords. Then, we searched with the keyword combination: each eye disease and ncRNA category name as complementary. After that, we selected published papers about the ED-related ncRNAs and extracted experimentally supported ncRNA-ED associations manually. All selected literature was reviewed by at least two researchers. In this step, we retrieved the ncRNA name, ncRNA category (e.g., miRNA, lncRNA, and circRNA), disease name, species, tissues/cell line, methods (e.g., microarray, qPCR, and Western blot), expression pattern (e.g., up-regulated, down-regulated), functional description and reference (PubMed ID, year of publication, title). In addition, we recorded whether the ncRNA was related to drugs according to the paper. Finally, we standardized the eye disease names refer to the MeSH term and searched the gene ID, Ensembl ID, and synonyms of each lncRNA from Ensembl (Zerbino et al., 2018) and NCBI Gene database (Brown et al., 2015).

After comprehensively reviewing more than 2400 published papers, a total of 7088 associations between 104 EDs and 4363 ncRNAs in eight species were manually collected. There were 132 of these ncRNAs were reported to be related with drugs in 14 EDs. Distribution of ncRNA-associated entries in each species and ncRNA category is listed in **Table 1**.

High-Throughput Transcriptome Datasets in EDs

A great number of studies based on high-throughput experiments have emerged in recent years (Liu X. et al., 2018;

TABLE 1 | Statistics for the ncRNA-ED entries in the Nc2Eye database.

Species	miRNA	lncRNA	circRNA	siRNA	shRNA	piRNA	snoRNA	snRNA	Total
Homo sapiens	3044	968	479	274	48	18	–	2	4833
Mus musculus	1016	165	2	137	41	–	4	1	1366
Rattus norvegicus	623	9	2	75	24	–	–	–	733
Canis familiaris	47	–	–	–	2	–	–	–	49
Macaca mulatta	17	5	–	14	3	–	–	–	39
Bos taurus	8	–	–	17	1	–	–	–	26
Oryctolagus cuniculus	1	–	–	21	–	–	–	–	22
Danio rerio	20	–	–	–	–	–	–	–	20
Total	4776	1147	483	538	119	18	4	3	7088

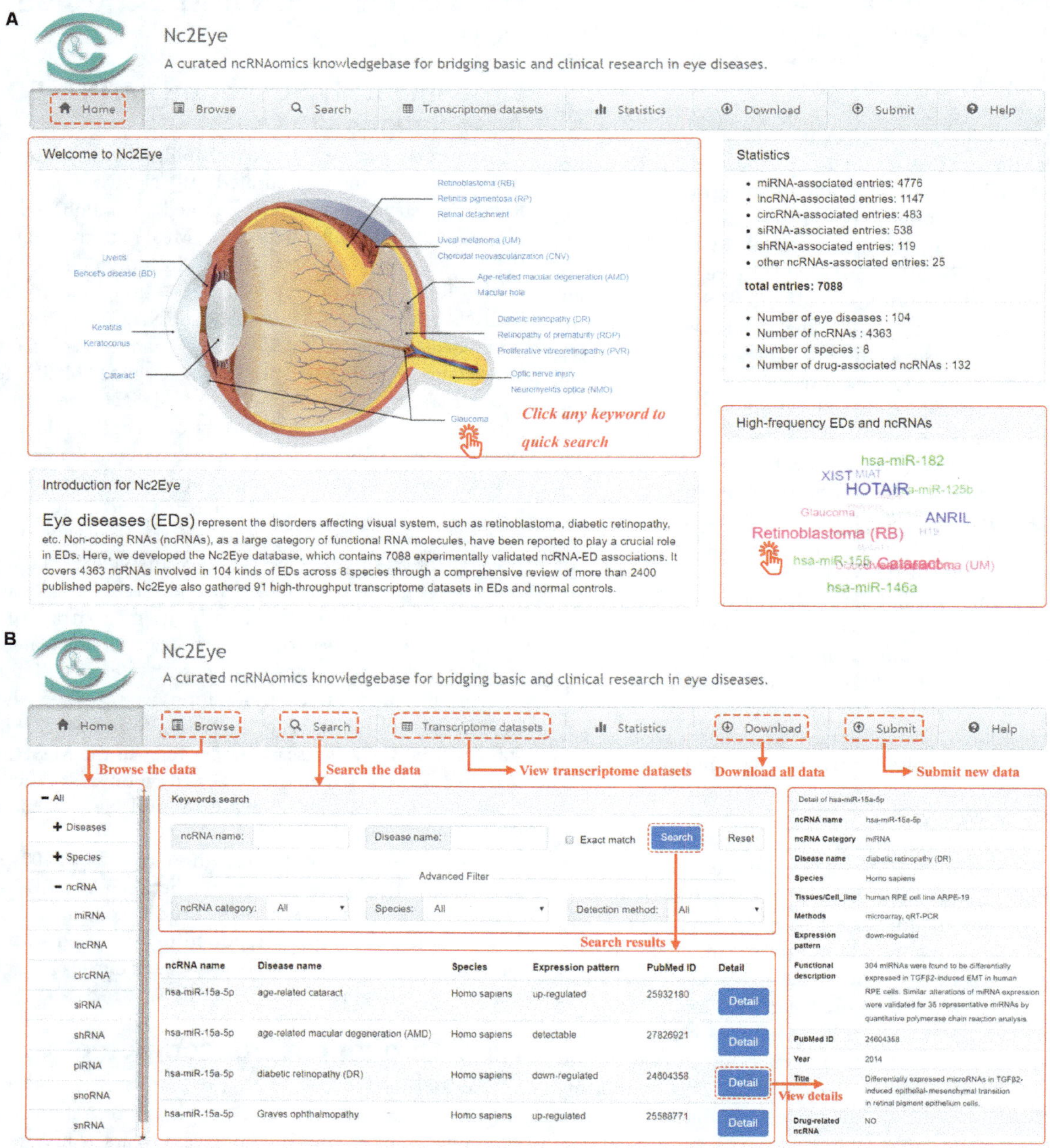

FIGURE 1 | A schematic workflow of Nc2Eye. **(A)** The 'Home' page allow to quick research for ncRNA-ED associations. **(B)** The 'Browse' and 'Search' pages allow the users to browse and search ncRNA-ED associations. The 'Transcriptome datasets' page shows public high-throughput transcriptome datasets. Users can download all ncRNA-ED association data in the 'Download' page and submit new ncRNA-ED association in the 'Submit' page.

Liu Y. et al., 2018; Xu et al., 2018). Mining and collecting high-throughput transcriptome datasets will help to investigate the underlying molecular mechanism of EDs. Nc2Eye gathered 91 microarray and next-generation sequencing datasets in EDs versus normal controls, most of which come from gene expression omnibus (GEO) database. Each entry contains "diseases name," "species," "sample type," "case/control description," "sample size," "data type," "accession ID," "platform," and "Pubmed ID." Users can conveniently browse and select transcriptome datasets according to their research requirements and click the GSE ID to jump to the GEO website for further exploration. GEO has developed several tools for data visualization and analysis which enable researchers to easily analyze this data and do not require to download any file (Clough and Barrett, 2016).

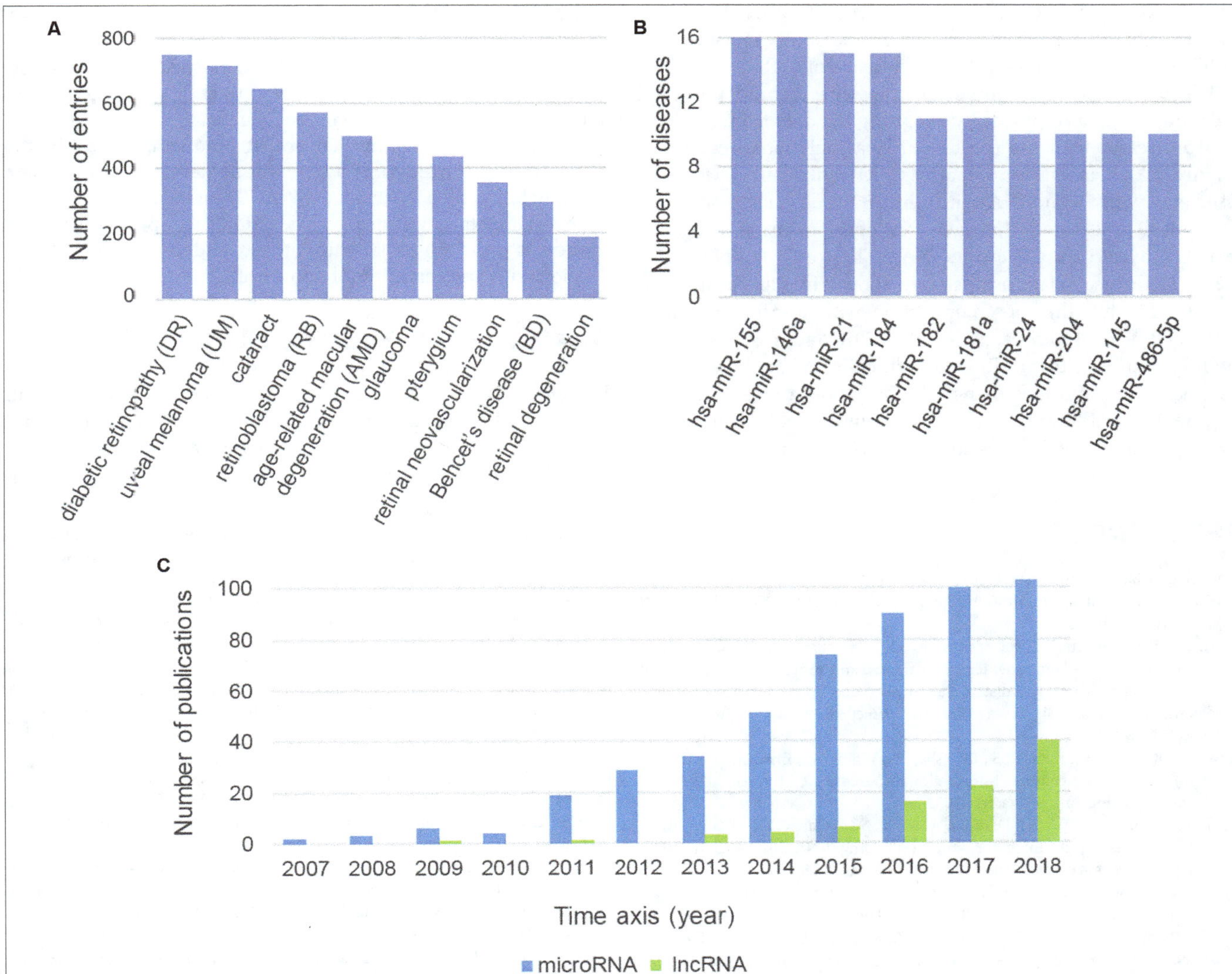

FIGURE 2 | (A) The top10 diseases with the most ncRNA associations. **(B)** The top10 ncRNAs with the most disease relationships. **(C)** The number of ncRNA-ED publications each year.

Finally, all data in Nc2Eye were organized using MySQL (version 5.7.25). The web interface was built in PHP and the web services were deployed using Apache (version 2.4.6). The Nc2Eye database is freely available at http://nc2eye.bio-data.cn/.

USER INTERFACE

Nc2Eye constructed a user-friendly web interface for convenient and flexible data browsing, querying, retrieving and submitting (**Figure 1**). In the "Home" page, users can click keywords in the eye anatomy and "high-frequency EDs and ncRNAs' to quickly research. In the "Browse" page, users can glance through Nc2Eye by clicking on a specific ED name, species or a class of ncRNA, and a list of corresponding entries will be displayed. Nc2Eye provides a "Search" page that enables users to search by ncRNA name, ED name or both. Defaulting to fuzzy search, and Nc2Eye also supports exact search. Moreover, users can use the "Advanced Filter" to filter the results by ncRNA category, species and detection method. In the "Transcriptome datasets" page, 91 expression profiles including EDs versus normal controls are listed and can be filtered by inputting keywords from any column. Nc2Eye also provides a submission interface that allows researchers to submit new ncRNA-ED association data which is not documented. At last, all ncRNA-ED association data in Nc2Eye can be downloaded in the "Download" page and a user tutorial of the website is available in the "Help" page.

DISCUSSION AND CONCLUSION

Eye diseases are a common group of disorders in the visual system, causing visual impairment and blindness. Emerging evidence demonstrated that the dysregulation of ncRNAs played critical roles in various EDs. We developed Nc2Eye, a curated knowledgebase of experimentally validated ncRNAs associated with EDs, which provides a global landscape of ncRNAs in EDs.

We could find some important messages behind the large and complex data resources by analyzing the data from Nc2Eye. Top10 diseases with the most ncRNA associations were listed (**Figure 2A**). Diabetic retinopathy (DR) ranked first, which is associated with 583 ncRNAs, including 32 drug-related ncRNAs. This result suggested that we can develop more drugs to treat DR by targeting these ncRNAs. The top10 ncRNAs with the most disease relationships were shown in **Figure 2B**. The *hsa-miR-155* has the most connection with diseases and it is associated with 16 diseases, such as DR and RB, indicating the importance of this miRNA in ophthalmopathy. In addition, we tracked the number of ncRNA-ED publications each year (**Figure 2C**) and found the research about lncRNA is increasing year by year which implies lncRNAs will become a hot topic in ophthalmopathy.

CONCLUSION

In conclusion, Nc2Eye, an eye disorders-specialized database, provides global insights into ncRNA functions in various EDs. We believe that Nc2Eye will be beneficial to researchers to dissect the underlying mechanism of ophthalmopathy. In the future, a confidence score system will be developed to estimate the reliability of a specific ncRNA-ED association according to experimental evidence. In addition, we plan to update the database every 3 months to extend newly ED-related relationships and make it more powerful.

AUTHOR CONTRIBUTIONS

HC and LX conceived and designed the experiments. YZ, ZX, and FY collected and analyzed the data. FG designed the website. YZ and LX wrote and revised the manuscript. All authors read and approved the final manuscript.

REFERENCES

Bhattacharya, S., Ha-Thuc, V., and Srinivasan, P. (2011). MeSH: a window into full text for document summarization. *Bioinformatics* 27, i120–i128. doi: 10.1093/bioinformatics/btr223

Bourne, R. R. A., Flaxman, S. R., Braithwaite, T., Cicinelli, M. V., Das, A., Jonas, J. B., et al. (2017). Magnitude, temporal trends, and projections of the global prevalence of blindness and distance and near vision impairment: a systematic review and meta-analysis. *Lancet Glob. Health* 5:e0888-97. doi: 10.1016/S2214-109X(17)30293-0

Brown, G. R., Hem, V., Katz, K. S., Ovetsky, M., Wallin, C., Ermolaeva, O., et al. (2015). Gene: a gene-centered information resource at NCBI. *Nucleic Acids Res.* 43, D36–D42. doi: 10.1093/nar/gku1055

Chen, G., Wang, Z., Wang, D., Qiu, C., Liu, M., Chen, X., et al. (2013). LncRNADisease: a database for long-non-coding RNA-associated diseases. *Nucleic Acids Res.* 41, D983–D986. doi: 10.1093/nar/gks1099

Clough, E., and Barrett, T. (2016). The gene expression omnibus database. *Methods Mol. Biol.* 1418, 93–110. doi: 10.1007/978-1-4939-3578-9-5

Cui, T., Zhang, L., Huang, Y., Yi, Y., Tan, P., Zhao, Y., et al. (2018). MNDR v2.0: an updated resource of ncRNA-disease associations in mammals. *Nucleic Acids Res.* 46, D371–D374. doi: 10.1093/nar/gkx1025

Esteller, M. (2011). Non-coding RNAs in human disease. *Nat. Rev. Genet.* 12, 861–874. doi: 10.1038/nrg3074

Jiang, Q., Wang, Y., Hao, Y., Juan, L., Teng, M., Zhang, X., et al. (2009). miR2Disease: a manually curated database for microRNA deregulation in human disease. *Nucleic Acids Res.* 37, D98–D104. doi: 10.1093/nar/gkn714

Kakrana, A., Yang, A., Anand, D., Djordjevic, D., Ramachandruni, D., Singh, A., et al. (2018). iSyTE 2.0: a database for expression-based gene discovery in the eye. *Nucleic Acids Res.* 46, D875–D885. doi: 10.1093/nar/gkx837

Karali, M., Peluso, I., Gennarino, V. A., Bilio, M., Verde, R., Lago, G., et al. (2010). miRNeye: a microRNA expression atlas of the mouse eye. *BMC Genom.* 11:715. doi: 10.1186/1471-2164-11-715

Kawamura, T., Ohtsubo, M., Mitsuyama, S., Ohno-Nakamura, S., Shimizu, N., and Minoshima, S. (2010). KMeyeDB: a graphical database of mutations in genes that cause eye diseases. *Hum. Mutat.* 31, 667–674. doi: 10.1002/humu.21240

Li, F., Wen, X., Zhang, H., and Fan, X. (2016). Novel insights into the role of long noncoding RNA in ocular diseases. *Int. J. Mol. Sci.* 17:478. doi: 10.3390/ijms17040478

Liu, C., Ge, H. M., Liu, B. H., Dong, R., Shan, K., Chen, X., et al. (2019). Targeting pericyte-endothelial cell crosstalk by circular RNA-cPWWP2A inhibition aggravates diabetes-induced microvascular dysfunction. *Proc. Natl. Acad. Sci. U.S.A.* 116, 7455–7464. doi: 10.1073/pnas.1814874116

Liu, X., Liu, B., Zhou, M., Fan, F., Yu, M., Gao, C., et al. (2018). Circular RNA HIPK3 regulates human lens epithelial cells proliferation and apoptosis by targeting the miR-193a/CRYAA axis. *Biochem. Biophys. Res. Commun.* 503, 2277–2285. doi: 10.1016/j.bbrc.2018.06.149

Liu, Y., Chen, Y., Wang, Y., Zhang, X., Gao, K., Chen, S., et al. (2018). microRNA profiling in glaucoma eyes with varying degrees of optic neuropathy by using next-generation sequencing. *Invest Ophthalmol. Vis. Sci.* 59, 2955–2966. doi: 10.1167/iovs.17-23599

Ran, X., Cai, W. J., Huang, X. F., Liu, Q., Lu, F., Qu, J., et al. (2014). 'RetinoGenetics': a comprehensive mutation database for genes related to inherited retinal degeneration. *Database* 2014:bau047. doi: 10.1093/database/bau047

Rassi, D. M., De Paiva, C. S., Dias, L. C., Modulo, C. M., Adriano, L., Fantucci, M. Z., et al. (2017). Review: MicroRNAS in ocular surface and dry eye diseases. *Ocul. Surf.* 15, 660–669. doi: 10.1016/j.jtos.2017.05.007

Sayers, E. W., Agarwala, R., Bolton, E. E., Brister, J. R., Canese, K., Clark, K., et al. (2019). Database resources of the national center for biotechnology information. *Nucleic Acids Res.* 47, D23–D28. doi: 10.1093/nar/gky1069

Sun, Q., Cong, R., Yan, H., Gu, H., Zeng, Y., Liu, N., et al. (2009). Genistein inhibits growth of human uveal melanoma cells and affects microRNA-27a and target gene expression. *Oncol. Rep.* 22, 563–567. doi: 10.3892/or-00000472

Venza, M., Dell'Aversana, C., Visalli, M., Altucci, L., Teti, D., and Venza, I. (2014). Identification of microRNA expression patterns in cutaneous and uveal melanoma cell lines. *Tumori* 100, e4–e7. doi: 10.1700/1430.15828

Wu, X. Z., Cui, H. P., Lv, H. J., and Feng, L. (2019). Knockdown of lncRNA PVT1 inhibits retinoblastoma progression by sponging miR-488-3p. *Biomed. Pharmacother.* 112:108627. doi: 10.1016/j.biopha.2019.108627

Xu, B., Ma, R., Ren, H., and Qian, J. (2018). Genome-wide analysis of uveal melanoma metastasis-associated lncrnas and their functional network. *DNA Cell. Biol.* 37, 99–108. doi: 10.1089/dna.2017.4015

Zerbino, D. R., Achuthan, P., Akanni, W., Amode, M. R., Barrell, D., Bhai, J., et al. (2018). Ensembl 2018. *Nucleic Acids Res.* 46, D754–D761. doi: 10.1093/nar/gkx1098

Zhang, S. J., Chen, X., Li, C. P., Li, X. M., Liu, C., Liu, B. H., et al. (2017). Identification and characterization of circular RNAs as a New Class of putative biomarkers in diabetes retinopathy. *Invest. Ophthalmol. Vis. Sci.* 58, 6500–6509. doi: 10.1167/iovs.17-22698

22

Optical Coherence Tomography Angiography (OCTA) in Multiple Sclerosis and Neuromyelitis Optica Spectrum Disorder

Iris Kleerekooper [1,2*†], *Sarah Houston* [3†], *Adam M. Dubis* [4], *S. Anand Trip* [2] and *Axel Petzold* [1,2,5]

[1] Department of Neuro-Ophthalmology, Moorfields Eye Hospital, London, United Kingdom, [2] Queen Square MS Centre, UCL Institute of Neurology and National Hospital for Neurology & Neurosurgery, London, United Kingdom, [3] Institute of Ophthalmology, University College London, London, United Kingdom, [4] National Institute for Health Research, Biomedical Resource Centre at University College London, Institute of Ophthalmology and Moorfields Eye Hospital National Health Service Trust, London, United Kingdom, [5] Dutch Expertise Centre of Neuro-Ophthalmology, Amsterdam UMC, Amsterdam, Netherlands

Correspondence:
Iris Kleerekooper
iris.kleerekooper.18@ucl.ac.uk

† These authors have contributed equally to this work

Vascular changes are increasingly recognized as important factors in the pathophysiology of neuroinflammatory disease, especially in multiple sclerosis (MS). The relatively novel technology of optical coherence tomography angiography (OCTA) images the retinal and choroidal vasculature non-invasively and in a depth-resolved manner. OCTA provides an alternative quantitative measure of retinal damage, by measuring vascular density instead of structural atrophy. Preliminary results suggest OCTA is sensitive to retinal damage in early disease stages, while also having less of a "floor-effect" compared with commonly used OCT metrics, meaning it can pick up further damage in a severely atrophied retina in later stages of disease. Furthermore, it may serve as a surrogate marker for vascular pathology in the central nervous system. Data to date consistently reveal lower densities of the retinal microvasculature in both MS and neuromyelitis optica spectrum disorder (NMOSD) compared with healthy controls, even in the absence of prior optic neuritis. Exploring the timing of vascular changes relative to structural atrophy may help answer important questions about the role of hypoperfusion in the pathophysiology of neuroinflammatory disease. Finally, qualitative characteristics of retinal microvasculature may help discriminate between different neuroinflammatory disorders. There are however still issues regarding image quality and development of standardized analysis methods before OCTA can be fully incorporated into clinical practice.

Keywords: OCTA, OCT, multiple sclerosis, NMOSD, optic neuritis, microvascular

INTRODUCTION

In addition to well-established immune mediated processes, vascular and metabolic factors are increasingly recognized to play important parts in the pathophysiology of neuroinflammatory disease, especially in multiple sclerosis (MS) (1). Optical coherence tomography angiography (OCTA) is a relatively novel technology that images the retinal and choroidal vasculature in a non-invasive and depth-resolved manner (2). OCTA technology is derived from additional processing of optical coherence tomography (OCT), a structural retinal imaging modality first used in 1991 that has since secured its place as a staple of neuro-ophthalmological clinical evaluation (3–5). Currently, some attention is diverted to the exciting potential that OCTA has in imaging the retinal vasculature using similar hardware and procedure.

Due to the design of the eye, the retina is one of the most easily accessible internal structures for imaging inside the human body. The retina is part of the central nervous system (CNS), as it contains the retinal nerve fiber layer (RNFL) and ganglion cell layer (GCL) which are formed of cells that relay visual information to the brain through the optic nerve (6, 7). Additionally, the anterior visual system is one of the most metabolically active structures in the human body and, accordingly, has a high perfusion rate which is rapidly adaptive to temporal changes in local demand (8–10).

The optic nerve is commonly injured in MS and neuromyelitis optica spectrum disorder (NMOSD) by optic neuritis (ON) (11–14). Demyelinating damage to the anterior visual system is virtually ubiquitous in postmortem studies of MS (15, 16). Thinning of the peripapillary RNFL (pRNFL) and GCL, as measured with OCT, have been shown to be markers of previous ON. However, retinal atrophy is also present in the absence of prior symptomatic ON and provides a valuable surrogate for more general, independent, CNS atrophy in neuroinflammatory disease (5, 11).

Even though immune mediated mechanisms are considered the most important drivers of neuroinflammatory disease, accumulating evidence indicates that CNS tissue energy failure, caused by hypoperfusion and hypoxia, is present in MS patients. This energy crisis may render neurons ineffective during an acute relapse and cause damage to oligodendrocytes which sets in action insidious processes of chronic demyelination and atrophy (1, 17). Neuropathologic studies of NMOSD affected tissue show that CNS lesions have a clear predilection for forming in perivascular locations (18). Furthermore, vessel walls in surrounding area are found to be fibrosed and hyalinised, a change in vessel morphology that can even be picked up on fundoscopy of NMOSD patients (19). In the acute clinical setting it can be difficult to differentiate between ON associated with MS and NMOSD, while the two diseases generally warrant different treatment decisions (13). Qualitative differences in vascular morphology picked up with OCTA may be diagnostically valuable in acute ON patients when differentiating between these conditions.

OCTA may be implemented in several interesting ways to advance the understanding of neuroinflammatory disease. Studies investigating OCTA in neuroinflammatory disease found that its findings are usually highly correlated to measurements of retinal layer thickness performed with the more consolidated technique of OCT (20–22). Therefore, OCTA can be an alternative quantitative measure of damage to the retina and optic nerve, as atrophied tissue requires less blood supply (20). Preliminary results in glaucoma research suggest that OCTA is sensitive to retinal damage in the earliest disease stages, while also being able to detect further damage in a severely atrophied retina, due to its low "floor-effect" (23, 24). In early-stage glaucoma, vascular density loss is faster compared with GCL thinning (25). Furthermore, another study concluded that the OCTA may be a promising tool to follow-up patients with late-stage glaucoma, as the measurement floor is lower compared with commonly used OCT metrics (26).

Additionally, OCTA may provide an avenue for investigations into vascular changes in the CNS. Preliminary OCTA research shows the retinal microvasculature is affected in both MS and NMOSD, even in eyes unaffected by ON and in some cases in the absence of structural retinal atrophy (20, 27). Investigating when vascular changes occur relative to thinning of retinal layers in neuroinflammatory disease may help answer important questions about the role of hypoperfusion in their pathophysiology (10). Finally, certain qualitative characteristics of the retinal microvasculature on OCTA may provide information for diagnostic discrimination between different causes of ON (28), similar to how the "central vein sign" on high-field MRI is a valuable diagnostic marker for MS (29). However, issues remain regarding image quality and the lack of standardization in image collection and analysis, which must be addressed before OCTA can be fully incorporated into clinical practice similar to what a network approach achieved for OCT (30).

In this review, we will discuss the potential value of OCTA in advancing research and clinical care in neuroinflammatory disease. First, we give an overview of the technical background of OCTA and the anatomy of retinal vasculature. Subsequently, we elaborate on the role of vascular alterations, particularly in the retina, in neuroinflammatory disease and we summarize research using OCTA in MS and NMOSD until now and finally, we discuss future prospects and the advantages as well as disadvantages of OCTA.

TECHNICAL BACKGROUND OCTA

OCT uses a technique that can be described as an optical analog to ultrasound-based imaging technology. OCT creates *in-vivo* structural images from biological tissue based on interferometry of low-coherence, near infrared light that is split into a reference arm, reflecting off a reference mirror, and a sample arm, reflecting from the investigated tissue. A strong interference occurs when both reflected beams recombine and a pattern of interference allows us to create a reflectivity profile, which is used to construct the OCT images (3). Currently, several generations of commercially available OCT devices are available and widely used.

OCTA expands on this technique by looking at temporal changes in the quality of backscattered light to distinguish locations of static tissues from blood flow. It detects blood vessels based on differences in amplitude, intensity, or phase variance between sequential OCT B-scans in the same position of the retina. Sequential B-scans are taken at the same transverse location and compared. The difference in signal between images reflects blood cells flowing through vessel lumen. Therefore, blood movement is used as an intrinsic contrast agent to create a vascular map (see **Figure 1**). Because of its reliance on picking up tiny temporal changes, a high sampling frequency is necessary to create sufficient quality OCTA images (31, 32). It is important

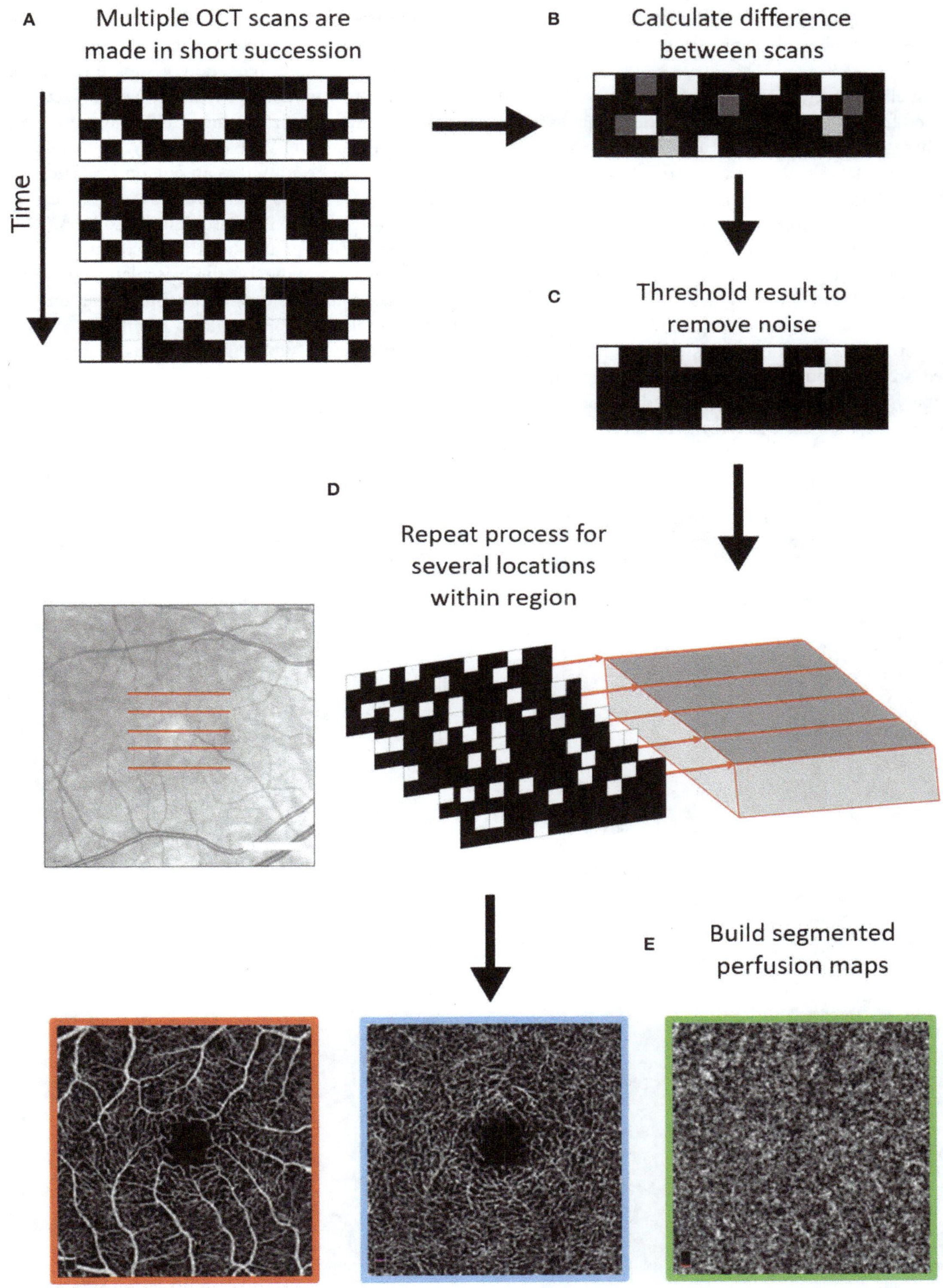

FIGURE 1 | Schematic of general optical coherence tomography angiography (OCTA) scanning technique. First, multiple OCT scans are repeated with a high frequency at the same location **(A)**, and based on differences between these scans in the phase, amplitude, and/or intensity of the backscattered light, areas with moving particles are differentiated from static tissue **(B,C)**. This process is repeated over several locations **(D)** and using a segmentation protocol perfusion maps are created for the different vascular plexi **(E)**. The example scans shown below are the superficial vascular plexus (red), the deep vascular plexus (blue), and the choroid (green) as obtained with the Heidelberg Engineering OCT2 system.

to remember that as a result of this technique, there is a floor to detectable OCTA signal that is slightly higher than slowest physiological flow, although the minimal detectable flow speed is not known.

Scans are visualized as en-face images of individual vascular layers, segmented from the volumetric map. The retinal vascular plexi are usually segmented in OCTA as a superficial layer, which consists of the superficial vascular plexus, and a deep layer, which takes the inner and deep vascular plexi together. But importantly, not all OCTA systems use the same segmentation algorithm for the superficial and deep vascular layers (33). Anatomical constraints and offsets from structural boundaries may vary between instruments (**Table 1**) (33).

OCTA images are generally analyzed by determining vessel density as the percentage of white pixels (representing vessels) in a segmented area. Although simple and easily implemented, this form of analysis is significantly influenced by the presence of artifacts, which are discussed later in this review. Most look at the vascular densities within a circular or square area around the fovea or optic disc. Densities of the macular SVP, DVP, and choroidal plexus are quantified separately in prespecified areas of investigation, generally a square of 3x3 or 6x6 mm. A separate outcome measure is the "foveal avascular zone" (FAZ), that estimates the size of the circular area in the center of the macula that has no SVP blood supply. The size and shape of the FAZ have both been used as an outcome, particularly in diabetes mellitus (DM) (34, 35). The FAZ has not yet been widely used as an outcome measure in neurological disorders.

A key feature of the healthy microvasculature is its fractal pattern, where shape of the vasculature is similar at every scale, fractal analysis has been gaining traction as an additional analysis tool (36, 37). This kind of analysis could be especially useful in cases of subtle microvascular change where there are no large regions of capillary dropout, but the highly specific pattern of the retina is altered due to the selective loss of small vessels.

TABLE 1 | OCTA platforms and segmentation of vascular plexi.

Platform	Instrument specifics	Vascular plexus	Slab boundary	Anatomic basis	Offset, μm
PLEX® Elite 9000 (Carl Zeiss Meditec)	Version 2018 v1.7 (Native seg); Version 2020 v2.1 (MLS)	Superficial (Native seg)	Top	ILM	0
			Bottom	IPL= ILM + 0.7·(OPL-ILM)	0
		Superficial (MLS)	Top	IML	0
			Bottom	IPL	−10
		Deep (Native seg)	Top	IPL	0
			Bottom	OPL (RPEFit – 110 μm)	0
		Deep (MLS)	Top	IPL	−10
			Bottom	OPL	0
CIRRUS™ HD-OCT 5000 with AngioPlex® (Carl Zeiss Meditec)	Version 9.5.0.8712; firmware 1.100.0.8; engine 6.5.0.8523	Superficial	Top	ILM	0
			Bottom	IPL= ILM + 0.7·(OPL-ILM)	0
		Deep	Top	IPL	0
			Bottom	OPL= RPEFit – 110 μm	0
RTVue XR Avanti (Optovue)	Version 2016.1.0.2	Superficial	Top	ILM	3
			Bottom	IPL	15
		Deep	Top	IPL	15
			Bottom	IPL	71
Triton DRI OCT (Topcon Medical Systems)	Version 10.07.003.03; IMAGEnet 6 version 1.14.8741	Superficial	Top	ILM	2.6
			Bottom	IPL/INL	15.6
		Deep	Top	IPL/INL	15.6
			Bottom	IPL/INL	70.2
Spectralis HRA OCTA (Heidelberg Engineering)	Version HEYEX V6.4a	Superficial	Top	ILM	0
			Bottom	IPL	0
		Deep	Top	IPL	0
			Bottom	IPL	0

ILM, inner limiting membrane; IPL, inner plexiform layer; OPL, outer plexiform layer; RPE, retinal pigmented epithelium; INL, inner nuclear layer.

ANATOMY RETINAL VASCULATURE

Retinal and optic nerve circulation has the challenging goal of supplying nourishment and removing waste without compromising vision. There are two discrete vascular systems in the retina; the retinal and choroidal vessels. Blood supply for both systems comes from the ophthalmic artery, a branch of the internal carotid artery. The ophthalmic artery in turn branches out in two main vessel types that supply the retina, the central retinal artery and the posterior ciliary arteries (**Figure 2**). The central retinal artery runs with the optic nerve inside the optic nerve sheath and enters the globe through the optic disc after which it branches out to supply the inner retina. The anatomy of the retinal microvasculature plexi is largely determined by constraints that are created by the anatomical organization of different regions in the retina. The three permeating retinal vascular plexi are organized based around the three cellular nuclear layers, the GCL, the inner nuclear layer (INL) and the outer nuclear layer (ONL) (**Figure 3**). The larger of the plexi, the superficial vascular plexus, mainly supplies the GCL, and roughly is located between the inner limiting membrane and the INL. The intermediate vascular plexus is located around the INL, while the deep vascular plexus is located primarily in the ONL (6, 7). The retinal venous system is interdigitated with the arterial vasculature and venous blood leaves the retina via the central retinal vein.

Retinal capillaries are formed of a layer of endothelial cells encapsulated by a basement membrane in which pericytes are embedded. Retinal capillaries are an important element of the blood-retinal barrier (BRB), the tightly controlled boundary between the intravascular and extravascular environment in the retina (38). Pericytes are essential for contractile function, endothelial barrier integrity and endothelial cell proliferation (38). Fluid and waste are drained from the eye through perivenous spaces, which are part of the ocular glymphatic drainage system (39). Beyond the lamina cribrosa there is no autonomic control of the retinal vasculature, therefore retinal capillaries are dependent on pericytes for local autoregulation of blood flow. Pericytes respond effectively to local tissue needs, and this relationship between local neural activity and changes in blood flow is known as neurovascular coupling. There is an approximate 1:1 ratio of pericytes to endothelial cells allowing for specific neurovascular coupling (40). The basement membrane between pericytes and endothelial cells is also very thin, allowing for increased communication between the two.

In the most common anatomical variant there are typically two posterior ciliary artery branches that run in parallel, but outside of the optic nerve sheath within the orbit. The posterior ciliary arteries supply the choroidal vascular plexus, which receives ~65–85% of the total ocular blood flow. The choroid is responsible for the oxygen supply of the outermost retinal layers, particularly the photoreceptors and retinal pigment epithelium. The choroid is also the source of oxygen for the foveal avascular zone. Finally, the posterior ciliary arteries give rise to the capillary network supplying the exterior optic nerve head in the annulus of Zinn (6, 7).

OCTA IN NEUROINFLAMMATORY DISEASE

Multiple Sclerosis

Vascular Pathology and MS

MS is an immune mediated demyelinating disease of the CNS and is one of the most common neurological causes for permanent disability in young adults (41, 42). Although many advances have been made in the field of MS over the last years, its pathophysiology has not yet been fully elucidated. Recently, increasing evidence indicates that energy failure, due to hypoxia and hypoperfusion, may be an important causal factor in

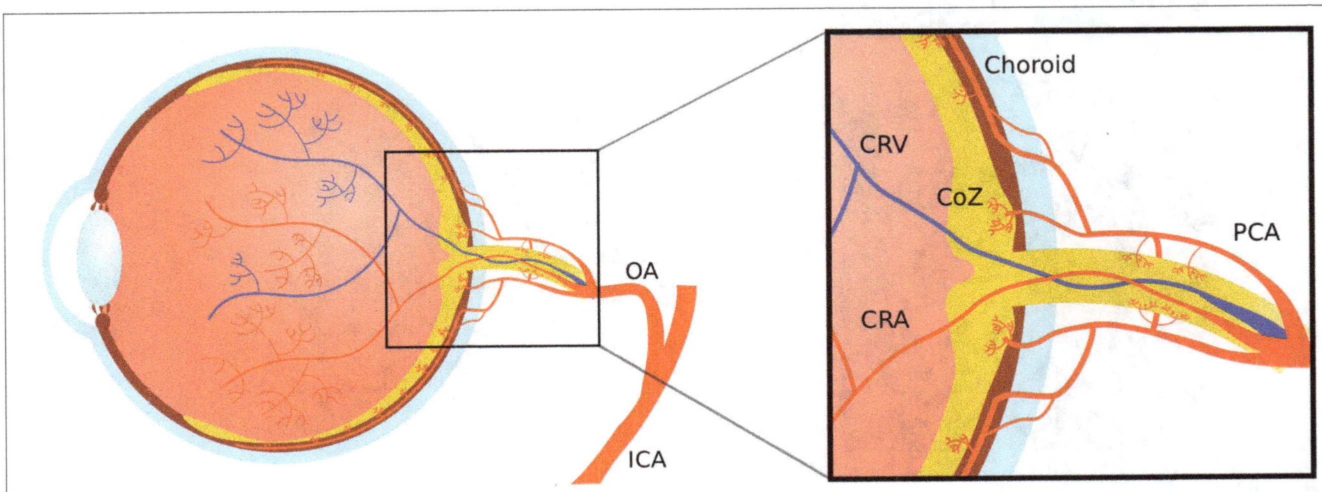

FIGURE 2 | Macrovascular anatomy of the blood supply to the eye. ICA, internal carotid artery; OA, ophthalmic artery; PCA, posterior choroidal artery; CRV, central retinal vein; CRA, central retinal artery; CoZ, circle of Zinn.

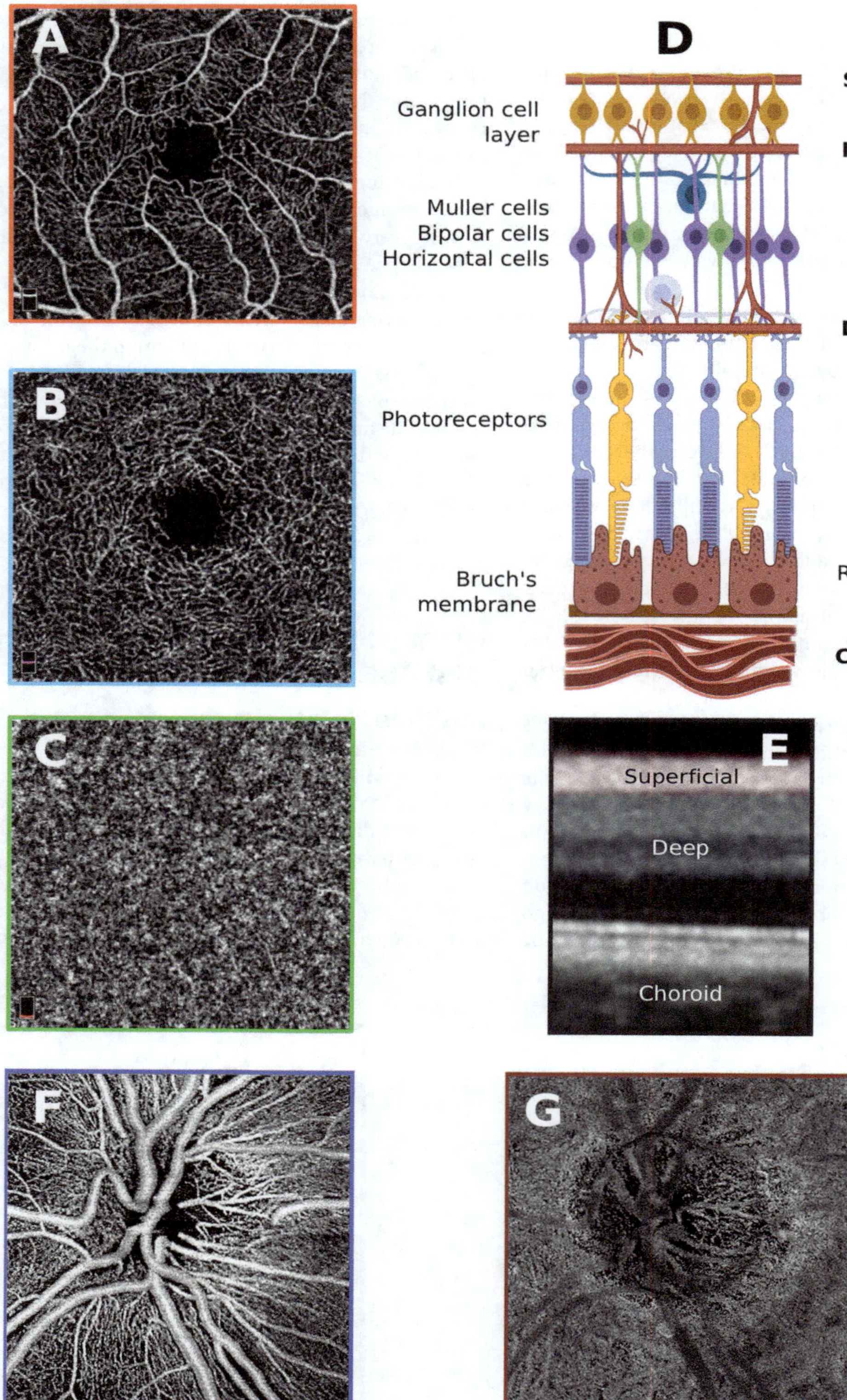

FIGURE 3 | Anatomy of the retinal vascular plexi. **(A)** Macular superficial vascular plexus centered around the fovea. **(B)** Macular deep vascular plexus. **(C)** Macular choroid. **(D)** Locations of the vascular plexi relative to the various cell types that construct the anatomy of the retina. Created with biorender.com. **(E)** Superficial and deep vascular plexi as well as choroid slabs overlain on OCT scan. **(F)** Superficial vascular plexus of the optic nerve head. **(G)** Choroid of the optic nerve head.

MS. Many studies have demonstrated the presence of hypoxia and hypoperfusion in the CNS of MS affected individuals clinically, radiologically, and histologically (1, 10). For example, cerebral type-III MS lesions histologically frequently resemble hypoxic insult and MS lesions tend to form in watershed areas of the areas of the brain, suggesting a role for hypoxia in its pathophysiology (18, 43). Several studies found a reduction in cerebral blood flow in MS affected individuals, even in the absence of structural damage (44, 45). Cerebral circulation times are increased from a mean of 2.8 s in controls to 4.9 s in all types of MS (46). Hypoperfusion in MS can be identified from very early in its disease course, as perfusion rates in patients with clinically isolated syndrome (CIS) have been found to be reduced (47). Additionally, a study which used near-infrared spectroscopy (NIRS) showed that almost half of MS patients had hemoglobin saturation values that were significantly reduced compared with healthy controls (48). Anemia more than doubles the risk of developing MS and also doubles the risk of experiencing a relapse in MS (49). Furthermore, patients with MS have an increased risk of ischaemic heart disease and stroke, suggesting further susceptibility to microvascular damage (50).

Interestingly, one exploratory case study found evidence for transient reduced blood flow focally in the optic nerve during acute MSON (51). Preliminary data suggests that blood flow in the retinal microcirculation is reduced in patients with relapsing-remitting MS compared with healthy controls (52, 53).

Animal work with experimental autoimmune encephalomyelitis (EAE) revealed that the inflamed spinal cord of affected animals was indeed severely hypoxic and hypoperfused (54–57). The level of hypoxia was temporally and spatially related to the clinical deficit, and predicted subsequent demyelinating damage. Investigations indicated that the hypoxia was caused by insufficient perfusion of the CNS, creating a shortage of oxygen delivery in the inflamed area (54). Accordingly, it was found that therapeutic approaches aimed at alleviating hypoxia, with inspired oxygen, or alleviating hypoperfusion, with vasodilating agents, were related to improved neurologic outcome and reduced later stage demyelination in the affected animals (17). These findings suggest that hypoxia and hypoperfusion may render nerve cells inexcitable through depolarization, causing disability in the acute stage, but also damage oligodendrocytes, causing subsequent demyelination.

Although hypoperfusion is increasingly recognized as a possible important component in the multifactorial etiology of MS, interpretation of its role is controversial. Ambiguity remains if it is a primary process, representing a causal factor in the disease mechanism, or a secondary process, representing the result of lower metabolic demand in atrophied tissue (1). As many existing methods for investigating CNS perfusion are invasive, time-consuming, or laborious, little follow-up data is available to discern the temporal patterns of vascular changes in neuroinflammatory disease. Combining OCT and OCTA may offer ways to explore temporal patterns in vascular changes and structural atrophy of the retinal layers, which might provide important insights into the pathophysiological processes that underlie MS.

OCTA in MS

With OCTA being a relatively novel technique, there is a high level of variability in choice of outcome metrics and OCTA system used in studies investigating the microvasculature in MS. Although the variability in test metrics and OCTA systems makes it difficult to make direct comparisons between studies, all currently published studies found a significant reduction in retinal vessel density, in the macular area, the peripapillary area, or both, in MS patients compared with controls. Most also identified clear correlations between structural retinal layer thickness OCT measurements and vessel density (20–22, 58, 59).

The largest study cohort to date consists of 111 RRMS or high-risk CIS patients, who were compared to 50 healthy controls using a Heidelberg Spectralis OCTA (20). This study focused on the macular microvasculature, and found a significant reduction in SVP vessel density from 29.1% in controls to 24.1% in MS eyes ($p < 0.001$), while the DVP was unaffected. Furthermore, MS eyes affected by ON (MSON) had a lower SVP vessel density at 21.7% compared with non-ON (MSNON) eyes at 26.0% ($p < 0.001$). Finally, the difference between vessel densities in MSNON eyes and control eyes just reached significance ($p = 0.03$). Reduced SVP density was related to combined GCL and inner plexiform layer (GCIPL) and pRNFL layer atrophy, while lower DVP densities were related to GCIPL and inner nuclear layer thickness. All analyses were adjusted for age, sex, ON history and within-subject inter-eye correlations. Interestingly, these changes were evident in a cohort of relatively early stage MS, with a mean EDSS scores of 1.5.

These results are corroborated by several smaller studies that recruited 20 to 50 MS patients and similar numbers of healthy controls, that identified reduced macular SVP vessel densities in eyes of MS patients compared with controls (21, 22, 58, 60), with a significant reduction in SVP vessel density in MSON compared with MSNON eyes being identified in the two larger cohort (21, 60). Two studies identified an additional significant reduction in DVP vessel density, one in MS compared with controls (21) and one only in MSON compared with MSNON (22) (**Figure 4**). However, not all studies have replicated the finding of reduced macular SVP vessel density in MS (61).

In two smaller cohorts of 35 and 45 patients with relatively more advanced MS, vessel density around the optic nerve head (ONH) was reduced in MS eyes compared to control eyes, as well as in MSON eyes compared with MSNON (61, 62). One study identified reduced vessel densities specifically in the inferior and nasal sections around the ONH in MS patients compared with controls (58), while another study found reductions only in the temporal zone (21). The finding of reduced vessel densities around the ONH has been classified as "capillary dropout" (61).

A recent study developed a novel metric, called volumetric vessel density (VVD), by dividing the macular vessel densities of the SVP and DVP by the tissue volume of the corresponding retinal layers (59). In a large cohort of 80 RRMS patients and

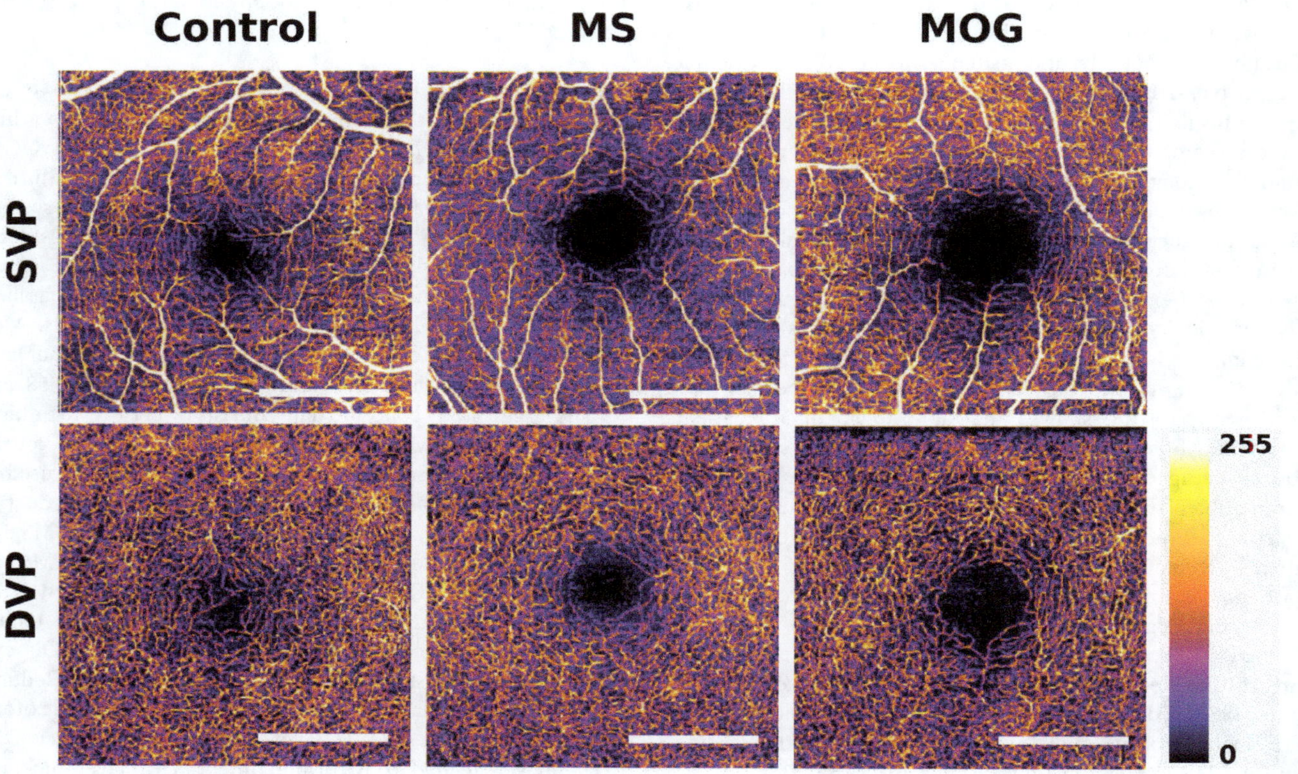

FIGURE 4 | Example of macular superficial vascular plexus (SVP) and deep vascular plexus (DVP) changes in MS and MOG-Ab seropositive NMOSD compared with a healthy control. The scans of MS and MOG-Ab seropositive NMOSD patients are made from eyes without prior optic neuritis. The foveal avascular zones (FAZ) of the MS and NMOSD eyes are greater than these in the healthy control. Scale bar: 1 mm. Scans are 3x3 mm and obtained with the Heidelberg Engineering OCT2 system.

99 matched controls, the VVD of the DVP was higher in MS patients compared with controls. Additionally, the VVD of the DVP and SVP of MSON eyes were significantly higher compared with MSNON eyes (59). This is an interesting new metric that combines structural and microvascular changes in the retina. However, one could argue that it might be clearer to estimate structural and microvascular measures independently, as the VVD is determined to a high degree by changes in retinal thickness. Therefore, the observed increase of the VVD might still reflect a strong decrease in vascular structure density that is obscured by a more pronounced decrease in retinal thickness. This seems not unlikely, as the volume of vascular structures is smaller compared with their corresponding retinal layers and structural retinal atrophy is severe after MSON. This appears to be affirmed by the fact that VVD measures were strongly and negatively correlated with analyzed tissue volumes. However, the VVD is an important step toward incorporating data as we look at the full integrated structural and functional system going forward.

The size and shape of the foveal avascular zone, readily visible using OCTA, has been used as an outcome metric in studies of diabetic retinopathy (63). The foveal avascular zone (FAZ) was used as the outcome metric in one study of MS, and found that neither the area nor perimeter of the FAZ differed between MS patients and healthy controls, even though the FAZ size was negatively related to the vessel density of the SVP and DVP (21).

OCTA data captured in the acute stages of ON is currently lacking, although one small case series of seven MSON patients with good clinical recovery did find significantly reduced SVP macular and ONH vessel densities in affected compared with unaffected eyes 2–8 months after the episode (64). These changes in vessel density were in all cases accompanied by structural thickness loss of the macular GCL layers. Prospective studies investigating the hyperacute stages of MSON might be able to delineate the temporal relationships between structural and vascular changes, which could further the understanding of the role of hypoperfusion in the pathophysiology of MS. The challenge here however will be disc swelling which limts OCTA signal strength.

Just one study has collected longitudinal OCTA data in MS patients to date. One-year follow-up OCTA scans were performed in a cohort of 50 MS patients (mean EDSS 3.5 and average disease duration of 11 years) who had stable disease and were on disease modifying treatment. Interestingly, parafoveal vessel densities increased slightly, a finding just reaching significance ($p = 0.035$), while structural thickness of the pRNFL and GCL remained stable (65). This provides some evidence for possible vascular regeneration or increase of lumen thickness in chronic disease, but additional longitudinal data on the microvasculature in MS, including in its earlier stages, are needed to interpret these findings. Future longitudinal data are required to identify if OCTA can function as a biomarker to predict and monitor disease progression in MS and other neurodegenerative disease (66).

Finally, although glaucoma research suggests that vascular density loss is faster in early-stage disease and has a lower floor-effect in late-stage disease compared with common structural OCT measurements, this has not yet been demonstrated in studies of MS patients (23, 25, 26).

Correlation OCTA With Clinical Measures in MS

A lower vessel density of the macular SVP was found to be related to a higher EDSS score and lower low-contrast visual acuity in MS patients (20). Interestingly, in this study results of other clinical outcomes like the 9-hole peg test, the timed 25-foot walk test and the multiple sclerosis functional composite (MSFC) were related to macular SVP vessel density, while combined GCL and inner plexiform layer thickness was not. Another study describes an inverse correlation between visual evoked potential latency times and vessel density of the SVP and DVP (21). Additional, smaller, studies identify no relationship between vascular metrics and clinical or visual outcomes (62). Interestingly, increased vessel density of the macular choriocapillaris has been found to be associated with higher inflammatory disease activity prior to the OCTA examination, suggesting another possible OCTA biomarker in MS (22). Finally, VVD of the macular SVP was positively related to EDSS and disease duration, while being negatively related to low-contrast letter acuity (59).

Neuromyelitis Optica Spectrum Disorder (NMOSD)

Vascular Pathology and NMOSD

The autoimmune inflammatory conditions of NMOSD share cardinal features of ON, longitudinally extensive transverse myelitis and area postrema syndrome that are often relapsing (12, 67). Although attention for vascular changes in neuroinflammatory disease has been primarily focused on MS, there is also evidence that NMOSD pathophysiology is in part vascularly mediated (68, 69). In most cases NMOSD is caused by the pathogenic effects of auto-antibodies targeting the water channel protein aquaporin-4 (AQP4), for which the majority of patients test positive. As AQP4 is predominantly expressed on perivascular astrocytic foot processes in the spinal cord and by Müller cells in the retina, NMOSD has a predilection for the anterior visual system and the spinal cord (70). Approximately 40% of NMOSD patients that test negative for AQP4 antibodies, test positive for antibodies against myelin oligodendrocyte glycoprotein (MOG) (67).

Neuropathology of AQP4-antibody seropositive NMOSD lesions show a perivascular pattern (71, 72), with rim deposits of activated complement components and macrophages found around thickened, fibrosed, and hyalinised vessels (73). Active spinal cord lesions may have an increased density of vascular structures (71). Similar to MS lesions predominantly forming in watershed areas of the brain with poor perfusion, AQP4-Ab seropositive NMOSD lesions preferentially form in the hypo-perfused posterior and lateral spinal columns (74). Interestingly, the choroid plexus expresses AQP4 to a high degree, and immunoreactivity of choroidal plexus epithelial cells is profoundly affected or even lost in NMOSD, even though the choroidal plexus remained structurally intact in neuropathological investigation (75). AQP4 is expressed in a vasculocentric pattern in the optic nerve and spinal cord (72).

Importantly, the predominantly perivascular location of is one of the key neuropathological features that can distinguish AQP4-antibody associated NMOSD from MS lesions at autopsy (72). One study found that retinal vascular changes identified through fundoscopy, such as attenuation of the peripapillary vascular tree (present in 3/40 MS eyes and 22/32 NMOSD eyes; $p = 0.001$) and focal arteriolar narrowing (present in 0/40 MS eyes and 9/32 NMOSD eyes; $p < 0.001$) could successfully distinguish NMOSD from MS patients (19). OCTA may be diagnostically useful tool capable of picking up these vascular differences more easily and systematically. To become clinically useful the aim will be to get high diagnostic sensitivity and specificity levels.

Neuropathological studies of CNS lesions in MOG-antibody seropositive patients reveal distinctly different features compared with AQP4-antibody associated lesions. Although MOG associated lesions have a predilection for perivascular locations, this is less profound compared with AQP4-associated pathology. MOG lesions were found to share pathological characteristics with immunotype II and III MS lesions (76). Type III pattern of demyelination shows similar tissue changes as observed in early stage white matter ischemia, and is therefore hypothesized to potentially be caused in part by hypoxia (77).

OCTA in NMOSD

Although there is currently a very limited number of studies published on OCTA in NMOSD, all available data suggest profound decreases in microvascular densities in affected individuals exist (27, 78, 79). A recent study investigating differences in structural thickness and microvascular retinal density of 27 AQP4-antibody seropositive NMOSD patients and 31 healthy controls found a significant difference in vessel density of the peripapillary region and the macular SVP between patients with NMOSD and controls. Interestingly, there were also significant reductions in vessel density in the macular and ONH region when comparing NMOSD patient without previous ON to controls ($p = 0.023$ and $p = 0.029$), while retinal thickness measures of the macular GCL and pRNFL were similar in these groups (27). These findings were replicated by a second study, that also found that vascular densities in the macula and ONH were reduced in NMOSD patients without ON compared with healthy controls, while pRNFL and macular GCL were not (78). This suggests OCTA may be more sensitive to ON-independent damage to the anterior visual system in NMOSD compared with structural OCT (**Figure 4**).

Additionally, these findings of vascular dropout in the absence of structural thinning argue against the hypothesis that reductions in microvascular density are a result of reduced demand in atrophied tissue and, if replicated, may provide evidence for a role of microvascular dysfunction as an independent disease process in NMOSD.

Both the densities of the macular SVP and DVP have been found to be negatively correlated to visual acuity measures in NMOSD (79).

Given that neuropathological research suggests that vascular vessel walls seem to be affected by fibrosis and thickening in NMOSD, it is important to consider that OCTA depicts as a vessel is actually moving blood within a vascular lumen. Therefore, OCTA can depict vessel thinning and capillary dropout, but not the unmoving vessel wall itself. In order to visualize these changes *in-vivo*, devices capable of high-resolution imaging which are not dependent on motion contrast are required, such as adaptive optics coupled ophthalmoscopy. The potentially more profound vascular changes in the anterior visual system of NMOSD patients compared with MS might be the result of the reduced metabolic demand associated with more severe structural atrophy in NMOSD related ON, although the reduction in vascular density in the absence of atrophy argue against this. Furthermore, the vascular pathology might be a result of more mechanical constriction at the ONH due to more severe papilledema during ON. Although there is some evidence for more profound papilledema in ON associated with NMOSD compared with MS, the fact that vascular density reductions are also identifiable in patients without ON is incongruous.

Data on OCTA alterations observed in MOG associated disease and in MOG associated ON specifically is currently lacking. Finally, future research is needed to investigate if certain distinctive qualitative or quantitative differences in retinal microvascular changes exist between MS and NMOSD that might provide valuable additions to the diagnostic arsenal.

PRACTICAL SOURCES OF BIAS

There are several important practical factors that should be taken into account when designing an OCTA study, as these may influence outcome metrics and thereby confound findings (23). First, there are various demographic factors that are associated with differences in OCTA results. For example, older age is associated with reduced macular and peripapillary vessel density (80, 81). Furthermore, in glaucoma research, eyes of people from European descent have been identified to have lower vessel density measures compared with eyes of people from African descent (23). Both hypertension and diabetes mellitus are related with decreased macular vessel density, also in the absence of a retinopathy. Chronic use of topical beta-blockers may lead to some reduction in macular SVP density (81).

Myopia is another important factor that is related to significant reductions in vessel density measurements. Highly myopic individuals have been found to have significantly lower vessel densities in the peripapillary region compared with emmetropic eyes. Myopic glaucomatous eyes have more severely reduced vessel densities compared with emmetropic glaucomatous eyes (82, 83). Image magnification in myopic eyes may be in part responsible for these effects (23). On the other hand, a greater disc size was not related to changes in peripapillary vessel density in one cross-sectional study (84).

Besides these demographic factors, there are also some important considerations regarding the timing of OCTA measurements. One study reported that in a small cohort of 13 healthy subjects, vessel density decreased significantly after strenuous physical activity (85). Retinal vessel calibers vary slightly with the cardiac cycle (86). Preliminary data suggests that increases in heart rate and blood pressure are related to higher macular SVP density measurements (87). The same study showed no important diurnal changes in OCTA vessel density.

Interestingly, multiple studies have found that vessel densities were reduced in OCTA scans with lower signal strength (84, 85, 87, 88). This is important since low image quality and motion artifacts are common in OCTA, mainly due to the relatively long acquisition time. As the OCTA signal is based on a threshold of change (movement) detected across the volume, when signal is reduced, vessels are harder to detect leading to reduced vessel density in poor scan quality volumes. Small pupillary size can interfere with image acquisition and generally pupil dilation is necessary for high quality images (89). Finally, media opacities in the lens or especially in the vitreous, can significantly reduce image quality.

Glaucoma research has shown that intra- and intervisit variability of OCTA vessel density measures is between 2.5 and 6.6% in the peripapillary region and between 3.4 and 5.6% in the macular SVP (88, 90). This intra- and intervisit variability of vessel density measures is more than is reported for OCT structural measures of the pRNFL and GCL thicknesses, which is ~1.5%. Importantly, glaucoma affected eyes had worse intervisit repeatability compared with healthy eyes, an effect that can be expected to occur in ON affected eyes as well due to problems with focusing (91). Future developments improving image acquisition speeds and eye-tracking of commercial OCTA systems are needed to bring intra- and intervisit repeatability into a range closer to OCT.

ADVANTAGES AND DISADVANTAGES OF OCTA

There are opportunities as well as obstacles when using OCTA in neuroinflammatory disease. Compared to other types of retinal vascular imaging, such as fluorescein angiography, OCTA is quick and non-invasive, with no intravenous dyes required. Most devices are user-friendly and require limited training to perform standard imaging. The speed at which OCTA can be obtained means it could be easily integrated into a clinical setting, especially where OCT is already performed and a multimodal retinal imaging setup is available.

The real strength of OCTA is in its multifunctional capacity. As it uses the change in the structural OCT images to map blood flow, both forms of imaging are collected simultaneously. Some studies have combined the information on tissue structure and vascular density to elucidate the vascular impact of multiple sclerosis, increasing diagnostic accuracy. Coupling structural information from retinal thicknesses with vascular density allows for a more complete picture of individual patients, which is highly useful especially in a disease with such variable presentation as MS.

OCTA also has certain disadvantages, namely imaging artifacts and inability to detect dynamic vessel related changes such as leakage or venous sheathing (92). There are yet no consensus quality control criteria similar to what has been achieved for OCT (30). Additionally, OCTA creates a binary 3D figure of moving components to static retinal tissue, but it cannot quantify retinal perfusion as it cannot measure blood velocity. It does not differentiate between areas of high and low flow. Multi-modal imaging approaches which combine Doppler OCT and OCTA are able to add this information, by adding velocimetry to the depth encoded OCTA image (93). In addition, novel high dynamic range OCTA systems are a promising extension to the technology that are sensitive to flow speeds, and are not compromised by angle issues present in Doppler OCT systems (94).

Imaging artifacts are a well-documented limitation to OCTA (95) which are further compounded by visual loss and nystagmus in neuroinflammatory disease (96). Small movements can have profound effects on an OCTA image. As the laser is scanned across the retina, small transverse motions of the eye in respect to that laser can lead to mass displacement of locations in the resulting image, causing a motion artifact. In order to choose the correct location for OCTA imaging, patients are required to fixate on a small target either internal or external to the imaging device. Patients with a history of ON may have poor fixation and are therefore more prone to these motion artifacts. These problems are enhanced in acute ON, where impact on the retinal vasculature may be most profound. Small eye movements can be compounded by larger movements caused by postural difficulties, especially in situations where the standard OCT set up is uncomfortable for the patient. Adjustments can be made but unfortunately there is not yet a handheld OCTA device commercially available to allow for complete accessibility for children and less mobile patients, especially in the later stages of disease. Fast and efficient scanning of the retina to avoid making patients sit or fixate for too long could rectify this issue of motion artifacts.

Segmentation of vascular layers, allowing the user to distinguish individual vessel networks, is a unique ability of OCTA. However, automated segmentation by the device is not always accurate, leading to segmentation artifacts in images which can appear as vessel dropout. Initial identification of the artifact is crucial, and segmentation can be manually adjusted by the user, but there is no consensus currently as to how these artifacts should be identified and remedied.

Ocular complications of MS can also lead to image artifacts. Media opacity, as found in uveitis, greatly diminishes the quality of imaging possible using OCTA. Changes in the optical pathway, such as that caused by microcystic macular oedema (MMO) that occur in MS and NMOSD, could also lead to distortions in the resulting signal.

Overall; motion artifacts, segmentation artifacts and opacity issues can have a profound impact in image quality in OCTA. The importance of quality control of OCT images has been widely accepted in recent times, as evidenced by the OSCAR-IB criteria being integrated into many clinical trials (97–99). Quality control of OCTA images is essential and should be stressed in both the design and interpretation of studies using OCTA in MS. The creation of a set of quality control criteria for OCTA may be very helpful for the standardization of methods between different studies.

The field of view available on OCTA devices is limited, with the largest scanning area available using commercial OCTA is 8x8 mm, a field of view of ~30 degrees. Images may be collected separately and "stitched" together, but this extends the image collection time and this montaging capability is not available on all devices (**Figure 5**). Peripheral changes in the vasculature, such as those caused by vasculitis, are not likely to be detected using even the largest available field of view. Wide-field OCTA when available would be of great benefit to studying the retinal microvasculature in MS.

Each device has its own machine-specific algorithm to measure the difference between B-scans in order to build a picture of the retinal vessels with specific detection thresholds. Many instances where blood flow is altered, such as in leaking vessels, microaneurysms, and polypoidal lesions, will not be detected since they are below this threshold. Interesting vascular features that occur in neuroinflammatory disease, such as venous sheathing or vascular leakage, will not be picked up by OCTA.

FUTURE OUTLOOK

As discussed in this review, OCTA has only just started to be utilized in research into neuroinflammatory disease. Preliminary studies suggest that the microvascular network in the macula and the peripapillary area is less dense in MS patients, and while prior MSON insult exacerbates this finding it is also present in the absence of MSON. Similar findings are identified in the first studies reporting on AQP4-antibody seropositive NMOSD patients. Interestingly, reduced vascular densities are even identified prior to structural atrophy of retinal layers in NMOSD. Larger cohorts of ON patients in the acute stage are necessary to elucidate the timing of vascular relative to structural changes, to identify if OCTA is indeed more sensitive to early-stage damage and to find if disparities in timing of these two factors may be of diagnostic value in differentiating NMOSD and MS related ON. Furthermore, glaucoma research shows that OCTA has a lower "floor-effect" compared with OCT, being able to pick up further damage in a severely structurally atrophied retina (23–26). If research in neuroinflammatory disease could identify a similar effect, OCTA vascular densities may be more suitable outcome measures in clinical trials where participants

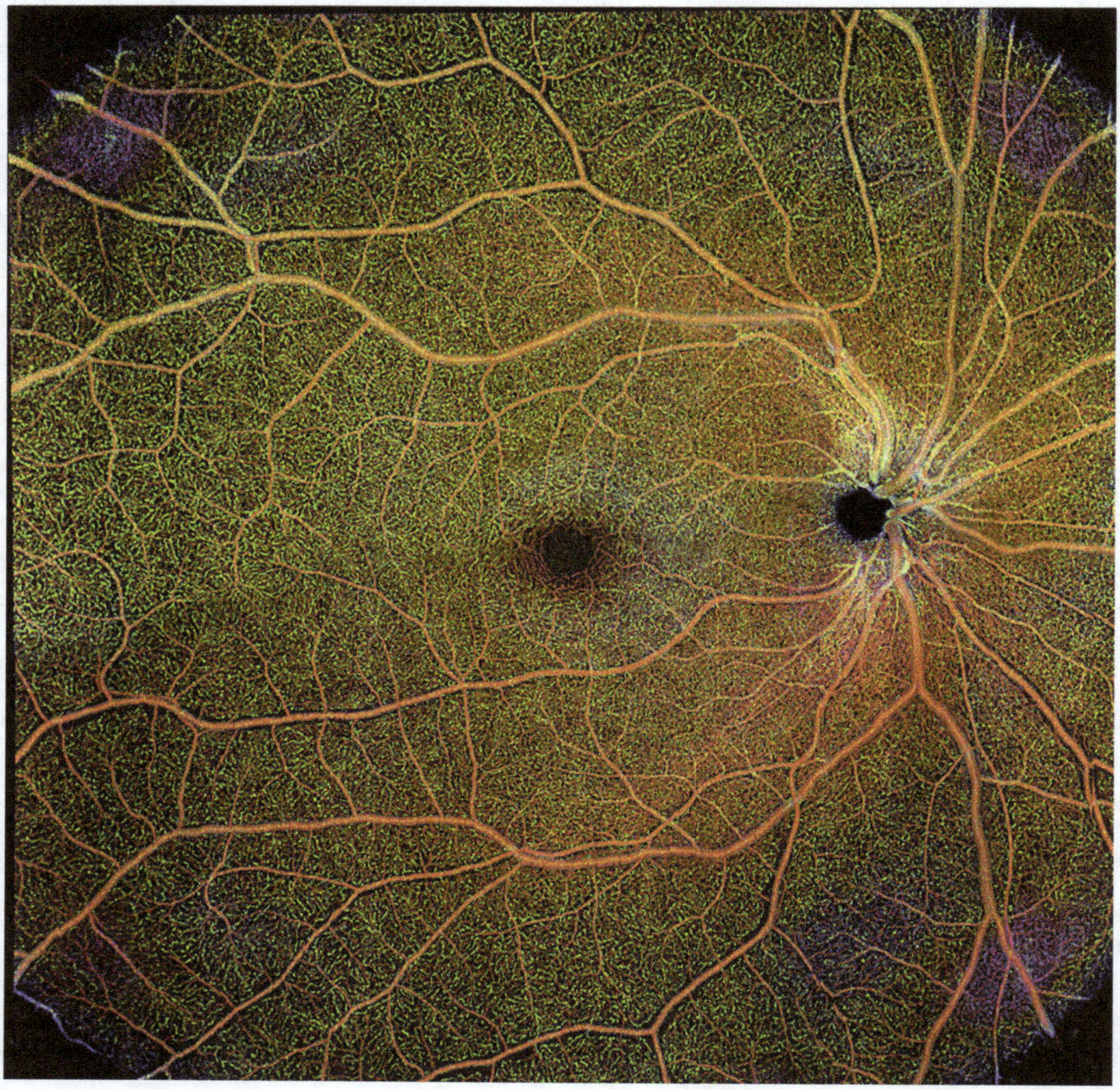

FIGURE 5 | Composite of wide-field optical coherence tomography angiography (OCTA) scan in healthy eye. Scan sample obtained with the Plex Elite 9000 (Carl Zeiss Meditec). Figure is a reprint from Kleerekooper et al. (10).

have advanced (progressive) disease or have suffered retinal insult due to prior ON compared with OCT. Additionally, choroidal density measures may be a valuable biomarker for disease activity.

The biggest cohort to date studying OCTA in MS (20) found that vascular density correlated with more clinical outcome measures compared with structural OCT metrics. This seems to suggest that the association between certain clinical parameters may be stronger with OCTA compared with OCT thickness measures, which is in line with results in glaucoma research (23). More data is necessary to see if OCTA may provide a more relevant outcome metric that is just as easily obtainable as OCT.

As mentioned before, the possibility to elucidate the timing of vascular relative to structural insult to the retina after acute ON may help to understand the role of hypoperfusion and energy failure in MS pathophysiology. If vascular damage occurs before structural atrophy can be identified, this would give argument to the important role of hypoperfusion in MS related damage. However, if vascular density loss occurs after thinning of retinal layers, this suggests that vascular supply may be reduced due to lower local metabolic demand. This is an important question, given the potential therapeutic possibilities that may reduce MS disability accrual by alleviating hypoperfusion, that OCTA might help answer (17).

Most research has focused on the peripapillary vascular layers and the macular SVP and DVP. As alluded to shortly in this review, there may be benefit to looking into the other retinal vascular layers, such as the choroidal layer. One study identified that a more dense choroidal plexus was related to more severe disease activity in the time before, suggesting it may provide an interesting biomarker (22). However, caution needs to be taken when looking at layers situated more deeply, as it is difficult to accurately interpret the meaning of imaged data. As light travels deeper through retinal tissue, it is more distorted and affected by absorption at different levels, producing a less reliable image.

From personal experience, we know that MS patients may have abnormal phenotypes of the FAZ on OCTA (see **Figure 6** for unpublished observations). However, similar FAZ abnormalities are sometimes also observed in healthy controls, and additional study is required to see if these are more common in MS.

Finally, OCTA may be able to pick up temporal and spatial differences in the choroidal blood supply, that is highly

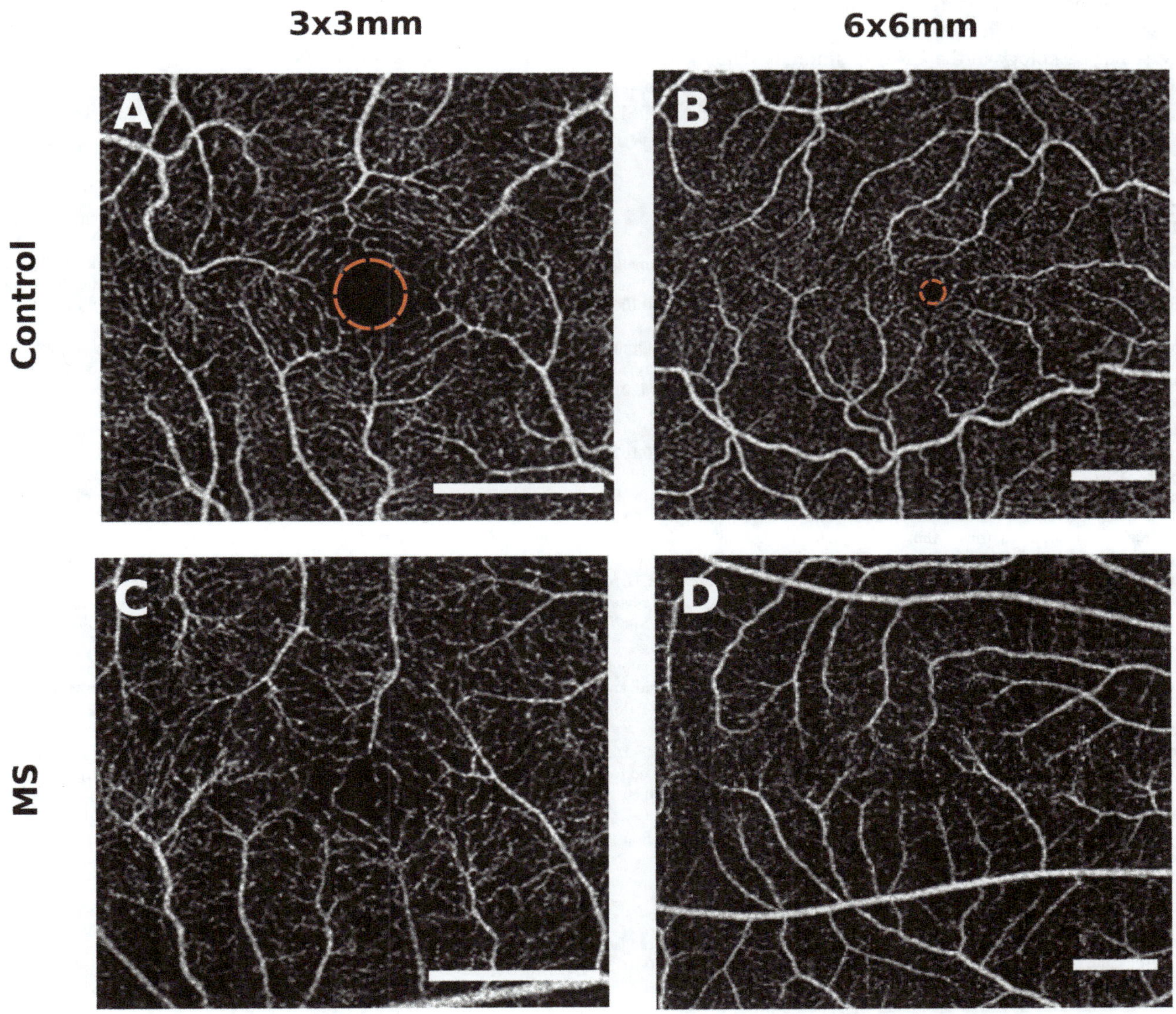

FIGURE 6 | Example of a foveal avascular zone (FAZ) abnormality in a patient with multiple sclerosis (MS). These figures represent an unpublished observation from the authors. However, abnormal FAZ phenotypes are also sometimes observed in healthy subjects, and additional research is necessary to investigate if these are more common in MS compared with healthy controls. **(A,B)** are from two different controls and show a symmetrical and round FAZ. **(C,D)** are from the same MS patient and show an asymmetric FAZ with vessels growing further into the center. Scale bar: 1 mm. The FAZ is delineated with a red circle in **(A,B)** (healthy control eyes).

adaptive to fluctuations in local demand. Preliminary animal studies have demonstrated spatial and temporal heterogeneity in retinal blood supply (8). OCTA may be used to investigate if neuroinflammatory disease decreases the adaptability of the ocular blood supply.

CONCLUSION

OCTA provides an alternative quantitative measure for retinal damage in MS and NMOSD. Early results suggest that in certain circumstances OCTA, compared with OCT, may be more sensitive to retinal changes both early in the disease process, making it useful for detection of disease, and late in the disease process, rendering it suitable for monitoring of disease. Furthermore, it may also serve as a surrogate measure for vascular pathology in the CNS. Preliminary data of patients both with and without optic neuritis consistently reveal lower densities of the retinal microvasculature in both MS and NMOSD compared with healthy controls. Exploring the temporality of vascular relative to structural changes may help answer important questions about the role of hypoperfusion in the pathophysiology of neuroinflammatory disease. Finally, qualitative characteristics of retinal microvasculature may help discriminate between different neuroinflammatory disorders. However, we have to be mindful of issues such as image quality and standardization before incorporating OCTA into clinical practice.

AUTHOR CONTRIBUTIONS

IK and SH: literature search, writing main text, and creating figures. AD, ST, and AP: manuscript writing and revision for intellectual content. All authors contributed to the article and approved the submitted version.

ACKNOWLEDGMENTS

We would like to thank the ECTRIMS for supporting IK through the ECTRIMS postdoctoral research fellowship.

REFERENCES

Martinez Sosa S, Smith KJ. Understanding a role for hypoxia in lesion formation and location in the deep and periventricular white matter in small vessel disease and multiple sclerosis. *Clin Sci.* (2017) 131:2503–24. doi: 10.1042/CS20170981

Koustenis A Jr, Harris A, Gross J, Januleviciene I, Shah A, Siesky B. Optical coherence tomography angiography : an overview of the technology and an assessment of applications for clinical research. *Br J Ophtalmol.* (2017) 101:16–20. doi: 10.1136/bjophthalmol-2016-309389

Huang D, Swanson EA, Lin CP, Schuman JS, Stinson WG, Chang W, et al. Optical coherence tomography. *Science.* (1991) 254:1178–81. doi: 10.1002/ccd.23385

Trip SA, Schlottmann PG, Jones SJ, Altmann DR, Garway-Heath DF, Thompson AJ, et al. Retinal nerve fiber layer axonal loss and visual dysfunction in optic neuritis. *Ann Neurol.* (2005) 58:383–91. doi: 10.1002/ana.20575

Petzold A, Balcer LJ, Calabresi PA, Costello F, Frohman TC, Frohman EM, et al. Retinal layer segmentation in multiple sclerosis: a systematic review and meta-analysis. *Lancet Neurol.* (2017) 16:797–812. doi: 10.1016/S1474-4422(17)30278-8

Joyal J, Gantner ML, Smith LEH. Retinal energy demands control vascular supply of the retina in development and disease: the role of neuronal lipid and glucose metabolism. *Prog Retin Eye Res.* (2018) 64:131–56. doi: 10.1016/j.preteyeres.2017.11.002

Campbell JP, Zhang M, Hwang TS, Bailey ST, Wilson DJ, Jia Y, et al. Detailed vascular anatomy of the human retina by projection- resolved optical coherence tomography angiography. *Sci Rep.* (2017) 7:1–11. doi: 10.1038/srep42201

Yu D, Cringle SJ, Yu PK, Balaratnasingam C, Mehnert A, Sarunic MV, et al. Retinal capillary perfusion: spatial and temporal heterogeneity. *Prog Retin Eye Res.* (2019). doi: 10.1016/j.preteyeres.2019.01.001

Wong-Riley M. Energy metabolism of the visual system. *Eye Brain.* (2010) 2:99–116. doi: 10.2147/EB.S9078

Kleerekooper I, Petzold A, Trip SA. Anterior visual system imaging to investigate energy failure in multiple sclerosis. *Brain.* (2020) 143:1999–2008. doi: 10.1093/brain/awaa049

Oertel FC, Zimmermann H, Paul F, Brandt AU. Optical coherence tomography in neuromyelitis optica spectrum disorders: potential advantages for individualized monitoring of progression and therapy. *EPMA J.* (2018) 9:21–33. doi: 10.1007/s13167-017-0123-5

Wingerchuk D, Banwell B, Bennett JL, Cabre P, Carroll W, Jacob A, et al. International consensus diagnostic criteria for neuromyelitis optica spectrum disorders. *Neurology.* (2015) 85:177–89. doi: 10.1212/WNL.0000000000001729

Toosy AT, Mason DF, Miller DH. Optic neuritis. *Lancet Neurol.* (2014) 13:83–99. doi: 10.1016/S1474-4422(13)70259-X

Petzold A, Woodhall M, Khaleeli Z, Tobin WO, Pittock SJ, Weinshenker BG, et al. Aquaporin-4 and myelin oligodendrocyte glycoprotein antibodies in immune-mediated optic neuritis at long-term follow-up. *J Neurol Neurosurg Psychiatry.* (2019) 90:1021–6. doi: 10.1136/jnnp-2019-320493

Toussaint D, Périer O, Verstappen A, Bervoets S. Clinicopathological study of the visual pathways, eyes, and cerebral hemispheres in 32 cases of disseminated sclerosis. *J Clin Neuroophthalmol.* (1983) 3:211–20.

Green AJ, McQuaid S, Hauser SL, Allen IV, Lyness R. Ocular pathology in multiple sclerosis: retinal atrophy and inflammation irrespective of disease duration. *Brain.* (2010) 133:1591–601. doi: 10.1093/brain/awq080

Desai RA, Davies AL, Del Rossi N, Tachrount M, Dyson A, Gustavson B, et al. Nimodipine reduces dysfunction and demyelination in models of multiple sclerosis. *Ann Neurol.* (2020) 88:123–36 doi: 10.1002/ana.25749

Haider L, Zrzavy T, Hametner S, Höftberger R, Bagnato F, Grabner G, et al. The topograpy of demyelination and neurodegeneration in the multiple sclerosis brain. *Brain.* (2016) 139:807–15. doi: 10.1093/brain/awv398

Green AJ, Cree BAC. Distinctive retinal nerve fibre layer and vascular changes in neuromyelitis optica following optic neuritis. *J Neurol Neurosurg Psychiatry.* (2009) 80:1002–5. doi: 10.1136/jnnp.2008.166207

Murphy OC, Kwakyi O, Iftikhar M, Zafar S, Lambe J, Pellegrini N, et al. Alterations in the retinal vasculature occur in multiple sclerosis and exhibit novel correlations with disability and visual function measures. *Mult Scler J.* (2019) 26:815–28. doi: 10.1177/1352458519845116

Yilmaz H, Ersoy A, Icel E. Assessments of vessel density and foveal avascular zone metrics in multiple sclerosis: an optical coherence tomography angiography study. *Eye.* (2020) 34:771–8. doi: 10.1038/s41433-019-0746-y

Feucht N, Maier M, Lepennetier G, Pettenkofer M, Wetzlmair C, Daltrozzo T, et al. Optical coherence tomography angiography indicates associations of the retinal vascular network and disease activity in multiple sclerosis. *Mult Scler J.* (2018) 25:224–34. doi: 10.1177/1352458517750009

Rao HL, Pradhan ZS, Suh MH, Moghimi S, Mansouri K, Weinreb RN. Optical coherence tomography angiography in glaucoma. *J Glaucoma.* (2020) 29:355–7. doi: 10.1097/IJG.0000000000001463

Van Melkebeke L, Barbosa-Breda J, Huygens M, Stalmans I. Optical coherence tomography angiography in glaucoma: a review. *Ophthalmic Res.* (2018) 60:139–51. doi: 10.1159/000488495

Hou H, Moghimi S, Proudfoot JA, Ghahari E, Penteado RC, Bowd C, et al. Ganglion cell complex thickness and macular vessel density loss in primary open-angle glaucoma. *Ophthalmology.* (2020) 127:1043–52. doi: 10.1016/j.ophtha.2019.12.030

Moghimi S, Bowd C, Zangwill LM, Penteado RC, Hasenstab K, Hou H, et al. Measurement floors and dynamic ranges of OCT and

OCT angiography in glaucoma. *Ophthalmology.* (2019) 126:980–8. doi: 10.1016/j.ophtha.2019.03.003

Chen Y, Shi C, Zhou L, Huang S, Shen M, He Z. The detection of retina microvascular density in subclinical aquaporin-4 antibody seropositive neuromyelitis optica spectrum disorders. *Front Neurol.* (2020) 11:35. doi: 10.3389/fneur.2020.00035

Petzold A, Wong S, Plant GT. Autoimmunity in visual loss. *Handb Clin Neurol.* (2016) 133:353–76. doi: 10.1016/B978-0-444-63432-0.00020-7

Sati P, Oh J, Todd Constable R, Evangelou N, Guttmann CRG, Henry RG, et al. The central vein sign and its clinical evaluation for the diagnosis of multiple sclerosis: a consensus statement from the North American Imaging in Multiple Sclerosis Cooperative. *Nat Rev Neurol.* (2016) 12:714–22. doi: 10.1038/nrneurol.2016.166

Tewarie P, Balk L, Costello F, Green A, Martin R, Schippling S. The OSCAR- IB consensus criteria for retinal OCT quality assessment. *PLoS ONE.* (2012) 7:e34823. doi: 10.1371/journal.pone.0034823

Kim DY, Fingler J, Werner JS, Schwartz DM, Fraser SE, Zawadzki RJ. *In vivo* volumetric imaging of human retinal circulation with phase- variance optical coherence tomography. *Biomed Opt Express.* (2011) 2:1504. doi: 10.1364/boe.2.001504

Schwartz DM, Fingler J, Kim DY, Zawadzki RJ, Morse LS, Park SS, et al. Phase-variance optical coherence tomography: a technique for noninvasive angiography. *Ophthalmology.* (2014) 121:180–7. doi: 10.1016/j.ophtha.2013.09.002

Spaide RF, Curcio CA. Evaluation of segmentation of the superficial and deep vascular layers of the retina by optical coherence tomography angiography instruments in normal eyes. *JAMA Ophthalmol.* (2017) 135:259– 62. doi: 10.1001/jamaophthalmol.2016.5327

Falavarjani KG, Shenazandi H, Naseri D, Anvar P, Kazemi P, Aghamohammadi F, et al. Foveal avascular zone and vessel density in healthy subjects: an optical coherence tomography angiography study. *J Ophthalmic Vis Res.* (2018) 12:260–5. doi: 10.4103/jovr.jovr

Lu Y, Simonett JM, Wang J, Zhang M, Hwang T, Hagag AM, et al. Evaluation of automatically quantified foveal avascular zone metrics for diagnosis of diabetic retinopathy using optical coherence tomography angiography. *Investig Ophthalmol Vis Sci.* (2018) 59:2212–21. doi: 10.1167/iovs.17-23498

Zahid S, Dolz-Marco R, Freund KB, Balaratnasingam C, Dansingani K, Gilani F, et al. Fractal dimensional analysis of optical coherence tomography angiography in eyes with diabetic retinopathy. *Investig Ophthalmol Vis Sci.* (2016) 57:4940–7. doi: 10.1167/iovs.16-19656

Lu CD, Lee B, Schottenhamml J, Maier A, Pugh EN Jr, Fujimoto JG. Photoreceptor layer thickness changes during dark adaptation observed with ultrahigh-resolution optical coherence tomography. *Investig Ophthalmol Vis Sci.* (2017) 1:4632–43. doi 10.1167/iovs.17-22171

Martin AR, Bailie JR, Robson T, McKeown SR, Al-Assar O, McFarland A, et al. Retinal pericytes control expression of nitric oxide synthase and endothelin-1 in microvascular endothelial cells. *Microvasc Res.* (2000) 59:131– 9. doi: 10.1006/mvre.1999.2208

Wang X, Lou N, Eberhardt A, Yang Y, Kusk P, Xu Q, et al. An ocular glymphatic clearance system removes β-amyloid from the rodent eye. *Sci Transl Med.* (2020) 12:eaaw3210. doi: 10.1126/scitranslmed.aaw3210

Frank RN, Turczyn TJ, Das A. Pericyte coverage of retinal and cerebral capillaries. *Investig Ophthalmol Vis Sci.* (1990) 31:999–1007.

Reich DS, Lucchinetti CF, Calabresi PA. Multiple sclerosis. *N Engl J Med.* (2018) 378:169–80. doi: 10.1056/NEJMra1401483

Thompson AJ, Baranzini SE, Geurts J, Hemmer B, Ciccarelli O. Multiple sclerosis. *Lancet.* (2018) 391:1622–36. doi: 10.1016/S0140-6736(18) 30481-1

Yang R, Dunn JF. Multiple sclerosis disease progression: contributions from a hypoxia–inflammation cycle. *Mult Scler J.* (2018) 25:1715–8. doi: 10.1177/1352458518791683

D'Haeseleer M, Hostenbach S, Peeters I, El Sankari S, Nagels G, De Keyser J, et al. Cerebral hypoperfusion: a new pathophysiologic concept in multiple sclerosis? *J Cereb Blood Flow Metab.* (2015) 35:1406–10. doi: 10.1038/jcbfm.2015.131

Juurlink BHJ. The evidence for hypoperfusion as a factor in multiple sclerosis lesion development. *Mult Scler Int.* (2013) 2013:1–6. doi: 10.1155/2013/598093

Monti L, Donati D, Menci E, Cioni S, Bellini M, Grazzini I, et al. Cerebral circulation time is prolonged and not correlated with EDSS in multiple sclerosis patients: a study using digital subtracted angiography. *PLoS ONE.* (2015) 10:e0116681. doi: 10.1371/journal.pone.0116681

Varga AW, Johnson G, Babb JS, Herbert J, Grossman RI, Inglese M. White matter hemodynamic abnormalities precede sub-cortical gray matter changes in multiple sclerosis. *J Neurol Sci.* (2009) 282:28–33. doi:10.1016/j.jns.2008.12.036

Yang R, Dunn JF. Reduced cortical microvascular oxygenation in multiple sclerosis: a blinded, case-controlled study using a novel quantitative near-infrared spectroscopy method. *Sci Rep.* (2015) 5:16477. doi:10.1038/srep16477

Tettey P, Siejka D, Simpson S, Taylor B, Blizzard L, Ponsonby AL, et al. Frequency of comorbidities and their association with clinical disability and relapse in multiple sclerosis. *Neuroepidemiology.* (2016) 46:106–13. doi: 10.1159/000442203

Jadidi E, Mohammadi M, Moradi T. High risk of cardiovascular diseases after diagnosis of multiple sclerosis. *Mult Scler J.* (2013) 19:1336–40. doi: 10.1177/1352458513475833

Haufschild T, Shaw SG, Kaiser HJ, Flammer J. Transient raise of endothelin-1 plasma level and reduction of ocular blood flow in a patient with optic neuritis. *Ophthalmologica.* (2003) 217:451–3. doi: 10.1159/000073079

Jiang H, Delgado S, Tan J, Liu C, Rammohan KW, DeBuc DC, et al. Impaired retinal microcirculation in multiple sclerosis. *Mult Scler.* (2016) 22:1812–20. doi: 10.1177/1352458516631035

Modrzejewska M, Karczewicz D, Wilk G. Assessment of blood flow velocity in eyeball arteries in multiple sclerosis patients with past retrobulbar optic neuritis in color doppler ultrasonography. *Klin Ocz.* (2007) 109:183–6.

Davies AL, Desai RA, Bloomfield PS, McIntosh PR, Chapple KJ, Linington C, et al. Neurological deficits caused by tissue hypoxia in neuroinflammatory disease. *Ann Neurol.* (2013) 74:815–25. doi: 10.1002/ana.24006

Nikić I, Merkler D, Sorbara C, Brinkoetter M, Kreutzfeldt M, Bareyre FM, et al. A reversible form of axon damage in experimental autoimmune encephalomyelitis and multiple sclerosis. *Nat Med.* (2011) 17:495–9. doi: 10.1038/nm.2324

Sadeghian M, Mastrolia V, Rezaei Haddad A, Mosley A, Mullali G, Schiza D, et al. Mitochondrial dysfunction is an important cause of neurological deficits in an inflammatory model of multiple sclerosis. *Sci Rep.* (2016) 6:33249. doi: 10.1038/srep33249

Nathoo N, Rogers JA, Yong VW, Dunn JF. Detecting deoxyhemoglobin in spinal cord vasculature of the experimental autoimmune encephalomyelitis mouse model of multiple sclerosis using susceptibility MRI and hyperoxygenation. *PLoS ONE.* (2015) 10:e0127033. doi:10.1371/journal.pone.0127033

Ulusoy MO, Horasanli B, Işik-Ulusoy S. Optical coherence tomography angiography findings of multiple sclerosis with or without optic neuritis. *Neurol Res.* (2020) 42:319–26. doi: 10.1080/01616412.2020.1726585

Jiang H, Gameiro GR, Liu Y, Lin Y, Hernandez J, Deng Y, et al. Visual function and disability are associated with increased retinal volumetric vessel density in patients with multiple sclerosis. *Am J Ophthalmol.* (2020) 213:34–45. doi: 10.1016/j.ajo.2019.12.021

Lanzillo R, Cennamo G, Criscuolo C, Carotenuto A, Velotti N, Sparnelli F, et al. Optical coherence tomography angiography retinal vascular network assessment in multiple sclerosis. *Mult Scler J.* (2017) 24:1–9. doi: 10.1177/1352458517729463

Wang X, Jia Y, Spain R, Potsaid B, Liu JJ, Baumann B, et al. Optical coherence tomography angiography of optic nerve head and parafovea in multiple sclerosis. *Br J Ophtalmol.* (2014) 98:1368–73. doi: 10.1136/bjophthalmol-2013-304547

Spain RI, Liu L, Zhang X, Jia Y, Tan O, Bourdette D, et al. Optical coherence tomography angiography enhances the detection of optic nerve damage in multiple sclerosis. *Br J Ophthalmol.* (2018) 102:520–4. doi: 10.1136/bjophthalmol-2017-310477

Mastropasqua R, Toto L, Mastropasqua A, Aloia R, De Nicola C, Mattei PA, et al. Foveal avascular zone area and parafoveal vessel density measurements in different stages of diabetic retinopathy by optical coherence tomography angiography. *Int J Ophthalmol.* (2017) 10:1545–51. doi:10.18240/ijo.2017.10.11

Higashiyama T, Nishida Y, Ohji M. Optical coherence tomography angiography in eyes with good visual acuity recovery after treatment for optic neuritis. *PLoS ONE.* (2017) 12:e0172168. doi: 10.1371/journal.pone.0172168

Lanzillo R, Moccia M, Criscuolo C, Cennamo G. Optical coherence tomography angiography detects retinal vascular alterations in different phases of multiple sclerosis. *Mult Scler J.* (2019) 25:300–1. doi: 10.1177/1352458518768060

Tsokolas G, Tsaousis KT, Diakonis VF, Matsou A, Tyradellis S. Optical coherence tomography angiography in neurodegenerative diseases: a review. *Eye Brain.* (2020) 12:73–87. doi: 10.2147/EB.S193026

Sato DK, Callegaro D, Aurelio Lana-Peixoto M, Waters PJ, De Haidar FM, Takahashi T, et al. Distinction between MOG antibody- positive and AQP4 antibody-positive NMO spectrum disorders. *Neurology.* (2014) 82:474–81. doi:10.1212/WNL.0000000000000101

Marignier R, Nicolle A, Watrin C, Touret M, Confavreux C. Oligodendrocytes are damaged by neuromyelitis optica immunoglobulin G via astrocyte injury. *Brain.* Springer (2010) 133:2578–91. doi: 10.1093/brain/awq177

Kawachi I, Lassmann H. Neurodegeneration in multiple sclerosis and neuromyelitis optica. *J Neurol Neurosurg Psychiatry.* (2017) 88:137–45. doi: 10.1136/jnnp-2016-313300

Amann B, Kleinwort KJH, Hirmer S, Sekundo W, Kremmer E, Hauck SM, et al. Expression and distribution pattern of aquaporin 4, 5 and 11 in retinas of 15 different species. *Int J Mol Sci.* (2016) 17:1–12. doi: 10.3390/ ijms17071145

Lucchinetti CF, Mandler RN, McGaver D, Bruck W, Gleich G, Ransohoff R, et al. A role for humoral mechanisms in the pathogenesis of Devic's neuromyelitis optica. *Brain.* (2002) 125:1450–61. doi: 10.1093/brain/awf151

Roemer SF, Parisi JE, Lennon VA, Benarroch EE, Lassmann H, Bruck W, et al. Pattern-specific loss of aquaporin-4 immunoreactivity distinguishes neuromyelitis optica from multiple sclerosis. *Brain.* (2007) 130:1194–205. doi: 10.1093/brain/awl371

Lefkowitz D, Angelo JN. Neuromyelitis optica with unusual vascular changes. *Arch Neurol.* (1984) 41:1103–5. doi: 10.1001/archneur.1984.04050210105027

Bradl M, Reindl M, Lassmann H. Mechanisms for lesion localization in neuromyelitis optica spectrum disorders. *Curr Opin Neurol.* (2018) 31:325–33. doi: 10.1097/WCO.0000000000000551

Guo Y, Weigand SD, Popescu BF, Lennon VA, Parisi JE, Pittock SJ, et al. Pathogenic implications of cerebrospinal fluid barrier pathology in neuromyelitis optica. *Acta Neuropathol.* (2017) 133:597–612. doi: 10.1007/s00401-017-1682-1

Höftberger R, Guo Y, Flanagan EP, Lopez-Chiriboga AS, Endmayr V, Hochmeister S, et al. The pathology of central nervous system inflammatory demyelinating disease accompanying myelin oligodendrocyte glycoprotein autoantibody. *Acta Neuropathol.* (2020) 139:875–92. doi: 10.1007/ s00401-020-02132-y

Lassmann H. Pathology and disease mechanisms in different stages of multiple sclerosis. *J Neurol Sci.* (2013) 333:1–4. doi: 10.1016/j.jns.2013.05.010

Huang Y, Zhou L, ZhangBao J, Cai T, Wang B, Li X, et al. Peripapillary and parafoveal vascular network assessment by optical coherence tomography angiography in aquaporin-4 antibody-positive neuromyelitis optica spectrum disorders. *Br J Ophthalmol.* (2019) 103:789–96. doi: 10.1136/ bjophthalmol-2018-312231

Kwapong WR, Peng C, He Z, Zhuang X, Shen M, Lu F. Altered macular microvasculature in neuromyelitis optica spectrum disorders. *Am J Ophthalmol.* (2018) 192:47–55. doi: 10.1016/j.ajo.2018.04.026

Chang R, Nelson AJ, LeTran V, Vu B, Burkemper B, Chu Z, et al. Systemic determinants of peripapillary vessel density in healthy African Americans: The African American eye disease study. *Am J Ophthalmol.* (2019) 207:240–7. doi: 10.1016/j.ajo.2019.06.014

Takusagawa HL, Liu L, Ma KN, Jia Y, Gao SS, Zhang M, et al. Projection-resolved optical coherence tomography angiography of macular retinal circulation in glaucoma. *Ophthalmology.* (2017) 124:1589–99. doi: 10.1016/j. ophtha.2017.06.002

Suwan Y, Aghsaei Fard M, Geyman LS, Tantraworasin A, Chui TY, Rosen RB, et al. Association of myopia with peripapillary perfused capillary density in patients with glaucoma an optical coherence tomography angiography study. *JAMA Ophthalmol.* (2018) 136:507–13. doi: 10.1001/jamaophthalmol.2018.0776

Wang X, Kong X, Jiang C, Li M, Yu J, Sun X. Is the peripapillary retinal perfusion related to myopia in healthy eyes? A prospective comparative study. *BMJ Open.* (2016) 6:1–7. doi: 10.1136/bmjopen-2015-010791

Rao HL, Pradhan ZS, Weinreb RN, Reddy HB, Riyazuddin M, Sachdeva S, et al. Determinants of peripapillary and macular vessel densities measured by optical coherence tomography angiography in normal eyes. *J Glaucoma.* (2017) 26:491–7. doi: 10.1097/IJG.0000000000000655

Alnawaiseh M, Lahme L, Treder M, Rosentreter A, Eter N. Short- Term effects of exercise on optic nerve and macular perfusion measured by optical coherence tomography angiography. *Retina.* (2017) 37:1642–6. doi: 10.1097/ IAE.0000000000001419

Hao H, Sasongko MB, Wong TY, Che Azemin MZ, Aliahmad B, Hodgson L, et al. Does retinal vascular geometry vary with cardiac cycle? *Investig Ophthalmol Vis Sci.* (2012) 53:5799–805. doi: 10.1167/iovs.11-9326

Müller VC, Storp JJ, Kerschke L, Nelis P, Eter N, Alnawaiseh M. Diurnal variations in flow density measured using optical coherence tomography angiography and the impact of heart rate, mean arterial pressure and intraocular pressure on flow density in primary open-angle glaucoma patients. *Acta Ophthalmol.* (2019) 97:e844–9. doi: 10.1111/aos.14089

Venugopal JP, Rao HL, Weinreb RN, Pradhan ZS, Dasari S, Riyazuddin M, et al. Repeatability of vessel density measurements of optical coherence tomography angiography in normal and glaucoma eyes. *Br J Ophthalmol.* (2018) 102:352–7. doi: 10.1136/bjophthalmol-2017-310637

Frost S, Gregory C, Robinson L, Yu S, Xiao D, Mehdizadeh M, et al. Effect of pupil dilation with tropicamide on retinal vascular caliber. *Ophthalmic Epidemiol.* (2019) 26:400–7. doi: 10.1080/09286586.2019.1639198

Holló G. Intrasession and between-visit variability of sector peripapillary angioflow vessel density values measured with the angiovue optical coherence tomograph in different retinal layers in ocular hypertension and glaucoma. *PLoS ONE.* (2016) 11:e0161631. doi: 10.1371/journal.pone.0161631

Manalastas PIC, Zangwill LM, Saunders LJ, Mansouri K, Belghith A, Suh MH, et al. Reproducibility of optical coherence tomography angiography macular and optic nerve head vascular density in glaucoma and healthy eyes. *J Glaucoma.* (2017) 26:851–9. doi: 10.1097/IJG.0000000000000768

Littlewood R, Mollan SP, Pepper IM, Hickman SJ. The Utility of Fundus Fluorescein Angiography in Neuro-Ophthalmology. *Neuro Ophthalmol.* (2019) 43:217–34. doi: 10.1080/01658107.2019.1604764

Braaf B, Gräfe MGO, Uribe-Patarroyo N, Bouma BE, Vakoc BJ, de Boer JF, et al. High resolution imaging in microscopy and ophthalmology: new frontiers in biomedical optics. In: Bille JF, editor. *OCT-Based Velocimetry for Blood Flow Quantification.* Cham: Springer (2019). p. 161–79. doi: 10.1007/978-3-030-16638-0_7

Wei X, Hormel TT, Pi S, Guo Y, Jian Y, Jia Y. High dynamic range optical coherence tomography angiography (HDR-OCTA). *Biomed Opt Express.* (2019) 10:3560. doi: 10.1364/boe.10.003560

Spaide RF, Klancnik JM, Cooney MJ. Retinal vascular layers imaged by fluorescein angiography and optical coherence tomography angiography. *JAMA Ophthalmol.* (2015) 133:45–50. doi: 10.1001/jamaophthalmol.2014. 3616

Iftikhar M, Zafar S, Gonzalez N, Murphy O, Ohemaa Kwakyi MS, Sydney Feldman BS, et al. Image artifacts in optical coherence tomography angiography among patients with multiple sclerosis. *Curr Eye Res.* (2019) 44:558–63. doi: 10.1080/02713683.2019.1565892

Sotirchos ES, Gonzalez Caldito N, Filippatou A, Fitzgerald KC, Murphy OC, Lambe J, et al. Progressive multiple sclerosis is associated with faster and specific retinal layer atrophy. *Ann Neurol.* (2020) 87:885–96. doi: 10.1002/ ana.25738

Saidha S, Al-Louzi O, Ratchford J, Bhargava P, Oh J, Newsome S, et al. Optical coherence tomography reflects brain atrophy in multiple sclerosis: a four-year study. *Ann Neurol.* (2015) 75:801–13. doi: 10.1016/j.physbeh. 2017.03.040

Pache F, Zimmermann H, Mikolajczak J, Schumacher S, Lacheta A, Oertel FC, et al. MOG-IgG in NMO and related disorders:a multicenter study of 50 patients. Part 4: afferent visual system damage after optic neuritis in MOG-IgG-seropositive versus AQP4-IgG-seropositive patients. *J Neuroinflammation.* (2016) 13:1–10. doi: 10.1186/s12974- 016-0720-6

Permissions

All chapters in this book were first published by Frontiers; hereby published with permission under the Creative Commons Attribution License or equivalent. Every chapter published in this book has been scrutinized by our experts. Their significance has been extensively debated. The topics covered herein carry significant findings which will fuel the growth of the discipline. They may even be implemented as practical applications or may be referred to as a beginning point for another development.

The contributors of this book come from diverse backgrounds, making this book a truly international effort. This book will bring forth new frontiers with its revolutionizing research information and detailed analysis of the nascent developments around the world.

We would like to thank all the contributing authors for lending their expertise to make the book truly unique. They have played a crucial role in the development of this book. Without their invaluable contributions this book wouldn't have been possible. They have made vital efforts to compile up to date information on the varied aspects of this subject to make this book a valuable addition to the collection of many professionals and students.

This book was conceptualized with the vision of imparting up-to-date information and advanced data in this field. To ensure the same, a matchless editorial board was set up. Every individual on the board went through rigorous rounds of assessment to prove their worth. After which they invested a large part of their time researching and compiling the most relevant data for our readers.

The editorial board has been involved in producing this book since its inception. They have spent rigorous hours researching and exploring the diverse topics which have resulted in the successful publishing of this book. They have passed on their knowledge of decades through this book. To expedite this challenging task, the publisher supported the team at every step. A small team of assistant editors was also appointed to further simplify the editing procedure and attain best results for the readers.

Apart from the editorial board, the designing team has also invested a significant amount of their time in understanding the subject and creating the most relevant covers. They scrutinized every image to scout for the most suitable representation of the subject and create an appropriate cover for the book.

The publishing team has been an ardent support to the editorial, designing and production team. Their endless efforts to recruit the best for this project, has resulted in the accomplishment of this book. They are a veteran in the field of academics and their pool of knowledge is as vast as their experience in printing. Their expertise and guidance has proved useful at every step. Their uncompromising quality standards have made this book an exceptional effort. Their encouragement from time to time has been an inspiration for everyone.

The publisher and the editorial board hope that this book will prove to be a valuable piece of knowledge for researchers, students, practitioners and scholars across the globe.

List of Contributors

Junhan Wei, Deying Kong, Xi Yu, Lili Wei, Yue Xiong, Jiawei Zhou and Zhifen He
State Key Laboratory of Ophthalmology, Optometry and Vision Science, School of Ophthalmology and Optometry, Affiliated Eye Hospital, Wenzhou Medical University, Wenzhou, China

Jinhua Bao
State Key Laboratory of Ophthalmology, Optometry and Vision Science, School of Ophthalmology and Optometry, Affiliated Eye Hospital, Wenzhou Medical University, Wenzhou, China
WEIRC, WMU-Essilor International Research Centre, Wenzhou, China

Adeline Yang, Björn Drobe and Yi Gao
WEIRC, WMU-Essilor International Research Centre, Wenzhou, China
R&D AMERA, Essilor International, Singapore, Singapore

Li Gu, Yiyao Wang, Saiqun Li, Mengwei Zhang, Qingqing Ye, Yijing Zhuang, Jinrong Li and Jin Yuan
State Key Laboratory of Ophthalmology, Zhongshan Ophthalmic Center, Sun Yat-sen University, Guangzhou, China

Zhong-Lin Lu
Division of Arts and Sciences, NYU Shanghai, Shanghai, China
Center for Neural Science, Department of Psychology, New York University, New York, NY, United States
NYU-ECNU Institute of Cognitive Neuroscience, NYU Shanghai, Shanghai, China

Peishan Dai, Xiaoyan Zhou, Yilin Ou, Tong Xiong, Jinlong Zhang, Zailiang Chen and Beiji Zou
School of Computer Science and Engineering, Central South University, Changsha, China
Hunan Engineering Research Center of Machine Vision and Intelligent Medicine, Central South University, Changsha, China

Xin Wei, Ying Wu and Manyi Xiao
Department of Ophthalmology, The Second Xiangya Hospital, Central South University, Changsha, China
Hunan Clinical Research Center of Ophthalmic Disease, Changsha, China

Anne Macnamara, Dimitrios Saredakis and Tobias Loetscher
Cognitive Ageing and Impairment Neurosciences Laboratory, UniSA Justice & Society, University of South Australia, Adelaide, SA, Australia

Celia Chen
College of Medicine and Public Health, Flinders Medical Centre, Flinders University, Adelaide, SA, Australia

Victor R. Schinazi
Department of Psychology, Faculty of Society & Design, Bond University, Gold Coast, QLD, Australia
Future Health Technologies, Singapore-ETH Centre, Campus for Research Excellence and Technological Enterprise (CREATE), Singapore, Singapore

Katelyn MacNeill, Amber Myatt, Kevin R. Duffy and Donald E. Mitchell
Department of Psychology and Neuroscience, Dalhousie University, Halifax, NS, Canada

Grace Lin, Raghda Al Ani and Ewa Niechwiej-Szwedo
Department of Kinesiology, University of Waterloo, Waterloo, ON, Canada

Xia Hu, Yi Qin, Xiaoxiao Ying, Junli Yuan, Xiaowei Ruan, Fan Lu and Fang Hou
School of Ophthalmology & Optometry and Eye Hospital, Wenzhou Medical University, Wenzhou, China

Rong Cui
Biosysen Ltd., Shenzhen, China

Xianghang He
School of Ophthalmology & Optometry and Eye Hospital, Wenzhou Medical University, Wenzhou, China
Fuzhou Aier Eye Hospital, Fuzhou, China

Tingting Peng, Meiping Xu, Fuhao Zheng, Junxiao Zhang, Shuang Chen, Jiangtao Lou, Chunxiao Wang and Yuwen Wang
The Eye Hospital, School of Ophthalmology and Optometry, Wenzhou Medical University, Wenzhou, China

Xinping Yu
The Eye Hospital, School of Ophthalmology and Optometry, Wenzhou Medical University, Wenzhou, China
State Key Laboratory of Ophthalmology, Zhongshan Ophthalmic Center, Sun Yat-sen University, Guangzhou, China

Jingchang Chen, Zixuan Xu and Shenglan Zhang
State Key Laboratory of Ophthalmology, Zhongshan Ophthalmic Center, Sun Yat-sen University, Guangzhou, China

Lily Y. L. Chan
State Key Laboratory of Ophthalmology, Zhongshan Ophthalmic Center, Sun Yat-sen University, Guangzhou, China
School of Optometry, The Hong Kong Polytechnic University, Hong Kong, China

Jingjing Xu, Xinjie Mao and Hao Chen
School of Ophthalmology and Optometry, Affiliated Eye Hospital, State Key Laboratory of Ophthalmology, Optometry and Vision Science, Wenzhou Medical University, Wenzhou, China
WEIRC, Wenzhou Medical University-Essilor International Research Center, Wenzhou, China

Chunwen Tao and Xin Lu
School of Ophthalmology and Optometry, Affiliated Eye Hospital, State Key Laboratory of Ophthalmology, Optometry and Vision Science, Wenzhou Medical University, Wenzhou, China

Chuan Hou and Gabriela Acevedo Munares
Smith-Kettlewell Eye Research Institute, San Francisco, CA, United States

Ruru Chen, Jianhui Mei, Pingping Huang and Bingzhen Chen
Eye Hospital, Wenzhou Medical University, Wenzhou, China

Guihua Liu, Yiyuan Wu, Biying Wang, Tianpu Gu, Bei Du and Ruihua Wei
Tianjin Key Laboratory of Retinal Functions and Diseases, Tianjin Branch of National Clinical Research Center for Ocular Disease, Eye Institute and School of Optometry, Tianjin Medical University Eye Hospital, Tianjin, China

Hua Bi
College of Optometry, Nova Southeastern University, Davie, FL, United States

Jianliang Tong
Doctor's Exchange of Georgia PC, Lawrenceville, GA, United States

Zitian Liu, Zidong Chen, Le Gao, Manli Liu, Yiru Huang, Lei Feng, Junpeng Yuan, Daming Deng and Minbin Yu
State Key Laboratory of Ophthalmology, Guangdong Provincial Key Laboratory of Ophthalmology and Visual Science, Zhongshan Ophthalmic Center, Sun Yat-sen University, Guangzhou, Guangdong, China

Chang-Bing Huang
Key Laboratory of Behavioral Science, Institute of Psychology, Chinese Academy of Sciences (CAS), Beijing, China
Department of Psychology, University of Chinese Academy of Sciences, Beijing, China

Fan Jiang, Xiaopeng Huang, Houxue Xia and Bingqi Wang
School of Ophthalmology and Optometry, Wenzhou Medical University, Wenzhou, China

Bin Zhang
College of Optometry, Nova Southeastern University, Fort Lauderdale, FL, United States

Jun Jiang
School of Ophthalmology and Optometry, Wenzhou Medical University, Wenzhou, China
Eye Hospital, Wenzhou Medical University, Wenzhou, China

Xueying He, Qian Wang, Ting Li, Xiaoxia Qu, Jing Liu, Wei Li, Lirong Zhang and Zhaohui Liu
Department of Radiology, Beijing Tongren Hospital, Capital Medical University, Beijing, China

Jie Hong, Yanan Guo and Jing Fu
Department of Ophthalmology, Beijing Tongren Hospital, Capital Medical University, Beijing, China

Pengjing Xu
College of Optometry, The Ohio State University, Columbus, OH, United States
Shanghai Technology Development Co., Ltd., Shanghai, China
Shanghai-Warsaw Joint Laboratory on Artificial Intelligence, Shanghai, China

Deyue Yu
College of Optometry, The Ohio State University, Columbus, OH, United States

Luis Andres Lesmes
Adaptive Sensory Technology, Inc., San Diego, CA, United States

Lin Xia, Jiong Dong, Sha Luo and Lixia Feng
Department of Ophthalmology, First Affiliated Hospital of Anhui Medical University, Hefei, China
Anhui Branch of National Clinical Research Center for Ocular Diseases, Hefei, China

He Chen
Hefei National Laboratory for Physical Sciences at Microscale, School of Life Sciences, University of Science and Technology of China, Hefei, China

Jie Ye, Meixiao Shen and Yilei Shao
School of Ophthalmology and Optometry, Wenzhou Medical University, Wenzhou, China

Pawan Sinha
Department of Brain and Cognitive Sciences, Massachusetts Institute of Technology, Cambridge, MA, United States

Pragnya R. Donthineni and Swapna S. Shanbhag
The Cornea Institute, L V Prasad Eye Institute, Hyderabad, India

Anthony V. Das
Department of eyeSmart EMR & AEye, L V Prasad Eye Institute, Hyderabad, India

Sayan Basu
The Cornea Institute, L V Prasad Eye Institute, Hyderabad, India
Center for Ocular Regeneration (CORE), L V Prasad Eye Institute, Hyderabad, India

Yan Zhang, Zhengbo Xue, Fangjie Guo, Fulong Yu and Liangde Xu
School of Biomedical Engineering, School of Ophthalmology and Optometry and Eye Hospital, Wenzhou Medical University, Wenzhou, China

Iris Kleerekooper
Department of Neuro-Ophthalmology, Moorfields Eye Hospital, London, United Kingdom
Queen Square MS Centre, UCL Institute of Neurology and National Hospital for Neurology & Neurosurgery, London, United Kingdom

S. Anand Trip
Queen Square MS Centre, UCL Institute of Neurology and National Hospital for Neurology & Neurosurgery, London, United Kingdom

Sarah Houston
Institute of Ophthalmology, University College London, London, United Kingdom

Adam M. Dubis
National Institute for Health Research, Biomedical Resource Centre at University College London, Institute of Ophthalmology and Moorfields Eye Hospital National Health Service Trust, London, United Kingdom

Axel Petzold
Department of Neuro-Ophthalmology, Moorfields Eye Hospital, London, United Kingdom
Queen Square MS Centre, UCL Institute of Neurology and National Hospital for Neurology & Neurosurgery, London, United Kingdom
Dutch Expertise Centre of Neuro-Ophthalmology, Amsterdam UMC, Amsterdam, Netherlands

Index